Administration and Supervision in Laboratory Medicine

Second Edition

Administration and Supervision in Laboratory Medicine

Second Edition

Edited by

John R. Snyder, PhD, MT(ASCP)SH
Associate Dean
Indiana University School of Medicine
Director and Associate Professor
Division of Allied Health Sciences
Indiana University Medical Center
Indianapolis, Indiana

Donald A. Senhauser, MD
Professor and Chairman
Department of Pathology
College of Medicine
The Ohio State University
Columbus, Ohio

with 36 contributors

J.B. Lippincott Company
Philadelphia
Cambridge, New York, St. Louis, San Francisco,
London, Singapore, Sydney, Tokyo

Acquisitions/Sponsoring Editor: Lisa A. Biello
Manuscript Editor: Lorraine D. Smith
Copy Editor: Jessie Raymond
Indexer: Alexandra Weir Nickerson
Senior Designer: Anita Curry
Production Coordinator: Pamela Milcos
Compositor: Digitype, Inc.
Printer/Binder: R. R. Donnelley & Sons Company

2nd Edition

1   3   5   6   4   2

Library of Congress Cataloging-in-Publication Data

Administration and supervision in laboratory
medicine.

   Includes bibliographies and index.
   1.   Medical   laboratories—Management.   I.
Snyder, John R.   II. Senhauser, Donald A. [DNLM:
1. Laboratories—organization & administration. QY
23 A238]
RB36.3.F55A35 1989   616.07′5   88-13309
ISBN 0-397-50857-3

The authors and publisher have exerted every effort
to ensure that drug selection and dosage set forth in
this text are in accord with current recommendations and practice at the time of publication. However, in view of ongoing research, changes in government regulations, and the constant flow of
information relating to drug therapy and drug reactions, the reader is urged to check the package in-
sert for each drug for any change in indications and
dosage and for added warnings and precautions.
This is particularly important when the recommended agent is a new or infrequently employed
drug.

This book is dedicated, on behalf of all contributing authors,

first, to our teachers, under whose initial guidance we sought to become administrators, supervisors, consultants, and proponents of quality laboratory medicine;

second, to our students, whose questions prompted serious investigation of the management literature in search of practical application to the clinical laboratory; and

finally, to our spouses and families, without whose support and understanding this writing would not have reached completion.

Preface

The success of any organization in meeting its goals and objectives depends largely on the quality of management within the organization. Management of medical laboratory services is no exception. The provision of quality laboratory analyses and efficient reporting of data rely heavily on the application of sound principles of administration and supervision.

The field of laboratory medicine has been slower than some other health services in acknowledging the need for administrative personnel with managerial preparation. While appropriate degrees and professional certification are a fairly reliable index of the laboratorian's technical competence, these alone do not ensure that the individual has the ability to manage. Quite often the challenge to stay abreast of our rapidly changing technology has received a higher priority than the development of managerial skills. This dilemma is compounded, since few authors have applied solid principles of management to administration of the clinical laboratory. The purpose of this text, therefore, is to bridge the gap between the theory of management and its application in the clinical laboratory setting.

Although only half a decade has elapsed since publication of the first edition of *Administration and Supervision in Laboratory Medicine,* the health-care industry has experienced dramatic changes in philosophy, size, structure, and payment mechanisms for health-service providers. At a time when medical knowledge and diagnostic technology are at an all-time high, clinical laboratory managers face tremendous challenges to meet both demands of consumers of laboratory services and

expectations of technical staff in a cost-containment environment.

This second edition of the text retains most of the distinguishing features of the first edition. These include an emphasis on the centrality of the laboratory manager's role in achieving organizational goals and objectives; the importance of understanding the responsibility of the manager for maximizing the human, physical, and financial resources entrusted to his care; annotated bibliographies and appropriate appendices; and the frequent use of examples and case studies to demonstrate the practical utility of management theory. Based on feedback from students, faculty, and other readers, this second edition also features an increased attention to employee involvement in work groups; a discussion of employee temperament styles and the importance of understanding these styles; new information on computers and laboratory information systems; suggestions for utilizing accreditation inspections as a management tool; guidance in marketing clinical laboratory services; increased attention to the financial aspects of human resources; and application of financial ratios for decision making. In addition, most chapters have been updated to reflect state-of-the-art laboratory management theory and practice. The net result is, we believe, a text that is interesting, readable, and relevant.

The text is directed to the basic–through–intermediate levels of management. It is written primarily for upper-division undergraduate students and postbaccalaureate medical technology students, graduate students in the clinical laboratory sciences and pathology, and pathology residents preparing for managerial roles in the medical laboratory. Since many laboratorians achieve management positions without the benefit of formal education in organizational theory and practice, this book will also be useful as a reference to practicing laboratory supervisors, chief or administrative technologists, and laboratory directors. Its major function is to provide a resource that explores basic principles and develops them into viable managerial processes within the constraints of the clinical laboratory.

The text is presented in five parts:

Part One consists of three chapters, which together address the basic fundamentals of managerial practice in the laboratory setting. The managerial functions of planning, organizing, and controlling are introduced, as well as decision making and problem solving.

Part Two includes seven chapters that focus on the concepts of managerial leadership—the human side of the directing function of laboratory administrators and supervisors. Separate chapters address managerial assumptions and their effects on motivation; communications within the laboratory organization; leadership styles and group effectiveness; employee-involvement work groups; authority and delegation; effective meeting techniques; and the management of conflict and change.

Part Three, which focuses on processes in personnel administration, discusses the practical procedures useful in the labor-intensive clinical laboratory setting. Considerations of interviewing techniques and employee selection are followed by a discussion of job descriptions and methods for staffing and scheduling. The focus then shifts to performance appraisal in the clinical setting and the preservice, inservice, and continuing education responsibilities of laboratory managers and supervisors. Since the context of personnel administration changes somewhat in the laboratory under union contract, a separate chapter is devoted to this subject.

Part Four includes ten chapters dealing with essential managerial activities for effective laboratory operation. Two chapters focus on the control of quality laboratory testing and method evaluation, and concepts of preventive maintenance for laboratory instrumentation. Effective communication between the medical laboratory and consumers of services is described, examples of laboratory requisitions and reports are provided, and computer applications are discussed. A separate chapter covers the basics of laboratory safety. External and internal control and evaluation of laboratory operations are described in terms of laboratory regulations, inspection, the peer review process in quality assurance, and medicolegal concerns in laboratory medicine.

Part Five consists of six chapters concerned with the principles of laboratory finance. The financial operation of the clinical laboratory is introduced, followed by a discussion of budgeting practices, cost accounting, wage and salary administration, work-load analysis, and financial ratios for decision making as management tools. The last chapter deals with cost containment through inventory control techniques.

The text reflects the special expertise of over 35 different contributors. We have been fortunate to work with such talented colleagues. We have not eliminated all redundancy or repetition among chapters; rather this has been encouraged when the effectiveness of a given topic was enhanced by such duplication of concepts.

Since managerial titles and responsibilities vary in laboratory medicine, the terms *director, administrator,* and *supervisor* are often used interchangeably to refer to individuals with managerial responsibility, regardless of institutional title. The terms *subordinates* and *staff* refer to the group of individuals for whom the manager is responsible. The reader should also recognize that throughout the text "his" also means "hers" and "he" also means "she."

Special thanks are due Lisa A. Biello, Eileen Rosen, and Lorraine D. Smith of the Lippincott organization for their editorial guidance and assistance, encouragement, and understanding. Phyllis Seidel and Tricia Arnett also deserve special appreciation for preparation of the manuscript.

John R. Snyder, PhD
Donald A. Senhauser, MD

Contributing Authors

LOUIS M. BRIGANDO, MBA
President
Personnel Management Technologies, Inc.
Hackensack, New Jersey

ROHN J. BUTTERFIELD, MBA
Administrator
Hospital Operations and Ambulatory Services
University Hospital
Cincinnati, Ohio

JANIE BROWN CRANE, BS, MT(ASCP)
Kalaheo, Hawaii

JUSTIN DOHENY, MHA
President
Wayne General Hospital
Wayne, New Jersey

DAVID J. FINE, MHA
Vice Provost for Health Affairs
Director, University Hospital and Health
  System
Cincinnati, Ohio

DAVID W. GLENN, BA, MT(ASCP)
Consulting Technologist
Pathology Services, P.C.
North Platte, Nebraska

SHARON S. GUTTERMAN, PhD
President, Gutterman Associates
Health Care Marketing and Training Services
Columbus, Ohio

CAROLYN C. HART, MS, MT(ASCP)
Marketing Manager
University Reference Laboratories, Inc.
The Ohio State University Hospitals
Columbus, Ohio

M. ROBERT HICKS, BS, MT(ASCP)
Department of Pathology and Microbiology
University of Nebraska Medical Center
Omaha, Nebraska

DORIS A. JOHNSON, MS, CLS
Instructor, Division of Medical Technology
School of Allied Health Professions
Administrative Technologist
University Health Center Clinical Laboratory
University of Nebraska Medical Center
Omaha, Nebraska

EDWARD A. JOHNSON, PhD
College of Business and Administration
University of Colorado
Boulder, Colorado

ANTHONY S. KUREC, MSH(ASCP)
Division of Clinical Pathology
State University of New York Health Science
    Center
Syracuse, New York

DANIEL I. LABOWITZ, JD, MFS
Attorney-at-Law
Pittsford, New York

ARDEN E. LARSEN, DVM, PhD, MT(ASCP)
Associate Professor
Pathology and Microbiology
College of Medicine
University of Nebraska Medical Center
Omaha, Nebraska

ARTHUR L. LARSEN, MD
Professor Emeritus, Pathology and
    Microbiology
College of Medicine
University of Nebraska Medical Center
Omaha, Nebraska

JOHN A. LOTT, PhD
Professor of Pathology
The Ohio State University
Director of Clinical Chemistry
The Ohio State University Medical Center
Columbus, Ohio

ROBERT V. LUCCHETTI
Director, Business Systems
Scientific Products Division
Baxter Health Care Corporation
McGaw Park, Illinois

PEGGY PRINZ LUEBBERT, MS, MT(ASCP)
Instructor in Medical Technology
University of Nebraska Medical Center
Omaha, Nebraska
Memorial Hospital of Dodge County
Fremont, Nebraska

BETTINA G. MARTIN, MS, MBA
Professor of Medical Technology
Laboratory Manager, Clinical Pathology
State University of New York Health Science
    Center
Syracuse, New York

DIANA MASS, MA, MT(ASCP), CLS (NCA)
Faculty Associate and Director
Clinical Laboratory Sciences Program
Department of Botany/Microbiology
College of Liberal Arts and Sciences
Arizona State University
Tempe, Arizona

KATHRYN R. MAXWELL, RN, BSN
Director, Quality Assurance/Utilization
    Review
The Ohio State University Hospitals
Columbus, Ohio

RICHARD L. MOORE II, EdD
Acting Vice Chancellor for Administration
    and Planning
University of North Carolina
Greensboro, North Carolina

JOHN C. NEFF, MD
Professor of Pathology
The Ohio State University Hospitals
Columbus, Ohio

LINDA L. OTIS, DDS, MS
Assistant Professor
Department of Diagnostic Sciences
School of Dentistry
University of Southern California
Los Angeles

BARBARA L. PARSONS
Assistant Professor of Management
Division of Commerce
Fairmont State College
Fairmont, West Virginia

DIETRICH L. SCHAUPP, DBA
Professor of Management
College of Business and Economics
West Virginia University
Morgantown, West Virginia

DONALD A. SENHAUSER, MD
Professor and Chairman
Department of Pathology
College of Medicine
The Ohio State University
Columbus, Ohio

JAMES SHARP, MD
Associate Pathologist
Northwest Community Hospital
Arlington Heights, Illinois

WALTON H. SHARP
Labor and Industrial Relations Institute
University of North Texas
Denton, Texas

JACK W. SMITH, MD, PhD
Assistant Professor
Department of Pathology
The Ohio State University
Columbus, Ohio

JOHN R. SNYDER, PhD, MT(ASCP)SH
Associate Dean
Indiana University School of Medicine
Director and Associate Professor
Division of Allied Health Sciences
Indiana University Medical Center
Indianapolis, Indiana

CARL E. SPEICHER, MD
Professor and Director of Clinical Laboratories
Department of Pathology

The Ohio State University
Columbus, Ohio

THOMAS STEVENSON, MD
Peer Review Sections
The Ohio State University Hospitals
Columbus, Ohio

JOHN R. SVIRBELY, MD
Assistant Professor
Department of Pathology
The Ohio State University
Columbus, Ohio

JUDITH THOMPSON, MS
Marketing Manager
Laboratory UF and Specialty Membrane
Amicon Division, W. R. Grace
Danvers, Massachusetts

JANA WILSON WOLFGANG, MS, MT(ASCP)
Wolfgang Associates
Portland, Oregon

Contents

PART 1
FUNDAMENTALS OF
LABORATORY MANAGEMENT

one
The Nature of Management
in the Clinical Laboratory   **3**
John R. Snyder, Donald A. Senhauser
Administration — Art or Science?   *4*
Managerial Duties and Responsibilities   *5*
The Administrative Process   *7*
Making the Transition to Laboratory
   Management   *10*
Challenges for Today's Laboratory Manager   *16*
Bridging the Gap — An Approach   *18*

two
Laboratory Planning, Organization,
and Control   **21**
John R. Snyder
Strategic Management and Planning   *21*
Planning at the Departmental Level   *23*
Establishing Policies and Procedures   *23*
Design of Clinical Laboratory Floor Plan and
   Work Flow   *25*
Laboratory Organizational Structure   *32*
Controlling Operations in the Laboratory   *38*

three
Problem Solving —
The Decision-making Process   **45**
John R. Snyder

Areas of Concern in Decision-making   *45*
Decision-making — Approaches and Effects   *46*
Human Factors in Decision-making   *50*
Quantitative Tools for Decision-making   *50*
Steps in the Problem-solving Process   *51*
Choosing a Management Decision Style Based on
   the Situation   *53*
Problem-solving and Decision-making With
   Proficiency Data   *56*

PART 2
CONCEPTS IN MANAGERIAL
LEADERSHIP

four
Motivation — Managerial
Assumptions and Effects   **61**
Diana Mass
Nature of Motivation   *61*
Motivational Theories   *62*
Responsibilities of Management   *68*
Group Dynamics   *69*
Motivating into the 1990s   *70*
Summary   *71*

five
Managerial - Organizational Communications   **73**
Edward A. Johnson
Interpersonal Communication Within
   the Laboratory   *73*

Interpersonal Communication—A Transactional
    Process   78
Organizational Communication Systems   81
Organizational and Interpersonal Communication
    Barriers   84
Improving Managerial Communication   86

six
Leadership Styles and Group Effectiveness   **93**
John R. Snyder
Measures of Group Effectiveness   94
The Climate Reflecting Leader Behavior   95
The Leadership Role of Managers and
    Supervisors   96
Bases of Power and Influence   97
Factors Influencing Leadership Styles   99
Leadership Styles: The Leader Dimension   100
Linking Leadership Style to Followership   103
Leadership and the Situation   113
Diagnosing the Situation   116
Management by Objectives   118
Leadership Behavior in Need of Change   119

seven
Employee-Involvement Work Groups   **123**
Dietrich L. Schaupp, Barbara L. Parsons
Why Employee Involvement?   123
Quality Circles Approach   124
The Quality of Work Life Approach   129
Autonomous Work Teams   133
Conclusions and Summary   134

eight
Authority and Delegation   **137**
Arthur L. Larsen, Arden E. Larsen
Sources of Authority   137
Types of Authority   137
Delegation   138

nine
Conducting Effective Meetings   **143**
Janie Brown Crane
Meeting Purposes   143
Planning   144
Conducting the Meeting   146
Follow-up   147
Avoiding Nonproductive Meetings   149
Effective Leadership   150

ten
Management of Conflict and Change   **153**
Dietrich L. Schaupp, Barbara L. Parsons
Change and Conflict Are Natural   153

The Laboratory as an Organizational Entity   154
Trying To Understand Change and Conflict   155
A Final Note   172

PART 3
PROCESSES IN PERSONNEL
ADMINISTRATION

eleven
Interviewing and Employee Selection   **177**
John R. Snyder, Stephen L. Wilson, Linda L. Otis
Recruitment   178
Legal Aspects of Interviewing and
    Employee Selection   178
The Application Form   181
Reference Checks   182
Conducting the Interview   182
The Selection Process   194
Transfer and Promotion   194

twelve
Staffing and Scheduling of
    Laboratory Personnel   **199**
Bettina G. Martin, Anthony S. Kurec
Staff Planning   199
Responsibility and Importance of Scheduling
    and Staffing   200
Historic Changes in Staffing and Scheduling   200
Criteria-based Job Description   201
Scheduling for Efficient Service   207
Staffing and Scheduling Guides   208
Available Resources   210
Innovative Approaches in Scheduling   211

thirteen
Standards and Appraisal of
    Laboratory Performance   **217**
Jana Wilson Wolfgang, Louis M. Brigando
Performance Appraisals—Definition
    and Purposes   217
Essentials of Meaningful Performance
    Appraisals   218
Designing Performance Appraisals   219
Performance Appraisals in the Context of
    Performance Management   223

fourteen
Educational Responsibilities of
    Managers and Supervisors   **233**
Richard L. Moore, II, John R. Snyder
Lifelong Learning   234

Educational Issues 235
Staff Development 236
Approaches to Educational Activities 237
*The Process of Developing Educational
    Activities 240*

fifteen
Labor Relations and the Clinical Laboratory **245**
Walton H. Sharp
Background 245
Labor Law and the Public Employee 245
Labor Law and the Private-sector Employee 247
Unions 250

PART 4
ESSENTIALS OF EFFECTIVE
LABORATORY OPERATION

sixteen
Quality Control and Method Evaluation **261**
John A. Lott
*Quality Control of Clinical Laboratory
    Performance 261*
Allowable Error in the Medical Needs Context 269
Interlaboratory Surveys 272
Resolving Analytical Surveys 274
Laboratory Mistakes 277
Method Evaluation 279

seventeen
Laboratory Requisitions and
    Reporting of Results **285**
Doris A. Johnson
The Request 285
The Report 292

eighteen
Computers and Laboratory
    Information Systems **299**
John R. Svirbely, Jack W. Smith, Carl Speicher
*Problems in Information Handling Prior
    to Computerization 299*
Overview of Computer Systems 300
The Fundamental Functions of the LIS 301
*Current and Future Requirements for Laboratory
    Information Systems 308*
Choosing a LIS 312

nineteen
Concepts of Preventive Maintenance
    for Laboratory Instrumentation **315**
Judith Thompson, Peggy Prinz Luebbert

*Government and Accrediting Agency
    Requirements 315*
Instrument Selection and Implementation 316
Documentation 316
Performance Responsibility 319
Benefits of Preventive Maintenance 322

twenty
Basics of Clinical Laboratory Safety **323**
M. Robert Hicks
Hazards of the Workplace 323
*Blood and Body Fluids Precautions
    for Laboratories 326*
Safety Precautions 330

twenty-one
Laboratory Accreditation, Licensure,
    and Regulation **339**
Donald A. Senhauser
Definitions 339
*Inspection and Accreditation of Clinical
    Laboratories 341*
*Federal and State Regulation of Clinical
    Laboratories 343*

twenty-two
Laboratory Inspection as a Management Tool **349**
John C. Neff
*Accrediting Agencies That Inspect Clinical
    Laboratories 349*
CAP Laboratory Accreditation Program 350
Quality Assurance — A Comment 354
Preparing for an Accreditation Inspection 355
Appendix 22-A 356
Appendix 22-B 360

twenty-three
Quality Assurance and Peer Review
    in the Clinical Laboratory **369**
Kathryn R. Maxwell, Thomas D. Stevenson
Defining Quality Assurance 370
*Monitoring Important Aspects of Care
    and Outcomes 371*
*Implementation of the Quality-Assurance
    Program 374*
Future Perspectives 376

twenty-four
Medicolegal Concerns in Laboratory Medicine **379**
Daniel I. Labowitz
Legal Liability 379
The Subpoena 385

The Technologist as Witness *386*
Records *388*

twenty-five
Marketing Clinical Laboratory Services **391**
Carolyn C. Hart, Sharon S. Gutterman
Defining the Marketing Concept *391*
Market Research *392*
Market Segmentation *393*
The Marketing Environment *393*
The Marketing Mix: The Controllables *394*
The Marketing Plan *395*

PART 5
PRINCIPLES OF
LABORATORY FINANCE

twenty-six
Basic Elements of Laboratory
  Financial Management **403**
David J. Fine, Rohn J. Butterfield, Justin E. Doheny
Financing Health Care *403*
Cost, Volume, and Revenue Relationships *407*
The Clinical Laboratory in Hospital Context *414*

twenty-seven
Budgeting Laboratory Financial Resources **417**
David J. Fine, Rohn J. Butterfield, Justin E. Doheny
The Operating Expense Budget *417*
Types of Budget *419*
Capital Decision-making *425*
Revenue Budget and Rate-setting *434*

twenty-eight
Wage and Salary Administration **439**
John R. Snyder
The Reward System: Compensation and
  Noncompensation Dimensions *439*
Legislation Governing Compensation
  Administration *441*
Human Resource Cost Accounting *442*
Personnel Budgeting *444*
Financial Compensation for Laboratory
  Staff *445*
Employee Benefits and Services *448*
Employee Incentive Systems Based on Merit *450*
Payroll Accounting *451*
Arrangements for Compensating Physicians *452*

twenty-nine
Laboratory Cost-Accounting
  and Work-Load Analysis **457**
David W. Glenn
Work-Load Recording *457*
Cost Accounting and Work-Load Statistics *460*
Other Uses of Work-Load Analysis *467*

thirty
Financial Ratios for Laboratory
  Management Decision-making **475**
James W. Sharp
New Goals and Challenges *475*
The Three-Step Process *476*

thirty-one
Inventory Management and Cost Containment **487**
Robert V. Lucchetti, John R. Snyder
Scientific Inventory Management *487*
Technical Description of Inventory
  Replenishment Systems *489*

Index **510**

Administration and Supervision in Laboratory Medicine

Second Edition

part one

Fundamentals of Laboratory Management

one

The Nature of Management in the Clinical Laboratory

John R. Snyder, Ph.D.
Donald A. Senhauser, M.D.

The American health-care system is large, complex, and diverse.[16] In 1981, expenditures totaled $287 billion, comprising 9.8% of the nation's gross national product (GNP).[27] Estimated spending by the year 2000 will be approximately 15% of the GNP. Complexity in the system is reflected by a diversity of providers, both physician and nonphysician; organized in a variety of ways—private practice, group practice, health maintenance organizations; and functioning in a variety of settings—different kinds and sizes of hospitals, clinics, nursing homes, and other agencies. It is estimated that approximately $16 billion of the nation's total health expenditures is for clinical laboratory services.[18] About 7000 hospital laboratories and tens of thousands of doctors' office laboratories perform most analyses, about 75%; the remaining 25% are performed in approximately 6500 independent laboratories.[18]

The most significant change in health care and laboratory medicine has resulted from the widely held notion that health-care costs are out of control. Thus, the expansionary climate of the seventies has abruptly given way to universal concerns over cost containment, and indeed, cost abatement of health-care spending.[23] These concerns have been reflected by the cascade of federal legislation, including Tax Equity and Fiscal Responsibility Act (TEFRA) in 1982, the introduction of Prospective Payment Systems (PPSs), including diagnosis-related groups (DRGs), in 1983, and the Medicare Provisions in the Budget Reduction Act of 1984. In 1985, the Comprehensive Omnibus Budget Reconciliation Act (COBRA) and the 1986 Omnibus Budget Reconciliation Act (OBRA) placed even greater fiscal constraints on the hospitals, and through the early 1990s we are promised more of the same—in the face of demands for the same standards of entry and quality.[22] Not only the public sector has been concerned with cost containment; American industry, which spent over $70 billion in health-insurance premiums in 1985, also has lent its support to cost-containment measures. For the first time in 20 years, health-care providers find themselves in a serious adversarial position with *both* government and industry and, in turn, with third-party insurers.[19]

Perhaps the most significant change affecting hospital laboratory administration today is the PPS, which became effective on October 1, 1983. Under PPS regulation a lump sum payment is made to most hospitals for Medicare admissions that is based not on the actual cost of the services provided, but rather on the discharge diagnosis. Under this system, all discharges are classified or grouped under DRGs, with payment based on a predetermined amount for each DRG. Before the introduction of this system, clinical laboratories were considered

3

revenue-generating centers in the hospital budget, since at least a portion of the costs to perform tests was reimbursable. Under prospective payment, each test performed becomes a cost charged against the lump sum payment for the DRG; hence the laboratory is now a cost center for the hospital. With the full implementation of the PPS, well-managed laboratories that were profit centers and primarily concerned with high levels of service and quality will become loss leaders to the hospitals. *Cost containment* and *competition* have become the watchwords of laboratory medicine in the 1980s.

This new climate of socioeconomic and regulatory restraint has put significant stresses on laboratory management. Cost-effective delivery of laboratory services rests more firmly than ever on the sound practice of administration and supervision, as described by McLendon and Reich:[15]

> The efficient operation of a clinical laboratory and the effective delivery of medical laboratory services to clinicians and their patients require a complex interdigitation of expertise in medical, scientific, and technical areas. . . . Although the medical, scientific, and technical expertise . . . are essential prerequisite(s) for the provision of medical laboratory services, success in applying these techniques to benefit patient care is vitally dependent on the management and communication skills of laboratory directors, supervisors, and technologists.

This concept may be criticized by those who contend that administration is an ancillary activity, and that quality laboratory services result directly from the performance of competent laboratory scientists; but the key element of a successful operation lies in the delivery of such services, a highly complex management activity. Laboratory management's task is to integrate and coordinate organizational resources (*e.g.,* personnel, equipment, money, time, and space) so that quality laboratory services can be provided as effectively and efficiently as possible. The successful administration of today's clinical laboratory, like any other organization or institution, requires a vast array of skills founded on sound principles of management science.

ADMINISTRATION — ART OR SCIENCE?

Laboratory professionals are often reluctant to consider management as a science. Our educational background, laden with courses in the exacting sciences of chemistry, physics, and biology, tends to bias our acceptance of the disciplines we allow to be classified as sciences. Our laboratory activities, incumbent on Gaussian statistics and predictive diagnostic value, create a mindset limiting the parameters by which we tend to judge the "true" sciences.

Administration can, however, qualify as a science comparable to economics, psychology, and sociology, in that there exists an organized body of knowledge unique to the domain. Koontz and O'Donnel proposed more than 50 truths or principles to define the science of administration.[9] The search for professionalism in management led to the excesses of the secular-rationalist approach to management in the 1960s,[17] which attempted to discard the human element from management science, because "human behavior complicates immensely the task of explaining and predicting phenomena."[20]

Administration is indeed a science that, like its sister disciplines psychology and sociology, is inexact *because* it must deal to a large extent with the human element. Thus, any proposed principles of administration will be characterized by some softness and variability due to human behavior in the organization. The new wave of management theory, expressed by Peters and Waterman,[17] recognizes the variability and change human relations bring to the science of administration.

Any proposed principles for the study of administration will be characterized by variables and change. All science is, in fact, dynamic. We are more accepting of the fact that laboratory medicine as a science is constantly changing as research continues to push back the frontier of the unknown. Likewise, the science of administration continues to change as the variables inherent in the management process stimulate research and modification of generalizations into new knowledge.

Still other laboratory professionals perceive administration as an art, requiring only native ability or common sense. Art by definition is creative adaptation, and a component of the management process does require native ability. In the practice of laboratory medicine, decisions are often contingent upon the specific situation. The art inherent in laboratory medicine is the application of knowledge based on perceived contingencies. In management it is the skill that comes with experience, observation, and study of the situation.

Thus, administration can be considered both a science and an art. The management process requires the art of creativity based on and conditioned by an understanding of the principles of management science.

DEFINITION OF ADMINISTRATION

In this book, the terms *administration* and *management* are used interchangeably. Administration of the clinical laboratory is generally viewed as an all-inclusive concept covering the managerial skills necessary for personnel from the laboratory director to the bench supervisor. At all levels, management involves the coordination and integration of resources to accomplish specific results. Management has been viewed differently by many authorities; and their various perceptions, schools of managerial thought, and experiences have resulted in nearly as many definitions as there are people who have attempted to define the term. Included are such definitions as "the process by which individual and group effort is coordinated toward superordinate goals"; "a social process comprising a series of actions that lead to the accomplishment of objectives"; "getting from where we are to where we want to be with the least expenditure of time, money, and effort"; and "the universal process of efficiently getting activities completed with and through other people."[1,9,20,21]

The most universally accepted definition bantered about has been simply "getting things done through other people." This is a fine rule for the practicing manager but leaves something to be desired from the academician's point of view. When a joint meeting was called with the primary purpose of defining *management* in terms that both the educators and executives could live with, the following definition resulted:[1]

> Management is the guiding of human and physical resources into dynamic organization units that attain their objectives to the satisfaction of those served and with a high degree of morale and sense of attainment on the part of those rendering the service.

This definition is perhaps a bit flowery, but it can serve as a place to begin and as a measuring stick for evaluation. The definition contains four basic elements identified by Kast and Rosenzweig:[7] (1) "toward objectives," (2) "through people," (3) "using techniques," and (4) "in an organization." The definition proposed by the educators and executives is the most comprehensive and perhaps the best suited as a working model for the clinical laboratory:

Toward objectives—goals and purposes consistent with efficient delivery of laboratory services for quality health care

Through people—guiding people (leading and directing) in such a manner that these professional laboratorians feel a sense of responsibility and attainment (achievement)

Using techniques—physical resources, such as laboratory equipment, computers, space, and so forth

In an organization—into dynamic organizational units implying division of labor, specialization, protocols and procedures, and functional processing units

It must be pointed out that management is an activity. It is not letting each day take care of itself; rather, it is making things happen. Too often laboratory managers fall into the trap of "fighting fires" on a daily basis. For administration to be effective, it must be in control, planning ahead the steps that will ensure efficient operation of the laboratory.

Figure 1-1 graphically displays this definition of administration.[20] Laboratory managers are entrusted with three categories of resources (input): *financial*—operating and capital budget; *physical*—space, equipment, and supplies; and *human*—technical and support staff. As a result of the managerial role and fulfilling certain functions—*i.e.,* planning, organizing, leading, and evaluating—three categories of output are expected: *satisfactory performance*—accurate and timely testing in a cost-effective manner; *products*—legible and interpretable laboratory reports to the physician when needed; and *self-serving behavior*—a sense of accomplishment among the staff doing the work. Note also that there are many external and organizational forces that influence the administrative process in any given institution.

MANAGERIAL DUTIES AND RESPONSIBILITIES

The terms *director, administrator, manager,* and *supervisor* are sometimes used interchangeably. Comte and Lee have delineated each in the following manner:[3]

A *director* directs the affairs of an organization by establishing goals and priorities that determine the direction the organization will take. The director might not directly supervise or manage in a technical sense, since his role is primarily one of broad policy-making.

An *administrator* administers or runs an organization within the framework of the various directives and policies given to him. Strictly speak-

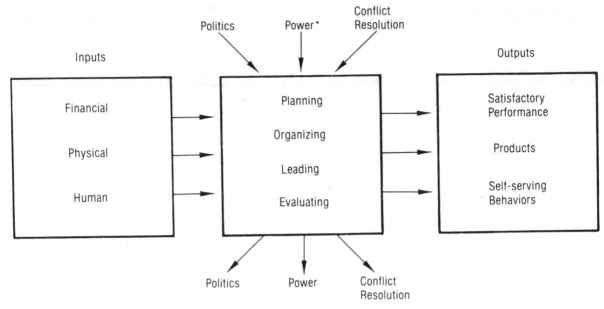

FIGURE 1-1. Advanced descriptive administrative model. (From Robbins SP: The Administrative Process, p 57. Englewood Cliffs, Prentice Hall, 1976. Reprinted by permission of publisher)

ing, he is not the person who establishes the larger goals, but a technician who knows how to make the organization move efficiently to achieve its purpose.

A *manager* takes charge of the management or oversees the functioning of an activity to achieve a set goal or purpose. His strength is in his ability to use all of these resources to get things done properly.

A *supervisor* oversees the activities of others to help them to accomplish specific tasks or to perform scheduled activities most efficiently.

There is considerable overlap in terms of duties and responsibilities among these members of the management team.[13] In the clinical laboratory, the administrative skills needed for each of these positions are largely the same. The differences rest in the amount of expertise that each member of the management team must possess. For example, the laboratory director will probably possess the greatest expertise in the overall function of the laboratory in the delivery of quality medical care, the manager in inspection and accreditation, and the supervisor in the technology, scheduling, and staffing of a given laboratory section.

There are several key concepts that enable distinction of three levels in the management team of the laboratory. *Laboratory directors* and *administrators* retain ultimate responsibility for seeing that the organization moves toward achievement of its goals. Changes in technology, capital investments, and services rendered are finalized by this level of laboratory management. *Laboratory managers,* sometimes termed *administrative* or *chief technologists,* create and maintain an environment designed so that other laboratory professionals can function efficiently. Laboratory managers plan, organize, direct, and control jobs. *Laboratory supervisors,* conversely, are managers whose major activities focus on people and operational provision of laboratory services. All levels of management have supervisory functions, but the first-line laboratory supervisor's major function is working with and through staff (bench-level) technologists and technicians to meet the needs of these employees and the objectives of the department.

Since personnel costs constitute the major portion of the laboratory budget, laboratory medicine is appropriately categorized as a labor-intensive "industry." Some laboratory managers contend that the only manager who needs human relations skills is the line supervisor. This simply is not true. Figure

1-2 shows three management levels within the clinical laboratory and corresponding blocks of administrative skills needed and exercised. The bench-level supervisor is called on to exercise a substantial number of technical skills in the performance of laboratory testing: instrument repair, trouble-shooting, new procedure selection, and development. The laboratory director or administrator, conversely, exercises fewer technical skills; rather, the emphasis shifts at this level to conceptual skills, such as long-range planning, goal-setting, and innovating in response to change. The administrative or chief technologist in the middle is required to exercise skills in both the technical and conceptual areas. But notice the block of interpersonal skills: all three levels of laboratory management need to be equally adept in this area. Human relations skills in a labor-intensive industry are of critical importance to managerial effectiveness.

It is noteworthy to comment on the key concept of *leader* versus *boss*. The clinical laboratory is staffed by individuals with a wide variety of backgrounds and educational preparation, from unit clerk through doctorate-level clinical associate. The cohesion of this group as a health-care team is essential for effective management. The clinical laboratory administrator is a manager of professionals. For this reason, the concept of a supervisor as a boss is inappropriate. Today's laboratory supervisor is a leader who promotes a climate of cooperation and respect so that the staff laboratorian will want to be led and possibly lead and direct himself.[8] One manages *things*, but leads *people*.

THE ADMINISTRATIVE PROCESS

Laboratory management's task is to integrate and coordinate resources toward accomplishment of a goal. The task is thus a process comprising a series of actions, which some authors like to call the five functions of a manager. The effective use of input resources to achieve output through administrative functions is shown in Figure 1-3. Regardless of the title given the activities, the administrative process includes *planning, organizing, directing,* and *controlling.* These terms are introduced here as part of the process and are elaborated on in later chapters.

FIGURE 1-2. Leadership skills needed/exercised at various managerial levels. (Adapted from Beam LK: Relating people and tasks: Managing your administrative and instructional staff. In Langerman PD, Smith DH (eds): Managing Adult and Continuing Education Programs and Staff, p 289. Washington, National Association for Public Continuing and Adult Education, 1979)

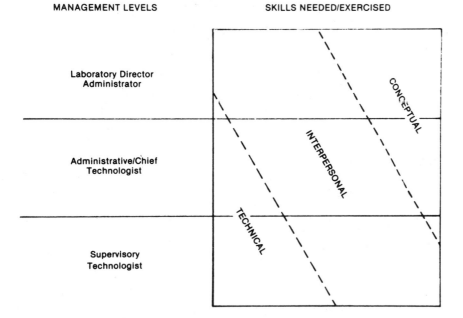

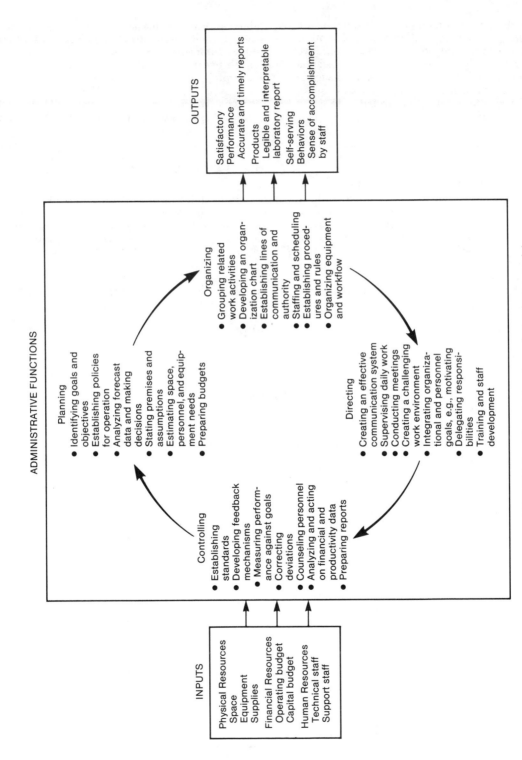

FIGURE 1-3. Clinical laboratory administration model.

Planning

A key function of managers at all levels is the planning of activities under their direction. In the medical laboratory, both long-range and short-range plans are drawn up. A laboratory director will probably be responsible for long-range planning concerned with growth potential or degree of expansion. For example, the director may wish to bring in house a battery of analyses previously sent to a reference laboratory. His planning steps would include identifying sufficient equipment, space, and personnel; a series of written protocols and procedures; cost-per-test analysis; and so forth. The laboratory director will no doubt involve the appropriate chief technologist and supervisor in some short-range planning. Short-range planning includes setting specific objectives to aid in reaching long-range goals. In this example, the supervisor may be responsible for planning a variety of steps to establish protocols and procedures (*e.g.,* method comparison research and development within the department; ordering of supplies and reagents; scheduling personnel based on the frequency with which the test is to be performed; and so forth). All levels of laboratory management should be involved in various phases of both long- and short-range planning—a crucial activity in the administration process. Most management failure is due to a failure in communication.

Organizing

The organizing function involves developing a structure to facilitate the coordination of resources to achieve completion of long- and short-range plans. A division of labor is created in which various units or departments are responsible for particular activities or phases of operation. A spectrum of working relationships must then be delineated to include such things as lines of authority or responsibility and work flow for the optimal functioning of the interrelated units.

Directing

The directing function is best described as managerial leadership. Managers in the clinical laboratory, as in any organization, must be concerned with the human element. Successful managerial leadership creates a climate in which both the needs of the individual and the goals of the organization can be met. This most crucial managerial function and the

parameters that increase or decrease its effectiveness will be discussed more fully in Part II of this book.

Controlling

The wrap-up function in the administrative process is controlling, which ensures that the end-product of organized and directed events conforms to plans. Supervisors of the clinical laboratory are ever aware of the importance of good quality control. In the administrative process, controlling is equally important and includes many of the same activities: defining standards and criteria for acceptable performance, developing a reporting system, and taking corrective action when and where needed.

Decision-Making

An activity that is inherent in all other administrative process activities is decision-making. This is the part of the process that ties everything together. Decisions must be made as part of planning, organizing, directing, and controlling. Because of its importance in all other process functions, we have devoted an entire chapter (Chap. 3) to the consideration of the decision-making process. Although many steps and concerns must be considered, the process itself generally includes problem analysis, development and analysis of alternative courses of action, and decision implementation and control.

The advent of prospective payment for reimbursement of laboratory services provided by hospitals has prompted top-level administration to closely scrutinize cost-effective management of clinical laboratories. As profit centers under cost reimbursement, clinical laboratories were allowed considerable latitude in their operations. And many laboratory administrators survived through the "cost be damned" attitude. Today, as a *cost* center, laboratory administrators must lead and manage. New skills under each of the traditional functions are now needed. As part of planning, for example, laboratory managers are called upon to accurately forecast cost/benefit ratios, to analyze new opportunities, and market to new entities such as health maintenance organizations (HMOs). When considering the laboratory's organization, managers must modify the structure for efficiency and redesign jobs, perhaps creating career ladders for technical staff. To increase productivity under the directing function, managers need to create a work environment characterized by responsibility and participative management. Under the controlling function, laboratory managers must implement cost-containment measures through reduction in overuse of testing, inventory control, and financial ratio analysis, a form of "economic grand rounds" in the laboratory.

MAKING THE TRANSITION TO LABORATORY MANAGEMENT

One of the most difficult hurdles for the new manager or supervisor is the transition from staff responsibilities to administrative responsibilities. This transition includes a shift in the focus from direct service responsibility to new relationships, new responsibilities of managing versus doing (delegation), and a new realm of influence (leadership).

Dual Hierarchy in Hospitals

Typical organizational hierarchies are bureaucratic pyramids (see Chap. 2) with specific lines of communication and authority. However, as hospitals developed over the last century, a unique governance structure evolved with them. The medical staff of the hospital (consisting of physicians with admitting privileges), who were the "users" of hospital services, including the laboratory, formed into a separate organization with an independent, but also an interdependent, relationship to the administrative structure of the hospital, thus creating a dual hierarchical structure. While the hospital administration was perceived to be primarily concerned with providing safe and efficient care for *all* of its patients, the major role of the medical staff was seen as ensuring the quality of care for the *individual* patient by controlling admission to the medical staff (credentialling) as well as the scope of privileges granted to a staff physician practicing within the hospital. The governance of the medical staff in its role of monitoring standards of medical practice within the institution was thought to be quite independent of the hospital administration and the governing board. The standards of performance of this dual hierarchy were mandated and monitored by outside accrediting agencies such as the Joint Commission on Accreditation of Hospitals—the JCAH (see Annotated Bibliography).

During the last decade, and due to radical changes in the legal and economic environment in which hospitals and their medical staffs operate, there has been a significant and major increase in the role and responsibilities of the governing board for the governance of the hospital. That body is now directly responsible for "establishing policy, maintaining the quality of patient care and providing for

institutional management and planning" (JCAH Manual for Accreditation of Hospitals, 1988). Under the pressures of these increased responsibilities, the governing boards of hospitals have moved vigorously to force both arms of the dual administrative hierarchy to become more responsive to the board itself. Thus the hospital administrator and the chief of the medical staff both report directly, but separately, to the governing board and board members sit on many hospital and medical staff committees. In turn, members of the executive committee of the medical staff are assigned to key subcommittees of the governing body (Fig. 1–4).

Under the new administrative pattern, the medical directors of the professional service departments (radiology, anesthesiology, and pathology [laboratory medicine]) are responsible to the governing board through the executive committee of the medical staff for all professional (medical care) activities. At the same time they are also responsible to the hospital administrative hierarchy, which may be more concerned with the management and fiscal issues of their departments, such as the laboratory, than in direct care to the individual patient (Fig. 1–4). This may place the medical director in a conflict situation, attempting to be responsive to the needs of the medical staff, which is primarily concerned with quality of patient care and outcomes, as well as to management demands of hospital administration.

In some institutions, especially the larger hospitals, this conflict situation may be minimized by the creation of two director/manager positions—a medical director for physician/patient affairs (usually a pathologist) and a laboratory manager for laboratory administration and technical services (usually a medical technologist with additional education and experience in management). In such an arrangement, matters of professional services and quality assurance are left to the pathologist/medical director, while the laboratory manager handles the day-to-day administrative affairs of the laboratory, reporting to hospital administration. Obviously the potential for conflict still exists under this arrangement, but may be better resolved between two laboratorians who share the mutual goal of maintaining excellence in the clinical laboratory.

The increasing demand for accountability of the governing body of the hospital for matters of cost containment, utilization review, and quality assurance by the courts, governmental agencies, and accrediting bodies such as the Joint Commission on Accreditation of Health Organizations (JCAHO) will require continuing modification of the hierarchical structures discussed above. It is almost certain that the governing body will become more and

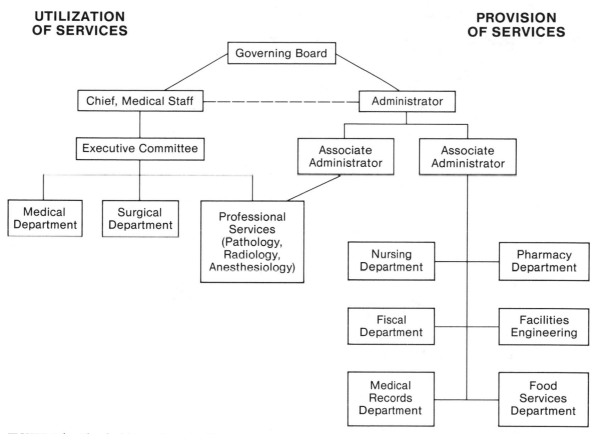

FIGURE 1-4. The dual hierarchy in health care.

more influential in the management of hospitals and other health care organizations.

New Relationships

To be effective, the laboratory director/manager must understand individual and professional outlooks and balance his respective interests while interacting with both sides of the dual hierarchy.[12] Table 1-1 shows differences in professional "cultures" among health-care professional groups. Contrast, for example, the differences in viewing resources: hospital administrators (health services management) focus on allocating scarce resources, whereas the attending physician perceives that all required resources should be available to maximize the quality of patient care.

The new laboratory director or manager also finds himself faced with a host of new relationships and variables to be balanced.[13,26] Figure 1-5 shows "top down" demands and requests of the organization for comprehensive services and efficiency, and

productivity and cost-containment expectations from his immediate supervisor. While handling these, the manager must balance demands and requests by subordinates for higher pay and factors to enhance job satisfaction in the laboratory setting. On either side, peer department managers expect coordination of efforts and cooperation. Stress and conflict resolution will play an increasing role in successful laboratory management.

Managing Versus Doing

One of the most difficult hurdles for the new supervisor is the transition period between staff responsibilities and management responsibilities. In past years, when a supervisor was needed, the common method was to evaluate the staff members within the department for the best-performing technologist. This individual was then appointed supervisor on the assumption that because he performed well at the bench, he would automatically make a good supervisor. Although it is true that a good laboratory

Table 1-1
Differences in Professional Cultures Among Health-Care Profession Groups

Attribute	Health Services Management	Clinical Laboratory Technical Staff	Physicians and Pathologists
Basis of knowledge	Social and management sciences	Combination of biomedical and social sciences	Primarily biomedical sciences
Patient focus	All patients in the larger community	Patients represented by specimen samples clustered by type of laboratory analyses requested	Individual patients categorized by type of disease
Exposure to clients while in training	The clients are primarily nurses and physicians. Relatively little exposure to them during graduate school training	Clients are attending physicians and nurses, to whom limited exposure is possible	Great deal of exposure but not necessarily what they will see in practice
Time frame of action	Medium to long range; gather information, analyze data; engage in long-range strategic planning	Short range with emphasis on timely results and quick turnaround of data	Generally short range; cause–effect relationships, although varies by specialty
View of resources	Limited; main challenge is one of allocating scarce resources	Recognize some limitations but more narrowly than the administrator	Resources essentially unlimited; resources should be available to maximize the quality of patient care
Professional identity	Less cohesive	Somewhat cohesive	Most cohesive

(Adapted with permission from Shortell SM: Theory Z: Implications and relevance for health care management. Health Care Management Review, Fall 1982.)

supervisor must know every facet of the department for which he is responsible, he may or may not possess the potential for managerial skills. The new supervisor's perception of his responsibilities are a good indication of how successful he will become, as illustrated by the following case history adapted from Scanlon.[21]

Case Study

A number of years ago, two medical technologists with essentially the same educational backgrounds, experience, and tenure in a large laboratory were placed in management positions at about the same time. As opposed to being paid for performing their

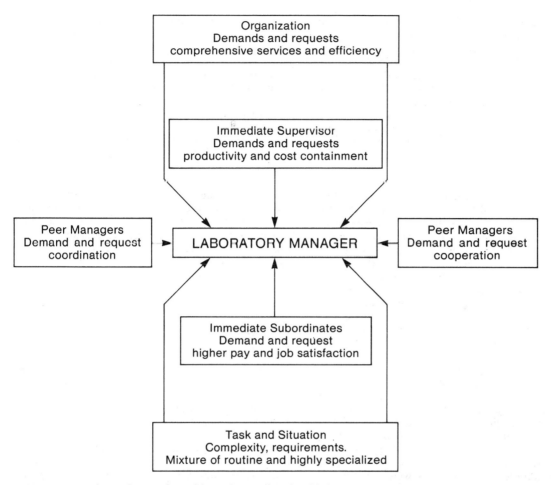

FIGURE 1-5. Relationships and variables to be perceived and balanced by a laboratory manager.

technical specialty, they were now being paid for being technical administrators, or supervisors of departments in which clinical laboratory testing was performed. At the end of the first 6 months, one of them was experiencing considerable success and enjoying his new managerial job. The other was not so successful. He was experiencing problems in meeting schedules and test report deadlines, there was a degree of unrest among the technologists in his department, and he himself was becoming discouraged and frustrated. Higher level management was becoming concerned about the situation.

The first man had obviously adapted well to his new role. He realized that, in a way, he was embarking on a new and different career within the laboratory organization and had adjusted accordingly. More specifically, whether it was because of his own

personal insight or because he received help from his superior, he perceived his role and function to be different from what it used to be. Among the many things he did after being appointed a manager was to take inventory of the department in terms of the work that had to be done and the people he had available to do it. He concerned himself not only with the number of people available but also with their individual skills and abilities, strengths, and weaknesses. He reviewed the work flow in the department; and using this as a base, formulated priorities and schedules. Through individual and departmental meetings, he communicated to his people the teamwork approach to health care and the interrelationship that the department shared with other departments and the medical center as a whole. In addition, he gave his technologists a clear picture of where the department stood with respect to what was expected and the present status of performance. He shared and discussed with them some of the problems that he thought were inhibiting better departmental performance and obtained their ideas on what could be done to improve things. Beyond this, he took an active interest in each technologist individually and worked with him or her in a coaching capacity to set goals, help improve performance, and provide more satisfaction from the job. In other words, he *managed:* he planned, made decisions, organized, directed, and controlled.

The other man became somewhat overawed by his new role. As soon as he realized he was no longer expected to do actual laboratory testing, he became confused. He had to spend his time some way, so he began by making a point of checking every test result before it left the department. When he found an error, which he was bound to do, he was quick to call it to the attention of the technologist in question. He made the corrections himself. He became convinced that more checking was needed; it almost became a challenge to find something wrong. This led him to spending more time to make sure things were done right. Frequently he would watch a technologist having trouble with a procedure so he could point out the flaw in the technique. He thought that all of the special procedures and research and development, as well as the CAP check sample, demanded his personal attention. Often he worked on these projects until late at night and on weekends. Because he became so involved in working alone on these "special" projects, other responsibilities were neglected. Workload-recording reports and employee evaluations were not filed on time. At a laboratory supervisors' meeting, he was unable to give an adequate breakdown on the status of the entire department's workflow or comment on why the turnaround time in reporting of results was increasing. In addition, his staff assumed less responsibility for their work. They became passive. One of

the more experienced technologists resigned, and two others requested transfers to other departments. This man was not *managing;* he was *doing.* He was doing what he had always done: practicing his technical specialty. In management he had found something strange and different to which he could not adjust. He was not able to become a supervisor and gain satisfaction in the accomplishments of others. He could not let go of the pipet, the test tube, and all the other laboratory apparatus with which he worked. Eventually he failed as a manager and returned to his specialty.

It is obvious from this case history that there is little direct relationship between technical and managerial skills. A supervisor requires a unique set of knowledge, skills, abilities, and attitudes. During this transitional phase, the new supervisor must recognize the shift from operational duties to supervisory duties. Inability to delegate is the most common downfall of the new manager.

The Supervisor's Circle of Influence

Although all levels of management have supervisory functions, the largest number of individuals involved in laboratory management are supervisors, so some additional attention to them is warranted. Successful supervisors are the key to successful laboratory administration.

The laboratory supervisor is undoubtedly the most significant member of the management team in influencing staff personnel. Not only the supervisor's perception of his new responsibilities but also his manner and attitude in dealing with his staff are important. Consider the effect of the supervisor's attitude (Fig. 1-6). Suppose a supervisor must find a way to schedule staff for holiday coverage of the laboratory; rather than discussing various options with his people, he arbitrarily assigns them, confi-

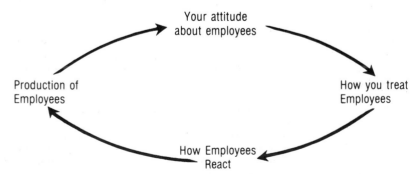

Your attitude about employees

How you treat Employees

How Employees React

Production of Employees

FIGURE 1-6. The supervisor's circle of influence.

dent that they would merely fight among themselves if he did not. As could be expected, the staff begins to grumble over the decision. On the third scheduled holiday, the supervisor receives a call at home informing him that one member of this staff has called in sick. This episode heretofore had been unheard of. In a rage, the supervisor reaffirms in his mind that this is typical of how inept the staff would have been in determining their own schedule and vows to continue making decisions without their input. The supervisor has fallen into the trap of the self-reinforcing cycle. His attitude about the staff dictated his manner of treating employees. How the employees were treated affected how the employees reacted. This reaction is reflected in their response or production, which in turn reinforces the supervisor's attitude. A vicious cycle is created, one to which each supervisor should be sensitive.

The supervisor has the ability to create an environment conducive to effective and efficient operations. It is up to the supervisor to develop surroundings in which people will want to work to their full potential.[8] In the clinical laboratory, as in any organization, there are those who are only interested in picking up their paychecks. Most employees, however, would like to get something more out of their daily jobs. The supervisor has the responsibility of acting as a catalyst in causing efficient and rewarding performance. Fulmer has described six contributions that can be particularly important in creating an environment to encourage maximum accomplishment:

1. A worker's job must define goals. These objectives must be carefully outlined and explained so that they are clearly understood by everyone involved. A person simply cannot work well toward an end that is not understood.
2. Surroundings should give workers a definite, clear idea of their roles in the organization. Not only must they understand goals; they must also recognize the kinds of personal judgment they can apply to the operation. In addition, the workers must have access to the information and tools necessary for the job.
3. The supervisor should try to remove any obstacles that might stand in the way of the worker's effective performance. If a supervisor cannot solve critical problems, he should ask for help from an immediate superior.
4. Ideally, the working environment should encourage personnel to do their jobs as the supervisors want them to be done. It must be clear that certain procedures are preferred because they are most effective.
5. The worker must have a sense of being a vital part of the organization, rather than a cog in a huge machine. The supervisor must always be aware that subordinates are people with needs and desires to be considered.
6. The supervisor should realize that some of his workers may have useful ideas for solutions to current problems. The working surroundings should stimulate them to express these ideas so that more answers can be found and more people can participate in making decisions.

EDUCATING LABORATORY ADMINISTRATORS

Many laboratory supervisors and managers have been promoted into their positions on the strength of their technical abilities; and, more often than not, their training has been received on the job.[4,14] Robbins has contrasted the concept of training to education:[20]

Training is the process of learning a sequence of programmed behaviors. We train bricklayers, television repairmen, typists, and hospital admission clerks. The activities of these jobs can be precisely defined, broken down, analyzed, and a "one best way" determined. Training is the application of knowledge. It gives people an awareness of the rules and procedures to guide their behavior.

In contrast, education instills sound reasoning processes rather than merely imparting a body of serial facts. Education is the understanding and interpretation of knowledge. It does not provide definitive answers, but rather develops a logical and rational mind that can determine relationships among pertinent variables and thereby understand phenomena.

This statement might lead us to believe that laboratory administrators can be educated in the classroom alone. Although the classroom setting is adequate to introduce the principles of management science and the basic techniques of effective supervision, it does not provide a complete preparation for administrative responsibilities. The introductory experiences of applying these principles and techniques within specific situations are missing. We know that academic grades are incomplete predictors of success for performing laboratory analysis. The same is true of a classroom exposure to laboratory administration. There exists no substitute for some type of trial experience or externship as part of the educational process. Indeed, if we were to survey laboratory administrators, it would be evident "that many outstanding administrators have never had a formal course in administration, whereas many incompetents have a long list of impressive academic accomplishments,"[19] as has been proven in industry.

Facilitating the development of technical managers requires an understanding of what technical managers need to learn and a sense of when they are most ready to learn.[10] When new supervisors were polled by Bittel to determine their feelings of need as they began new careers, the following results were obtained:[2]

89% wanted more knowledge of human relations

59% needed better communications techniques

40% felt deficient in personnel procedures and record-keeping

39% needed help in operations planning

27% wanted better methods of staff development

Notice that most of the specified needs were for effective methods of dealing with people. This knowledge is not easily or simply obtained and probably is best realized through practice in the working setting. Once again, no substitute exists for experiencing these forces as part of the educational process.

CHALLENGES FOR TODAY'S LABORATORY MANAGER

A host of external forces has prompted clinical laboratories to change in recent years. Governmental intervention, cost-containment initiatives, prospective reimbursement, increasing competition, and societal demands for access to complex diagnostic services are just a few of the forces driving change. These changes, coupled with characteristics inherent in laboratory medicine, pose a significant challenge for the laboratory manager.[25]

Subsequent chapters dissect laboratory administration and supervision by functions and tasks in an effort to thoroughly analyze strategies for effective management. Before this dissection is begun, it is appropriate to again recognize that management is a process and that functions and tasks overlap.

One helpful tool for maintaining the interrelatedness of management function is a system analysis.[25] Leavitt proposed a systems model focusing on four interactive components or dimensions of an organization:[11] *task,* the mission, goals, and objectives of the laboratory; *structure,* characteristics of the organizational chart, including lines of authority and communication, division of labor, and workflow; *technology,* tools and instrumentation available for accomplishing the goals; and *people,* laboratory employees' knowledge, skills, attitudes, and expectations. Figure 1-7 illustrates the interactive nature of each dimension with double-ended arrows. The systems model is helpful in viewing the laboratory from a holistic perspective and predicting how modifying one dimension of the system is likely to have an impact on other dimensions. For example, if the mission of the laboratory was expanded (task dimension) to include services to an HMO in the community, this change would probably have an impact on the workflow (structure dimension), the demands on testing equipment and data processing (technology dimension), and personnel requirements needed for the increased volume.

The figure displays selected negative characteristics of laboratory medicine influencing each of these dimensions that make managing a clinical laboratory difficult.[6] The task dimension is buffeted and responsive to demands in the marketplace for increased numbers of diagnostic procedures in opposition to cost-containment efforts. Managers are challenged to deal with the problem of poor image and lack of identity by laboratory staff in the structure dimension. In this dimension also, a lack of uniform personnel standards has technologists doing technician-level work, and *vice versa.* The organizational chart in many laboratories allows limited opportunities for career advancement. Rapid advances in the technology dimension have been a mixed blessing. While adding to the accuracy, efficiency, and cost-effectiveness of many analyses, they have prompted task repetition and significant variability between departments and settings. Laboratory work, even with advances in technology, remains stressful. Managers must also deal with dissatisfaction on the part of technical staff members when expectations for more challenging work are not realized and salaries remain mediocre in contrast to those of other health-care professionals. Interpersonal conflict among personnel often smolders as a result of allegiance to different professional organizations.

Although this list is far from conclusive, the sampling of characteristics discussed should be sufficient to heighten the awareness of the laboratory manager to the challenges inherent in administering the clinical laboratory. In addition, the systems analysis perspective shows how interactive the components of the clinical laboratory are.

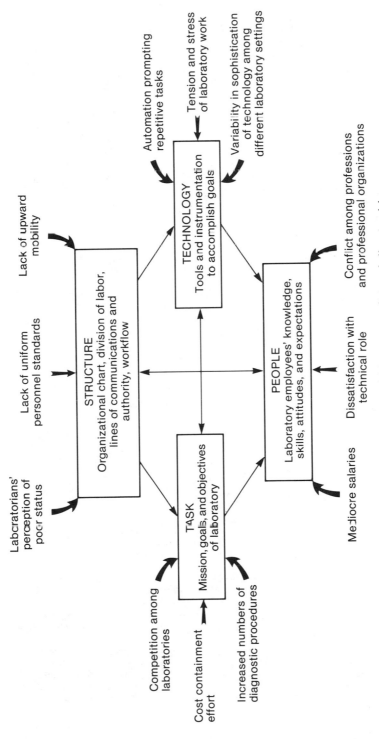

FIGURE 1-7. Select characteristics of laboratory medicine challenging laboratory managers

Finally, as Leavitt[11] has pointed out, the managing process is an interactive flow of three variables: pathfinding, decision-making, and implementing. The successful manager understands that the three variables are interconnected, and in the complexity described above, he must be able to make decisions and implement them, often in the face of inadequate information.

BRIDGING THE GAP—AN APPROACH

Sufficient background is provided herein on the science of management in order to apply and develop a variety of managerial skills essential for effective laboratory administration. We have purposely avoided recording the research that led to the establishment of various principles. Accordingly, the development and differentiation of different schools of administrative thought have not been explored. The emphasis is on bridging the gap between the theory and the practice of management for clinical laboratory administrators.

REFERENCES

1. Appley LA: The Nature of Management, Film One in a series. In Supervisory Management Course—Part One. New York, American Management Association, 1968
2. Bittel L: What Every Supervisor Should Know, 3rd ed, p 18. New York, McGraw-Hill, 1974
3. Comte RF, Lee LW: Management Procedures, p 16. Indianapolis, Bobbs-Merrill, 1975
4. Florane RK: Marketability of medical technologists with a graduate degree in administration and supervision. J Med Technol 2:453–458, 1985
5. Fulmer RM: Supervision: Principles of Professional Management, p 6. Beverly Hills, Glencoe Press, 1976
6. Karni KR: Clinical laboratories—a survey. In Karni KR, Viskochil KR, Amos PA (eds): Clinical Laboratory Management: A Guide for Clinical Laboratory Scientists, pp 3–40. Boston, Little, Brown, 1982
7. Kast FE, Rosenzweig JE: Organization and Management: A Systems Approach, 2nd ed, p 6. New York, McGraw-Hill, 1974
8. King EC: A design for laboratory managers to encourage staff motivation. Laboratory Management 16(3):45–48, 1978
9. Koontz H, O'Donnel C: Principles of Management, 5th ed. New York, McGraw-Hill, 1972
10. Krembs PK: Making managers of technical gurus. Training and Development Journal 37(9):36–41, 1983
11. Leavitt HJ: Applied organizational change in industry: Structural, technological and humanistic approaches. In March TG (ed): Handbook of Organizations, pp 1144–1170. New York, Rand McNally, 1965
12. Levey S, Loomba NP: Health Care Administration: A Managerial Perspective, 2nd ed, pp 3–20, 58–60. Philadelphia, JB Lippincott, 1984
13. McBride K: Task analysis of medical technology administration and supervision. Am J Med Technol 44:688–695, 1978
14. McClure IL, Bayliss FT: Medical technologist supervisors: Are they prepared to manage? Am J Med Technol 44:97–111, 1978
15. McLendon WW, Reich MD: Organization and management of the clinical laboratory. In Henry JB (ed): Clinical Diagnosis and Management by Laboratory Methods, p 1977. Philadelphia, WB Saunders, 1979
16. Miller JR: Strategic management in health care. Lab Med 16:46–48, 1985
17. Peters TJ, Waterman RH Jr: In Search of Excellence. New York, Harper & Row, 1982
18. Peterson LJ: Trends in new laboratory arrangements. MLO 18(2):27–30, 1986
19. Relman AS: Cost control, doctors' ethics and patient care. Issues in Science and Technology, Winter:103–111, 1985
20. Robbins SP: The Administrative Process. Englewood Cliffs, Prentice-Hall, 1976
21. Scanlon BK: Management 18: A Short Course for Managers, pp 3–4. New York, John Wiley & Sons, 1974
22. Schwartz WB, Aron HJ: Health Care Costs: The Social Trade-offs. Issues in Science and Technology, Winter:39–44, 1985
23. Senhauser DA: Medical technology—the challenge to evolve. Laboratory Management 28:48–51, 1985
24. Shortell SM: Theory Z: Implications and relevance for health care management. Health Care Management Review, Fall 1982
25. Snyder JR, Hartzell RK: A systems analysis perspective for managing change in clinical laboratories. Lab Med 18:43–46, 1987
26. Umiker WO: The Effective Laboratory Supervisor, pp 2–11. Oradell, NJ, Medical Economics Company, 1982
27. U.S. Department of Health and Human Services, Health Care Financing Administration: Health Care Financing Review. Washington, D.C., U.S. Government Printing Office, September 1982

ANNOTATED BIBLIOGRAPHY

Joint Commission on Accreditation of Hospitals: Accreditation Manual for Hospitals. Chicago, Joint Commission on Accreditation of Hospitals, 1988.

> This manual should be a "must" reference source for all laboratory managers, as the standards set forth absolutely govern the administrative structure and function of all hospitals and hospital departments.

Bean-McBride K: Textbook of Clinical Laboratory Supervision. New York, Appleton-Century-Crofts, 1982

> This resource is targeted for medical technology undergraduate students or medical technologists who have recently been promoted to a clinical laboratory supervisor position. Components of the laboratory supervisor's role addressed in the text include (1) personnel supervision, (2) monitoring adherence to laboratory procedures, (3) preventive maintenance and troubleshooting of instruments, (4) instruction of medical technology students, (5) daily work scheduling, and (6) ordering reagents and equipment.

Bennington JL, Handmaker H, Freedman GS, et al (eds): Management and Cost Containment Control Techniques for the Clinical Laboratory. Baltimore, University Park Press, 1977
> Part One deals with management of people. Chapters 1, 2, and 3 describe the management team of the clinical laboratory and the interrelationships necessary for organization and effective operation.

Drucker PF: Management Tasks, Responsibilities, Practices. New York, Harper & Row, 1974
> Chapters 1 through 4 of this excellent reference provide a perceptual dimension concerning the history and importance of administration. Chapters 30 through 36 describe the preparation and ultimate role of a manager in today's organization.

Hodgetts RM, Cascio DM: Modern Health Care Administration. New York, Academic Press, 1983
> Recognizing the state of turmoil surrounding current health-care administration, these authors systematically analyze the role of the health-care manager during the decade of the 1980s. Particularly noteworthy chapters include Chapter 4, "Strategic Planning and Health Care"; Chapter 7, "Job Design"; Chapter 15, "Economics and Health Care"; and Chapter 16, "Health Care Marketing." Two short case studies are included at the end of each chapter, providing the reader with an opportunity to apply management principles.

Karni KR, Viskochil KR, Amos PA: Clinical Laboratory Management: A Guide for Clinical Laboratory Scientists. Boston, Little, Brown, 1982
> This resource provides a comprehensive view of clinical laboratory management. At the beginning of each chapter, key words and definitions help the reader to understand new concepts presented in the text. Of particular note is Chapter 1, which collates a wealth of data on the current status of clinical laboratories. This particular chapter ends with a section addressing special problems and challenges facing managers of clinical laboratories.

Levey S, Loomba NP: Health Care Administration: A Managerial Perspective, 2nd ed. Philadelphia, JB Lippincott, 1984
> The authors of this text provide a valuable contribution to the understanding of health care administration primarily from the administrator's perspective. The textbook is divided into three parts: The Framework of Health Care Systems," "Operations Planning," and "Operations Management." Each chapter includes a well-written introduction followed by well-chosen selections from the current literature. Readers will find Part 1 particularly helpful because it introduces a global perspective of the overall parameters of the health-care industry and a systems approach for analyzing various health issues and problems.

McConnell CR: The Effective Health Care Supervisor. Rockville, MD, Aspen Systems Corporation, 1982
> This valuable resource focuses on the key activities of a health-care supervisor. The text is divided into four parts: (1) "The Setting," (2) "The Supervisor Himself," (3) "The Supervisor and the Employee," and (4) "The Supervisor and the Task." While not specifically written for clinical laboratory supervisors, concepts are well presented, and case studies add to the reader's understanding.

Robbins SP: The Administrative Process. Englewood Cliffs, Prentice Hall, 1976
> Chapters 1 through 4 of this book provide an excellent perspective on the philosophy and development of administrative thought. The author provides a substantial background for understanding the forces contributing to current management thinking as well as differences in administrative models. Of particular interest throughout this text is the comparison of a large and small administrative structure through examples.

Shortell SM, Kaluzny AD: Health Care Management: A Text in Organizational Theory and Behavior, 2nd ed. New York, John Wiley & Sons, 1988
> Written from a health care administrator's perspective, this textbook emphasizes the centrality of the managerial role in relation to organization performance. The authors offer a broad exposure to the organizational theory and behavior literature while focusing on the commonality and differences in managing health services organizations. Many chapters include sets of managerial guidelines. Readers will find new information regarding multihospital systems and related organizational coalitions, networks, federations, and affiliations particularly useful. Of interest also will be the discussions about negotiation, bargaining, and conflict resolution managerial skills.

Timmreck T: Dictionary of Health Services Management. Owings Mills, MD, National Health Publishing, 1982
> Practitioners in health care recognize that the industry has always had its unique vocabulary. To help understand the vocabulary of health services management, this is a particularly valuable resource.

Umiker WO: The Effective Laboratory Supervisor. Oradell, NJ, Medical Economics Books, 1982
> This excellent resource is written specifically for laboratory supervisors. Its focus is on the practical applications of management functions and skills by the laboratory supervisor. The author, well known for his numerous contributions to the laboratory management literature, has prepared a clear, cohesive, comprehensive personnel management handbook.

two

Laboratory Planning, Organization, and Control

John R. Snyder

As described in Chapter 1, laboratory management is a complex process in which the manager is entrusted with certain physical, financial, and human resources (input) with the expectation that specific outcomes (quality results in a timely and efficient manner) will be forthcoming. It is important to view management as a *process*. For the purpose of study, laboratory management is often described in terms of four basic functions: planning, organization, direction, and control. In practice, the boundaries between these functions are often obscure because of an interdependence of each function on the other for effective management. This chapter provides a broad, integrative framework for the functions of planning, organization, and control with some specific managerial tools for each.

The key to the management process is goal formulation. The process begins with a specification of the goals of the laboratory and ends with an evaluation of whether they were reached. To carry out the management process, laboratory supervisors and directors determine objectives as part of the planning process, construct an organization able to do the work needed to fulfill the objectives, direct the activities of staff toward meeting the objectives, and compare actual results to measure success or failure in the achievement of the goals.

STRATEGIC MANAGEMENT AND PLANNING

Recent public and government pressure aimed at controlling health-care costs have prompted significant changes in management practices for service providers in the industry. One of the most notable changes is an emphasis on strategic management and planning with a focus on goal formulation and design of specific strategies to be competitive.

Strategic management is defined as the development and implementation of the laboratory's "grand design," or overall strategy, in relation to its current and future demands for service. Schendel and Hofer[22] describe six related major tasks in the strategic management process: (1) goal formulation, (2) environmental analysis, (3) strategy formulation, (4) strategy evaluation, (5) strategy implementation, and (6) strategic control (Fig. 2-1). Inherent in this process is a realization that clinical laboratories need to analyze the external environment, opportunities for growth and development in new service markets, as part of a strategic planning process.

Strategic planning is a related managerial activity that has become popular for clinical laboratories in the last two decades. *Strategic planning* is the process of deciding on objectives for the organiza-

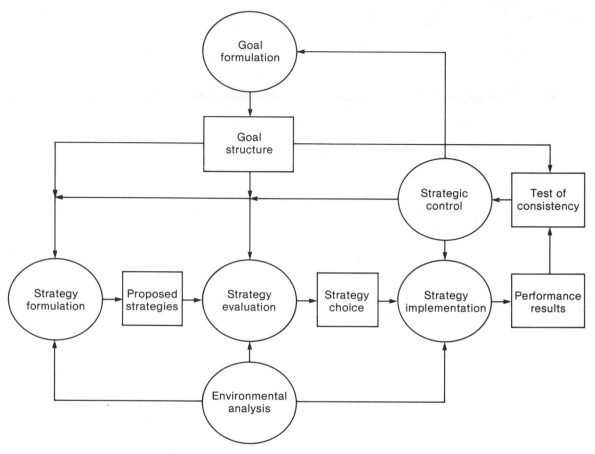

FIGURE 2-1. An overview of the strategic management process. (From Schendel D, Hofer CW: Strategic Management: A New View of Business Policy and Planning, p 15. Boston, Little, Brown & Co, 1979).

tion, on changes in these objectives, on the resources needed to obtain these objectives, and on the policies that are to govern the acquisition, use, and disposition of these resources."[2] Although many methods for doing strategic planning exist, a functional strategic planning process for the clinical laboratory should include defining the mission (goal formulation); developing baseline data; integrating long-range and short-range plans; involving key personnel; and managing in accordance with the objectives.[1] Laboratory managers are increasingly being involved in strategic planning at the institutional level. Albers and Vice offer the following example of a functional strategic planning process appropriate for use in a health-care facility:[1]

I. Strategic planning
  A. Review existing mission and goals using articles of incorporation, minutes of board meeting, etc.
  B. Develop baseline data
    1. Assess market demand using population trends, demographic trends, hospital fee trends, regulatory trends
    2. Estimate market share using utilization trends, medical staffing trends, competition trends, and projected market share trends
    3. Project resource utilization using data on admissions, outpatient visits, and average stay

4. Identify strategic issues including geographic, competitive, resource, medical staff, and patient mix
5. Determine financial status including payor-mix, inpatient capacity, and regulatory factors

C. Evaluate alternative courses of action and identify strategic directions for various market segments

II. Developmental planning
 A. Do market segment analysis
 B. Determine geographic alternatives
 C. Configure programs
 D. Determine financial feasibility
 E. Design construction, etc.
 F. Obtain certificate of need

III. Operational planning
 A. Identify management style, goals, etc.
 B. Establish operating budget
 C. Establish capital budget

IV. Implement the plans

V. Monitor performance

VI. Recycle annually or when significant new data are obtained

PLANNING AT THE DEPARTMENTAL LEVEL

The initial function of departmental management is planning. The laboratory manager must determine both laboratory goals and objectives, as well as the means for achieving them, before he can organize, direct, or control the results. Scanlon proposes that a systems approach to planning is most effective, in that it allows the manager to adapt to changing situations, using feedback information during the process.[14] In the systems approach, planning is divided into four phases:

1. Establishing the goals and objectives for the laboratory
2. Formulating policies to carry out objectives
3. Developing intermediate and short-range plans to implement policies
4. Stating detailed procedures for implementing each plan

This systems approach emphasizes establishing a clear direction (goal or objective) before the laboratory manager begins planning strategies. When policies are set with the goal in mind, constraints are in place to guide the planning strategies prior to the major plan-development stage. The third step is characterized by a plan for completion of a project as well as short-range, interim plans. Finally, the details necessary for the plan's implementation should be spelled out.

Since planning is the initial function in all administrative activities, separating it from organizing and controlling functions is difficult. Figure 2-2 shows the relationship of organizational hierarchy to general planning and control mechanisms. The pyramid structure is typical when describing a hierarchy. The inverted pyramid reflects the degree of detail in each of the mechanisms listed in the planning and control structure. The laboratory director will generally deal with the institution's objectives and goals, one example of which might be to increase the scope of specialized chemistry procedures that the laboratory would perform in house, rather than send to a reference center. The administrative technologist deals with operational policies, those rules for action that will contribute to the successful achievement of goals and objectives. In the example just mentioned, perhaps the administrative technologist would establish policy regarding cost/test ratios to determine which special tests would still be sent to a reference center. The supervisory technologist is responsible for implementing procedures. Procedures are the sequence of steps to implement the short-range plans established by operational policy. In the achievement of this specific goal, the supervisor would undoubtedly have the responsibility for evaluating and implementing the special analytic procedures as well as procedures governing the staffing and instrumentation required. Finally, the technical and clerical staff deal with the rules that govern everyday testing and the performance of the newly established special chemistry analyses of the example. The mechanisms in this figure, then, serve a dual and overlapping role with regard to planning and controlling.

ESTABLISHING POLICIES AND PROCEDURES

Planning has sometimes been referred to as preparation for *where* the organization is going. Establishing policies and procedures addresses the question of *how* the organization is going to achieve specific goals. As evidenced in Figure 2-2, planning mechanisms go from the abstract (general purpose objectives, strategies, goals) to the specific (rules). In between are the purposes, principles, and rules of action, known as policies and procedures, which guide an organization. Their purpose is to designate

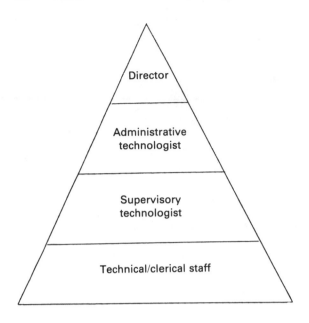

Organization hierarchy

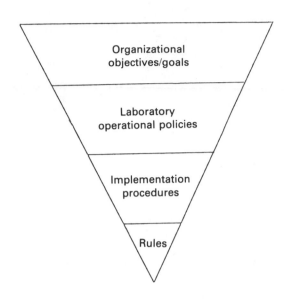

Planning and control mechanisms

FIGURE 2-2. Laboratory planning and control structures.

the aims and ends of an organization and the approximate means to be used in their accomplishment.*

Variations

Within the clinical laboratory, individual policies and procedures will vary according to purpose and application. Policies will vary in specificity. Some policies should be stated in general terms to allow flexibility by professionals in the department. For example, a policy dealing with time off for continuing education may be written in general terms. By contrast, a procedure written to protect against hepatitis will usually be quite detailed. The importance of policies will also vary. Some will be common sense but must be written for the individual who does not always exercise this trait. In some cases, the level of determination of a policy may be to

*This section considers all those directions, both explicit and implied, that qualify as policies and procedures related to the clinical laboratory organizational operations. That is to say that the term *procedures* here excludes the analytic steps and accompanying information that are traditionally found in a laboratory testing procedure manual.

serve as a guideline only, such as the number of weekends each technologist may be required to work. Other policies will be "hard and fast," such as termination for being under the influence of alcohol while on duty.

Another aspect of policies and procedures that will vary is the timing or frequency. Some policies always apply, as in the case of reporting to work on time. Others are less crucial, such as the acceptable manner of dress if a technologist is called in for emergency laboratory testing in the middle of the night.

Origin

Policies and procedures may originate from various stimuli. One source over which laboratory administrators have little control is government regulation. An obvious example is the impact the Occupational Safety and Health Administration (OSHA) has had on clinical laboratory procedures for health and safety. At times, formal decisions from above in the organizational hierarchy will become the origin of a policy or procedure, as in the case of mandatory compensatory time for weekends worked. If a laboratory functions under a union contract, bargaining agreements become the basis of many policies. In addition, most institutions can point to at least one policy or procedure that originated from tradition. As an example, the allowance of a floating holiday traditionally taken on an employee's birthday suddenly shows up as a written policy stating that the day off must be taken on the employee's birthday. Finally, some policies are initiated through precedent.

Characteristics

There is no magic formula for writing a policy, but several key points will be listed here. First, the policy must be reasonable. At times, laboratory managers become so engrossed in providing organizational guidance that this simple common-sense component is lacking. If a procedure is not followed, it is usually because it is not understood or was not properly communicated. Understanding generally hinges upon adequate two-way communication (discussion) before the policy or procedure is implemented. A policy or procedure also needs to be flexible, so that the policymaker has some latitude in its enforcement.

Some policies address the privileges of being associated with a particular institution or holding a specific position. The policymaker should be aware that such privileges may be perceived as rights. A prime example is the privilege to accumulate earned sick leave to be used in case of a major illness. The policy is laudable and functional until a healthy individual, about to leave the company, decides that it is his right to use his accrued sick hours as vacation days.

Policies and procedures for the operation of a clinical laboratory are typically developed in the form of a manual. A well-written, comprehensive policy and procedure manual can be an effective management tool to clarify management directives, reduce uncertainties, and save time and energy in dealing with personnel problems.[3] Consistent with the focus of strategic planning, the manual should begin with a broad objective, narrowing the focus to details for its accomplishment in the form of policies, procedures, methods, and rules. The following example by Barros shows this narrowing and integration:[3]

Objective: To provide optimum service in the laboratory department for both inpatients and outpatients.

Policy: It is the policy of the laboratory to maintain 24-hour service 7 days a week for inpatient testing and 8-hour service 5 days a week for all outpatient procedures, unless special arrangements are made.

Procedure: 1. Maintain sufficient laboratory staffing around the clock for all inpatient services.
2. Provide outpatient services between the hours of 8 AM and 4:30 PM Monday through Friday, and 8 AM to noon on Saturday.
3. Schedule appointments for all outpatients.

Method: 1. Laboratory staff will be assigned to the following shifts: 7 AM to 3:30 PM; 3 PM to 11 PM; 8 AM to 4:30 PM; 11 PM to 7 AM.
2. Obtain approval from medical director or administrative director to schedule outpatient procedures outside the regular assigned hours.
3. Daily work schedules and job assignments will be posted 2 weekdays in advance.

Rule: 1. All employees will report for duty at time assigned. Deviations from these hours without prior approval will be considered cause for possible disciplinary action.
2. Three reported incidents of unexcused tardiness of more than 10 minutes will result in a written and verbal warning.
3. Five reported incidents of unexcused tardiness of more than 10 minutes will result in 1-day suspension without pay.
4. Additional reported incidents of unexcused tardiness will result in termination.

DESIGN OF CLINICAL LABORATORY FLOOR PLAN AND WORK FLOW

An obvious example of integrating the planning, organizing, and controlling activities of laboratory administrators and supervisors is the design of laboratory facilities. Only rarely does the laboratory practitioner have the opportunity to participate in the structural planning of a new laboratory facility. For this reason, architectural planning of a clinical laboratory is not included in the scope of this book, and readers seeking such information are referred to several listings in the Bibliography. More frequently, a laboratory manager is asked to relocate a portion of the laboratory or to evaluate the efficiency of an existing section. In this planning, organizing, and controlling activity, several key pieces of information and techniques are useful.

Design of the clinical laboratory floor plan and work-flow pattern contains both quantitative and qualitative elements. Frequently, concerns focus only on the amount of space available and not on how efficiently the space is being used.[12]

Design of Laboratory Space

The question of size in planning a laboratory is always a foremost concern. Several factors need to be considered in determining the space required for an efficient laboratory. These include the scope of procedures to be performed, the intended operational approach for performing the procedure, the anticipated size of the laboratory staff, and the setting (e.g., a teaching versus a nonteaching institution).[11]

Space Allocation

When either relocation or a new facility is planned, the laboratory manager is usually provided information on how much space is allocated for the laboratory. Several terms are essential to convert this information to meaningful figures. The term used to describe the total area based on outside location or building dimensions is the gross area. By contrast, the net (useful) area is the portion between the walls available for laboratory work space excluding building support, mechanics (ventilation, shafts for communication and transport, stairways, and so forth), and support facilities (restrooms, custodial closets, storerooms). Another helpful term is use factor, which represents a percentage ratio of net useful area to gross area. The usual use factor for clinical laboratory facilities is 60%.

SCOPE OF SERVICES. The scope of procedures provided by the clinical laboratory reflects the type of hospital or facility it serves. Even so, it is inadequate to project laboratory volume on the basis of the number of hospital beds or annual admissions. Such a projection does not include services provided for outpatient departments, dispensaries, special clinics, or emergency departments. In light of the skyrocketing hospital costs, the number of procedures performed for patients from some type of ambulatory-care facility or department is bound to increase at a faster rate than other growth. By their nature, some types of hospitals, such as teaching medical centers with research programs, have increased tests over admission number predictions. Even daily census or percentage of occupancy figures are inadequate predictors owing to seasonal variations, competing providers of similar laboratory services, or the economic conditions of the community. With the expanding scope of procedures in laboratory medicine, it is estimated that an additional space allotment of 25% should be planned to accommodate steady growth.[12]

OPERATIONAL APPROACH. The amount of space required in a laboratory is partially dependent upon how the testing is to be performed. In the preautomated era (1953 to 1964) Rappoport and others compared technologist productivity with space utilization for manually performed hematology and chemistry procedures.[12] The data from these analyses estimated that 45 to 50 total tests per year could be performed per net square foot of laboratory space. With the advent of automation, these figures changed and vary with the type of instrument used and its test/hour capacity. In the latter part of the 1960s Rappoport compared the effect of test automation and electronic data processing on space utilization in his chemistry laboratory as an example. With semiautomation, 91 tests per square foot were being performed. This increased to 252 tests per square foot under partial automation, and then to 1285 tests per square foot with total automation.[12] In designing laboratory space for an automated laboratory, the types and numbers of instruments should be identified early in the process. Once these decisions are made, space requirements can be predicted using instrument specifications.

SIZE OF STAFF. When planning laboratory space one must also consider the number of technical personnel who are to function in each area. The size of laboratory staff depends in part on the sophistication of instrumentation used. Rappoport also compared technologist productivity (tests performed annually per technologist) with automation and computerization. Semiautomation enabled technologists to perform 18,302 chemistry tests per year. With partial automation, that figure was boosted to 25,264 tests per year. And with total automation, technologist performance was raised to 285,562 chemistry tests per year. These figures provide an impression of the impact that automation has had on technologist productivity. Figures will change with different instrumentation, depending upon the tests per day capacity.[12]

The work volume is also an important consideration when one is determining the size of laboratory staff for planning space requirements. The College of American Pathologists (CAP) offers an approach to predicting and monitoring technologist productivity using the Computer Assisted Workload Recording System at its Computer Center in Traverse City, Michigan. In 1975, approximately 400 hospitals participated in this recording system, and the data collected should be helpful as rough guidelines to probable staffing requirements. Figure 2-3 contrasts technologist productivity by laboratory department and size and type of institution.[18] The high and low figures that were observed during the collection of this material should serve as a warning that laboratory staffing and planning are not exact sciences.

Using the CAP work unit as a basis and the type of instrumentation to be employed, a manager can make a reasonable prediction of the number of technical staff required. This information can then be used to plan the laboratory on a space-per-person requirement. Research by various individuals suggests that an estimated 228 square feet gross area per technologist should be allocated (approximately 152 square feet net area per technologist). When planning for all laboratory personnel, the suggested figure is 173 square feet gross, which reflects reduced requirements for clerical and administrative staff.[19] McCutchen studied space alloca-

FIGURE 2-3. Technologist productivity expressed in CAP work units. Each work unit represents 1 minute of technical and clerical time. The charts are expressed in work units per man hour. These data are a product of the Computer Assisted Workload Recording System, which is offered by the CAP. (Adapted from Thomas RG: Manual for Laboratory Planning and Design [rev], pp 181–182. Skokie, College of American Pathologists, 1977)

PRODUCTIVITY BY LABORATORY DEPARTMENT

Department	High	Median	Low
BLOOD BANK	92.5	42.5	20.3
CHEMISTRY	123.1	62.2	36.4
HEMATOLOGY	103.0	54.8	32.9
HISTOLOGY	80.9	43.8	25.7
IMMUNOLOGY	100.0	44.1	16.7
MICROBIOLOGY	88.6	47.1	24.3
MISCELLANEOUS	89.6	38.7	9.2
RADIOSOTOPES	55.0	28.4	14.4
SPECIMEN PROCUREMENT	130.3	47.6	23.2
URINE & FECES	105.7	40.6	21.2

MEDIAN PRODUCTIVITY FOR ALL LABORATORY DEPARTMENTS IN LABORATORIES OF DIFFERENT SIZES AND TYPES

Type or Bed Size	Median Productivity
Independent Lab	60.6
Under 50 Beds	Unavailable
50–74 Beds	Unavailable
75–99 Beds	59.5
100–149 Beds	62.6
150–199 Beds	54.5
200–299 Beds	54.9
300–399 Beds	50.7
Over 400 Beds	49.4

tions based on the CAP work-load recording and reporting system required by departments of laboratory medicine in three hospitals. She concluded that total department allocation, including anatomic and clinical pathology, should be 600 work units per square foot in institutions with a large teaching effort and 750 work units per square foot in institutions with a small teaching effort.[11]

Laboratory Structural Design

Medical laboratories follow two basic structural designs: modular and open. Both of these have advantages and disadvantages, and the choice of design will generally reflect the laboratory director's pref-

erence and philosophy of management. The key point is to recognize the positive and negative characteristics of each design in order to optimize efficiency and productivity. Indeed, it is possible to use a combination of the two designs within the same laboratory.

MODULAR LABORATORY DESIGN.   Figure 2-4 shows the floor plan of a modular laboratory. The emphasis is on departmentalization, with a separate room for each laboratory division. This creates a degree of ''turfdom.'' The separation of laboratories by walls has both good and bad effects on interdepartmental communication. Although discouraging needless visiting, the walls do not facilitate easy interaction

FIGURE 2-4.   Modular laboratory design. (From Thomas RG: Manual for Laboratory Planning and Design, p 103. Skokie, College of American Pathologists, 1977. Reprinted with permission of publisher)

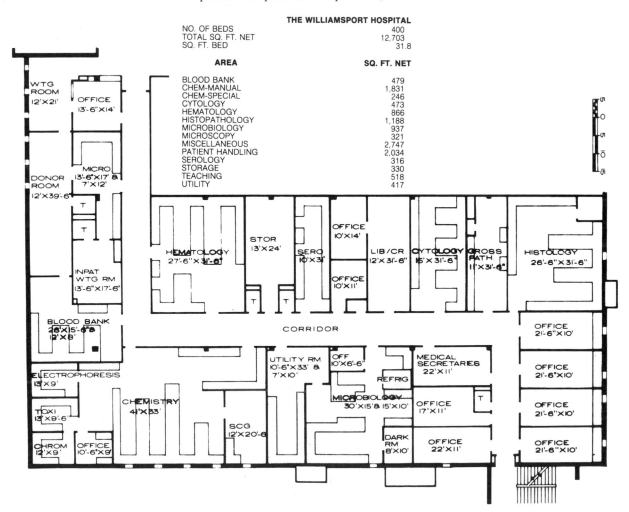

THE WILLIAMSPORT HOSPITAL	
NO. OF BEDS	400
TOTAL SQ. FT. NET	12,703
SQ. FT. BED	31.8

AREA	SQ. FT. NET
BLOOD BANK	479
CHEM-MANUAL	1,831
CHEM-SPECIAL	246
CYTOLOGY	473
HEMATOLOGY	866
HISTOPATHOLOGY	1,188
MICROBIOLOGY	937
MICROSCOPY	321
MISCELLANEOUS	2,747
PATIENT HANDLING	2,034
SEROLOGY	316
STORAGE	330
TEACHING	518
UTILITY	417

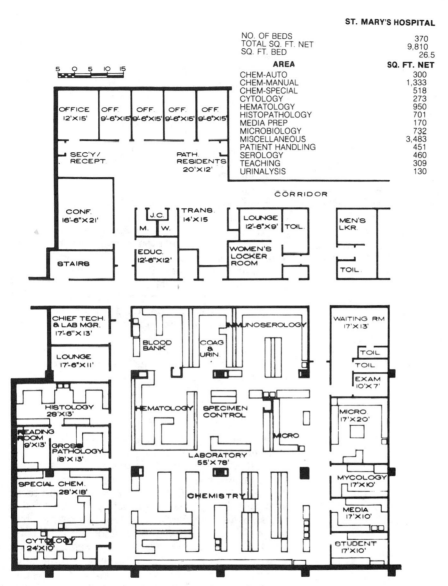

ST. MARY'S HOSPITAL	
NO. OF BEDS	370
TOTAL SQ. FT. NET	9,810
SQ. FT. BED	26.5
AREA	**SQ. FT. NET**
CHEM-AUTO	300
CHEM-MANUAL	1,333
CHEM-SPECIAL	518
CYTOLOGY	273
HEMATOLOGY	950
HISTOPATHOLOGY	701
MEDIA PREP	170
MICROBIOLOGY	732
MISCELLANEOUS	3,483
PATIENT HANDLING	451
SEROLOGY	460
TEACHING	309
URINALYSIS	130

FIGURE 2-5. Open laboratory design. (From Thomas RG: Manual for Laboratory Planning and Design, p 143. Skokie, College of American Pathologists, 1977. Reprinted with permission of publisher)

among divisions when it is appropriate. Although there is little sharing of laboratory equipment in a modular design, there is also little encroachment of space. The modular design appears to be less flexible if expansion is needed, although most walls are removable. There is some merit to the separation of areas from a visibility standpoint to discourage interdepartmental checks and criticism during workload peaks and valleys.

The noise level is reduced in those laboratories where loud instrumentation is not used. The modular design promotes safety in that contaminated specimens can be localized; and in case of fire, the modules would serve to contain the burning materials.

OPEN LABORATORY DESIGN. Figure 2-5 is an example of an open laboratory floor plan. With this design, many of the departments interface freely without dividing walls. For some laboratory administrators this approach is more aesthetically pleasing because it gives the feeling of roominess. The open floor plan promotes interaction between departments and fosters the concept of "one big happy family." This can have a negative effect if interaction between departments is allowed to interrupt the daily routine. Visiting is less controllable, and it becomes obvious to all when a particular department is slow. At the same time, a department that is short of staff will feel unjustly busy if personnel cannot be shared. The open floor plan lends itself well to the sharing of equipment, and expansion is easily accomplished within the confines of the laboratory by simply rearranging several benches or reallocating a bench to the expanding department. There is less control of noise and safety hazards in the open design, and planning for both of these concerns is important if this floor plan is adopted.

Design of Laboratory Work Flow

Several other key planning, organizing, and controlling strategies deal with the flow of specimens into the laboratory, through the department for analysis, and the return of the report to the requesting physician.[17]

Layout Flow Chart

Physical layout has important effects on the efficiency of work procedures.[10] The layout flow chart allows the laboratory manager to study physical layout in order to eliminate unnecessary steps. Following is an example of the benefit of studying the layout work flow of complete blood count (CBC) and coagulation procedures within a hematology department.

Before the study (Fig. 2-6), specimens entered the laboratory by passing the supervisor's area to be logged in by the recording clerk. The CBC specimen then was carried to a cell counter in the far corner of the laboratory, judiciously placed so that it would be away from excessive traffic. The specimen then traveled back to a sink area so that smears could be made and stained. Sometimes a routine test, such as a reticulocyte count or sedimentation rate, would briefly sidetrack the specimen before the differential was performed on the central island bench. The path of the CBC report, once the differential was complete, was relatively short, although the path of reporting immediate (*stat*) hemoglobin and hematocrit results from the cell counter fol-

lowed the same trip across the room as the specimen originally followed. Coagulation procedures were also placed away from traffic, but this necessitated taking the specimen from the clerk's area, around the end of the central island bench to the far area of the laboratory, and then returning along the same route with the report.

A rearrangement of analytic equipment, which was done after the layout work flow was studied, is shown in Figure 2-7. The clerk responsible for logging-in specimens and reporting results was moved closer to the specimen point-of-entry into the department. The supervisor was relocated to the corner alcove, since the routine specimen flow did not require his interaction. The path traveled by the CBC specimen was shortened considerably by placing the cell counter on the central island bench and relocating the coagulation testing on the same bench as the clerk. Reporting of stat hemoglobin and hematocrit values, CBC results, and coagulation procedures was facilitated by these relocations. Technical staffing was improved, too. The person operating the cell counter could perform stat coagulation tests with the instrument located directly behind him. The technologists performing differentials took advantage of the opportunity to stand up and stretch when taking stacks of completed CBCs back to the clerk for reporting.

Operational Flow Chart

Another helpful tool in assessing the efficiency of laboratory testing is the operational flow chart. The *flow chart* is a symbolic representation of a system broken down into its sequential component steps. A process is first reduced to its basic steps, and these steps are then placed in proper sequence. Finally, the steps are graphically displayed in a flow chart emphasizing decision points and alternate pathways. This technique is especially useful if several individuals must share in the operation of a given process. It can also be used to emphasize decision-making modes and describe the degree of responsibility and authority the technical staff has in deciding how a specimen is processed. Figure 2-8*A* shows some of the symbols frequently used in flow-charting, and Figure 2-8*B* is a flow chart for the process of urinalysis.[4]

Network Analysis

At times, a laboratory manager may wish to add a time and efficiency dimension to the operational flow chart, which is best accomplished by using a

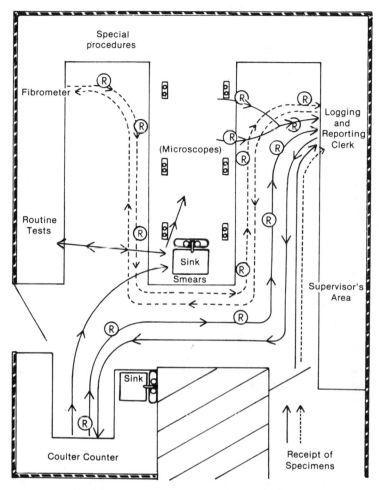

Key: —— Path of CBC with differential
  - - - Path of coagulation tests
  (R) Report Path

FIGURE 2-6. Laboratory layout flow chart before work-flow study.

network analysis technique. Bennington defines *network analysis* as a "schematic and mathematical approach to the planning of a project which shows the relationships among different activities and how their timing will affect the overall project."[5] Several components of a project are evaluated, including the shortest possible completion time, activities with delay potential, and extra-effort-to-cost-benefit analysis.

The two most commonly used network analysis approaches are the Program Evaluation Review Technique (PERT) and Critical Path Method (CPM). PERT is appropriate when one or more of the completion points must be reached at a specific time or in planning a project where a high degree of uncertainty exists (a totally new project, for example). The CPM technique, while similar, does not require a specific point completion time as in PERT.

The basis of network analysis includes construction of activities and events (Fig. 2-9). An *activity* is an operation requiring time between two events, such as drawing blood. An *event* is a time when one or more activities commence or are completed. For example, the receipt of the requisition in the laboratory (event) must precede the blood-drawing (activity). The *critical path* is defined as the chain of events and the total time all of these together require for completion of a project. The *noncritical path* is a chain of events leading to completion of the project but exclusive of some events

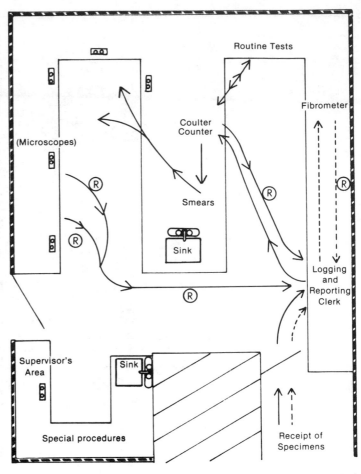

FIGURE 2-7. Laboratory layout flow chart after work-flow study.

Key: —— Path of CBC with differential
      - - - Path of coagulation tests
      Ⓡ Report Path

FIGURE 2-8 A. Flow-charting symbols.

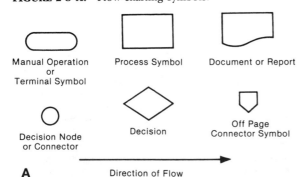

Manual Operation
or
Terminal Symbol

Process Symbol

Document or Report

Decision Node
or Connector

Decision

Off Page
Connector Symbol

A   Direction of Flow

in the overall project. *Float* is a term for spare time (slack) resulting from the difference between the times to accomplish the critical path and the noncritical path. Two activities can branch from a given event, thus creating concurrent activities within the project.

Additional information concerning these planning and evaluation tools can be found under appropriate references listed in the Annotated Bibliography at the end of this chapter.

LABORATORY ORGANIZATIONAL STRUCTURE

Organization in the clinical laboratory refers to both structure and process.[6] *Structure* exemplifies

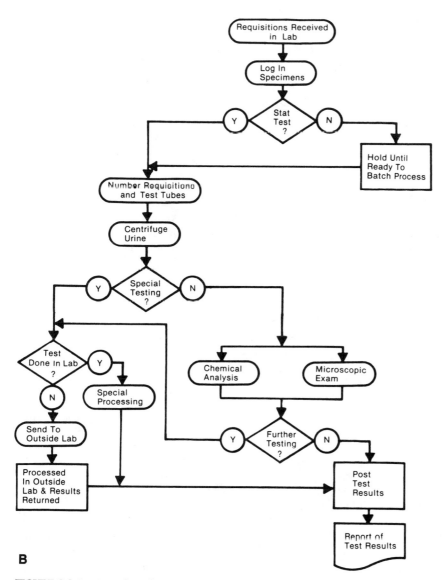

B

FIGURE 2-8 B. Urinalysis flow chart. (From Bennington JL: Management and Cost Control Techniques for the Clinical Laboratory, pp 228, 232–233. Baltimore, University Park Press, 1977. Reprinted with permission of publisher)

stated relationships or framework, while *process* deals with interaction. The three key elements of organization are the tasks to be performed, the individuals who are to perform the tasks, and the clinical laboratory as a workplace.

Organization of the Pathology Laboratory

Figure 2-10 is an example of an organization chart for a department of pathology. Although a standard fixture in most organizations, the chart serves only

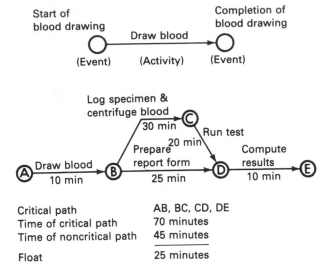

FIGURE 2-9. Network analysis—critical path method. (From Bennington JL: Management and Cost Control Techniques for the Clinical Laboratory, pp 242, 244. Baltimore, University Park Press, 1977. Reprinted with permission of publisher)

Critical path	AB, BC, CD, DE
Time of critical path	70 minutes
Time of noncritical path	45 minutes
Float	25 minutes

limited functions, one of which is providing visualization of who is doing what and the chain of command. Townsend advocates the use of an organizational chart solely as an administrative tool—not for everyone's consumption.[19] As he has pointed out, organization charts tend to demoralize people because nobody likes to think of himself as being below other people.

Organization plays an important role in the effectiveness of the clinical laboratory by defining the relationship between tasks, individuals, and the workplace. The basis for this relationship is authority, responsibility, and accountability. A laboratory manager possesses *authority* within the organization if he has the right to issue instructions that others are expected to follow. Authority is generally attached to a position, and its location on the organizational chart implies a degree of consent. *Responsibility* refers to the group of tasks or duties assigned an individual or position in the organizational structure, and *accountability* is the obligation to a higher authority for the successful fulfillment of assigned tasks. The organizational structure serves as a visual aid for evaluating each of these basics. For example, in investigating the difficulty a laboratory supervisor is experiencing in maintaining sufficient inventory (responsibility), the laboratory director may realize that the problem is in the purchasing system, which does not accept the supervisor's signature on a requisition (authority).

The organization chart also attempts to show relationships between line and staff. In this organizational concept, a *line position* is one in which a superior exercises direct supervision over a subordinate. A *staff position* is advisory, supportive, or auxiliary. These terms were defined in industry, and health-care institutions seldom use the same connotation. When a laboratory manager speaks of his staff, he generally is referring to his technical personnel, who are in fact serving in line positions. Individuals involved solely in academic instruction and research would be defined as staff to the functioning anatomic and clinical laboratories (Fig. 2-10). Another component of the structure, more visibly staff, is the administrative section. Its role is supportive to the primary laboratory-testing function. There are times when line–staff conflicts occur, stemming primarily from a failure to define clearly the operational difference between the two.[9] The pathology administrator in Figure 2-10 is faced with a dual authority situation. The position is line within the administrative section but staff in its relationship to each of the clinical laboratories. This may produce a conflict when the rightful prerogative of a line supervisor is usurped by a staff administrator.

Sometimes it is helpful to map out the relationships in an organizational structure from several standpoints. Gallamore has contrasted the change in relationships and roles that occurs when both administrative and technical structures are delineated (Fig. 2-11).[8] Consider the changing role of the laboratory manager in the two structures. In the administrative structure, he serves in a line position, while in the technical structure, his position is staff.

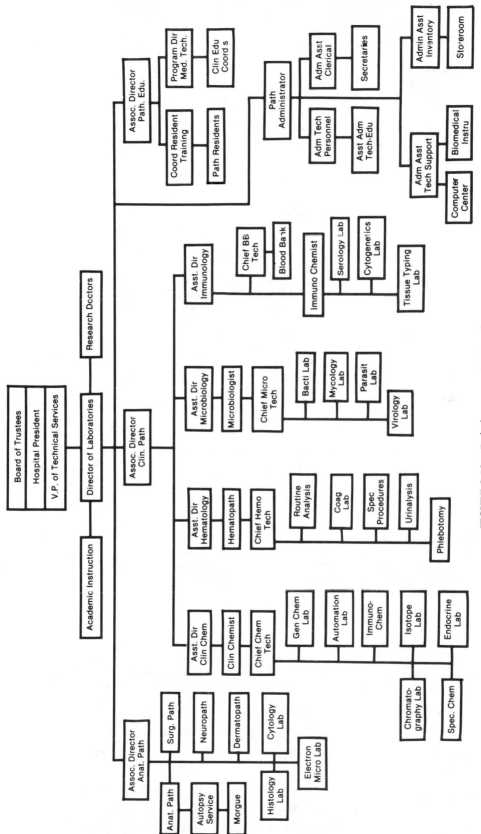

FIGURE 2-10. Pathology organization chart.

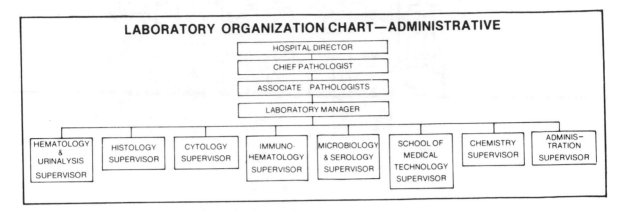

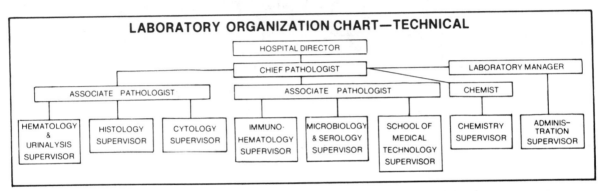

FIGURE 2-11. Laboratory organization chart—administrative versus technical structure. (From Gallamore C: The evolving role of the laboratory manager. Laboratory Management 13:45, 1975. Reprinted with the permission of publisher)

Organizational Design and Hierarchy

An organizational hierarchy is a multileveled, vertical structure signifying who outranks whom. In designing or evaluating a laboratory organizational hierarchy, there are several characteristics that should be considered.

Departmentation/Specialization

The design of all organizational structures includes a division of labor. Overall goals are divided into activities. These activities are subsequently separated into departments to achieve a degree of specialization. In the medical laboratory, departments have reflected uniformity of technique (chemical analysis), uniformity of specimen required (whole blood for hematologic analysis), uniformity of function (administrative support), or uniformity of patient services (stat laboratory). In any large labora-

tory, it is obvious that specialization has a positive effect on efficiency. At the same time, the technical staff generally suffers from a degree of boredom with its limited scope of analytic procedures.

Scalar Principle

Organizational structures reflect a scalar chain or line of authority from the ultimate superiors in the laboratory (directors) down to the lowest rank, sometimes referred to as the chain of command. Authority throughout the hierarchy implies that decisions are being made at numerous levels.

Unity of Direction

If goals are to be achieved, coordination is essential. Unity of direction requires that a single laboratory manager be responsible for coordinating the activities necessary for achieving these goals, as well as

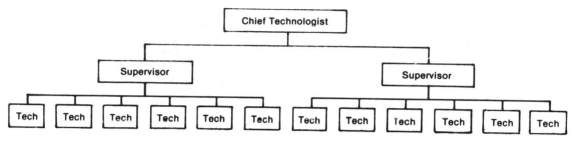

FIGURE 2-12. Flat organizational structure.

for the technical and support staff assigned to his department. By scrutinizing the organizational structure, it should be possible to eliminate overlapping managerial responsibilities.

Unity of Command

Not only must a single manager have coordinating responsibility for specific activities and personnel, he must also have the authority to carry these out. Another way of stating this concept is to say that a worker should receive orders from only one superior and be accountable only to him.

Span of Control

Effective control necessitates a limitation on the number of subordinates a manager is to supervise. Bennington states that four to six subordinates is thought to be an appropriate number.[6] The ideal number of subordinates probably varies with an individual manager's skills.

Depending on the institution and philosophy of the laboratory director, most organization charts will fall into one of two basic designs. Figure 2-12 is an example of a flat organizational structure with few levels of hierarchy. By contrast, Figure 2-13 is a tall organizational structure with numerous levels.

FIGURE 2-13. Tall organizational structure.

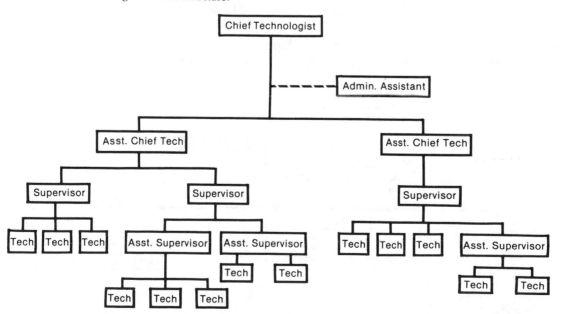

Without making a value judgment concerning which is better, consider some of their respective characteristics. The tall structure generally is used when there is increased specialization. Both the flat and tall structures exhibit the scalar chain of command, although the increased number of levels in the tall structure may prompt uncoordinated decisions and bypassing. The tall structure, by its inherent specialization, will generally permit a greater unity of direction. This can be negated if an assistant chief technologist in the structure insists on having a say in the supervisor's coordinating decisions, thus making the unity of command ineffective. In this case the technologists may think they must serve two masters. The flat structure is characterized by a broad span of control—many subordinates responsible to one superior—whereas the tall structure shows a short span of control. If the span of control is too broad, the manager may not have access to sufficient information to make quality decisions, or complaints may be made by the technologists that they cannot see their supervisor or get decisions made at all. If the span of control is too short, the manager may oversupervise by participating in day-to-day operations or offering unsolicited advice.

Organizational Myths and the Informal Structure

The organizational hierarchy, no matter how well designed, does not ensure total organization. Figure 2-14 shows the impact of the informal organization. It is not always true that decisions are made by the manager, with orders flowing down and feedback information flowing up. The broken lines, indicating routes of communication in the informal structure, may be substantially different from those planned in the formal structure. The organization chart may not show the true distinctions between line and staff or the influences that may affect decisions, as in the relationship between the administrative technologist and line technologist under Supervisor 3. Bypassing can occur, as reflected by the lines of communication and influence under Supervisor 1, whose assistant is totally missed. Supervisor 2 undoubtedly is affected by the influence two of his technologists have on his superiors, and it is certainly possible that the line technologist who influences the chief has more power in the structure than any other single technologist or supervisor. Lest one conclude that the informal organization is all bad, this simply is not the case.[13] Often information is communicated more abundantly and efficiently through informal channels than through those delineated in the formal structure. The informal organization is inevitable and has both positive and negative consequences. The laboratory manager must be aware of its existence and impact.

CONTROLLING OPERATIONS IN THE LABORATORY

The final management function of the laboratory administrator is controlling, that is, ensuring that plans are carried through the organizational and operational phases so that goals are met. Therein, the

FIGURE 2-14. Example of informal organizational structure. Broken lines indicate routes of communication and sources of influence not evident in the formal organizational structure.

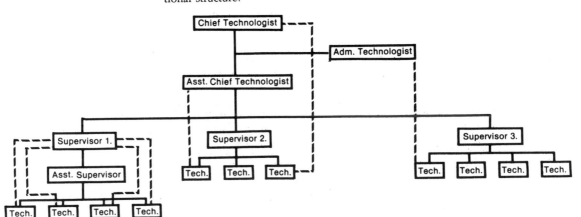

UNIVERSITY OF NEBRASKA MEDICAL CENTER
CLINICAL PATHOLOGY
PATIENT RESULTS

INTRALABORATORY COMMUNICATION
ABNORMAL and or QUESTIONABLE DATA

TO: Dr. Frost (Clinical Pathologist)
FROM: Susan B. (Medical Tech.)
*PATIENT'S NAME: John Citizen *HOSPITAL NUMBER 012345
(and Initials)
PATIENT'S DOCTOR: Dr. Doctor INPATIENT: X
(and Initials) OUTPATIENT:
  ROOM NUMBER 5433-1
DOCTOR'S TELEPHONE NUMBER 3033 WARD TELEPHONE NUMBER
*DATE/TIME 8-12-80
*REASON FOR COMMUNICATION:

↓ Anion Gap

*ESSENTIAL LAB DATA

Date	Time	TESTS						
		4-19 ANION GAP	8.4-10.4 CA++	6-8 TP	3.4-5.2 ALB	<3.1 GLOBIN		
8/6	0726			6.5	3.7	2.8		
8/12	0753	2	15.3					

ACTION TAKEN:

CONCLUSION: Malignant melanoma patient w/↑ Ca++

COMMENT Admission diagnosis — malignant melanoma
Patient running ↑ Ca++
H proteins

*MINIMAL REQUIREMENT IN EMERGENCIES: COMPLETE THESE ITEMS

8-13
Date

Signature (Clinical Pathologist)

FIGURE 2-15. Control mechanism for abnormal or questionable laboratory data.
(Reprinted with permission of the Chairman, Department of Pathology, University of
Nebraska Medical Center)

CONFIDENTIAL REPORT OF INCIDENT (Not part of medical record)

Name and address of person involved. Give medical record number. Use addressograph if available.	IDENTIFICATION	SEX	AGE	TIME LOST (Employees Only)	NURSES STA. NO.
	☐ 1 - Patient ☐ 2 - Employee ☐ 3 - Visitor	☐ 1 - Female ☐ 2 - Male		☐ 1 - Yes (If unknown, check "No".) ☐ 2 - No	
	(19)	(20)	(21-23)	(24)	(25 - 29)

	INCIDENT DATE	REPORT DATE	INCIDENT SHIFT	TIME	HOSPITAL CODE NOS.
	(Digits Only)	(Digits Only)	☐ 01 - 1st ☐ 02 - 2nd ☐ 03 - 3rd	: A.M. : P.M.	STATE (2 Digits) HOSP. NUMBER (3 Digits)
(1 - 18)	(30 - 35)	(36 - 41)	(42 - 43)		(44 - 48)

CONDITION BEFORE (Patients Only)	BED ADJUSTMENT (Not Bed Rails) (Patients Only)	LOCATION OF INCIDENT	NATURE OF INJURY (Injury sustained as a result of incident)
☐ 1 - Normal ☐ 2 - Senile ☐ 3 - Disoriented ☐ 4 - Sedated ☐ 5 - Unconscious ☐ 6 - Other ☐ 7 - Behavior	☐ 1 - Not Applicable ☐ 2 - Up ☐ 3 - Down	☐ 400 Admitting ☐ 410 Offices ☐ 420 Elevators ☐ 430 Corridors ☐ 440 Stairs ☐ 450 General Premises - Interior ☐ 460 Housekeeping ☐ 470 Dietary ☐ 480 Laundry ☐ 490 Eng. & Maint. ☐ 500 Patient's Room	☐ 510 Patients Bathroom ☐ 520 Nurses Station ☐ 530 Surgery & Recovery ☐ 540 Delivery, Labor & Recovery ☐ 550 Central Supply ☐ 560 Laboratory ☐ 570 Pharmacy ☐ 580 X - Ray ☐ 590 Physical Therapy ☐ 600 Emergency ☐ 610 Parking Lots & Sidewalks ☐ 620 General Premises - Exterior	☐ 100 Asphyxia, Strangulation, Inhalation ☐ 110 Burn or Scald ☐ 120 Chemical Burn ☐ 130 Concussion ☐ 140 Contagious or Infectious Disease ☐ 150 Contusion, Cut, Laceration ☐ 160 Fracture or Dislocation ☐ 170 Viscera Injury ☐ 180 Sprain or Strain ☐ 190 No Injury ☐ 200 No Apparent Injury ☐ 210 Other - Not Classified
(49)	(50)	(51 - 53)	(54 - 56)

INCIDENT CAUSE (57 - 58) If more than one cause, check predominating one and describe others in lower part of report.
*Do not use for employee or visitor incidents.

A - Falls	B - Medication	C - Other	
☐ 1-Bed, Rail Up ☐ 2-Bed, Rail Down ☐ 3-From Chair or Equip. ☐ 4-From Different Level ☐ 5-On Same Level ☐ 6-Fainting	☐ 7-Patient Identification ☐ 8-Dosage ☐ 9-Route ☐ 10-Unordered ☐ 11-Duplication ☐ 12-Omission	☐ 13-Transcription ☐ 14-Transfusion ☐ 15-Wrong Medication ☐ 16-Labeling ☐ 17-Time Given ☐ 18-Other ☐ 19-I.V. or Injection Tech.	☐ 20-Struck by Patient ☐ 21-Struck by Equipment ☐ 22-Struck Equipment ☐ 23-Struck by Tool or Object ☐ 24-Overexertion-Handling Pt. ☐ 25-Lifting or Moving ☐ 26-Loss of Personal Property	☐ 27-Patient Care - Nurses ☐ 28-Patient Care - Others ☐ 29-Anesthesia ☐ 30-Sponge, etc. Count ☐ 31-Patient Identification ☐ 32-Caught, In, On, or Between ☐ 33-Misc. ☐ 34-Needle Puncture

IF PATIENT	IF EMPLOYEE	IF VISITOR
Out-of-Bed Privileges? ☐ Yes ☐ No Cause for Hospitalization: _____ Room No.: ___ Attending Physician: ___	Dept: _____ Job Title: _____ Date returned to work: _____ ☐ First Aid Only	Reason for presence: _____ Home Phone: _____ Occupation: _____

GIVE BRIEF DESCRIPTION OF INCIDENT, INCLUDING PREDOMINATING AND CONTRIBUTING CAUSES. _____

EQUIPMENT INVOLVED: _____ MANUFACTURER: _____ SERIAL NO.: _____

STATE CORRECTIVE ACTION TAKEN TO PREVENT RECURRENCE. INDICATE IF FURTHER INVESTIGATION IS NECESSARY. _____

List all patients in the room. Give names and addresses of witnesses. _____

Was person seen by a physician? ☐ Yes ☐ No If "Yes", time seen: _____ A.M./_____ P.M.	PHYSICIAN'S NAME (PRINT)	PHYSICIAN'S SIGNATURE

PHYSICIAN'S FINDINGS _____

Name and Address of HOSPITAL	Name and title of person preparing the report.
	Supervisor's Signature

(C - 2682 - H) 6-77

HOSPITAL USE

CAT. 450707
PRINTED IN U.S.A.

FIGURE 2-16. Incident report form. (Reprinted with permission of the Chancellor, University of Nebraska Medical Center)

control process is closely linked to both planning and organizational structure (Fig. 2-2).

The control process involves three steps: (1) establishing standards; (2) measuring performance against these standards; and (3) correcting deviations from standards and plans.[7] Controlling involves locating operational weaknesses—those factors having a negative impact on the economical, effective, and efficient achievement of goals—and taking the appropriate action to ensure desired results.

Standards may be determined in several ways. Within the clinical laboratory, standards are mathematically determined to control the quality of any given analytic process (see Chap. 16). Standards may also be determined by past experience or competitive operations, as, for example, in controlling the turn-around time acceptable for stat procedures. Finally, standards may be suggested or mandated by an accrediting body or governmental agency.

An excellent example of control within the clinical laboratory is the technique of self-study or evaluation preceding an accreditation inspection. The standards have been specified by the accrediting body. The operation of the laboratory is compared to these standards, and corrective action is implemented.

The clinical laboratory, by its departmentalized nature, poses a problem of controlling medical data. Intralaboratory communications are essential for the correlation of patient results. Figure 2-15 is an example of a control mechanism for investigating patient results that are either abnormal (beyond established acceptable parameters) or have a questionable correlation. The use of such a communications form may prompt a chart review or discussion with the attending physician to ensure the release of quality data.

Control is also applicable in the management of human resources for the clinical laboratory. Personnel policies and procedures are the established standards against which performance is measured. Chapter 13 describes performance evaluation techniques and approaches. Control of deviations from established policy must be recorded in order to investigate the problem and take corrective action. Even many routine activities covered by personnel policy are best controlled using some form of documentation. Figure 2-16 is a general incident report form used to assist in recording deviations from

FIGURE 2-17. Absence report form. (Reprinted with permission of the Chancellor, University of Nebraska Medical Center)

UNIVERSITY OF NEBRASKA MEDICAL CENTER

ABSENCE REPORT

Submit to the Personnel Department to Report All Absences

Name ______________________________ **Date** ______________

Soc. Sec. ______________________________ ☐ **Monthly**

Department Name: ______________ **Dept. No.** ______________ ☐ **Bi-Weekly**

I request that my absence of ________ **hours from** ______________ **thru** ______________ **inclusive be charged to:**

Vacation	☐	**Leave of Absence**	☐	**Military Leave**	☐	**Work Comp. Injury**	☐
Sick Leave	☐	**Funeral Leave**	☐	**Jury Duty**	☐	**Other**	☐
						Reason ______________	

I have made arrangements with ______________ **or** ______________ ______________
Supervisor Staff Alternate

to discharge my duties and responsibilities during the period of my absence.

This absence is to be **with** / **without** **pay.**

FOR PERSONNEL USE ONLY

____ ____ **hours to be paid**

PE-60 9/78

____
Signature of Employee

Recommended: ______________________________
Dept. or Administrative Head

Approved: ______________________________
Director of Personnel

routine, and Figure 2-17 is an example of staffing control by ensuring adequate coverage before an absence is granted and written documentation of the exercised policy.

The control process includes correction of deviations, a topic in itself when considering human resources. The single most important resource of the laboratory manager is his technical staff, and discipline (the corrective phase of the control process) must be justly executed. The process is positively influenced if the supervisor creates an atmosphere where employees abide by rules they consider fair. When necessary, discipline should be exercised in a gradual manner: first an oral reprimand, then written warnings, and finally suspension. The disciplinary sequence usually includes a statement and description of the problem, collection of facts, decision regarding the penalty and application thereof, and follow-up. Discipline should only be applied as a last resort. Indeed, the laboratory manager faces a dilemma when discipline is necessary. The climate of cooperation and trust is threatened. Douglas McGregor encourages the use of the "red hot stove rule" to preserve a cooperative and fair working environment. Under this rule, discipline is immediate, consistent, and impersonal. The manager must not procrastinate his decision to punish. The decision to punish must be made every time the deviation occurs, and the act should be punished, not the individual. This analogy between touching a hot stove and discipline allows no room for favoritism, waiting until punishment is more convenient, or applying a penalty inconsistent with the offense—all of which would promote unfairness.[16]

REFERENCES

1. Albers J, Vice JL: Strategic planning. Am J Med Technol 49:411–414, 1983
2. Anthony RN: Planning and Control Systems: A Framework for Analysis, p 16. Boston, Harvard Graduate School of Business Administration, 1965
3. Barros A: Developing an effective policy and procedure manual. MLO 17(6):29–33, 1985
4. Bennington JL: Flow charting. In Bennington JL, Handmaker H, Freedman GS, et al (eds): Management and Cost Control Techniques for the Clinical Laboratory, pp 225–237. Baltimore, University Park Press, 1977
5. Bennington JL: Network analysis. In Bennington JL, et al (eds): Management and Cost Control Techniques for the Clinical Laboratory, pp 239–257. Baltimore, University Park Press, 1977
6. Bennington JL: Organization and management. In Bennington JL, et al (eds): Management and Cost Control Techniques for the Clinical Laboratory, pp 31–42. Baltimore, University Park Press, 1977
7. Fulmer RM: Supervision: Principles of Professional Management, pp 235–253. Beverly Hills, Glencoe Press, 1976
8. Gallamore C: The evolving role of the laboratory manager. Laboratory Management 13:45, 1975
9. Kast FE, Rosenzweig JE: Organization and Management: A Systems Approach, 2nd ed, pp 213–217. New York, McGraw-Hill, 1974
10. Mayer RW: Designing a more productive laboratory. MLO 17(7):67–71, 1985
11. McCutheon G: Space allocation guidelines for the clinical laboratory. J Med Technol 2:772–777, 1985
12. Rappoport AE: Laboratory design. In Race GJ (ed): Laboratory Medicine, Vol IV (rev), pp 1–30. Hagerstown, Harper & Row, 1979
13. Roseman E: Tune in to the informal organization in your lab. MLO 14(7):102–108, 1982
14. Scanlon BK: Management 18—A Short Course for Managers, pp 17–28. New York, John Wiley & Sons, 1974
15. Schendel D, Hofer CW: Strategic Management: A New View of Business Policy and Planning, p 15. Boston, Little, Brown, 1979
16. Strauss G, Sayles LR: Personnl: the human problems of management, 3rd ed, pp 267–276. Englewood Cliffs, Prentice-Hall, 1972
17. Teeple KL, Snyder JR, Swanson F: Using planning tools for reorganization. MLO 19(4):59–64, 1987
18. Thomas RG: Manual for Laboratory Planning and Design (rev). Skokie, College of American Pathology, 1977
19. Townsend R: Up the Organization, p 116. Greenwich, Fawcett Publications, 1970

ANNOTATED BIBLIOGRAPHY

Brown M, Lewis HL: Hospital Management Systems. Germantown, Maryland, Aspen Systems Corporation, 1976

To gain an appreciation of the organization of the clinical laboratory and its ability to deliver effective health care, it is sometimes advantageous to view the hospital or health-care-delivery system as a whole. This reference provides an insight into the integration of health-care-delivery systems in numerous institutions throughout the country.

Charms MP, Schaefer MJ: Health Care Organizations: A Model for Management. Englewood Cliffs, Prentice-Hall, Inc., 1983

While building upon general theories of organization and management, this textbook addresses the unique characteristics of the health care environment, its institutions, history, and practices. The authors describe a conceptual organization model based on the analysis of work, and make explicit distinction between management and direct (or clinical) work. Both Chapter 4, "Purposes and Goals," and Chapter 6, "Organization Structure," will be of particular interest to readers.

Laliberty R, Christopher WI: Enhancing Productivity in Health Care Facilities. Owings Mills, MD, National Health and Law Publishing Corp, 1984

Focusing on human resource management, these authors describe specific managerial strategies related to planning, organization and control. Readers may wish to focus on four chapters: "Analyzing the Job," "Work Distribution," "Workflow Process Analysis," and "Improving Productivity through Creative Scheduling and Alternate Work Schedules."

Liebler JG, Levine RE, Dervitz HL: Management Principles for Health Professionals. Rockville, MD, Aspen Systems Corporation, 1984

While addressing management principles generic for many health professions, these authors provide excellent contributions to the managerial functions of planning, organization, and control. The planning chapter provides guidance for the creation of goals, objectives, policies, and procedures. The organizing chapter provides a fundamental discussion of concepts and principles related to the process of organizing. Separate chapters on controlling and work sampling include qualitative and quantitative techniques such as the Gantt Chart, the Pert Network, the flow chart, the flow process chart, and the work distribution chart.

Lynch RM, Williamson RW: Accounting for Management Planning and Control, 2nd ed. New York, McGraw-Hill, 1976.

This text is an excellent reference for managerial planning and controlling from an accounting perspective. Section 1 serves as the foundation for the remainder of the book by introducing basic accounting techniques. Section 2 addresses planning in terms of cost-volume-profit analysis and the use of budgets. Section 3 stresses the use of accounting practices appropriate for control, including standard material and labor costs and overhead variance analysis. The final section of this book investigates several accounting techniques appropriate for special management decisions.

Rakich JS, Longest BB, O'Donovan TR: Managing Health Care Organizations. Philadelphia, WB Saunders, 1977

This reference applies management theory to the practices of general institutions providing health care. The entire scope of management is covered, with numerous examples from specific health-care organizations. Part 2, dealing with output-input determination (decision-making and planning), and Part 3, dealing with organizational design and structure, are particularly informative. One chapter in Part 5 deals with control and control techniques from a process viewpoint.

Selbst PL: Modern Health Care Forms. Boston, Warren, Gorham & Lamont, 1976

Planning, organization, and control are often enhanced by proper documentation techniques and forms. This book contains a plethora of forms that can be used as guides in designing records for specific situations and institutions. Appropriate forms are displayed for organization and management, financial management, personnel and labor relations, medical and professional affairs, physical facilities, and support services.

Taylor JK: Quality Assurance of Chemical Measurements. Chelsea, MI, Lewis Publishers, 1987

This resource describes a systematic approach to measurement and attainment of statistical control of the measurement process by quality control procedures. Chapter 14, describing control charts, and Chapter 19, entitled "Quality Audits," provide valuable information. In addition, Chapter 26, entitled "The Quality Assurance Program," offers a good discussion on the development of a quality assurance program.

Thomas RG: Manual for Laboratory Planning and Design (rev). Skokie, College of American Pathology, 1977

This reference is essential for designing an efficient laboratory. Part 2 addresses architectural considerations of the laboratory in general, while Part 3 describes parameters for specific laboratory departments. Of considerable interest, Part 4 contains floor plans and specifications of 51 different clinical laboratories.

The Prentice-Hall Editorial Staff: Encyclopedic Dictionary of Systems and Procedures. Englewood Cliffs, Prentice-Hall, 1966

This text, as the name implies, is an encyclopedic dictionary. For the new supervisor or experienced laboratory administrator, it will serve as a valuable resource for basic information on "management operations, methods, and practices developed by systems and procedures techniques."

three

Problem-solving — The Decision-making Process

John R. Snyder

While a multitude of specific managerial skills have an impact on the effectiveness of a laboratory administrator or supervisor, the most important is his decision-making ability. The decision is the core of administrative action. Any administrative activity — planning, organizing, directing, or controlling — requires the manager to be a decision-maker. In fact, all organizational activity can be looked at as a series of decisions.

A great temptation for all managers is to rely on past experience and common sense as the basis for their decision-making skill. Unfortunately, this does not always suffice, because management in laboratory medicine evolves with nearly the rapidity of technical advances in the field. Decisions about personnel administration, electronic data processing, and method evaluation, to name just a few, are areas that require specific new judgment skills.[5] Today's laboratory manager faces an ever-changing environment. Scanlon summarizes this concern by stating that "decisions based solely on intuition and past experience are becoming less effective in dealing with organizational problems because things are changing at too rapid a pace and because yesterday's experience does not always mirror tomorrow's problem."[12] To decide means to pass judgment and determine a course of action. Perhaps the most complete definition is that managerial decision-making is the selection of a preferred course of action from two or more alternatives after weighing the effects of the various alternatives in light of organizational goals. This definition adds two important facts: (1) consideration of the results if one alternative is chosen over another, and (2) the impact the chosen alternate will have in achieving organizational goals. These concepts are further delineated later in this chapter when we discuss the problem-solving process.

AREAS OF CONCERN IN DECISION-MAKING

Before attempting to make any management decision, there are several general areas of concern to which a laboratory manager must be sensitive:[2]

Quality of the Decision

In order to make a quality decision, the manager must determine whether he has all of the appropriate information available. Often the creative talents of several people are beneficial in generating possible alternatives. The manager may need to seek out information regarding specific skills necessary to complement a given alternative. The practice of "bouncing ideas off" peers, subordinates, and superiors is an excellent practice for gaining a broader point of view.

Acceptance of and Commitment to the Decision

This concern is fundamental to management which must get things done through people. It is important to consider not only the degree of acceptance by the subordinates affected directly by the decision but also the degree of acceptance at other levels of management within the organization. It must be remembered that a group of employees' acceptance of a decision (with or without verbal and nonverbal reaction) does not ensure commitment. Commitment on the part of those who must implement the decision is essential. Sometimes commitment hinges on the attitude employees have about how the decision was made. There are times when it is appropriate to involve the laboratory staff in the decision-making process because it gives added quality to the decision and increases the acceptance and commitment to the alternative chosen. Finally, consideration must be given to the acceptance the decision will receive outside the organization: How will other departments in the hospital be affected?

The Speed of the Decision

The time element must obviously be considered. If the decision needs to be made immediately, it is unlikely that staff can be involved. Even if it is not essential that the decision be a quick one, the laboratory manager must consider the length of time it will take to involve appropriate parties. If the decision process must be accelerated, there is generally a trade-off in quality and acceptance of the decision.

The Nature of the Value Judgments in the Decision

All decisions involve a value judgment in terms of what is beneficial or nonbeneficial and important or nonimportant in projecting the probable outcomes of the decision. Chapter 9 describes these as hidden agendas for people attending meetings. The laboratory manager must recognize the impact these hidden forces may have on the acceptance and commitment to the decision. There are times when individual goals and organizational goals do not mesh because of differing value judgments. At these times the manager must consider the nature of the value judgments when making a decision.

The Cost of the Decision

The use of organizational resources to make decisions costs money. This must be considered when the decision is reached, because the time of the people involved in the decision is an important component. Often it is difficult to quantitate the appropriate costs that will yield the best decision in terms of quality, acceptance, speed, and values.

DECISION-MAKING — APPROACHES AND EFFECTS

There is a variety of what may be termed "decision-making management styles," ranging from total dictatorship to total abdication. These are addressed here as approaches to decision-making, because style implies a degree of consistency.

Management in the clinical laboratory is full of decisions. There are those supervisors who think their managerial role is somewhat routine because few if any of their decisions would be considered major. In fact, all of the decisions they render are for routine situations, and hence they have a lack of concern about approaches to decision-making. Perhaps these supervisors more than any others need to examine the decision-making process and the effect various approaches have on quality, acceptance, speed, value, and cost.

Making wise management decisions is not an intuitive skill. Supervisors who are new in their positions will attest to this. It is common for a fledgling supervisor to falter when faced with this newfound responsibility. This skill perhaps more than any other management skill requires an experiential learning period. Some laboratory managers never become good decision-makers. Roseman categorized a variety of dangerous decision-making habits he had observed in laboratory managers (Fig. 3-1).[9] Perhaps if one considers first some pitfalls in the decision-making approaches, other more appropriate approaches will be easier to adopt.

The breathless decision, as the name implies, is made on the spur of the moment. While the laboratory supervisor cannot always prevent the need for a hurried decision, making too many is also a bad sign. These may signal a failure to plan, resulting in crisis management—putting out fires. Characteristic of the breathless decision is an oversimplification of the facts and a frantic effort to rapidly come up with *any* alternative, which ultimately becomes the decision.

Contrasted with the breathless decision are the trade-off and hold-off decision habits. The laboratory supervisor who practices the trade-off habit tends to solve the easy problems—find the ready-made and obvious solutions—but to shelve the rest. Those that are shelved are put off so that the supervisor can avoid confrontation. This habit is an attempt to keep everything in harmony by trading off

Breathless decisions	
What You Do	Why
Act without thinking	Submit to time pressure
Limit alternatives	Succumb to emotion
Overreact	Avoid pain
Oversimplify	Avoid thinking
Solve the wrong problem	
Trade-off decisions	
What You Do	Why
Placate others	Seek harmony
Submit to authority	Focus on tasks, not goals
Solve easy problems	Think short-range
Tolerate partial solutions	Hope to reduce risk of failure
Repeat past mistakes	Desire to conform
Hold-off decisions	
What You Do	Why
Generate multiple, superficial alternatives	Fear of unknown
	Accept unworkable constraints
Gather irrelevant facts	
Fight the problem	Wait for more favorable conditions
Hop from problem to problem	
	Wait for someone else to act
Rationalize delay	

FIGURE 3-1. Dangerous decision-making habits. (From Roseman E: How to sharpen your decision-making. MLO 7:84, November 1975. Reprinted with permission of publisher)

successful decisions (the easy ones) for half-successes or even failures. The supervisor who practices hold-off decisions looks at the trade-off habit and proposes that failures on tough problems are not necessary. If the decision is not made, then the situation will either resolve itself or an obvious good alternative will surface. These supervisors work very hard at postponing decision-making by generating endless superficial alternatives. Unfortunately, this rationalizing of delay tactics tends to gather so much data that even relevant facts become hidden in a mass of irrelevancies. All of these dangerous decision-making habits are characteristic of the weak decision-maker. Table 3-1 shows how decision-making is related to the four basic functions of a manager: planning, organizing, directing, and controlling.[16] It also contrasts four typical decision-making approaches along the spectrum from dictatorship to abdication.

Authoritarian

Some laboratory managers use the authoritarian decision-making approach with regularity. This manager views himself as a central authority, more knowledgeable than his staff because he has access to the big picture of the laboratory. His communication is one-way—down the organizational structure. He shuns opportunities to interact with his technical staff and pays little attention to their ideas, proposals, or suggestions for alternatives. Of the identified major areas of concern in decision-making, this approach elicits a decision of the poorest quality, least acceptance and commitment, and least concern for value factors. The true worth of this approach lies in the speed at which a decision is reached. Because no one other than the laboratory manager is involved, a decision is able to be rendered with speed.

Table 3-1
Approaches to Decision-making

	Authoritarian	Democratic	Consensus	Laissez-Faire
Planning	All determination of policy by the supervisor	All policies a matter of group discussion and decision, encouraged and assisted by the supervisor	All policies a matter of group discussion and decision with supervisor insisting that all members be satisfied	Complete freedom for group or individual decision with a minimum of supervisor participation
Organizing	The supervisor usually dictates the particular work task and work companion of each member	The members are free to work with whomever they choose and the division of tasks is left up to the group	Division of duties and tasks are responsibility of all members of the group such that all members agree with structure	Complete nonparticipation of the supervisor
Directing	Techniques and activity steps dictated by the supervisor, one at a time, so that future steps are uncertain to a large degree	Activity perspective gained during discussion period. General steps to group goal sketched, and when technical advice is needed, the supervisor suggests two or more alternative procedures from which choice could be made	General group discussion of techniques and activities. All group members must agree on the approach to be followed. Supervisor actively seeks agreement through discussion, justification, and compromise	Various materials supplied by the supervisor, who makes it clear that he will supply information when asked. He takes no other part in work discussion
Controlling	The supervisor tends to be personal in his praise and criticism of the work of each member, remains aloof from active group participation except when demonstrating	The supervisor is objective or fact-minded in his praise and criticism and tries to be a regular group member in spirit without doing too much of the work	The supervisor insists on uniform, harmonious peer review	Supervisor makes infrequent spontaneous comments on member activities unless questioned, and no attempt is made to appraise or regulate the course of events

(Adapted from White R, Lippitt R: Autocracy and Democracy, pp 26–27. New York, Harper & Row, 1960. By permission of Harper & Row.)

Democratic

In a democratic society, the laboratory manager feels most comfortable attempting to reach decisions by majority vote. This does not mean that the manager polls the staff in his laboratory to determine the decision, but rather that he personally makes the decision after taking a straw vote. He perceives that this is best because the majority then will be committed to following through to implement the decision. The quality, acceptance, and staff feelings about this decision-making process are improved over the authoritarian approach, but those who spoke against the decision will generally feel ignored and disgruntled to some extent. Obviously the time taken to reach such a decision will be longer, because the manager has taken the time to poll his subordinates.

Consensus

When the laboratory manager uses the consensus approach to decision-making, he works hard at getting all members of his staff to at least partially agree with the decision made. He approaches the alternatives from a logical point of view and avoids arguing his own viewpoint. All staff members are encouraged to voice their opinions and to describe the reasoning behind their choice.[1] These differences of opinion are viewed by the manager as a help, rather than a hindrance, in decision-making. He also avoids any conflict reducing techniques such as majority vote, averaging, or trading. Of the three decision-making approaches described thus far, the consensus format yields the highest quality decision, since everyone not only provides information and creativity but must explain the rationale for his favored alternative. The staff will feel good about the approach employed, and this generally will result in increased acceptance and commitment.[11] On the contrary, this approach can be time-consuming.

Laissez-Faire

The laboratory manager who employs this approach has nearly abdicated from his administrative responsibility. He sees his role as merely inputting into the decision process—a supportive effort—but leaves the planning, organizing, directing, and control of the process up to his staff. From this decision-making approach, it would appear that the laboratory manager is only a figurehead, with his staff in control. This is by far the least effective approach. If a quality decision is reached, it will usually be because of the presence of an informal leader. Most members of the laboratory staff will fault the manager for using this approach and not feel satisfied with the process. With no manager directing, the wait for a decision to be made could drag on for extended periods of time.

Various levels of participation by subordinates in the decision-making process have a direct impact on how successful the manager will be in implementing the decision.[3] This is summarized in Figure 3-2. Resistance toward implementation is diminished with increased participation, but the trade-off is time.

No single decision-making approach is best for all situations. To be effective, a laboratory manager should vary his decision-making approach depending on the situation.[6] A laboratory supervisor may find the authoritarian approach to be best when making routine decisions about procedures, and certainly it is appropriate in an emergency situation. The democratic approach can be effectively used if the laboratory manager is deciding on a color scheme for new laboratory furniture. When deciding who should work various scheduled holidays, a

FIGURE 3-2.   The effects of various levels of participation on the decision-making process. Participation lowers resistance to decisions but increases the time required to implement them.

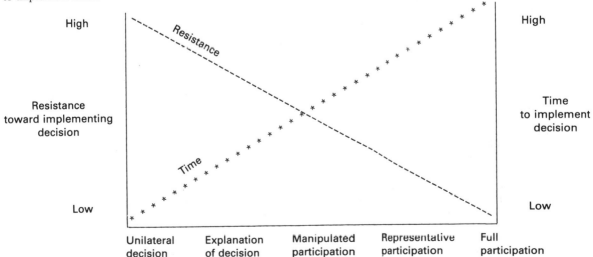

laboratory supervisor can employ the consensus method quite effectively. Abdicating, as in the laissez-faire approach, is perhaps only in order when decisions regarding the laboratory's annual holiday party are being generated.

Whether the approach is authoritarian, democratic, or consensus, the effective laboratory manager must always make the final decision.[7] He must make it as an individual and accept responsibility for it as an individual. If he relies solely on majority opinion or a consensus approach, he is not a manager; he is a presiding officer.

HUMAN FACTORS IN DECISION-MAKING

Managers do not make decisions following any single pattern. Rather, they respond to a variety of complex factors including economic, social, cultural, and political pressures.[4] Another group of influences worthy of mention consists of the human factors that affect the manager's approach to decision-making. Robbins described five such human factors and the impact each would carry.[8] The first has to do with the manager's personal value systems. The administrator's attitudes, biases, and personal beliefs, based on what society has told us is right or wrong, will have a significant impact on which decisions he considers major and on the array of alternatives that he will create. According to Robbins, the manager's perception of the situation will also play a role in decision-making. Indeed, the manager's judgment and creativity will reflect how he perceives the problem or situation requiring a choice. The third factor involves the limitations in human processing of information. Different managers have differing capacities for mentally storing and sorting out bits and pieces of information related to the decision at hand. Rarely does the decision-maker have all the information necessary far enough in advance to spend excessive time sorting out specifics, and this then becomes the limitation. A decision-maker is also conscious of and responsive to political and power behaviors relative to any given selection. The manager may be concerned with warding off challenges to his decision-making power as a means of protecting his own self-interests. The fifth human factor affecting the decision-maker is the constraint of time. A limitation on the time available for the manager to assess and study the situation before making a decision is characteristic of today's administrative environment. Hence, the decision-maker, subject to an interaction of organizational influences and human factors, attempts to make the best possible choice. Obviously, the optimum decision is not always made. Sometimes the factors influencing a decision are so complex that analysis of the rationale is impossible. This phenomenon has been so widely substantiated that Rowe states it as a rule: "In any complex decision where personal or behavior factors apply, the individual's preference will dominate the results."[10]

QUANTITATIVE TOOLS FOR DECISION-MAKING

Seeking selection of the best alternative is sometimes fraught with difficulties. There exist several quantitative techniques for better assessment of each alternative. These are briefly mentioned here, and the reader is encouraged to seek additional information if a technique appears appropriate for a given situation. Other techniques not discussed here, such as return on investment (ROI), marginal analysis, and break-even models, may also be helpful.

Queuing Theory

This technique is frequently referred to as the waiting-line theory. Its objective is to balance the cost of having a waiting line against the cost of enough personnel to eliminate that line. Queuing theory could be used to determine the number of phlebotomists required to draw blood in an outpatient clinic when the flow of patients varies such that lines occur at certain times.[13]

Linear Programming

When there exists a linear relationship between problem and objective, certain graphic, algebraic, or simplex techniques may be used. Linear programming is often used when there are two activities competing for limited resources. This technique may be employed in determining which of several chemistry-profiling instruments would be best for a given laboratory work load.

Probability Theory

This technique generally is used to assist the decision-maker in reducing risk on the basis of statistics. In the blood bank laboratory, a statistical probability of the number of specimens requiring use of antibody identification panels may be used to predict the inventory of reagents necessary to avoid a stockout or oversupply.

STEPS IN THE PROBLEM-SOLVING PROCESS

Problem-solving and decision-making are not synonymous activities. While they are similar, problem-solving has several facets that separate it as a managerial skill from typical decision-making. The primary difference is in determining precisely that for which a decision needs to be rendered. Figure 3-3 graphically describes a brief but comprehensive flow of events in the problem-solving process. Each of the steps in the problem-solving cycle could be expanded with substeps and detail similar to a massive decision tree. The simple, seven-step approach described here allows the manager the flexibility to modify when necessary but still have some basic guideline to follow.

Step 1. Definition of the Problem

As in the treatment of disease, therapy is only effective if it is appropriate for the diagnosis. The manager must learn to look beyond the symptoms of the problem and focus on the real issue. Often it is a symptom, such as absenteeism, which calls attention to the fact that a problem exists. Scanlon defines *symptoms* as "adverse events or things which are present in an operation but have not yet developed to the point of emerging as basic deviations."[12] The *basic deviations* are problems that are referred to as "glaring mistakes," as contrasted to *effect problems* (surface problems), or *causal problems* (root problems). The manager who focuses his attention on an effect problem is attempting to achieve a temporary solution, whereas addressing a causal problem should prevent recurrence of the deviation.

One pitfall that many managers encountered as they begin a problem-solving process is the temptation to hypothesize about what should have been done earlier so the problem would not have developed. Some problems will be inherited, some resulting from decisions made elsewhere in the organizational hierarchy, and still others from one's own doing. Regardless of the origin of the problem, the solution must still be made within the framework of the situation.

Step 2. Fact-Gathering

Once the problem has been identified, the manager can begin to gather information needed for developing alternative solutions. Facts surrounding the decision situation are important to seek out, as are constraints and assumptions. *Constraints* are factors that limit the scope of alternatives. *Assumptions* are applied to factors in an effort to simplify the problem and make it solvable. Fact-gathering requires a search for pertinent information from persons directly involved in the problem, from books and printed materials, from other people, and from experts and experimental work.

Step 3. Development of Alternative Solutions

The generation of possible solutions calls for creative thinking. Often when faced with this step, a manager will draw on his past experience; and in most cases, this will be adequate. On the basis of similarities with, and differences from past experiences, the manager can adjust past alternatives that have proven successful. Past experience, however, can never be fully sufficient in developing alternatives; rather, its most useful purpose is to act as a guide. Today's manager must supplement his creativity by seeking information from others who have

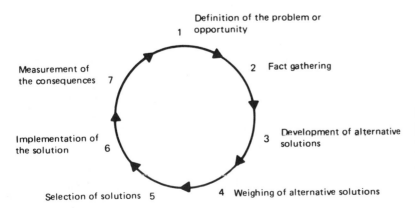

FIGURE 3-3. Flow of events in the problem-solving process. (From Knudson HR, Woodworth RT, Bell CH: Management: An Experiential Approach, p 239. New York, McGraw-Hill, 1973. Reprinted with permission of publisher)

solved a similar problem or from individuals directly involved in the situation. It is wise to keep an open mind and not prejudge ideas as they are generated.

Step 4. Weighing of Alternative Solutions

This step requires the analysis of alternative solutions by stating the advantages and disadvantages of each possible course of action. For some problems, this may be a simple and straightforward task; for other situations, the analysis may be a complex and detailed procedure. This step also requires the consideration of each alternative as to how effectively it will accomplish the objectives and requirements of a satisfactory solution. The manager must consider the ramifications of each potential solution. Finally, consideration should be given the question of whether a chosen alternative will eliminate reoccurrence of the problem or generate another in its place.

Step 5. Selection of Solutions

Choosing the best possible course of action is obviously not an isolated event, but rather an integrated process. Considerable fact-gathering and planning has already occurred. Even though alternatives have been scrutinized, any single approach is not always "best." There is generally more than one way to solve a problem; and in choosing a solution, trade-offs in quality, acceptance, speed, value, or cost may be necessary. When the decision is made, it is often wise to discuss it with someone who has considerable problem-solving skills.

Step 6. Implementation of the Solution

Of all the steps in the problem-solving process, the implementation step is usually the most time-consuming. At the same time, even the best decision, if not properly implemented, is useless. This step is critical. As in the decision-making process, implementation must involve those who are directly affected by the solution to the problem. Scanlon identified three essential aspects of effective implementation[12]: (1) a questioning attitude concerning every detail of the decision and the development of necessary procedures; (2) a plan for communicating the decision to those involved in and affected by it; and (3) participation by all levels—management and employees alike.

Step 7. Measurement of the Consequences

As depicted in Figure 3-3, once the solution to a problem has been implemented, the cycle is not complete. Evaluation of the consequences is appropriate. Not all decisions rendered will have the effect that was planned. An analysis of what occurred, whether predicted or not, provides an ever-increasing basis of experience from which future problems can be solved. Perhaps in the analysis and measurement of consequences, the problem-solving process will be started over again.

Problem-solving as a management skill is probably best developed through repeated exposure with guidance in the laboratory setting. Consider the following problem described by a laboratory supervisor in a small laboratory:*

> I have a lot of trouble keeping experienced personnel. I know that the problem isn't that our technologists are bored with their work but that they are dissatisfied with the amount they are paid. Our hospital has a policy of keeping salaries down by hiring inexperienced personnel for the lab rather than employing experienced technologists at rates that are competitive with other hospitals in the area.
>
> Recently, I lost a technologist who had assumed a great deal of responsibility in running the lab. I had been trying to get the hospital to appoint her my assistant supervisor for a year, but they refused. Their reasoning was that it would cost too much money and that I did not need an assistant. Nevertheless, for a year she acted as my assistant without the recognition or money that would normally accompany this role. When I had to be away from the lab, I could depend on her to keep things running smoothly, but finally, when the hospital continually refused to raise her salary or give her a promotion, she left.
>
> Last week, when I was sick for three days, the lab had a lot of problems that could not be solved by the inexperienced technologists who make up our staff.
>
> What can I do?

The first step for the laboratory supervisor in this case is to define the problem. He must sort through a variety of symptoms surrounding the high turnover rate. He has ruled out job boredom and focused on staff salaries. The underlying problem, on the basis of information presented, is that the administration is unaware of the value—or is unwilling to recognize the value—of experienced technologists who require more pay.

*MLO, p 28. New York, United Business Publications, January 1976. Reprinted with permission of the editors.

In resolving this problem, there is considerable information to be gathered. The supervisor could survey the community to determine the standard for technologist's salaries and benefits. Certainly a record of the increased turnover would be essential. Some type of analysis of the cost of training or orienting a new technologist should be carried out. Perhaps the supervisor should document the feasibility of reducing the total staff if all technologists were experienced. And finally, some information should be gathered about potential legal ramifications of having nonsupervisory, inexperienced staff in charge.

Several alternatives could be developed and analyzed before a selection is made. This may include an attempt to resolve the problem within the laboratory, perhaps by trying a rotating supervisor in the absence of the designated management technologist. Perhaps a more comprehensive orientation is appropriate for the inexperienced technologists. The best solution may be a meeting with the hospital administrator describing the problem and presenting the data gathered. While it is generally difficult to explain the technical insufficiencies that result from inexperienced personnel, hospital administration can appreciate productivity figures and bottom-line profits and losses.

CHOOSING A MANAGEMENT DECISION STYLE BASED ON THE SITUATION

It should be apparent at this point that decision-making is an integral part of a laboratory manager's daily practice. Furthermore, there is little doubt that the effectiveness of a laboratory manager is largely based on his past history of making the right decisions.

The clinical laboratory is a highly complex environment in which management decision styles may promote or detract from the effectiveness of the organization. Although it is impossible to create a totally reliable formula for determining which decision style to use at which time, Vroom has proposed a normative model based on the complexities of any given situation.[15]

The conceptual basis of the model rests on distinguishing among three classes of outcomes, which bears on the ultimate effectiveness of decisions. These include the quality or rationality of the decision, the acceptance and commitment on the part of subordinates to execute the decision, and the amount of time required to make the decision. The manager works through a decision tree (Fig. 3-4) answering a series of questions that will have an impact on decision effectiveness. The end-result is a descriptive management decision style based on the situation.

Problem Attributes Assessment

Vroom's model requires the laboratory manager to evaluate the situation and possible effects of differing decision styles using seven parameters called problem attributes:

1. Quality—the importance of the quality of the decision made. The manager must decide whether a quality requirement exists so that one solution is likely to be more rational than another.
2. Manager's information—the extent to which the leader possesses sufficient information and expertise to make a high-quality decision by himself.
3. Problem structure—the extent to which the problem is structured. The manager decides whether there is a planned approach based on previous experience. If so, this may provide a map for solving the problem at hand.
4. Acceptance—the extent to which acceptance or commitment on the part of subordinates is critical to the effective implementation of the decision.
5. Prior probability of acceptance—the extent to which the leader's autocratic decision can be expected to receive acceptance by subordinates. The manager evaluates the situation to determine whether it can be reasonably certain that a decision will be accepted by his subordinates if he makes it himself.
6. Goal congruence—the extent to which the subordinates are motivated to attain the organizational goals as represented in the objectives explicit in the statement of the problem. Essentially, the manager determines whether his subordinates want to solve the problem and whether they will achieve some personal goals in the process.
7. Conflict—the extent to which subordinates are likely to be in conflict over preferred solutions.

Types of Management Decision Styles

When the manager completes an evaluation of the situation by using the decision tree (Fig. 3-4), he

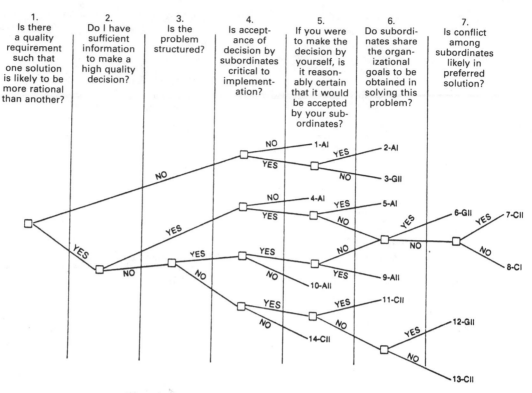

FIGURE 3-4. Decision process flow chart. (From Vroom VH: A new look at managerial decision making. Organizational Dynamics 1:5, Spring 1973. Reprinted with permission of publisher. All rights reserved)

has identified the problem type. Using Table 3-2, he can then determine the acceptable decision-making method(s). These decision-making processes are keyed on the basis of autocratic (A), consultative (C), or group involvement (G), with the following variations:

AI— The manager solves the problem himself, using information available at the time.

AII— The manager obtains the necessary information from his subordinate(s), then decides on the solution to the problem himself. He may or may not tell his subordinates what the problem is in getting information from them. The role played by the subordinates in making the decision is clearly one of providing the necessary information to the manager, rather than generating or evaluating alternative solutions.

CI— The manager shares the problem with relevant subordinates individually, getting their ideas and suggestions without bringing them to-

gether as a group. The manager then makes the decision, which may or may not reflect his subordinates' influence.

CII— The manager shares the problem with his subordinates as a group, collectively obtaining their ideas and suggestions. He then makes the decision, which may or may not reflect his subordinates' influence.

GII— The manager shares the problem with his subordinates as a group. Together they generate and evaluate alternatives and attempt to reach agreement (consensus) on a solution. The manager's role is much like that of a chairman. He does not try to influence the group to adopt his solution, and he is willing to accept and implement any solution that has the support of the entire group.

Consider the following case as an example of how Vroom's model can be applied to a decision-making situation in the laboratory:

Table 3-2
Problem Types and the Feasible Set of Decision Processes

Problem Type	Acceptable Methods
1	AI, AII, CI, CII, GII
2	AI, AII, CI, CII, GII
3	GII
4	AI, AII, CI, CII, GII*
5	AI, AII, CI, CII, GII*
6	GII
7	CII
8	CI, CII
9	AII, CI, CII, GII*
10	AII, CI, CII, GII*
11	CII, GII*
12	GII
13	CII
14	CII, GII*

*Within the feasible set only when the answer to question 6 in Fig. 3-4 is YES.
(Adapted from Vroom VH: A new look at managerial decision making. Organizational Dynamics 1:2–7, Spring 1973. Adapted with permission of publisher.)

You are the administrative technologist of special chemistry in a large commercial laboratory. The company's management has always been searching for ways to increase efficiency, especially in terms of turnaround time. They have recently installed a new computer employing a modified on-line reporting system. To the surprise of everyone, including yourself, the expected decrease in turnaround time has not been realized. In fact, the time required from specimen entry to report availability has increased slightly overall, an increase in clerical report errors has been noted, and a number of employee requests for transfer have resulted.

You do not believe there is anything wrong with the new computer system. You have had reports from other laboratories using the system, and they confirm this opinion. You have also had representatives from the firm that built the computer system go over it, and they report that it is operating at peak efficiency.

You suspect that some programming in the new computer system may be responsible for the problems. This view, however, is not widely shared among your immediate subordinates, who are four first-line supervisors, each in charge of a section, and the department's quality-control coordinator. The increase in turnaround time has been variously attributed to poor orientation of the technical staff, lack of an adequate system of financial incentives, and poor morale. Clearly this is an issue about which there is considerable depth of feeling and potential disagreement among your subordinates.

This morning you receive a phone call from the director of operations. He has just received your delayed report figures for the last four weeks and is calling to express his concern. He indicates that the problem is yours to solve in any way that you think best but that he would like to know by tomorrow what steps you plan to take.

You share the operations manager's concern with the increased turnaround time and know that your technical staff is also concerned. The problem is to decide what steps to take to rectify the situation.

Decision Strategy Analysis

Applying Vroom's model in this case, the administrative technologist attempts to answer the following diagnostic questions to assess problem attributes:

1. Is there a quality requirement such that one solution is likely to be more rational than another? YES (direct impact on efficiency).
2. Does the administrative technologist have sufficient information to make a high-quality decision? NO (unsure of exact problem).
3. Is the problem structured? NO (problem not solved before).
4. Is acceptance of the decision by subordinates critical to effective implementation? YES (implementation to be carried out by subordinates).
5. If the decision is made by the administrative technologist himself, is it reasonably certain that it would be accepted by his subordinates? NO (different decisions perceived as appropriate).
6. Do the subordinates share the organizational goals to be reached in solving this problem? YES (all concerned with problem).
7. Is conflict among subordinates likely in preferred solutions? YES (concerned that they are not faulted in the problem).

Using Figure 3-4, the administrative technologist identifies the problem type as 12; the management decision style indicated in Table 3-2 is GII. The problem should be shared with the supervisors and quality-control coordinator as a group. Together they should identify the problem, generate and evaluate alternatives, and attempt to reach a consensus agreement on the best solution. The solution agreed upon by the whole group must then be implemented.

PROBLEM-SOLVING AND DECISION-MAKING WITH PROFICIENCY DATA

Analysis of proficiency survey results can often help in troubleshooting procedural problems and improve the instrument and procedure selection process.[14] Data from proficiency studies can aid both in the definition of the problem and in fact-gathering steps. Unfortunately, most laboratory managers peruse these data quickly to be sure that no obvious problems exist without gaining the maximum value of this decision-making and troubleshooting resource. With approximately 7000 laboratories in the United States contributing to the CAP data base, this resource can serve as a valuable technical and managerial tool for troubleshooting.

In most cases, if a problem exists with a procedure or instrument, it will be identified in the summaries of performance by all participants. For example, in recent slide tests for rheumatoid factor, more than 97% of the participants reported a survey specimen negative. But most laboratories using one manufacturer's procedure reported the specimen positive, disagreeing with all other procedures and the consensus. The conclusion can be drawn that there is difficulty with this particular procedure.

The laboratory should compare its own unacceptable results with results on previous surveys to see whether the problem is an ongoing one. The unacceptable results should also be compared with daily quality control records for determining whether a systematic error exists. Because the CAP often includes values from very low normals to very high normals for each constituent, the laboratory should verify the linearity of each procedure.

Survey data can spotlight a number of specific problems. For example, evaluations of most urinalysis dipstick results are based on consensus of survey participants. Because the ketone portion of the dipstick is the first to become insensitive to trace amounts of a positive constituent, false-negative results in a particular laboratory may indicate that the sticks have been exposed to too much humidity and should be replaced.

No other resource provides as much information as the CAP's quarterly participant summaries about how a given method or instrument has performed in the hands of so many laboratories. For this reason, they are an excellent shopping guide. A laboratory can use them to compare its current instruments with products under consideration for purchase. Mean results give one a reasonable idea of an instrument's future accuracy, and coefficients of variation will reveal its future reliability or precision.

One chemistry analyzer consistently demonstrated accuracy and precision for blood urea nitrogen (BUN) when the proficiency sample was in the normal range. When an abnormal BUN of 51 mg/dL was tested, however, the acceptable range of responses (± 2 standard deviations) was 36 to 64 mg/dL.

If one is planning a purchase, one should personally check the product's track record against others in the survey.

REFERENCES

1. Birchall D, Wild R, Carnall D: Redesigning a way to worker participation. Personnel Management 8(8):26–28, 1976
2. Knudson HR, Woodworth RT, Bell CH: Management: An Experiential Approach, p 239. New York, McGraw-Hill, 1973
3. Likert R, Likert JG: A method for coping with conflict in problem-solving groups. Group and Organizational Studies 3:427–434, 1978
4. McFarland DE: Management: Principles and Practices, 3rd ed, pp 75–133. New York, Macmillan, 1970
5. McFarland DE: Managerial Innovation in the Metropolitan Hospital. New York, Praeger Publishers, 1979
6. Michael SR: The contingency manager: Doing what comes naturally. Management Review 65(11):20–31, 1976
7. Ray JJ: Do authoritarians hold authoritarian attitudes? Human Relations 29(4):301–325, 1976
8. Robbins SP: The Administrative Process, pp 165–167. Englewood Cliffs, Prentice-Hall, 1976
9. Roseman E: How to sharpen your decision-making. MLO 7:84, 1975
10. Rowe AJ: The myth of the rational decision maker. International Management, pp 38–40, August 1974
11. Rubinstein SP: Participative problem solving: How to increase organization effectiveness. Personnel 54:30–39, 1977
12. Scanlon BK: Management 18: A Short Course for Managers, pp 35–49. New York, John Wiley & Sons, 1974
13. Schober A: We applied queing theory to our outpatient lab service. MLO 9(12):69–77, 1977
14. Snyder JR, Glenn DW: Problem solving and decision making with proficiency data. MLO 18(2):46–49, 1986
15. Vroom VH: A new look at managerial decision making. Organizational Dynamics, pp 2–7. New York, AMACOM, Spring 1973
16. White R, Lippitt R: Autocracy and Democracy, pp 26–27. New York, Harper & Row, 1960

ANNOTATED BIBLIOGRAPHY

Anundsen K (ed): Participative Decision Making. New York, AMACOM, 1974.

   This reference contains selected articles from AMACOM publications dealing with involvement in decision making. The scope of articles includes problem solving through organizational development and management by objectives.

Bennett AC: Improving Management Performance in Health Care Institutions. Chicago, American Hospital Corporation, 1978

Part 4 is a process-oriented section dealing with problem solving and employee participation. Both Chapter 11, ''The Manager as a Problem Solver,'' and Chapter 12, ''Gaining Employee Participation,'' include sections on the appropriate questions a manager should ask in gathering information for making a quality decision.

Fitzgibbon RJ, Snyder JR: The Laboratory Manager's Problem Solver. Oradell, NJ, Medical Economics Books, 1985

This resource provides practical answers to more than 400 management problems that trouble clinical laboratory managers and supervisors. A panel of experienced laboratory managers have offered their solutions to questions received from practitioners in the field. This textbook is a rich source of provocative questions for discussion by current supervisors and potential supervisors.

Flippo EB: Principles of Personnel Management, 4th ed. New York, McGraw-Hill, 1976

A comprehensive text on personnel management, this book contains 22 case studies that are excellent examples of the decision-making process in action.

Longest BB: Management Practices for the Health Professional. Reston, Virginia, Reston Publishing Co, 1976

This book addresses each of the functions of a manager. Of particular value is the creation of appropriate relationships between the functions. Chapter 4 specifically deals with decision-making tools for the practice of management.

Margerison CJ: Managerial Problem Solving. London, McGraw-Hill, 1974

This reference addresses each step of the problem-solving process in detail. The true science and art of decision-making are emphasized through the description of strategies and solutions as well as behavior and expression in the problem-solving process.

Maskowitz H, Wright GP: Operations Research Techniques for Management. Englewood Cliffs, New Jersey, Prentice-Hall, 1979

A compendium of statistical tools and concepts of probability, this book emphasizes the integration of operations research in managerial decision-making. This reference is replete with numerous techniques for decision analysis, programming models (linear, network, goal, etc.), and applications of operations research.

Rappoport A (ed): Information Decision Making: Quantitative and Behavior Dimensions. Englewood Cliffs, New Jersey, Prentice-Hall, 1970

This book describes various techniques and strategies for acquiring and dealing with data (information) in the decision-making process. Of particular value is Section 3, ''Behavioral Aspects of Information''; in this section, emphasis is placed on motivation, quality, acceptance, and effects of alternatives in decision-making.

part two

Concepts in Managerial Leadership

four

Motivation — Managerial Assumptions and Effects

Diana Mass

In addition to sound leadership and organizational skills, a successful laboratory manager must also have the ability to motivate or instill self-motivation in employees. Because motivation must be directed toward a constructive outcome compatible with the goals of the organization, the prudent manager is one who minimizes discrepancies between individual and organizational goals. Once this is accomplished, the manager will support and reinforce those character traits that lead to the fulfillment of shared goals. This chapter examines some assumptions about human behavior, the theories of motivation that have evolved from them, and how managers can use those theories to motivate employees.

NATURE OF MOTIVATION

When different people perform the same job, invariably some do it better than others. If one can quantify each worker's contribution, one may find that the best person in each group is contributing two, five, or perhaps ten times as much as the poorest performer. What causes these differences in performance? One answer is that these differences reflect individual differences in skill or ability. Another answer is that differences in performance reflect differences in motivation. At any given time, people vary in the extent to which they are willing to direct their energies toward the attainment of

organizational goals. The problem of motivating workers is as old as organized activity itself, but only within the last half century has it been scientifically studied. This relatively brief period has seen the beginning of attempts to apply the tools of the behavioral sciences, particularly psychology, to the relationship between an individual's motivation and his work.[10,20]

Defining Motivation

Before examining the nature of motivation, we must agree on a meaning for the term. Motivation is not a simple concept, and its definition must refer to desires, goals, plans, intents, impulses, and purposes. Some of these terms imply deliberate and calculated processes that involve reason, and others imply spontaneity. In general, the strength of a person's motivation depends on the strength of his individual motives. Motives are the causes that direct a given type of behavior. Thus, motives are the mainsprings of action.[10,11] Motivated behavior has these essential features:

1. Motivated behavior is purposeful, or goal-directed.
2. The motivated individual expects that specific behaviors will lead to the attainment of goals.
3. Motivation is assumed to be selective or

directional and requires that energy be involved to propel the individual to a level that enables the performance of the appropriate behavior.

4. Motivation involves the persistence of behavior over time so that effort can be sustained even if setbacks occur.[11]

It is easy to see, then, that motivation is a complex concept and an explanation thereof must include a discussion of personality, for the effectiveness of motivators varies among individuals.

Personality

Personality can be defined as the aggregate of an individual's behaviors. The development of personality is affected by many things: the individual's genetic and physical makeup; his family size, composition, and style of interactions; the culture in which he is raised; the types of groups to which he belongs; the nature and amount of his education; and so forth. The great number of possible combinations of these elements gives rise to individuals with different needs and, thus, a variety of motivation techniques are necessary.

Behavior constantly changes in response to the situations and the kinds of people one encounters. An individual's behavior is a function of his personality. Components of personality include needs, drives, motivation, perceptual approaches, past experiences, attitudes, values, and particular types of relations with others, all of which affect the individual's performance on the job.[11]

Motivation Process

The process of motivation is depicted in Figure 4-1. Because all behavior is motivated, either consciously or unconsciously, a cause-and-effect relationship exists. This phenomenon has often been called the path goals approach to fulfillment of unsatisfied needs. The first step in the path goals cycle involves the sensing or realization of an unsatisfied need. This is followed by establishing goals that are intended to fulfill the need and then developing behavior in the attempt to accomplish those goals. Motivation should not be confused with satisfaction. If action is viewed as a process, one can easily see that motivation describes the force that pushes people to perform, while satisfaction describes the feeling of contentment and achievement experienced after a goal is met. That is, people are motivated to seek satisfaction.[3]

Many of the early management scholars emphasized financial incentives as prime means for motivating individuals. Today money is still an important motivator; however, psychologists now agree that people seek to satisfy needs other than purely economic ones. There is a wide difference of opinion as to what these needs and their relative importance are. Most, however, take a pluralistic approach, which emphasizes that there are many different types of needs, each of which may be defined by the satisfaction it brings. Understanding that unsatisfied needs motivate people to alter their behavior to achieve their goals has led to the development of motivational theories. Four of the most well-known motivational theories are (1) the *need-hierarchy* theory; (2) the *two-factor* theory; (3) the *preference–expectation* theory; and (4) *theories X and Y*. A discussion of these theories and their relevance to today's organizational setting follows.

MOTIVATIONAL THEORIES

Need-Hierarchy Theory

One of the most widely adopted theories of human motivation was proposed in the early 1940s by Abraham Maslow. Maslow described a hierarchy of needs as a predictor and descriptor of human motivation. His theory of motivation is based on two premises: (1) Needs depend on what one already has. That is, needs that are not satisfied can influence behavior, but satisfied needs will not act as motivators. (2) Needs are arranged in a hierarchy of importance. When one need is satisfied, a higher-level need emerges and demands satisfaction.

FIGURE 4-1. Path goals cycle.

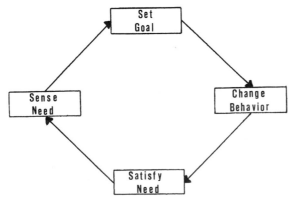

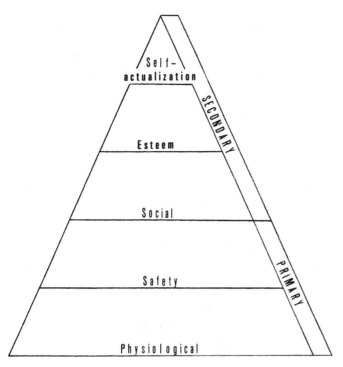

FIGURE 4-2. Hierarchy of needs.

The various needs are described in a framework referred to as the hierarchy of needs (Fig. 4-2). According to Maslow, five general categories, or levels, of needs can be found in any individual: (1) physiologic, or survival, needs; (2) safety, or security, needs; (3) social needs; (4) esteem, or ego, needs; and (5) self-actualization, or self-fulfillment, needs.

These five categories of needs are arranged in a hierarchy ranging from the lowest-order needs (physiologic) to the highest-order (self-actualization). This hierarchy determines priority. According to Maslow, behavior is always determined by the lowest-order level of need remaining unsatisfied, and unsatisfied needs are the important motivators. Therefore, when selecting effective motivators in the organizational setting, it is important to recognize whether a certain motivator is directed toward satisfying a previously unsatisfied need or one that no longer exists.[3,4,6,9,10,12,13,18,20] We can now examine the five need levels and relate them to a modern organizational setting.

Physiologic Needs

Food, clothing, and shelter constitute the primary needs, and thus are the prime motivators. In terms of the work environment, the satisfaction of physiologic needs is usually associated with money. What money can buy satisfies a person's physiologic needs. It should also be noted that money is useful not only as a satisfier of physiologic needs but also in the satisfaction of needs at any level.[3,4,6,9,10,12,13,18,20]

Safety Needs

With the physiologic needs fulfilled, the next level of needs assumes priority. Safety needs include protection from physical harm, ill health, and economic disaster. In a work setting, this category has been broadened to include needs such as job security and greater financial support. If an employee senses that management makes fair judgments regarding all subordinates, he is not likely to feel threatened. If, however, management's policies reflect favoritism and arbitrary discrimination, the employee may insist strongly on job security. This is evidenced by stronger demands from labor unions regarding job security and legal cases resulting from dismissal of an employee without sufficient justification. With regard to protection from physical harm, the Occupational Safety and Health Administration (OSHA) has been active in attempting to eliminate many of the dangerous elements of various jobs. Management's attention to safety in order to minimize these dangers serves as a strong motivator.[3,4,6,9,10,12,13,18,20]

Social Needs

After the safety and security needs have been satisfied, social needs have an influence on behavior. These include needs for both giving and receiving affection and love; the need to accept, associate with, and be accepted by others; and the need to belong or to feel oneself a part of social groups. In essence, one needs to be liked by and to like one's co-workers. The fulfillment of social needs manifests itself in the formation of informal groups within organizations. Research has shown that in many cases individuals seek affiliation because they desire to have their beliefs confirmed; *i.e.*, people tend to seek out others who share similar beliefs. Under proper direction, this natural activity can help in the formulation of a cooperative and constructive group. Unfortunately, management may fear that the group will develop consolidated attributes in opposition to the organization's goals. Hence, the social needs of the employee are often downgraded, leading to frustration and resentment.[3,4,6,9,10,12,13,18,20]

Esteem Needs

Maslow's fourth level consists of the esteem or ego needs; that is, the need to be recognized for what one does. This category includes the need for respect from others; the feeling of achievement, appreciation, recognition, and status; and, generally, a feeling of worthiness. These needs could be subdivided into two groups: self-esteem and esteem from others. Self-esteem refers to the development of self-confidence and self-respect. This often takes the form of mastery of an area of knowledge or competency in a technical skill. Currently management's tool to help develop the employee's self-confidence usually takes the form of constructive appraisals of the employee. From the employee's viewpoint, knowing that a job is done well increases self-confidence. In addition, recognition by management and others leads to the development of self-respect.[3,4,6,9,10,12,13,18,20]

Self-Actualization Needs

The highest hierarchical need is for self-actualization, or self-fulfillment. Maslow defines it as the need "to become everything one is capable of becoming." In attempting to satisfy this need, an employee becomes less concerned about recognition and more concerned about the pleasure and sense of satisfaction obtained from performing a job. Self-actualization describes a potential for self-development. Unfortunately, rarely does an individual have the financial and emotional freedom to pursue ultimate self-development and total creativity.[3,4,6,9,10,12,13,18,20] In 1962 Maslow estimated that only 10% of self-fulfillment needs were satisfied, compared with 85% of the physiologic needs.[4] In keeping with his premises of a hierarchy, Maslow argues that the satisfaction of self-actualization needs is possible only after the satisfaction of all other needs in the hierarchy. As Maslow perceives it, the hierarchy-of-needs theory is applicable to most people in most situations. However, some individuals, because of their unique personality or situation, establish a different hierarchy of needs. For example, a great composer or artist might thrive on fulfillment of the higher-level needs while caring little about his physical sustenance.[3,4,6,9,10,12,13,18,20]

For the sake of definition, the needs are separated into five categories. In reality, however, they interact within the individual. Lower-level needs never remain fully satisfied, and once the needs for esteem and self-actualization become important, a person seeks continuously for more satisfaction of them. In fact, people can never fully satisfy all of their needs. The need-hierarchy model essentially says that needs that are satisfied are no longer motivators. In essence, people are motivated by what they seek much more than by what they already have.[3,4,6,9,10,12,13,18,20]

Management's task in the application of this theory is to create situations within the organization that allow employees to satisfy their needs. Most organizations satisfy the lower-level needs. Salaries and fringe benefits satisfy physiologic needs and security needs, respectively; interactions and associations on the job provide satisfaction of social needs. Typically, however, little opportunity exists for the satisfaction of higher-level needs. Unsatisfied needs produce tension within the individual regardless of the level at which the need occurs. When an individual is unable to satisfy a particular need, frustration results.[12]

Frustration is a feeling that arises when one encounters certain kinds of blocks to need fulfillment. These feelings arise when the blocks seem insurmountable and when failure to overcome them threatens personal well-being. The reaction to frustration varies according to the person and the situation. Frustration can lead to behavior that is positive and constructive or negative and defensive. A useful model to describe the relationship existing between needs and constructive destructive behaviors is shown in Figure 4-3.[3,12]

Figure 4-3 shows that unsatisfied needs contribute to tension within the individual, motivating a search for ways of relief. If one is successful in achieving a goal, the next unsatisfied need emerges. If attempts to satisfy needs are frustrated, a person may engage in either constructive or defensive types of behavior. For example, an employee who is frustrated in attempts to satisfy a need for recognition on the job may direct that frustration in a positive direction by seeking recognition off the job, temporarily satisfying the need and allowing job performance to remain intact. However, the organization will eventually be forced to deal with his need-frustration.

Conversely, destructive behaviors may consist of withdrawal, aggression, substitution, or rationalization. Withdrawal may be physical (quitting the job), but it is more likely that it will be internalized and manifested in apathy. Such individuals may have excessive absences or latenesses. Sometimes frustration leads to aggression. In certain rare situations, the frustrated employee may be aggressive toward his superior, but in most instances the employee is more inclined to become aggressive toward other persons or objects. Substitution takes place when an individual puts something in the place of an original object. For example, an individual's frustration in not getting a promotion may result in his trying to achieve leadership in an informal group whose objectives are to resist and frustrate management policies.[3,12]

It is important for the manager to recognize and understand frustration. Frustration may occur when an employee has a strong need for esteem but the job is such that it cannot satisfy this need. It is up to management to restructure the job so that such needs can be met.

Two-Factor Theory

Maslow's need-hierarchy theory is a basic model upon which many theories of motivation have been built. One of these is the two-factor (motivator-hygiene) theory developed by Frederick Herzberg in 1959 as a result of research to determine what affects employee motivation in work settings. The basic premise of Herzberg's theory is that employees are motivated to produce at high levels if they perceive that the result will satisfy their needs. Herzberg concluded that people's needs can be classified into two categories that are independent of each other and affect behavior in different ways.

Using a critical incident study, Herzberg interviewed 200 engineers and accountants. Each individual was asked to recount a time when he felt exceptionally good and a time when he felt exceptionally bad about his job and to describe the conditions that seemed to cause those feelings. The types of conditions that caused good feelings were rarely the same conditions that, when absent, caused bad feelings.

Good feelings were generally associated with the content of the job itself. Five factors seemed especially important: (1) opportunity for achievement; (2) recognition for accomplishment; (3) challenging work; (4) more responsibility; and (5) advancement. These factors, called motivators or satisfiers, contribute greatly to motivation and job satisfaction; but their absence from the organization does not necessarily prove to be highly dissatisfying.

Bad feelings, conversely, were usually related to the environment surrounding the job. Lack of the following factors promoted dissatisfaction: (1) effective company policies; (2) competent technical supervision; (3) good interpersonal relations; (4) satisfactory salary, security, and status; and (5) appropriate working conditions. These environmental

FIGURE 4-3. Behavioral response.

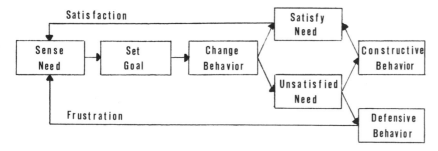

dimensions of the job are referred to as maintenance or hygiene factors because they are vitally necessary for maintaining a reasonable level of satisfaction. The term *hygiene* is used in the sense that proper hygiene prevents infection; and by analogy, good psychologic hygiene prevents dissatisfaction. The accountants and engineers in the study expected these factors to be present and saw them as basic to the work situation. Their absence served as strong dissatisfiers, although their presence did little to promote good feelings. The hygiene factors are necessary prerequisites for motivation, but by themselves they neither increase motivation nor cause satisfaction. Conversely, the hygiene factors, coupled with satisfiers, result in strong motivation of employees.[3,4,6,9,10,12,13,18,20]

Herzberg's theory suggests that job satisfaction and dissatisfaction are not opposites. Instead, the opposite of dissatisfaction is simply the absence of dissatisfaction. This distinction is important when related to levels of job performance. A neutral or zero point in performance levels exists where employees are neither dissatisfied nor satisfied with their jobs (Fig. 4-4). At this point, employees simply perform at the minimal acceptable level necessary to maintain their jobs and employment. What Herzberg emphasizes is that job satisfaction and dissatisfaction are influenced by different factors and exert different effects upon employees. The hygiene factors tend to affect dissatisfaction, and their absence promotes performance below acceptable levels. Motivators tend to affect job satisfaction and motivation; and when they are present, they promote performance above acceptable levels.[12]

There is some similarity between Herzberg's and Maslow's work. While they both study what motivates human behavior, Maslow looks at the human needs of the individual, whereas Herzberg focuses on how job conditions affect the individual's basic needs. The relationship between the two theories is shown in Figure 4-5. Money and benefits satisfy needs at the physiologic and security levels; interpersonal relations and supervision are examples of hygiene factors that tend to satisfy social needs; whereas increased responsibility, challenging work, growth, and development are motivators that tend to satisfy needs at the esteem and self-actualization levels.

The basic advance of Herzberg's theory over Maslow's is that Herzberg distinguishes between maintenance and motivational factors. Herzberg shows that motivation derives mostly from the work itself. Herzberg encourages management to build into the work environment an opportunity to satisfy the motivators by enriching the job. Job enrichment refers to increasing the scope of responsibility and challenge in work, not, Herzberg emphasized, simply increasing the number of tasks. It is a way for management to provide employees an opportunity to grow and at the same time receive achievement and recognition. It is a way to make the work itself a more rewarding experience.[3,12]

Preference – Expectation Theory

In 1964 Victor H. Vroom developed a motivational model that is more an explanation of the motivation phenomenon than a description of what motivates. The Vroom model views motivation as a process governing choices. According to this theory, an employee's motivation to perform effectively is determined by two variables, preference and expectation. Vroom believed that people subjectively assign preferences to all expected outcomes. In addition, he believed that the degree of motivation was a product of both the goals that people wanted to achieve and the degree to which they believed or expected that their own actions were instrumental in accomplishing their goals:

$$\text{Motivation} = \text{Goal preference} \times \text{Effectiveness of actions}$$

Furthermore, Vroom proposed that the level of performance was equal to the product of the degree of motivation and the individual's own inherent abilities.

$$\text{Performance} = \text{Motivation} \times \text{Ability}$$

FIGURE 4-4. Relationship among job satisfaction, dissatisfaction, and performance.

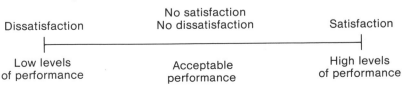

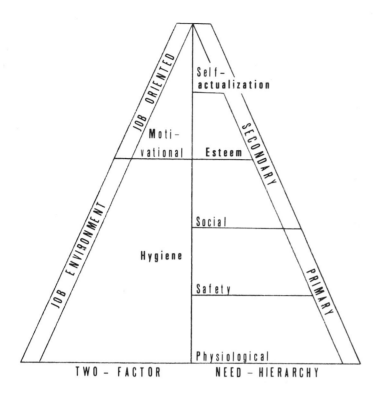

FIGURE 4-5. Comparison of two-factor and need-hierarchy theories.

If the two determinants of motivation nullify each other, there is no motivation, and the individual will not be motivated to increase performance. For example, if an employee values being promoted to departmental supervisor but realizes that even exceptional performance will not earn the position, the employee will not be motivated. Because there is no reason to increase performance, the employee does not. Vroom's model emphasizes that the motivational process is lodged within the individual. It depends upon the individual having a specific, preferred outcome coupled with a belief or expectation that certain activities or behaviors will bring about the desired outcome. This model adds additional insight into the study of motivation because it attempts to explain how individual goals influence individual efforts.[4,6,9,18,20]

Theories X and Y

In 1960 Douglas McGregor published *The Human Side of Enterprise*, which attempted to demonstrate that management's basic attitude toward employees had a significant impact on employee job performance.[14] He described two basic management attitudes: Theory X and Theory Y. These attitudes are reflected in management styles based upon different assumptions regarding human behavior (Table 4-1).[10,14] Theory X managers assume that employees are lazy; that they would rather be directed than left to their own initiative; that they do not want responsibility; that they only seek safety and security. Theory X managers attempt to structure, control, and closely supervise their personnel. They believe that people are motivated by money, fringe benefits, and the threat of punishment. These assumptions of Theory X are similar to Herzberg's hygiene factors or dissatisfiers.

McGregor argued that the close supervision exercised by Theory X managers resulted in less than satisfactory job performance. He believed that closely supervised employees would resist the restrictions and do only the required minimum. McGregor also believed individuals would not demonstrate any drive, initiative, or creativity to accomplish organizational goals under Theory X management. Consequently, he proposed Theory Y, a more positive set of assumptions regarding human behavior. These management practices are based on a more accurate understanding of human nature and motivation.[3,6,7,10,12,13,20]

Table 4-1
Theory X and Theory Y Assumption About Human Behavior and Motivation

Theory X	Theory Y
Work is inherently distasteful to most people.	Work is as natural as play if the conditions are favorable.
Most people are not ambitious, have little desire for responsibility, and prefer to be directed.	Self-control is often indispensable in achieving organizational goals.
Most people have little capacity for creativity in solving organizational problems.	The capacity for creativity in solving organizational problems is widely distributed in the population.
Motivation occurs only at the physiologic and safety levels.	Motivation occurs at the social, esteem, and self-actualization levels, as well as physiologic and security levels.
Most people must be loosely controlled and often ordered to achieve organizational objectives.	People can be self-directed and creative at work if properly motivated.

Theory Y managers help their employees grow by allowing them to direct and control themselves. In this way employees are able to satisfy their social, esteem, and self-actualization needs. According to McGregor, Theory Y managers create climates that allow employees to achieve both individual and organizational goals, thus enriching all aspects of the job, as Herzberg advocates.

Theory-Y thinking has given rise to the "participative" management style. Participative managers allow for decentralized decision-making and delegate responsibility and authority to employees. The participative manager serves as a resource person for the employees, who exercise independent judgment in getting the job done. This style is most applicable when dealing with highly skilled employees (such as clinical laboratory scientists), when individual or group participation is advantageous, and when problems need to be solved. In the long run, this style of management elicits the greatest productivity for the organization.[6,12]

RESPONSIBILITIES OF MANAGEMENT

Because human motivation and behavior are extremely complex, it is not surprising that the theories are too simplistic to yield a model that is beyond reproach. Nevertheless, each theory does offer some insight into human behavior. It is management's responsibility to understand the shortcomings and strong points of each theory and synthesize the workable philosophies of motivation into concrete actions and policies.

The following are management behaviors that stimulate motivation:

- Provide an open communication system. Individuals should be a part of the communication system and should be allowed to contribute to the decision-making process. In this way, the goals of employees will become integrated with the goals of management. An open communication system allows for trust, reciprocity, and growth on the part of individuals and at the same time decreases the effectiveness of informal groups and grapevines, which frustrate organizational goals. Part of good communication includes active listening. Active listening requires that managers give explicit responses to employees speaking to them. This process facilitates problem solving.
- Provide an integration of individual needs with the organization's goals. Organizational goals are met by employees who expect to meet their needs and are satisfied by their outcomes. A mechanism for accomplishing this is jointly establishing performance objectives. Individuals who understand the purpose of their work and are allowed to develop their job objectives will give their best efforts to achieving objectives, while at the same time developing strong feelings of

identification with organizational goals. Management must be sure that the objectives are specific, clearly understood, and measurable. Objectives should be difficult but achievable. Objectives that are too easy or too difficult do not motivate people. Achievable goals, when achieved, build self-confidence and self-esteem. In addition, specific dates should be set for reviewing progress, because this process maintains motivation by initiating employees to make reportable progress by the predetermined dates.

- Delegate responsibility and authority. A good manager must trust others to accomplish organizational goals. Once employees demonstrate ability, they should be given the freedom to make decisions, implement actions, make mistakes, take corrective actions, and achieve goals without constant supervision. This process provides opportunities for enrichment.

- Develop employees' self-esteem. In general, the higher an employee's self-esteem, the better the employee performs. Management can promote employees' confidence in themselves by praising good work and expecting their best efforts. This can be accomplished by the application of the reinforcement principle: Reward behavior that is desirable, because people tend to repeat rewarded behavior. Additional points regarding this principle are: Reward is most effective when applied immediately after behavior. Apply more reward at the onset of desired behavior than after the pattern is established. Ensure that the reward is acknowledged as such by the employee. For some employees the reward may be a bonus; for others, it may be public recognition.

- Maintain contact. Successful leaders in any organization maintain personal contact with their colleagues. This allows for a better understanding of their personality characteristics, abilities, and potential capabilities. Through this contact managers will understand the individual better and thus provide job enrichment opportunities that lead to job satisfaction.

- Analyze the problem, not the person, and take corrective action. Managers should never presume that performance deficiencies are attitudinal problems. If managers unwisely evaluate the person and not the work, then a lowering of self-esteem will result, which ultimately adds to the problem. If the problem is one of a personal nature, then active listening is required to solve the problem. When dealing with the negative aspect of an employee's performance, the manager should communicate in private and take corrective action. It is always important to maintain an employee's self-esteem.

It is management's responsibility to create an environment to encourage motivation. Furthermore, to apply the knowledge of motivational theory means to anticipate the factors most likely to have motivational effect on work. An effective manager understands his employees' needs and endeavors to involve them in accomplishing the organization's goals.[15]

GROUP DYNAMICS

The major thrust of this chapter thus far has been directed to understanding individual motivation as a means of improving an organization's productivity. When ideas and individual abilities are combined in a group effort, productivity increases.

Group Structure

It is inevitable that groups will form in any organization. For example, management might deliberately appoint several individuals to a committee charged with performing a specific function. This is referred to as a formal group. Conversely, an informal group is developed by several individuals who have shared mutual esteem and goals.

Groups, whether formal or informal, serve several functions. Formal groups allow the spreading of responsibility for decisions among many individuals and allow a broader range of participation in decision-making. Additionally, they provide a formal division of labor to study specific problems and general issues; and they arrive at more satisfactory and longer-lasting decisions through discussion and compromise.

Informal groups allow the development of mutual benefit. Each individual possesses skills and knowledge and uses these to help other members perform their duties more satisfactorily. Additionally, informal friendship groups strengthen the individual's commitment to the organization, while at the same time reducing the level of unproductive competition. Thus, management should encourage group formation.

There are various assumptions about small-group behavior of which management must be cognizant. The following assumptions concerning group behavior will show how individuals act within groups and how groups function. This overview of group dynamics is presented to demonstrate the impact groups have on employee motivation and productivity.[6]

Motivational Assumptions

We can assume that the working group has an important psychologic function. Development of feelings of satisfaction and competence can be profound, especially when they are reinforced informally by co-workers. A sincere and personal recognition of good performance by one's peers is often more meaningful than a general statement of approval by distant supervisors.

The second assumption follows as a natural outgrowth of the first. Most people wish to be accepted by the people surrounding them and will work to gain their approval. The desire for acceptance stimulates people to interact cooperatively with each other, thus increasing the effectiveness of the group as a whole.[9] If the element of approval centers around positive or constructive behavior, it stands to reason that management should approve this type of group interaction.

The third assumption deals with the relationship of the formal group leader and the members. An effective leader knows that he or she cannot do all things at all times. The supervisor must rely on the group members working together to carry out directives so that the department operates smoothly, even in the supervisor's absence. In other words, it is assumed that the effectiveness of the group is related to the cooperative attitude of its members toward the formal leader.

The fourth assumption deals with the emotions of individuals. Suppressed feelings tend to eat away at an individual, rarely having a positive effect. It is generally assumed that an individual who is able to express emotion is likely to have better mental health. This presumably results in a better employee. However, great care must be taken with regard to how emotions are expressed. The ability to handle emotions objectively and rationally is a skill that is not developed overnight. Nevertheless, if group skills in this area are refined, the rewards can be staggering. Group morale and problem-solving capabilities can be greatly improved. Conversely, if emotions are vented irrationally, it is likely to have the opposite effect, causing disruption and conflict among the group members.

The fifth assumption of consequence to managers is that the previously discussed qualities are usually inadequately developed. Rarely in any group situation is there a perfect example of interpersonal trust, cooperation, or acceptance. Similarly, few people can claim to be in control of themselves in all aspects, at all times, in all situations; even the most level-headed occasionally lose their temper. Knowing that there is always room for improvement, management should strive to continually upgrade the positive aspects of human group behavior.

The sixth assumption states that resolution of problems is more effective and longer lasting if both sides involved are willing to work together. If management issues an ultimatum regarding a certain change without discussion or consultation with employees, the resistance will be pronounced. Conversely, if management and employees have the philosophy of working together with the goal of becoming mutually effective, resistance will be minimized.[5]

Clearly, these currently accepted assumptions regarding human group behavior are intricately involved in the motivational process. Thus, it follows that management must use leadership styles and managerial philosophies that benefit the individual as well as the organization.

MOTIVATING INTO THE 1990s

In his book *The Third Wave*, Alvin Toffler[19] forecasts that workers will seek more responsibility and will have more commitment to work that fully uses their talents. In recent times, the economics of laboratory operation have led to cost-cutting measures that have, in many cases, created an increasingly mechanized work environment. A major consequence has been the underutilization of the laboratory professional's talent—creating a negative motivational environment. One approach to circumvent this inevitable consequence is in the use of quality circles.[1,2,8,16,17]

Established in Japan, quality circles have succeeded in harnessing the ingenuity and energy of the work force to the solving of problems within the organization. Fostered by management, quality circles involve employees voluntarily meeting in groups of 8 to 12 to identify, analyze, and provide solutions to problems in their work area. These individuals meet weekly, with their supervisor as the circle leader. Initially, the group receives training in techniques of problem-solving, data-gathering, and problem analysis. Solutions to problems are conveyed to management, which commits itself to responding to the circle within a stated length of time. Quality circles give the employee opportunity for involvement, participation in work improvement, challenge, and opportunity for personal growth.[1,2,8,16,17]

The benefits of quality circles are rooted firmly in the motivational theories discussed in this chapter. Today's employee is viewed as one who brings a whole set of needs to the job and hopes to satisfy many of them on the job. Finding solutions to problems through a quality circle program provides personal as well as group gratification. The presentation to management offers individuals the opportunity to satisfy their highest goals of esteem and self-actualization as identified by Maslow. Through this interaction the employee gains recognition.

The opportunity to do interesting and meaningful problem-solving provides the work challenge described by Herzberg. Job enrichment through redesigning work routines is often limited by physical and other factors. Quality circles may not alter the entire job, but the effect of 1 hour a week involving Herzberg's motivators can have a dramatic effect on the other 39 hours.[1,2,8]

The design of quality circles provides a vehicle for implementing McGregor's ideas by allowing employees to exercise self-direction and become more involved in working toward organizational objectives. Through quality circles, an employee gains the opportunity to be part of a team seeking common goals, matching his needs to the organization's goals. Quality-circle solutions have produced savings that can be calculated in terms of increased production, cost containment, and reduction in employee turnover. Improvements in attitude and morale have also resulted.[1,8]

The continued technologic and economic changes in the health-care field will no doubt take their toll on laboratory employees. Greater demands will be placed on laboratory professionals to increase their knowledge and to maintain their skills, while at the same time dedicating their energies to improving productivity. This type of work environment may stifle motivation. However, employees want fulfilling and meaningful work experiences characterized by knowledge, care, respect, and responsibility. To ensure these outcomes, management must invest in the maintenance of human productivity. Laboratory management must consider how their employees' work can be enriched and the quality of their lives improved. The quality circles concept provides an invaluable means to achieve these ends. Quality circles provide employees the opportunity to use their creative problem-solving, technical, and professional abilities in the identifi-

cation and solution of problems. In these ways, quality circles serve a multi-beneficial function: they enhance the quality of the employee, the organization, and health-care delivery in general. The quality circles solution is a process of working smarter, not harder, that yields an increase in productivity — the key to financial security.[1,2,8,16,17]

SUMMARY

Management is encouraged to make the individual's job more challenging and responsible, thus allowing for individual advancement and growth. With the fundamental understanding that motivation is closely related to needs and individual personality, it is management's responsibility to create opportunities that allow satisfaction of those needs in a manner compatible with both the individual's personality and the organization's goals. These must include attitudes, policies, and management styles that are supportive of the motivational process. If this is successful, management and employees will work together in a cohesive fashion to accomplish mutual goals and to increase individual satisfaction.

REFERENCES

1. Baird JE Jr: Positive Personnel Practices; Quality Circles, Leaders Manual. Prospect Heights, IL, Waveland Press, 1982
2. Dewar DL: The Quality Circle Handbook. Ref Bluff, CA, Quality Circle Institute, 1980
3. Donnelly JH Jr, Gibson JL, Ivancevich JM: Fundamentals of Management: Functions, Behavior, Models. Austin, Business Publications, 1971
4. Filley AC, House RJ: Managerial Process and Organizational Behavior. Glenview, Scott, Foresman, 1969
5. Frech WL, Bell CH Jr: Organization Development. Englewood Cliffs, Prentice-Hall, 1973
6. Fulmer RM: Management and Organization. New York, Harper & Row, 1979
7. Gellerman SW: Management by Motivation. New York, American Management Association, 1968
8. Goldberg AM, Pegels CC: Quality Circles in Health Care Facilities. Rockville, MD, Aspen Publications, 1984
9. Gustafson DH, Doyle J, May JJ: Employee Incentive System for Hospitals. Washington, DC, U.S. Department of Health, Education, and Welfare, Publication No. HSM 72-6705, 1972
10. Hershey P, Blanchard KH: Management of Organizational Behavior; Utilizing Human Behavior. Englewood Cliffs, Prentice-Hall, 1972
11. Jung J: Understanding Human Motivation. New York, Macmillan, 1978
12. Koehler JW, Anatol K, Applbaum KL: Organizational Communication. New York, Holt, Rinehart and Winston, 1981
13. Lobovitz GH: Motivational Dynamics Unit I: Mainsprings of Motivation. Minneapolis, Control Data Corporation, 1975
14. McGregor D: The Human Side of Enterprise. New York, McGraw-Hill, 1960

15. Meredith GG, Nelson RE, Nech PA: The Practice of Entrepreneurship. Geneva, International Labour Organization, 1982
16. Orlikoff JE, Snow A: Assessing Quality Circles in Health Care Settings: A Guide for Management. Chicago, American Hospital Publishing, 1984
17. Patchin RI: The Management and Maintenance of Quality Circles. Homewood, IL, Dow Jones-Irwin, 1983
18. Steers RM, Porter LW: Motivation and Work Behavior. New York, McGraw-Hill, 1975
19. Toffler A: The Third Wave. New York, William Morrow 1980
20. Vroom VH, Edward LD: Management and Motivation. New York, Penguin Books, 1982

five

Managerial – Organizational Communications

Edward A. Johnson

A supervisor of any clinical laboratory facility must perform a variety of important management activities, such as planning, organizing, staffing, directing, and controlling. In order to carry out successfully such managerial responsibilities, the supervisor must have a clear understanding of two kinds of communication: interpersonal and organizational.

Interpersonal communication can be defined as a process of exchanging information and transmitting meaning between two individuals or in a small group of individuals.[12] *Organizational communication* can be viewed as a process by which managers develop a system to provide information and transmit meaning to large numbers of individuals within an organization and to relevant individuals and institutions outside the organization.[12] A supervisor who is able to deal effectively with his subordinates, his peers, his manager, and others within his organization recognizes that both processes of communication are essential to management because management is highly dependent on communication for its success.

INTERPERSONAL COMMUNICATION WITHIN THE LABORATORY

What does a clinical supervisor do when he communicates with his subordinates and others with whom he interacts in the process of managing his unit? To help provide an answer to such a question, two models related to the process of interpersonal communication will be examined.[21] The focus will be primarily on communication patterns between the supervisor and the subordinate, rather than between the supervisor and his peers or his superior.

A Simplistic View of Interpersonal Communication — Model I

One common way of representing the process of interpersonal communication is to view it as a source transmitting a message to a receiver, which results in some action taking place (Fig. 5-1)[27] For example, assume that the chief technologist—administrative in the organization chart shown in Figure 5-2 thinks that he has several ideas for improving the work of the general bacteriology unit, and he wants these ideas implemented immediately. According to the model depicted in Figure 5-1, the chief technologist—administrative (the source) would convey these ideas both orally and in writing. The supervisor of general bacteriology (the receiver) would hear these ideas, and as a result of understanding them, would proceed immediately to implement them.

Any clinical supervisor who believes that the process of interpersonal communication functions

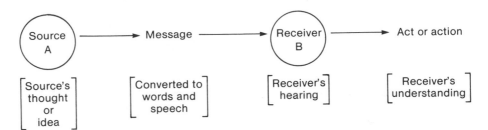

FIGURE 5-1. A simplistic view of interpersonal communication.

in such a simplistic fashion is, of course, in for considerable difficulty in performing his job. Unfortunately, however, there are a number of supervisors today who do, in fact, subscribe to such a view.

The model depicted in Figure 5-1 simply fails to tell enough about the nature and complexity of interpersonal communication. It depicts what David K. Berlo refers to as a "conveyor theory of communication."[3] According to this theory, the process of interpersonal communication is viewed primarily as a transportation problem. In the example cited above, the chief technologist—administrative is concerned only that the data move from point A to point B (Fig. 5-1). Communication takes place when the chief technologist—administrative speaks to the supervisor of general bacteriology, but it cannot be assumed that *successful* communication automatically takes place whenever two individuals get together.[25]

A More Realistic Model of Interpersonal Communication—Model II

In reality, the process of interpersonal communication is much more complicated than that portrayed in figure 5-1. The model presented in Figure 5-3 attempts to reflect the view of contemporary communication theory and to present in a more realistic fashion the major variables and relationships that characterize the situations faced by most supervisors of clinical laboratories. The model depicts the process of interpersonal communication as being dynamic, continuous, and complex. Each component of the model is discussed below separately. However, it is extremely important to recognize that these components are strongly interrelated.

Source

Interpersonal communication is generated by a source.[28] Interpersonal communication takes place because an individual wants to respond in some way to his environment.[17] For example, let us suppose that the supervisor of hematology (Fig. 5-2) is dissatisfied with the work of one of the medical technologists in his department. As the situation becomes increasingly more disturbing and uncomfortable to the supervisor, he seeks some way to convey his concern to the medical technologist. He is, in effect, responding to his environment and seeking to initiate some type of communication.[17]

Encoding

In interpersonal communication, the source (individual) engages in what is known as encoding. The *encoding process* takes place when the idea to be transmitted is transformed by the individual into written or spoken language.[17] In encoding the source must search for appropriate ways to convey his meaning. If the message is not clear, the probability of communication failure will be high.

For example, if the supervisor of hematology cited in the previous example is to communicate to the medical technologist that he is dissatisfied with the medical technologist's work, he must translate his thought into language that the medical technologist can understand. The supervisor may succeed and select appropriate language, or he may fail and select language that is confusing to the medical technologist.

Message

The end result of the encoding process is a *message*. The primary function of a message is to express the purpose of the source.[17] In a sense, a message is somewhat like a coin: it has two sides. There is the message as perceived by the source, and there is the message as perceived by the receiver. The two are not always the same.[28] For example, in the case of the supervisor of hematology and the medical technologist, the interpretation of the message may vary

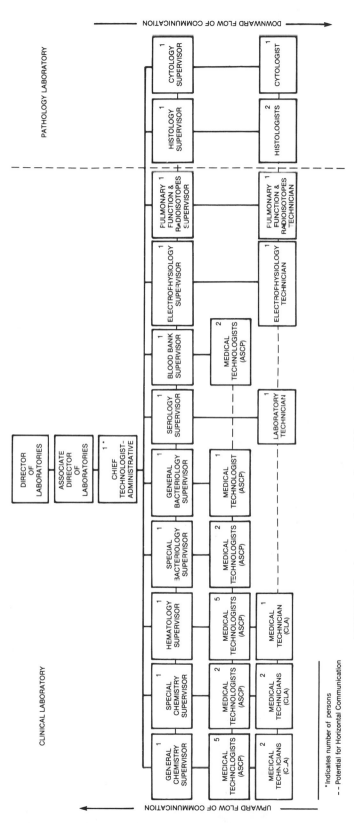

FIGURE 5-2 An example of a clinical laboratory/pathology laboratory organization chart.

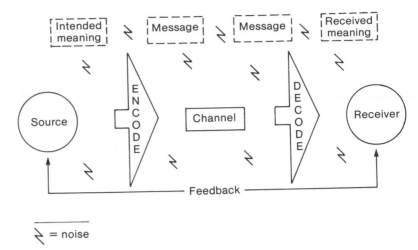

FIGURE 5-3. A realistic model of interpersonal communication. (Adapted from Hicks HG, Arnold KK: Communication for supervisors. In Newport MG (ed): Tools and Techniques, p 158. St Paul, West Publishing Co, 1976)

substantially because of the different perspectives of the two individuals.

Channel

A *channel* is the medium by which a message is transmitted[17]; it connects the source to the receiver. There are many types of channels; several may be appropriate for any given situation. Channels can be verbal (telephone calls or meetings) or nonverbal (letters, memoranda, and formal reports). Under the proper set of circumstances, any of the many types of channels can be effective.[28]

The channel-choice decision is especially important, because it has implications for what type of encoding-decoding will be required, as well as for the ultimate success of the communication effort.[28] The supervisor of hematology in the example cited above could use any number of channels to transmit his dissatisfaction (the intended message) to the medical technologist (Fig. 5-4). Some alternatives are discussed below[30]:

The supervisor may want to meet with the medical technologist and *tell* him that he is dissatisfied. In this case, message is encoded in the form of direct verbal communication. The medical technologist must then decode the message, interpreting what the supervisor means. If the supervisor says, "I am dissatisfied with your work," the medical technologist may still have to decide, for example, whether that means that the supervisor likes to frighten the medical technologist now and then or whether he is on the verge of being fired.

The supervisor may decide to *telephone* the medical technologist about his dissatisfaction. In this instance, the supervisor encodes his message into an indirect verbal communication, and the telephone operates as a channel to the receiver.

If the supervisor wants to be more specific, he may choose to *write* his message in a memorandum adding impact to his message, because the medical technologist will be able to look at the well-chosen words and reread them. In this case, the supervisor again encodes the message in written rather than spoken language.

Another way the supervisor could send his message would be to frown. He would be *using body language*, encoding his message into a frown, which the medical technologist might then decode as meaning that the supervisor is dissatisfied with the medical technologist's work. The medical technologist might not know the reason; so the message is a rather vague one, but it has nevertheless been transmitted.

Another possibility would be silence. When the medical technologist says, "Good morning," the supervisor might fail to respond. After a few mornings of this, the medical technologist might begin to get the message that the supervisor is dissatisfied. The message has been *encoded* into another form, still understandable to the medical technologist.

The supervisor could also use visual communication. He could enclose a "pink slip" with the medical technologist's paycheck. The medical technologist, understanding this as a dismissal notice, will most certainly receive the message

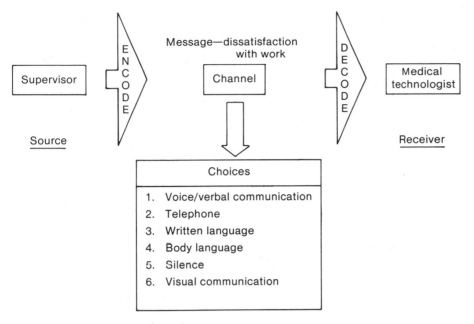

FIGURE 5-4. Some examples of channel choice. (Adapted from Wright J: The Communication Process: A Look at How Messages Are Sent, pp 13–19. Syracuse, Center for Instructional Development, Syracuse University, 1973)

that the supervisor is dissatisfied even before taking the time to read the words printed on the slip.

Decoding

For the process of interpersonal communication to function properly, the receiver must decode the message in such a fashion that he derives a meaning from it that is approximately the same as that transmitted by the source. Decoding is really encoding in reverse.[17]

It is extremely important to note that it is not sufficient for the receiver to decode a message by simply attaching some meaning to it. Successful communication takes place only when the meaning that the receiver derives from a message is similar to that intended by the source. A failure to understand the intended meaning of a message is probably the greatest source of problems in interpersonal communication.[17]

Again using the example of the supervisor of hematology, the message, "I am dissatisfied with your work," may be decoded by the medical technologist to mean any of the following messages:

He must be dissatisfied because I was late three or four times during the past several weeks.

He must be dissatisfied because I was imprecise on the results of several blood workups during the past week.

He must be dissatisfied because I could not solve that problem he mentioned.

Differences in meaning occur because most sources and receivers have different backgrounds, experiences, values, needs, goals, expectations, attitudes, knowledge, and emotional constitution. Such factors determine the meanings that individuals give to certain words or actions. These factors can never be exactly the same for any two individuals; thus, no two individuals will ever attach precisely the same meaning to a particular set of words or actions. However, the greater the similarities among these factors, the greater the likelihood of successful communication.[17]

Feedback

Up to this point, the discussion has focused on communication of messages from the source to the receiver. Another important component of the communication process is feedback.

Feedback refers to a response from the receiver. In the process of providing feedback, the receiver encodes and sends a message through some channel to the original source, who is now in the position of being a receiver. In this way, the source can tell whether the original message did get through to the receiver. If the feedback indicates that the receiver understood the intended meaning of the message, additional communication can take place. If the message was unclear, however, the source might have to alter the encoding of the message until the feedback indicates that the receiver has understood the intended meaning.[17]

Looking at the case of the supervisor of hematology and the medical technologist, the medical technologist's reaction or response to the message, "I am dissatisfied with your work," will let the supervisor know whether or not the intended meaning was decoded. Suppose that the medical technologist did agree. If the medical technologist says, "I know; let's talk about it," he lets the supervisor know that he derived the intended meaning from the message. Conversely, if the medical technologist's response is, "What's the matter? The demands of your job must be getting to you," he is telling the supervisor that he did not derive the intended meaning from the message.

Feedback does not always have to be in the form of spoken or written words.[17] For example, if the supervisor sees a frown on the face of the medical technologist, he knows that the medical technologist either does not understand, disagrees, or is generally unhappy about the statement. If he sees a smile, he may think that the medical technologist assumes he is joking about what he has just said, or thinking about something that has nothing to do with his message. If he sees a blank face, he may believe the medical technologist is listening attentively or bored. All of these facial expressions are part of feedback.

As we see how complex interpersonal communication can become, it is easier to understand why messages sometimes have a difficult time getting through.

Noise

In communication theory, noise has a broader definition than the typical one relating to loud sounds. It pertains to anything that may reduce the accuracy or fidelity of communication.[17]

Noise is frequently inputted to the channel,[28] but it can be present in all of the components shown in Figure 5-3. Some illustrations of the impact of noise are provided below:[17]

Noise can exist if the source perceives an object or an activity in an incorrect way.

Noise can occur during the encoding process if the means selected do not adequately convey the appropriate mental perception of the source.

Noise can exist if the form or code of the message is not understandable to the receiver. This can take place, for example, if the source and the receiver speak different languages.

With respect to the channel, noise can prevent a message from getting through accurately. For example, it is extremely difficult to talk to someone in an exceptionally noisy environment.

Noise is present if the receiver does not decode the message correctly.

If the supervisor of hematology is dissatisfied with the medical technologist's work and wants improvement, he may select the wrong methods to encode his mental perception. If his office is noisy, the message may not be heard clearly by the medical technologist. The possibilities for miscommunication are numerous.

The same components of this interpersonal communication system can be used to analyze the communication process between the physician requesting a laboratory test and the technologist.[19] Figure 5-5 displays the process from the sender, the attending physician, encoding the service request, channeling the message to the laboratory, where the request is decoded before the actual analysis is performed. The communications loop is continued when the laboratory encodes the test result (report) for later interpretation by the requesting physician. The channels of communication, whether in written format, *i.e.,* requisition and report forms, or verbal, are susceptible to comparable errors resulting from poor encoding, decoding, and noise.

INTERPERSONAL COMMUNICATION — A TRANSACTIONAL PROCESS

A useful way for a clinical supervisor to analyze interpersonal communication is through an awareness of the concepts associated with *transactional analysis* (TA). TA represents an attempt to understand human behavior based on how individuals interact and relate to one another.[4,5,16]

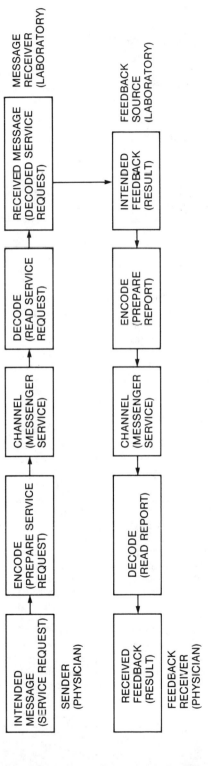

FIGURE 5-5. Communication process in the clinical laboratory.

The subject area of TA includes the following four components: (1) *structural analysis*—the analysis and understanding of the individual personality; (2) *transactional analysis*—the analysis of what people say to each other and how each responds; (3) *game analysis*—the analysis of motives, rewards, and tactics that individuals use to win in interpersonal communication; and (4) *script analysis*—the analysis of the patterns of habitual behavior or "scripts for life" that individuals consciously and unconsciously act out, making them winners, losers, delinquents, and so forth.[6]

Because of space limitations, the discussion that follows will focus on structural analysis and transactional analysis. However, the reader should become familiar with game analysis and script analysis by consulting Berne[4,5] and Harris[16] and the bibliography for this chapter.

Structural Analysis

According to TA, the personality of an individual contains three ego states: Parent, Adult, and Child.

The *Parent ego state* contains those parts of an individual that behave in the same manner as the individual's mother, father, or guardian. All the rules and laws that the individual heard from his parents are recorded in the individual's Parent. All the "should do's," "shouldn't do's," "must do's," and "mustn't do's" are included in this state. At times the Parent is nurturing and benevolent, whereas at other times it is judgmental and critical. In either case, the Parent exerts a powerful influence on an individual. Many objections and excuses originate from this state.[1]

The individual's *Adult ego state* functions like a logical, computerlike, rational decision-maker. It relies on facts to make decisions. It gathers, stores, and processes information from the Parent, Child, and Adult in an attempt to solve problems.[1]

The *Child ego state* in an individual represents what he was when he was young. It is the individual's emotions and feelings, his laughter and love, his fun-making and creativity. It also contains the individual's fears, frustrations, moodiness, aggressiveness, and defensiveness.[1]

Although none of the three ego states is necessarily superior to or more desirable than the others, an important ground rule for a clinical supervisor is that successful transactions and effective communication between the supervisor and subordinate(s) in the laboratory generally can only take place when both parties are operating in their Adult. This does not mean that the supervisor cannot transact with the subordinate's Parent or Child. However, when it comes to solving problems, the supervisor ideally should appeal to the subordinate's Adult.

Transactional Analysis

When a supervisor interacts with a subordinate, there are three basic types of communication transactions: (1) complementary transactions; (2) crossed transactions; and (3) ulterior transactions.

A *complementary transaction* can be defined as one that is "appropriate and expected and follows the natural order of healthy human relationships."[4] In such transactions the source can usually predict the type of response that will be received. Complementary transactions involve only two ego states, and the stimulus and response vectors are parallel (Fig. 5-6). Another way of identifying a complementary transaction is that "(a) the response comes from the same ego state as that to which the stimulus is directed, and (b) the response is directed to the same ego state from which the stimulus is initiated.[29]

When the lines of communication are not parallel and do not meet the conditions cited above, the *transaction is crossed*. Crossed transactions result in temporary communication breakdowns because the source receives a response that is unexpected (Fig. 5-7).[29] Crossed transactions are not desirable. Effective communication can be increased only if the frequency of crossed transactions are reduced. One method for eliminating crossed transactions would be for each individual to get in touch with each of his three ego states (Parent, Adult, Child) and respond to another individual's remark from the appropriate ego state. Another method would be for a person to become more or less locked into one ego state and respond from that frame of reference regardless of the stimulus behavior from another person.[29]

An *ulterior transaction* is generally more complicated than the two previous transactions because it involves more than two ego states and has a surface and a hidden meaning.[21] Such transactions can be angular (involving three ego states) or duplex (involving four ego states). In either case, multiple messages are communicated (Fig. 5-8).[22] Ulterior transactions tend to reduce effective communication and frequently weaken relationships between individuals. Because a person may not be aware of the mixed messages that he is transmitting, this method of analysis should make him more likely to identify his own ulterior transactions. Of course, an important step toward eliminating ulterior transac-

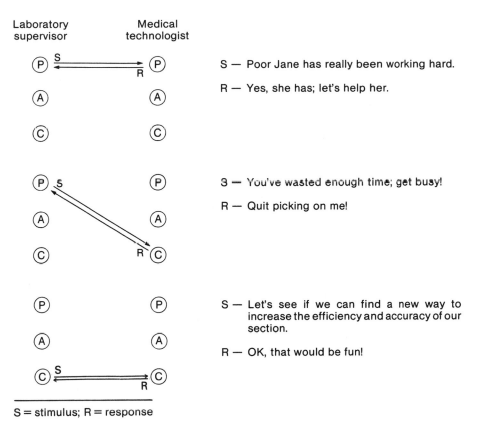

S = stimulus; R = response

FIGURE 5-6. Complementary transactions.

tions is to be able to recognize them when they occur.[22]

TA suggests that a supervisor of a clinical laboratory can eliminate or prevent many communication problems in his day-to-day relations with his subordinates if he learns to analyze his transactions. For example, if he learns to stay in the Adult, he is more likely to relate effectively to his subordinates than if he is locked into the Parent or Child response modes. TA is an important tool for clinical supervisors who wish to improve interpersonal communication.

ORGANIZATIONAL COMMUNICATION SYSTEMS

Three formal types of communication are found in most organizations. These are (1) downward communication, (2) upward communication, and (3) horizontal communication. The organization chart shown in Figure 5-2, in addition to showing lines of authority and accountability, serves as a diagram of an organization's formal communication network.

Downward Communication

This type of communication is probably the most frequently used channel in organizations.[21] It flows naturally from higher to lower levels of authority, and it has several basic purposes[18]:

1. To provide specific task directives (job instructions)
2. To provide information designed to produce an understanding of the task and its relation to other organizational tasks (job rationale)
3. To provide information about organizational procedures and practices
4. To provide feedback to the subordinate about his performance

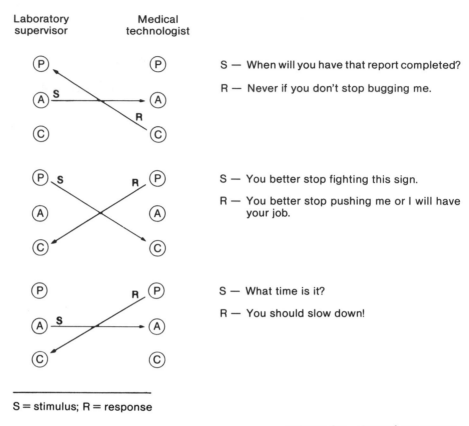

S = stimulus; R = response

FIGURE 5-7. Crossed transactions.

5. To provide information of an ideologic character to inculcate a sense of mission (indoctrination goals)

Downward communication also provides an opportunity for supervisors to spell out objectives, change attitudes, influence opinions, reduce fear and suspicion resulting from misinformation, prevent misunderstandings from lack of information, and help subordinates prepare for change.[21]

It is important to note, however, that downward communication can be misused, especially if a supervisor does not allow for any significant feedback from his subordinates. Just because a supervisor and a subordinate go through the *motions* of communicating with one another does not necessarily mean that they have actually communicated. Special efforts must be made on the part of a supervisor to make sure that instructions, orders, directions, and other types of downward communication are actually understood by subordinates.[17]

Upward Communication

The supervisor of any clinical laboratory facility who believes that downward communication is sufficient as an adequate channel for transmitting messages to subordinates will be in for a big disappointment. Most organizations provide, to some extent, for an upward flow of communication.[28] This is frequently referred to as feedback.

Encouraging upward communication is not an easy matter, especially since it runs contrary to the usual higher-to-lower flow of authority found in most organizations.[17,21,26] Yet upward communication is important, and the supervisor of a clinical laboratory who encourages it will (1) obtain a better picture of the work, accomplishments, problems, plans, attitudes, concerns, and feelings of those in his unit; (2) be in a better position to identify individuals, policies, actions, or assignments that are likely to cause trouble; (3) strengthen the only device he has for tapping ideas and help from his staff;

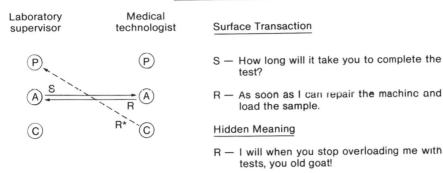

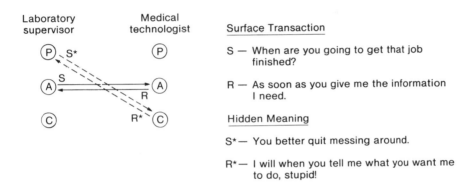

S = stimulus; R = response

FIGURE 5-8. Ulterior transactions.

(4) receive better answers to his problems; and (5) help the flow and acceptance of his own downward communication simply because good listening makes good listeners.[21]

The research cited by Lewis clearly demonstrates that two-way communication (downward and upward) is more accurate for developing understanding than one-way communication (downward).[21] With two-way communication, the receiver has the chance to test the information being sent by the source, and the source can change the message immediately if necessary for the purpose of achieving a better understanding.

However, two-way communication requires more time than one-way communication, and it can cause the source to feel under attack in a psychologic sense because the receiver can pick up mistakes or omissions and let the source know about them. Two-way communication can also be somewhat noisy and disorderly at times.

For the clinical supervisor who is interested primarily in speed, appearance, and the protection of his own seeming infallibility and power base, one-way communication is preferable, but the clinical supervisor who is interested in more accurate and valid communication will find that two-way communication can lead to more positive results.[21]

Horizontal Communication

Horizontal communication takes place between individuals who are at approximately the same level of authority in an organization.[17] It can be either formal or informal, depending on whether it is allowed for and shown on the organization chart.[21] The primary purpose of horizontal communication is to facilitate the solution of problems that arise from a division of labor and specialization.[17] The messages generally deal with task coordination, problem-solving, information-sharing, and conflict resolution.[13] For example, the supervisor of a special bacteriology unit and the supervisor of a general bacteriology unit in a certain clinical laboratory may find that the only way for a certain problem to be resolved is to have a closer coordination of the efforts of these two units (Fig. 5-2).

One way to accomplish this coordination would be to use horizontal communication. Some problems could occur if only horizontal communication took place throughout an organization. The authority structure could possibly be abolished, and too many messages could blow in all directions without screening or filtering. As a result, a compromise between the rigidity of zero horizontal communication and the anarchy of total horizontal communication is generally supported by most supervisors.[21]

Informal Communication Systems

Upward, downward, and horizontal communication systems comprise only part of the total communication flow in any organization. Another important component to consider is the informal communication system.[10,17]

Informal communication systems exist in any formal organization, but they cannot be identified by looking at authority relationships on a formal organizational chart.[11] They result from the social interaction of employees. They do not have any official sanction, and at times they contain considerable scuttlebutt.[7] An informal communication system is frequently referred to as the grapevine, since it

moves back and forth across organizational lines (Fig. 5-9). It can be either beneficial or detrimental to an organization, depending to a great extent upon the influence that a supervisor can exert on it.[17]

An informal communication system can be desirable because it provides insights into employee attitudes, it provides a safety valve for employee emotions, and it helps spread useful information. However, the dysfunctional aspects of such a system include its spreading of rumor and untruth, its nonresponsibleness, and its nonappearance on the organization chart, which contributes to uncontrollability. Two of its attributes that can work to either the good or detriment of an organization are its speed and influence.[21]

No supervisor in any laboratory facility should ever attempt to abolish such a system; it is a factor with which a supervisor must deal in the daily activities associated with managing his unit. The astute supervisor will attempt to understand it, analyze it, and consciously try to influence it.[11]

ORGANIZATIONAL AND INTERPERSONAL COMMUNICATION BARRIERS

If a clinical supervisor is to communicate successfully, he must learn what barriers or obstacles to effective communication stand in his way. Such barriers can be divided into organizational and interpersonal obstacles, although there obviously will be some overlapping.

Organizational Communication Barriers

Certain characteristics of any organization make communication especially difficult. Some of the more important ones are as follows[21]:

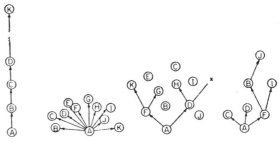

FIGURE 5-9. Grapevine methods of spreading information. (From Davis K: Management communication and the grapevine. Harvard Bus Rev 5:49, 1953)

SINGLE STRAND   GOSSIP   PROBABILITY   CLUSTER

An organization is a system comprised of overlapping and interdependent groups; as a result, if all things are somewhat equal, individuals will communicate more frequently with those individuals who are geographically closest to them.

Subgroups within an organization demand and expect allegiance and loyalty from their members, and they have their own immediate goals and methods to achieve them. Thus, when a given message is communicated to several subgroups within an organization, each group may interpret a rather different meaning from the one that was transmitted.

Organizational groups represent different subcultures. In a hospital setting, such subgroups as the clinical laboratory facility, the hospital administrative office, the emergency room, the nursing service unit, the radiology department, the dietary department, and the personnel department, establish and attempt to preserve their own value systems, idealized images, and traditions. Each group frequently develops its own jargon; for meaning to be transmitted between groups, then, each group must understand what the other group means when a certain word or phrase is used.

The members of an organization are comprised of various systems of relationships (*i.e.,* work, authority, status, prestige, friendship, and so forth). Each of these structures exerts an influence on the expectations that individuals have about who should communicate with whom and in what fashion.

In growing, dynamic organizations the relationships among members are in a constant state of change. Therefore, the problem for communicators frequently is to determine who is best to receive a particular message.

Interpersonal Communication Barriers

A basic problem in interpersonal communication is that the meaning that is actually received by an individual may not really be what the other individual intended to send. The source and the receiver are two separate individuals, and any number of barriers can distort the messages that pass between them. Examples of some of the more important interpersonal barriers are discussed below[25,26]:

1. A subordinate hears what he expects to hear. What a subordinate hears or understands when a supervisor talks to him is greatly influenced by the subordinate's own personal experience and background.

2. A subordinate frequently ignores information that conflicts with what he already knows or believes.

3. A subordinate evaluates the source. If a supervisor is perceived as trustworthy, friendly, and supportive, what is said is likely to be accepted and believed by the subordinate. Conversely, disliked or distrusted supervisors will find it difficult to communicate anything but the most banal facts to the subordinate. This represents an aspect of stereotyping.[8,13]

    A subordinate who trusts a supervisor is more likely to accept the information that the supervisor provides than a subordinate who does not trust a supervisor. Trust-building is important if the subordinate and the supervisor are to be able to participate in an open, honest fashion.

    Research has confirmed that when there is trust between two parties, there tends to be a much lower level of misunderstanding between them. Perhaps this is so because there is less defensiveness and therefore better listening and better understanding. Perhaps it is so because to trust an individual, one must first know the other person; and when one knows and understands the other person, there is a greater tendency to empathize, if not to move, at least to some degree, toward agreement. When the parties move toward agreement, communication naturally improves. Or maybe there are fewer misunderstandings because when two people know each other, they can make their messages congruent with the other person's frame of reference.[8,15]

4. The Halo Effect. One dimension of stereotyping and evaluating a source is for a receiver to ignore "gray areas" and react in terms of "black or white"—right or wrong. For example, much of what is said by a supervisor who is distrusted by a subordinate will be ignored. Conversely, much of what is said by a supervisor who is trusted will be accepted as good and correct. The halo effect occurs when a subordinate is not able to discriminate appropriately between the good and the bad that may be intermixed within a supervisor's comments.

5. The Semantic Problem. In a strict sense, meaning cannot be conveyed from a source to a receiver; all that the source can do is

convey words. However, the same words may suggest quite different meanings to different individuals. For example, it has been established that the word *run* has over 800 different uses, the word *round* has over 70 different uses, and the word *fast* can be just as confusing. In addition, the 500 most frequently used words have an average of 28 meanings per word.[21] The problem is especially difficult when one is dealing with abstract terms, but even simple, concrete words and phrases can lead to communication problems. To a supervisor, "as soon as you can" may mean immediately; to a subordinate it may mean as soon as it can be done without endangering the subordinate's other work. Unfortunately, confusion can result even when words are selected with great care.

6. Emotions. When a subordinate is insecure, worried, or fearful, what he hears and sees will generally appear to be more threatening or distressing than when he is secure. At the same time, when a subordinate is angry or depressed, he tends to reject what might otherwise appear to be a reasonable request or a good suggestion from his supervisor. Similarly, if the subordinate is in good spirits, he may not "hear" any problems or criticisms.

7. Tuning Out. Subordinates learn to tune out many things. For example, certain statements that a supervisor makes may be ignored, actually never heard by the subordinate, because they sound so much like what the supervisor always says: "Work efficiently," "Keep busy." "This test is stat," "Reduce costs." Thus before a subordinate can hear a message, he must learn to discriminate between background noise (what is always being said by the supervisor) and what is significant and relevant new information worthy of attention.

Improving Organizational and Interpersonal Communication

Both organizational and interpersonal barriers can hinder and restrict the communication efforts of any clinical supervisor. Probably the most important step that such a supervisor can take to improve communication within his unit is simply to be aware of the complexity of the communication process. It cannot be taken for granted, and it must be performed as accurately as possible. An improvement in communication can be achieved through a greater knowledge of how the communication process functions. By being aware of and sensitive to how barriers can affect the process, the supervisor can take steps to minimize them.[17]

IMPROVING MANAGERIAL COMMUNICATION

Improving managerial communication depends on a number of skills. Some of the more basic skills include (1) listening effectively, (2) demonstrating empathy, (3) monitoring feedback, and (4) recognizing nonverbal cues.

Listening

Successful listening (like communication) is an active, dynamic process. If a clinical laboratory supervisor is to be an effective listener, he cannot be passive. He must actively attempt to grasp facts and feelings in terms of what he has heard, and he must be willing to help his subordinates work out any problems.[20] Alertness at every point of the communication encounter is a prerequisite for the supervisor, as well as for the subordinate.[21]

Research indicates that most individuals listen at about 25% efficiency. In other words, an average person experiences a 75% loss of information over a short period of time because of poor listening skills. One of the primary reasons that listening-retention rates are so low is that the ability of the mind to think is four to six times as fast as the average person speaks (*i.e.,* 600–700 words per minute versus 125 words per minute). The receiver can easily tune in and out or divert his attention while the source is transmitting a message at a relatively slower speed. As a result, the receiver frequently indulges in a "skip-and-jump" listening pattern, pretending attention but giving way to distractions.[21] Because of this, most clinical supervisors will frequently face critical problems in terms of getting their messages through.

Some of the factors preventing the subordinate from being a good listener include the following:[12]

1. Faking attention when the topic is considered to be uninteresting (lack of interest)
2. Permitting diversion to take place because of emotional words or topics (evaluative/contrary attitudes)
3. Inefficient note-taking (getting swamped with details)
4. Allowing environmental noise to continue (interruptions)

5. Listening only for facts and allowing the mind to wander (bad listening techniques)

There are, however, several things that a clinical supervisor can do to aid a subordinate's listening:[21]

1. He should tailor information on the basis of the subordinate's point of view.
2. He should phrase words and couch statements in language that is on the subordinate's level; however, he should not talk down to the subordinate.
3. He should transmit information, instructions, and directives in small units. Large amounts of data tend to be threatening, whereas small amounts of information are more likely to be accepted by the subordinate.
4. He should provide ample opportunity for feedback from the subordinate. In other words, he should find out what the subordinate has heard and what he has understood.

It is important to note that listening is not something to be applied only when a supervisor is dealing with specific problems. It is a general attitude which a supervisor should apply when dealing with his subordinates. It is a matter of always being ready to listen to the subordinate's point of view and trying to take it into account before taking action.[26]

Skillful and effective listening is an art. It requires training and experience, and it can be learned through practice. Each supervisor must establish an approach that is comfortable for him and that is congruent with his personality, but it is recommended that he avoid using the same technique(s) with all subordinates and for all purposes.[26]

Regardless of what approach a supervisor does develop, however, the following suggestions should prove useful[12]:

1. Stop talking; show that you can also listen.
2. Establish rapport with the subordinate. Put him at ease.
3. Indicate a willingness to listen to the subordinate. Look interested. Show empathy.
4. Eliminate distractions. Hold telephone calls and select a quiet place to communicate. Do not engage in other activities.
5. Allow sufficient time for discussion. Listen patiently to the full message.
6. Keep your emotions under control. Do not get angry or lose your temper. Recognize and be sensitive to your emotional involvement in some topics and try not to argue or criticize.
7. When you are not sure of part of the message, restate what you thought you heard in the form of a question. When you think that something is missing, ask questions.

Listening can be contagious. If a laboratory supervisor wants his subordinates to listen to what he has to say, he must prove to them that he is an individual who consistently listens with understanding.[21]

Demonstrating Empathy

Empathy is sometimes defined as understanding, but it really goes beyond that. It includes understanding the feelings as well as the content of another individual's message. In a sense, empathy is seeing the world the way another individual sees the world or "getting inside the individual's skin and feeling the way that individual feels about something."[9]

A number of supervisors confuse empathy with sympathy. Sympathy goes beyond empathy and implies *agreeing* with what the other individual feels. Some supervisors are reluctant to develop the ability to empathize with a subordinate because they believe it implies that they are agreeing with the subordinate. Evidence suggests quite the contrary. Many people in a communication situation are simply seeking understanding and do not necessarily demand agreement with their viewpoint. In fact, there are many cases where a subordinate, once he has discovered that his supervisor really empathizes with (understands) his viewpoint, drops a difficult point or issue, or at least becomes less hostile and easier to deal with on that point or issue as well as on other matters.[9]

A clinical supervisor can show concern for a subordinate by standing in the subordinate's position, identifying with the subordinate's frame of reference, and helping to meet the subordinate's objectives. From this standpoint, empathy is an exceptionally strong component of effective communication.[2]

To empathize with a subordinate, a clinical supervisor should be able to answer a number of questions about the subordinate:[21]

1. What are his beliefs and values?
2. How does he see the world?
3. What disturbs and disrupts him?

4. Under what conditions will he accept or reject change?
5. Does he listen carefully and patiently to what is said, or is he more interested in who said it?
6. Does he weigh the evidence or simply go along with individuals he likes?

Answers to such questions cannot be obtained without the use of good interviewing skills, which are discussed more fully in Chapter 11.

Feedback

Any supervisor who does not provide for monitoring feedback from his subordinates will find his managerial and communication skills to be severely limited. If he does not encourage feedback from his subordinates, he may eventually become isolated or bypassed. A clinical supervisor who sincerely subscribes to the importance of feedback and wishes to monitor it more carefully should find Table 5-1 to be especially valuable. What the table suggests is that there are certain cues, sent both from the subordinate and from within the supervisor himself, which give the supervisor information concerning whether or not the subordinate and the supervisor understand each other.[23] These indicators represent danger signals, signs that the message may not be getting through. It is important for the supervisor to recognize these signals because they indicate that corrections are necessary.[23]

Nonverbal Communication

During the entire verbal communications process, the clinical supervisor and the subordinate communicate with each other in another way: nonverbally.[21,24] The nonverbal message a supervisor sends to a subordinate can cause the subordinate to tune out the supervisor, especially during the listening process. Beneficial or dangerous emotional environments can be created through nonverbal language, which can strengthen or destroy a subordinate's trust in a supervisor.[1]

A clinical supervisor must be able to recognize in a subordinate nonverbal cues such as nervousness, confidence, anger, openness, rejection, or defensiveness. If the supervisor is not aware of these cues, he shows a lack of sensitivity to the subordinate's feelings. This can also lead to a reduction in trust.

Three of the more important areas of nonverbal communication are body language, voice intonations, and proxemics.[1] Body language is a significant component of nonverbal communication. It is important for a clinical supervisor to become aware of both his own body projections and those of his subordinates. He can increase tension and decrease trust simply by projecting negative body language or by lacking sensitivity to a subordinate's body projection. Some of the major areas of interest in body language include the eyes, face, hands, arms, legs, body posture, and walk. These areas can be combined in different ways to indicate openness, evaluation, indifference, rejection, frustration, nervousness, or confidence.

Defensiveness, anger, or frustration on the part of a subordinate may be the direct result of a clinical supervisor's aggressive, dominant, or manipulative body language. A deterioration of trust can result from such postures.

Additional meanings can be derived from changing voice intonations. Voice qualities generally account for the way a subordinate speaks his words. These include such factors as stress, resonance, speed, inflection, clarity, rhythm, and volume. Simple changes in such voice qualities can change the meaning of the same group of words. A lack of emotional sensitivity on the part of a clinical supervisor to voice tones can reduce trust between the supervisor and the subordinate.

One of the most important things for a supervisor to keep in mind when paying attention to the voice intonations of the subordinate is to concentrate primarily on changes in the subordinate's voice qualities. Some subordinates naturally talk fast, softly, or resonantly. When a subordinate changes his normal voice qualities, however, the subordinate is communicating something extra.

Another component of nonverbal communication is *proxemics*, the study of personal distance and territoriality. All individuals have various distances of interaction. For example, a supervisor can generally get physically closer to members of his family than he can get to subordinates in his unit. When he gets too close to a subordinate, the subordinate will likely experience uneasiness and discomfort.

Research in proxemics indicates that there are four boundaries of interaction: the intimate (up to 2 ft); personal or casual (2 ft to 4 ft); social or consultative (4 ft to 12 ft); and public (12 ft or more).[14] During any interaction with a subordinate, a clinical supervisor probably would not want to work at all within the intimate space, nor initially within the personal space. The clinical supervisor can use proxemics to increase his trust with subordinates.

Knowledge about the entire area of nonverbal communication can increase the clinical supervi-

Table 5-1
Sources of Feedback and Approaches to Monitoring It

Indicators*	Feedback from the Subordinate	Feedback from Within the Supervisor
Examples of feedback that indicate the subordinate does not understand the supervisor	Subordinate changes subject abruptly.	Supervisor feels uncomfortable.
	Subordinate is apparently daydreaming or withdraws.	Supervisor talks too much (excessively long statements).
	Subordinate asks inappropriate follow-up questions.	Supervisor repeats himself.
	Facial expressions or posture	
	Misinformation	
	Subordinate gives irrelevant answers, especially to probe questions.	
	Subordinate shows signs of hostility.	
Examples of feedback that indicate the supervisor does not understand the subordinate	Subordinate's metamessage (words and voice or gestures) appears to be inconsistent with message.	Supervisor finds himself daydreaming.
	Subordinate's comments appear to be inconsistent with previous comments.	Supervisor interrupts repeatedly.
	Subordinate keeps repeating himself.	Supervisor desires to argue or defend.
	Subordinate's voice or gestures show frustration (more intense or forceful)	Supervisor feels uncomfortable or confused.
	Subordinate begins to use a higher level of abstraction, more qualifiers, more pronouns.	

*The indicators provided above are all examples of danger signals, indicators that the message may not be getting through. It is also possible to specify a set of indicators that the message *has* been received, but the danger signals are probably more important for the supervisor to recognize because they indicate that corrections are necessary.

(Adapted from Pyron HC: Communication and Negotiation for the Right of Way Professional, p 239. Culver City, International Right of Way Association, 1972.)

sor's awareness of and proficiency in communication. The supervisor can become more sensitive to the subordinate's feelings, which can help considerably in building a trustful relationship.[1] Communication skills are critical tools that any clinical supervisor needs in order to interact with a subordinate in an open, honest, and constructive manner. These skills allow the supervisor and the subordinate to develop and maintain trustful relationships, and they enable the supervisor to determine whether he is communicating effectively with the subordinate and whether the subordinate is communicating successfully with the supervisor.

REFERENCES

1. Allesandra AJ, Davis JW, Wexler PS: Non-manipulative selling: Removing pressure and still getting the sale. California Real Estate, Vol 57, p 40, January 1977
2. Berlo DK: Communicating Management's Point of View. A film from the Effective Communication Series. Rockville, Maryland, BNA Communications, 1965
3. Berlo DK: Meanings Are in People. A film from the Effective Communication Series. Rockville, Maryland, BNA Communications, 1965
4. Berne E: Games People Play: The Psychology of Human Relationships. New York, Grove Press, 1964
5. Berne E: Transactional Analysis in Psychotherapy: A Systematic Individual and Social Psychiatry. New York, Ballantine Books, 1961
6. Blubaugh JA: Advanced Communication Skills: Transactional Analysis for the Right of Way Professional (Workbook). Culver City, International Right of Way Association, 1978
7. Borman EG, Howell W, Nichols R: Interpersonal Communication in the Modern Organization. Englewood Cliffs, Prentice-Hall, 1969
8. Communications in Right of Way Acquisition, Course 1, Student Reference Manual (old version), p 51. Culver City, International Right of Way Association, 1973
9. Communications in Right of Way Acquisition, Course 201, Student Reference Manual (new version), p 28. Culver City, International Right of Way Association, 1981
10. Davis K: Human Behavior at Work, pp 261–270. New York, McGraw-Hill, 1972
11. Davis K: Management communication of the grapevine. Harvard Business Review 5:43–49, 1953
12. Glueck WF: Management, pp 238, 249–250. Hinsdale, Illinois, Dryden Press, 1977
13. Goldhaber GM: Organizational Communication, p 40. Dubuque, William C Brown, 1974
14. Hall ET: The Hidden Dimensions. Garden City, Doubleday, 1969
15. Hall J: Communication revisited. In Dupuy GM, Khambata DM, Ruth SR, et al: The Enlightened Manager, pp 264–274. Lexington, Massachusetts, Ginn Custom Publishing, 1979
16. Harris TA: I'm OK — You're OK. New York, Harper & Row, 1967
17. Hicks HG, Arnold KK: Communication for supervisors. In Newport MG (ed): Supervisory Management: Tools and Techniques, pp 157–170. St. Paul, West Publishing Co, 1976
18. Katz D, Kahn R: The Social Psychology of Organizations, p 239. New York, John Wiley and Sons, 1966
19. Krieg AF: Laboratory Communication, pp 3–24. Oradell, New Jersey, Medical Economics Co, 1978
20. Kumata H: Communication that gets results. Supervisory Management, pp 35 ff, February 1966
21. Lewis PV: Organizational Communications: The Essence of Effective Management, pp 19–20, 38–41, 74, 91–120, 150–165. Columbus, Ohio, Grid, 1975
22. Patton BR, Giffin K: Interpersonal Communication in Action, 2nd ed, pp 61–64 New York, Harper & Row, 1977
23. Pyron HC: Communication and Negotiation for the Right of Way Professional, pp 237–239. Los Angeles, American Right of Way Association, 1972
24. Rosenfeld LB, Civikly JM: With Words Unspoken: The Nonverbal Experience. New York, Holt, Rinehart, & Winston, 1976
25. Strauss G, Sayles LR: Personnel: The Human Problems of Management, 2nd ed, pp 223–232. Englewood Cliffs, Prentice-Hall, 1967
26. Strauss G, Sayles, LR: Personnel: The Human Problems of Management, 4th ed, pp 162–170, 184–188, 266–271. Englewood Cliffs, Prentice-Hall, 1980
27. Thayer L: Communication and Communication Systems, p 23. Homewood, Illinois, Richard D Irwin, 1968
28. Wofford JC, Gerloff EA, Cummins RC: Organizational Communication: The Keystone to Managerial Effectiveness, pp 25–32; 349. New York, McGraw-Hill, 1977
29. Woolams S, Brown M, Huige K: Transactional Analysis in Brief, p 17. Ann Arbor, Huron Valley Institute, 1974
30. Wright J: The communication Process: A Look at How Messages Are Sent, pp 13–19. Syracuse, Center for Instructional Development, Syracuse University, 1973

ANNOTATED BIBLIOGRAPHY

Baskin OW, Aronoff CE: Interpersonal communication in Organizations. Santa Monica, Goodyear Publishing Co, 1980

This book represents an interesting attempt at combining the bodies of theory and research surrounding both interpersonal communication and organizational behavior, although it does not presuppose a knowledge of either. Interpersonal communication is viewed by the authors as the medium through which relationships are established and maintained within organizations.

Bowman JP, Branchaw BP: Understanding and Using Communication in Business. San Francisco, Canfield Press, 1977

The objective of this book is to present information about why and how certain messages communicate and other messages do not. The book discusses the general principles and purposes of communication; written communication, including basic skills, letters, and reports; techniques for improving reading and listening skills; nonverbal and oral techniques of communicating; and the psychological principles of formal and informal relationships.

Goldhaber GM: Organizational Communication. Dubuque, William C Brown, 1974

This book discusses major theoretical findings related to organization theory and human relationships, and examines the flow of messages within three major interaction formats in an organization; the dyad, the small group, and the collective audience.

Useful methods, procedures, and techniques for designing and conducting research in organizations are discussed, along with applications for training and consulting.

Krieg AF: Laboratory Communication. Oradell, New Jersey, Medical Economics Company, 1978

This resource describes in detail the communication process between the attending physician and the laboratory. Specific chapters highlight the potential barriers and pitfalls in handling requests and reporting results. Excellent information is provided about physician-laboratory communications and systems analysis.

O'Connell SE: The Manager As Communicator. San Francisco, Harper & Row, 1979

This book provides managers with a number of practical techniques for improving face-to-face communication as it relates to management functions. The author centers on situations where effective interpersonal communication is critical, such as getting work done at meetings, explaining policies and procedures, discussing employee performance, and building open communication. Step-by-step directions are given for developing a better personal communication plan.

Mayerson EW: Shoptalk: Foundations of Managerial Communication. Philadelphia, WB Saunders, 1979

This book is a practical guide for managers who wish to improve communication between themselves and their subordinates. Among the topics covered are nonverbal communication, telephone communication, mediation of conflict, and decision-making and creativity in relation to group effort.

six

Leadership Styles and Group Effectiveness

John R. Snyder

The most comprehensive definition of management, perhaps, is that of the executives and academicians which states that the process of management is the "guiding of human and physical resources into dynamic organization units that attain their objectives to the satisfaction of those served and with a high degree of morale and sense of attainment of the part of those rendering the service."[1] This directing function of guiding resources to achieve both organizational and personal goals is critically important. Guiding is often referred to as *leadership*. Leadership is a very complex activity. Many management authors and critics have defined leadership in different ways, several of which will be offered throughout the course of this chapter.

The relationship of the directing function to other managerial functions is embodied in the following discussion regarding leadership:[10]

> Leadership is the ability to persuade others to seek defined objectives enthusiastically. It is the human factor which binds a group together and motivates it toward goals. Management activities such as planning, organizing, and decision-making are dormant cocoons until the leader triggers the power of motivation in people and guides them toward goals.

This definition includes two key elements of leadership: the ability to motivate and the ability to focus efforts on goal accomplishment. Administration and supervisors have the authority to lead and manage:

they do not always have the power to influence and motivate.[7] This definition also includes a focus on the leader or manager's ability to have the cooperation of staff workers to achieve organizational goals. Recall that one of the first steps in strategic management described in Chapter 2 was the definition of the laboratory's mission, goals, and objectives. The goals and plans for the laboratory need to be translated into departmental or divisional objectives if the laboratory is to achieve its mission. Likert referred to this critical leadership component as the "linking pin" function of the manager.[34] Figure 6-1 graphically displays the match between the creation of a missions statement, long-range goals, and strategic plans by top level administration. These directives are mobilized by performance objectives at lower levels. The laboratory manager plays a crucial role in linking his employees' efforts to where the organization and the laboratory are headed. In health-care institutions, like other multilevel organizations, goals and objectives are often formulated at the management team level, *i.e.*, in department head meeting. Too often these are not then shared with the staff who are ultimately responsible for implementation.

Within the clinical laboratory in the organizational context, there may exist two types of leaders: formal and informal. The formal leaders are those appointed to managerial positions of authority with responsibility for the laboratory analyses or func-

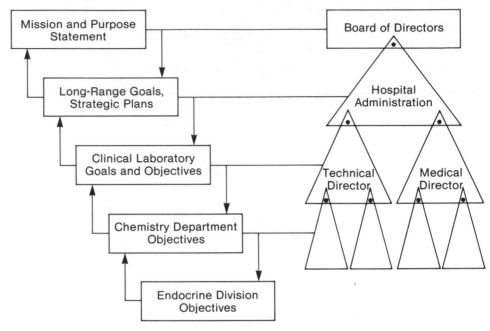

FIGURE 6-1. The "linking pin" function: involving employees in the goals and objectives of the laboratory.

tional tasks of those who report to them. Informal leaders may also be present, leaders whose influence is based on knowledge of the job, tenure with the laboratory, age, respect, or other characteristics. In some cases, conflict may arise when the two leaders in the same laboratory have different objectives for the same group of followers. Regardless of whether the functional leader is formally appointed or simply fills the role, still another definition of leadership sheds some light on this complex subject.[43]

> Leadership is the process by which one person designates "what is to be done" and influences (inspires, commands) the efforts of others in order to accomplish specific purposes (objectives and work tasks).

This definition contains four key elements: *acts, goals, influence,* and *acceptance.* Inherent in it is the fact that those who are to accomplish the task accept the leader's role and influence on them.

Early studies of leadership concentrated on the traits necessary to be an effective leader. Early hypotheses contended that a finite number of individual traits, whether intellectual, physical, emotional, or other personal characteristics, constituted effective leadership. Most of these physical, psychologic, and sociologic traits were thought to be inherent and perhaps could be used to discriminate leaders

from nonleaders. Many years of study have failed to pinpoint a single personality trait or set of qualities that was common to all leaders.[25] Rather, current philosophy suggests that leadership is a dynamic process in which there exists an interrelationship between the capabilities and inherent traits of the leader involved, the needs of the followers, and the characteristics and demands of the situation,[23,37] Schwartz has summed up the specific factors within these areas affecting the effectiveness of leadership behavior as the size of the organization, the interaction and personalities of group members, the congruence of personal and organizational goals, and the level of decision-making.[46]

The focus of this chapter, then, will be on leadership styles, the followers as a group to be effectively influenced, and situational variables. Since trait factors present at the time of birth are not the only determinant of effective leadership, a study of the various approaches to leadership with corresponding outcomes is appropriate.

MEASURES OF GROUP EFFECTIVENESS

Before considering leadership styles or leader behaviors, it is wise to identify the measuring tools that will indicate leadership effectiveness in dealing with followers. Gibson, Ivancevich, and Donnelly described three measures of short-run organizational or leadership effectiveness: production, efficiency, and satisfaction; and two measures of intermediate or long-term effectiveness: adaptiveness and development.[20] *Production* reflects the ability to perform the quantity and quality of laboratory analyses required by the institution. This measure excludes efficiency, looking only at output items such as test volumes and diversity of testing. *Efficiency* is defined as the ratio of outputs to inputs, focusing on the turn-around time for analyses, instrument downtime, technical staff unit production over a given block of time, and so forth. *Satisfaction* refers to the extent with which the laboratory is meeting the needs of its staff. A similar term, *morale,* reflects satisfaction as indicated by employee attitude surveys, absenteeism, turnover, and grievances. *Adaptiveness* is the ability of the laboratory section as a whole to respond to internal and external changes. There may exist a need to adapt practices or policies to alleviate problems associated with production, efficiency, or satisfaction. *Development* is a long-term measure of the ability to invest in the laboratory to enhance its operations. Examples of development measures taken to improve effectiveness include in-service programs, continuing education opportunities, and other growth-related activities. These measures of leadership effectiveness should be borne in mind by the reader during later discussions of leadership styles. Examples accompanying the styles should enable the reader to predict how these measures of leadership effectiveness would be influenced.

THE CLIMATE REFLECTING LEADER BEHAVIOR

Part of this complex issue of leadership is the joint function of the laboratory structure as an organization and its processes or procedures. This combination is termed the laboratory *climate*. The manager plays a key role in setting the working climate as defined (loosely or tightly) by the laboratory organizational structure and the usual mode of conducting the daily work. The climate that the laboratory manager establishes/supports/condones is, in turn, related to performance and job satisfaction. In a study of 300 scientists in 21 large research and development laboratories, Lawler, Hall, and Oldham report that process variables, rather than structural variables, have a greater impact on climate, and climate seems to have a greater effect on job satisfaction than on performance.[31]

Leader behavior analysis is the usual manner for studying leadership and group effectiveness. There are three dimensions that are fairly reliable indicators of the type of climate the leader is attempting to establish or foster: the degree of decision-making authority held by the manager, the manner of supervision, and the leader's interpersonal relationships.[43]

Degree of Decision-Making Authority Held by the Manager

The laboratory manager influences the climate by either involving subordinates in the decision process, soliciting their contributions before arriving at a decision, or totally excluding them. (The reader is referred to Chapter 3 for a discussion of the cost/benefit relationship in involving others in the decision-making or problem-solving process.) Because production was cited earlier as one measure of group effectiveness, a study by Taylor[53] on the impact of management style, most noticeably "allowing input and participation in decisions," on staff productivity in 12 clinical laboratories is insightful. Although the study has some recognized shortcomings, including a nonrandom sample and absence of testing for factors other than management style, that have an impact on productivity, Taylor did find a positive relationship. His study supports earlier research that found productivity increased as the manager involved employees more in the decision-making process.

Manner of Supervision

This dimension of leader behavior refers to how closely a manager oversees the predetermined work of his subordinates. This includes not only monitoring the quality and quantity of work but also specifically assigning tasks within the department. Some authors attempt to further define this leader behavior as "close" versus "distant" supervision or "direct" versus "indirect" supervision. Over-supervision can negatively affect the organizational climate; it is typified by the supervisor who "keeps pulling up the flowers to see how the roots are growing."[55] The technique of *management by exception* is based on the belief that staff can handle the majority of problems on their own (distant supervision). With this technique, the laboratory manager tells employees that two kinds of activities must be brought to his attention: any unusual occurrence, special problem, or other event they cannot cope with and a defined list of specific deviations from the routine. In the first category, a technologist should perhaps alert the supervisor if calibration on a piece of instrumentation begins fluctuating more than is typical. In the latter instance, the supervisor may determine a list of abnormal results that should be called to his attention before being reported. In later discussions about leadership styles, an individual's supervisory climate will be referred to as having differing emphasis on people or production concerns.

The Leader's Interpersonal Relationships

The climate of the clinical laboratory is definitely influenced by the nature of interpersonal relationships fostered by the manager between himself and subordinates. A manager may establish a "good buddy" personal relationship with each of his subordinates, or he may swing to the other extreme and have a totally nonpersonal relationship with his employees, treating them as he does the instruments and other assets of the department. Some laboratory managers foster a paternalistic relationship with their subordinates, referring to them as "my girls in the lab" or "the boys in my section." The intent is usually one of protection and care for the subordinates in return for loyalty. The climate for each of these three interpersonal relationship examples would be different. A close personal relationship may foster erosion of authority, a strictly nonpersonal relationship may result in high turnover, and a paternalistic relationship prevents the development of self-reliance in the group members.

These climatic influences are summarized in Table 6-1 as organizational variables and the characteristics that foster an organizational climate conducive to high productivity.[2]

The climate established by a leader's behavior has a major impact on the attitudes and sometimes the production of the laboratory. Much of the information related to communication and motivation in previous chapters, as well as discussions about leadership styles later in this chapter, shed light on factors that influence the working climate and whether or not these promote good production by happy employees. Two past presidents of the United States spoke of leadership in such a manner as to incorporate the key element of climate. Eisenhower defined leadership as "the art of getting someone else to do something you want done because he wants to do it"; while Theodore Roosevelt commented, "The best executive is the one who has sense enough to pick good men to do what he wants done, and self-restraint enough to keep from meddling with them while they do it."

Table 6-1
Factors Affecting Organizational Climate

Organizational Variables	That Require
Leadership processes	High confidence and trust
Motivational forces	Economic rewards based on compensation system developed through genuine participation
Communication processes	Free and valid flow of information at all levels
Interaction-influence processes	High degree of mutual confidence and trust
Decision-making	Wide involvement in decision-making and well-integrated through linking processes
Control processes	Wide responsibility for review and control at all levels

(Adapted from Argyris C: Management and Organizational Development, p 17. New York, McGraw-Hill, 1971. Used with permission.)

THE LEADERSHIP ROLE OF MANAGERS AND SUPERVISORS

The clinical laboratory supervisor may be called upon to assume a variety of leadership roles. In the following discussion, different viewpoints of the supervisor's role as postulated by Davis are linked to leadership functions.[11,54]

Often the supervisor is viewed as the key person in the laboratory because of his ability to significantly facilitate or hinder the production, morale, and flow of communications. As a key person, the supervisor serves as the hub of service in ensuring that laboratory tests are completed on time and the morale in the laboratory is at an acceptable level. The key-person concept can be displayed graphically as follows:

Key Person   **Laboratory Administration**
                          ↓   ↑
                     Supervisor
                          ↓   ↑
                Laboratory Staff

Sometimes the supervisor belongs to neither the staff nor management, but rather is caught in the middle to interact with and reconcile opposing goals and objectives. The major function of this type of supervisory role is to identify and solve problems. This author, while still a flegling supervisor, recalls the wise reminder of his chief technologist: "As a supervisor, you're not going to win any personality contests."

Person in the Middle

Laboratory Administration

↓

Supervisor

↑

Laboratory Staff

Some unfortunate supervisors are empowered only symbolically. Staff bypass them on their way to a higher level in the organizational hierarchy. The laboratory administration holds these supervisors responsible for the laboratory's performance but confines their authority. These supervisors appear powerless and ineffective as leaders, and the reason can be seen in the following diagram:

Marginal Person

Laboratory Administration

Supervisor

Laboratory Staff

The legal status of most supervisors is that they are part of the administrative team. Often, the laboratory supervisor will be a "working supervisor," performing a mixture of both analytic and administrative responsibilities. With relation to their staff subordinates, these supervisors provide an initiating function of "thinking up" ideas, planning, and conceptualizing. An important concept about this role of the clinical laboratory manager is that, as a supervisor of professionals, he serves as a leader among equals.

Another Staff Member

Laboratory Administration

Supervisor ⇌ Laboratory Staff

Some supervisors are expected to serve as staff specialists concerned with caring for the human side of the laboratory operation. The primary function of these supervisors as leaders is giving advice, information, or counsel.

Human Relations Specialist

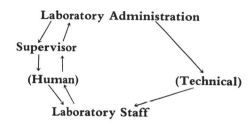

This discussion of the leadership role is not intended to categorize supervisors, but rather to show the differing perceptions with which a supervisor may be functionally considered. The supervisor has a unique position in the laboratory organizational hierarchy, synthesizing many parts of the roles described above. He serves a key position in influencing productivity while being held accountable from both above and below. While performing side by side with other technical professionals, he fills a leadership role that is best termed a leader among equals, responsible for maintaining the interpersonal relations and morale of the laboratory section. In summary, the laboratory supervisor's role is often supportive in nature, similar to that advocated by Townsend: to carry water for the troops.[55]

BASES OF POWER AND INFLUENCE

The ability to effectively lead implies acceptance by the followers of the leader's power. If one considers power in terms of who makes the decisions in a laboratory, the individual with power has the ability to limit alternatives of choice. In doing this, he has influenced the actions of those following.

The power to influence followers in the laboratory setting is not always a function of title or position, whether laboratory director, administrator, manager, or supervisor. Position-related power grants the manager only the authority to influence. There are other personal and positional attributes that provide the leader with a much stronger base of power. The following bases of power may be used:[17]

Coercive power is based upon fear. The supervisor who threatens to record negative incidents and place them in a subordinate's personnel file is exercising coercive power.

Reward power is based upon the expectation of receiving tangible or intangible rewards. A laboratory supervisor might exercise reward power by offering to grant additional time off for volunteers who cover an emergency situation.

Expert power is based upon special skills or knowledge. An assistant supervisor may influence the preventive maintenance practices of an entire department based upon his special skills in trouble-shooting certain instruments.

Referent power stems from a leader's ability to inspire by personality alone. This type of power is often referred to as charismatic power. An informal leader in the laboratory setting may move colleagues emotionally or psychologically through the use of referent power. For example, this leader may prompt an entire section to believe a particular policy is unfair by using persuasive personality skills.

Sanctioned power results from a leader's ability to negotiate and "trade-off" favors. This is similar to reward power except that influence in sanctioned power can be exerted beyond the realm of one's duly authorized reward system. For example, a supervisor may influence the actions of other supervisors at a departmental meeting on the bases of premeeting negotiations to vote a particular direction on one item for a return-favor vote on another item.

Legitimate power is derived from an individual's position in the laboratory organizational structure. The supervisor, by designation, has legitimate power over specific laboratory staff members. A supervisor may exercise legitimate power in assigning staff members to cover the 3 PM to 11 PM shift every eighth week, for example.

Information power results from the control of some portion of the communication process or control of information itself. The laboratory administrator who refuses to disclose the percent salary increase to be granted on an annual merit review is exercising information power.

The phenomenon of power plays a definite role in how effective a laboratory manager is perceived. Seldom, if ever, will the manager possess all forms of power just described. Recalling the managerial role as a leader among equals, the astute laboratory manager will determine where the various types of power are held in the organization. The manager who relies solely on his legitimate power to influence subordinates will be a less effective leader than one who enlists the support of all staff members possessing power. For example, seeking the

opinion of the staff member with expert power will increase the likelihood that the leader will be able to achieve group cooperation. Further, Reichman and Levy suggest that enlisting support decreases natural competitive tendencies and allows a compromise to achieve cooperation.[45]

Knudson, Woodworth, and Bell have described some of the trade-offs to be considered when a manager chooses not to exercise leadership influence through legitimate power.[29] The term *trade-offs* is not used here in a negative sense, but rather refers to those areas that may be affected when different power sources are allowed to exert influence. Trade-off areas include

Quality of decision. What powers can be used effectively in arriving at the highest quality decision? Should expert power be used?

Acceptability of a decision. The use of which powers will prompt the most universal acceptance of a decision? Will legitimate power suffice?

Motivation of those over whom the manager has power. What effect on motivation will result from the use of certain types of power? Will coercive power be counterproductive?

Existing organizational relationships. What effect does the exercise of sanctioned power, for example, have on relationships now present in the laboratory?

Control of activities/responsibility. How might the supervisor's control of operations be affected by not totally exercising legitimate power in a particular situation?

Communication patterns. Will the use of information power, for example, adversely affect upward communication?

Need to maintain a position of power. Will the invitation to share leadership influence with others who possess different types of power threaten the manager's ability to exercise legitimate power at a later date?

The ability to provide leadership that is effective in influencing group behavior often includes the application of some type of power. The laboratory manager needs to consider the cost/benefit result of exercising power personally or of inviting others with power to share in his leadership role. Regardless, the phenomenon of power is a very real entity in the laboratory organization and deserves careful consideration.

FACTORS INFLUENCING LEADERSHIP STYLES

Most laboratory managers achieve administrative positions, whether first-line supervisory or directorship, without the benefit of advanced degrees in business or management. This does not imply, however, that these managers began without some form of leadership style. Earlier in this chapter, the concept of leadership based solely on intellectual, psychologic, or sociologic traits was discounted. Undoubtedly, any reader can call to mind an example of someone he thought was an outstanding leader in the clinical laboratory or someone who was a particularly poor laboratory leader. A person's leadership style is defined through behaviors exhibited in the directing function that reflect assumptions and beliefs about the leader's position, his followers, and the salient components and beliefs about the leader's position, his followers, and the salient components of the situation.[21] It may be informative at this point to investigate the influences that prompt the difference between an individual's effective (outstanding) or ineffective (poor) leadership style.

Leader-Influencing Factors

Much of what constitutes a leader's frame of reference from previous experiences influences his actions. This may include educational courses or seminars attended and the actions of past supervisors whom the individual perceived as outstanding leaders (role models). Past experiences also include the leadership methods a person has tried in the past after he has sorted out that which was effective from that which was ineffective.

There is little doubt that some personal traits influence a person's leadership style. His readiness to show fear or anger, for example, plays an influential role. His goals for himself, for his followers, and expectations of outcomes become a powerful influential force. How competent he feels as a manager influences his leadership behavior. This is supported by Mitchell, Larson, and Green, who report that leaders' perceptions of their own good behavior increases followers' ratings of leader behavior.[37]

In support of all the researchers who have attempted to isolate the trait or traits that comprise effective leadership, there does appear to exist an indefinable ingredient in leadership:

> There exists somewhere the gist of the manager, his soul, his philosophy of life, his basic approach to life and other human beings. This weightless component cannot be bought, sold, or built into an individual. If he *has* it, it can be nurtured and cultivated. If he doesn't have it, all the leadership training courses in the world can't make him a leader.[18]

Follower-Influencing Factors

The perceived characteristics of a group of subordinates influences a person's leadership style. The personality of the group may be perceived as openly receptive or adversely hostile, for example. Bias may be built into a leader's perception of his followers in such areas as the age of the personnel to be led. Contrast the belief that a group of subordinates is from the "old school," and therefore has to be told everything to do, with a "new school" philosophy, where the supervisor might wish to ask everyone's opinion before making any decision. These types of assumptions influence an individual's leadership behavior.

Frequently, in the laboratory setting, a leader's behavior will shift with his perception of his subordinates' backgrounds and levels of development. The misconception exists that people who are less educated or are doing more routine tasks should be led differently from others with more education. For example, contrast the leadership style generally employed with a group of phlebotomists or specimen preparation clerks with the leadership style used for a group of special chemistry technologists.

Situational-Influencing Factors

Undoubtedly the greatest number of factors influencing a leader's style has to do with his interpretation of the situation or problem. The type of organization itself plays a substantial role: supervisors lead differently if serving in a proprietary commercial laboratory than if working in a nonprofit hospital laboratory, government, or religious institution. The policies established within each of these differing environments limit or expand the leader's ability to influence the work climate. The size of the laboratory department will undoubtedly affect the leadership style as the manager attempts to deal with the span of control. Similarly, the nature of the communication process may cause the leader to be very close to his subordinates or very distant. Control, or lack thereof, of the departmental budget and the rewards system is often perceived as an influence dictating a leader's behavior with subordinates. Certainly the presence or absence of a union influences a leader's style. These concerns and others account for situational influences based on the characteristics of the institution that affect leadership style.[9]

Other situational factors as perceived by the supervisor regarding his position also influence the leader's style. A supervisor can only lead within the realm of his authority. It is possible to predict many laboratory supervisors' leadership styles on the basis of the pathologist's leadership style. It is unlikely that a supervisor will be very employee-concern oriented if his immediate supervisor is a pathologist whose interest is strictly in production. The supervisor's circle of influence would predict that these two styles would be in conflict. Finally, no discussion of situational factors would be complete without identifying time as a critical component that influences leadership style.

This is by no means an exhaustive list of those factors which stimulate, detract from, or in some other fashion influence the basis for differing leadership behaviors. The factors identified are not all quantitative criteria. Likert verifies the fact that there is an important human angle in leadership styles to be considered.[33] This discussion is intended to prompt the reader to critical self-evaluation of those factors influencing his leadership style.

LEADERSHIP STYLES: THE LEADER DIMENSION

Theory X and Theory Y

Many behavioral scientists have attempted to study leadership behavior and its effects on subordinate productivity. Douglas McGregor's "Theory X–Theory Y" is perhaps one of the most well-known hypotheses.[36] According to McGregor, managers' assumptions about human nature and human motivation influence their perception of the organization environment; and this, in turn, prompts characteristic leader behavior. At one end of the spectrum are those managers who focus on the aspects of superior–subordinate organizational structure with centralized decision-making and strict external control. This leadership style is labeled *Theory X*. The Theory-X assumptions about employee behavior are summarized in Chapter 4, Table 4-1. Within the clinical laboratory, a Theory-X manager assumes that most of his staff prefer to be directed, desiring as little responsibility as possible. In the Theory-X manager's perception, staff members would rather have their supervisor exercise strict control in checking all results prior to reporting. The laboratory may be permeated by a feeling of fear, reflecting the leader's belief that staff members must be coerced to perform or intimidated into following the direction of the leader. Within the laboratory of the Theory-X manager, all decisions for change are made in an authoritarian manner, seeking little or no input from staff members. As a rule, the Theory-X manager also suffers from the lack of solicited information from staff members, since even crucial information that should be flowing up the organization is never communicated.

After concluding his description of Theory X, McGregor questioned these assumptions of human nature in light of current levels of education and the democratic society in which we live. Drawing heavily on Maslow's hierarchy of needs (see Chap. 4), McGregor described an alternate theory of leadership called Theory Y. The assumptions concerning human nature and motivation that characterize Theory Y are listed in Table 4-1. A comparison of assumptions that underline Theory-X and Theory-Y leadership styles illuminates the two ends of the spectrum of manager behaviors as described by McGregor.

A laboratory that functions under Theory-Y leadership most likely has all levels of laboratory professionals sharing responsibility for their activities. A subsection supervisor, for example, makes decisions regarding the selection and purchase of specific reagents for his area. Technologists share the responsibility with the supervisor for creating a holiday schedule and decreasing overtime in the laboratory. This reflects the assumption that the technical staff is creative and is willing to put these talents to use. Often the rewards system is directly linked with productivity and personal-growth goals. In this fashion, the Theory-Y manager attempts to reward the full range of individual needs while recognizing that personnel can be properly motivated to accomplish organizational goals through the achievement of their own goals.

Lest one gain the impression from this discussion that Theory X is "bad" and Theory Y is "good," that simply is not the case. McGregor's definitions imply that most people under Theory Y have the *potential* to be mature and self-motivated, given managers who are supportive, but a distinction must be drawn between attitude and behavior. Argyris recognized the difference between these two in his comparisons of A and B behavior patterns.[3] Theory-X assumptions are revealed in A-pattern interpersonal behavior and group dynamics. Theory-Y assumptions are reflected in B-pattern behavior. While it may be true that the best possible set of attitudes (assumptions) toward people may be Theory Y, there may be some individuals who best function when the leader demonstrates Type-A behavior. This, of course, will depend upon the situation and the need to foster a more mature disposition of the employee.

Continuum of Leadership Behavior

McGregor has been widely criticized for the creation of a dichotomous, either–or situation. However, his work points toward two opposing poles in a continuum of leadership behavior.

Tannenbaum and Schmidt have defined the continuum by contrasting the use of authority by the leader of a group with the amount of freedom allowed the group regarding decision-making (Fig. 6-2) [52] At one end of the continuum, the leader makes decisions without input from the group; at the other end of the continuum, the problem is focused by the leader, but the followers play a major role in investigating alternatives and proposing solutions. The shift from autocratic leadership behavior at one extreme (Theory X) is gradual as a leader changes behavior toward a more democratic approach (Theory Y) at the other extreme:

Autocratic. The manager makes decisions alone.

Persuasive. The manager solely makes decisions, then attempts to influence followers by selling his idea, gathering support for his idea, and stirring enthusiasm among subordinates.

Consultative. The manager confers with subordinates to gather information, then makes the decision himself.

Democratic. The manager solicits not only information from subordinates, but also requests their involvement in the generation of alternatives and selection of a decision.

This continuum is often extended beyond the democratic pole to include a *laissez-faire* style. This style is one of abdication, the absence of formal leadership characterized by the lack of procedures and policies, with subordinates influenced only by informal leaders.

A well-known measurement tool to assess leadership patterns along this continuum was developed by Likert.[33] The following four categories reflect characteristics of highest- and lowest-producing departments:

FIGURE 6-2. Continuum of leadership behavior. (Adapted from Tannenbaum R, Schmidt WH: How to choose a leadership pattern. Harvard Bus Rev 51:166, 1973. Used with permission of the publisher)

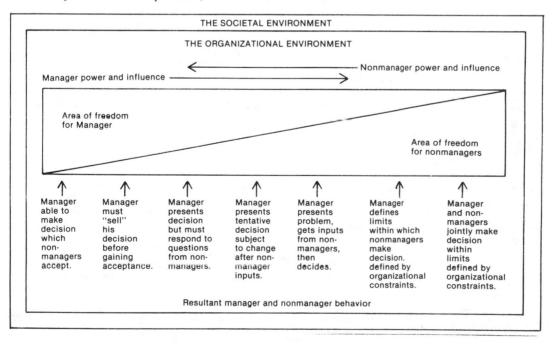

1. Exploitative–Autocratic—typified by low trust, no participation
2. Benevolent–Autocratic—typified by condescension and token participation
3. Participative—typified by substantial trust and participation but with control and decision-making retained by the leader
4. Democratic—typified by complete confidence and democratic decision-making

Lilkert's research supports the fact that a democratic leadership style, while not always being the most efficient, fosters higher productivity.

Initiating Structure and Consideration—the Ohio State Studies

The Bureau of Business Research at Ohio State University, in attempting to identify various dimensions of leader behavior, considered two dimensions: initiating structure and consideration.[51] *Initiating structure* refers to "the leader's behavior in delineating the relationship between himself and members of the work group and in endeavoring to establish well-defined patterns of organization, channels of communication, and methods of procedures." *Consideration* refers to "behavior indicative of friendship, mutual trust, respect, and warmth in the relationship between the leader and members of his staff."[22] Two data-gathering devices, the Leader Behavior Description Questionnaire (LDBQ) and the leader Opinion Questionnaire (LOQ) were used to substantiate that these were, in fact, separate and distinct dimensions.

In assessing results from the LBDQ and LOQ, leader behavior was plotted on two axes, one for each dimension (Fig. 6-3). It was noted that a high score in one dimension did not preclude a high score in the other dimension. Laboratory managers exhibiting high consideration (relationship behavior) are leaders who are friendly toward their subordinates, who encourage a sharing of subordinates' concerns, who are willing to listen, and who are receptive to change. A laboratory manager characterized by high initiating structure (task behavior) is intent on making specific assignments with detailed guidelines telling subordinates exactly what is expected of them.

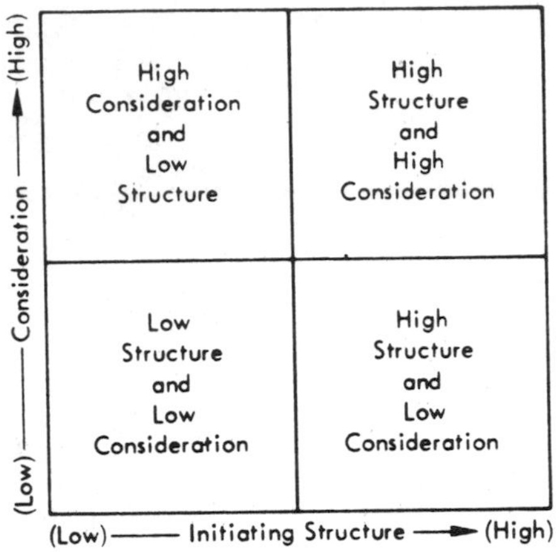

Blake and Mouton's Managerial Grid

While the Ohio State conceptual model examines leader behaviors predominantly perceived by

FIGURE 6-3. The Ohio State leadership quadrants. (From Stogdill RM, Coons AE [eds]: Leader Behavior: Its Description and Measurement. Research Monograph No. 88. Columbus, OH, Bureau of Business Research, The Ohio State University, 1975)

others, Blake and Mouton's Managerial Grid measures the predispositions of managers in terms of (1) concern for people and (2) concern for production.[5] Although similarities in the two models exist in terms of relationship emphasis and task emphasis, the Managerial Grid stresses that this is an unnecessary dichotomy. Rather than being mutually exclusive, Blake and Mouton contend that people and production concerns are complementary and must be integrated to achieve effective leadership.[4]

The Managerial Grid (Fig. 6-4) theoretically contains 81 possible positions or leadership styles. For discussion purposes, the focus usually centers around five basic styles:

1. *1,1 Impoverished.* A laboratory manager with this leadership style has probably abdicated many of his responsibilities, encouraging subordinates "not to make waves" but to do the minimum to keep the lab going.
2. *1,9 Country Club.* This leadership style would be reflected in the manager's inclination toward keeping the laboratory staff happy. Scheduled breaks are never violated, and frequent social gatherings take priority over laboratory productivity.
3. *9,1 Task.* The major emphasis by a laboratory manager with this orientation is one of work before all else. Development of a department with high productivity and efficiency is

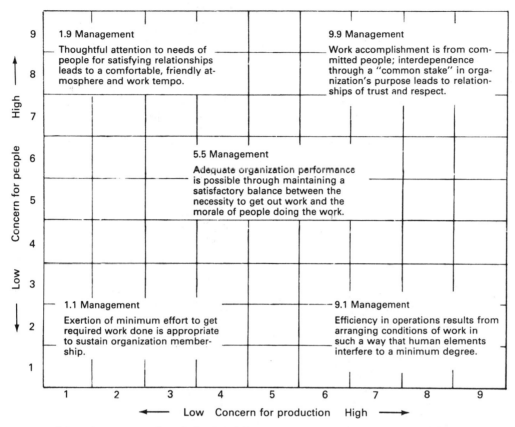

FIGURE 6-4. The managerial grid. (From Blake RR, Mouton JS: The Managerial Grid, p 10. Houston, Gulf Publishing Company, 1964)

reflected in the manager's attitude that everyone is there, being paid, to work.

4. *5,5 Middle of the Road.* This leadership style incorporates both a concern for the volume and efficiency of laboratory testing as well as concern for the morale of the department.
5. *9,9 Team.* A laboratory manager with this leadership style attempts to integrate laboratory and personal goals within the department. This manager enlists the participation of the staff in decision-making and serves as a coach for the testing function (productivity) of the laboratory.

Blake and Mouton have used the concepts embodied in the Managerial Grid rather extensively for organization and management development. A recent publication highlights the value of the grid concept after 20 years of experience with it by the authors.[6] They report that specific conditions in a manager's childhood experiences prompt his inclination to a given grid orientation. The advocated 9,9 Team leadership is supported as the best possible orientation in terms of profitability, career success, and personal health. The publication outlines grid orientations that are correlated with heart attacks, asthma, ulcers, and cancer, among other diseases.

LINKING LEADERSHIP STYLE TO FOLLOWERSHIP

We have defined some dimensions of effectivess and contrasted several leadership styles. A logical question arises: Is there a most effective leadership style? Leavitt provides the following answer:[32]

There is no such thing as the right way for a manager to operate or behave. There are only ways that are appropriate for specific tasks of specific enterprises under specific conditions, faced by managers of specific temperaments and styles.

The most effective leadership styles for a laboratory manager must include consideration of the leader's ability, the follower's motivations and; characteristics, and the dimensions of the situation.[24,47,48] While the 9,9 Team approach may seem the best possible for all situations, it is often difficult to sustain the team effort over time. The team approach is certainly preferred if the situation is one in which everyone has a stake in the outcome, such as the generation of policies and goals or overall evaluation of a laboratory section.

The 1,9 Country Club quadrant of leadership style is appropriate and, in fact, most effective when dealing with a situation in which motivation is based on personal interaction. External activities related to laboratory public relations, for example, often are not directly tied to the organization's reward systems. Consider the leading of a group of staff members in designing and implementing a weekend career day for high school students interested in becoming medical technologists. The most effective leadership style recognizes that the feeling of making a contribution toward the future of the profession is an intrinsic motivation. A leadership style emphasizing people concerns is the best approach.

Similarly, a 9,1 Task orientation is appropriate and effective when deadlines are pressing. A laboratory manager may be faced with an emergency surrounded by chaos, for example. In this case, a leadership style reflective of an orientation toward work and immediate problem resolution is most effective. In addition to situations in which time is crucial, critical, or short, a task orientation is often appropriate for assigning very simple tasks.

Even the 1,1 Impoverished Leadership style may be appropriate for some situations. Consider a situation in which subordinates need to exercise flexibility and creativity, such as in certain types of problem resolution or research.[21] The wise manager will be there for support or assistance but does not attempt to influence the group's productivity. Often this leadership style may be appropriate for the administrative technologist when his subordinates (supervisors) are attempting to resolve problems within their sections. During his days as a newly appointed supervisor, this author recalls the leadership style exercised by his superior, the chief technologist: "You make the decision and I'll stand behind you, but you'd better be ready to come explain your rationale to me."

In real-life situations, it is often quite difficult to choose the most effective leadership style. Maintaining an optimum balance between concern for people and concern for production is at best a herculean task. An example follows:

Case Study

The Leadership Dilemma

I know a man who is a boss — not a big boss and not a very bossy boss. But he does have a title on his door (Administrative Director of Laboratories) and plush carpet on his floor and he takes his job very seriously and personally. Which, of course, is his problem.

You see, when this administrator took courses in graduate school he was taught that management was a question of profits and losses. Now he spends a great deal of time worrying about the cost-accounting of personnel problems — personal personnel problems.

Moreover, he says, it's going around. He keeps reading articles about "corporate irresponsibility" toward private lives. He hears how often an individual's work plays the heavy role in family crisis. But from where he's sitting . . . in a corner office looking down on the rest of the medical center . . . he sees something else.

He sees employees who want to be treated strictly professionally one moment and then treated personally the next. He sees the conflicts faced by his employees, but also the conflicts of being a boss. He is often in a no-win situation.

The administrator had three stories to tell me. The first was about his secretary. Last month when he interviewed her, he was warned by the personnel office to keep the questions strictly professional. On pain of lawsuit, he could not quiz her on her marital status or child care. So he stuck to the facts, just the facts . . . steno, typing, and work experience. Then, after hiring her, when one of her children got sick, he was expected to understand why she had to be home. He saw the situation this way: one month he wasn't allowed to ask if she had children, the next month he was supposed to care that they were sick.

Then there was the supervisor he wanted to promote. The technologist was clearly ambitious and good. The administrator had judged her on the basis of her work and management potential. He'd groomed her and watched her. Sent her away to attend management seminars, talked with her about taking on a higher level management position when one became available. Then he'd handed her the big promotion to Chief Technologist of the Stat laboratory. But the supervisor asked to be excused. She didn't want to make this change, because she just couldn't accept the responsibility for weekend and evening coverage. But, said the administrator, the supervisor had never described herself as inflexible on account of teen-age children with extracurricular activities. Now, the administrator was to make allowances.

The third story was somewhat ironic, because it happened at the laboratory administration level itself. The administrative assistant in charge of personnel was a man who conducted the most careful, scientific, professional human resources program the administrator had ever seen. He screened people in and out of the laboratory, up and down the hierarchy, on the basis of multiple questions.

But now this man himself had just gotten custody of two small children. He had come in to ask for flexible hours. Under the circumstances, he wanted to know whether he could make some special arrangement that would help his personal life.

This particular administrator isn't a Simon Legree. Not is he the sort of man who treats people like interchangeable plastic parts. So he adjusted to his secretary. He adjusted to his supervisor. He adjusted to the administrative assistant. He did it because, well, a happy employee is probably a productive employee and all that.

He did it because a person's private life is a factor in his professional life and all that. He did it because he believed that a laboratory should be more flexible. To a point. But he feels a certain frustration. People want him to treat them professionally when it's to their advantage and personally when it's to their advantage. While he understands the family–work conflict, he also understands the conflict that comes with the title ''boss.''

Every day this administrator had to decide at what point the best interests of his employees conflict with the best interests of his laboratory. Where is it writ, he asks, that institutions increasingly have to deal with personal personnel problems and issues? How do you balance the needs of the institution and the needs of the workers?

Sometimes this man is afraid that he's running a family agency instead of a medical center department. Other times he's afraid he's being a heel. The boss does not expect any sympathy. People don't sympathize with the boss anyway, he says, because it's hard to sympathize with someone who has the power to hire and fire you. He understands that. But the fact is that he's responsible for 150 lives and one departmental balance sheet. And he takes both of these jobs very personally.*

*Adapted from an article © 1978 The Boston Globe Newspaper Company/The Washington Post Writers Group. Used with permission.

The dilemma is not resolved. The scenario is included here to heighten the awareness of the reader regarding the complexity of the leadership issue.

Participative Leadership

Many management authors support the 9,9 Team approach to leadership as the ultimate style for which a manager should strive. The term participative leadership reflects the equally high emphasis placed on both production concerns and people concerns.

Many investigators have attempted to substantiate the value and acceptance of participative leadership.[35] Murnigham and Leung report that individuals led by a more-involved leader produce more than those led by a less-involved superior.[38] Cherrington and Cherrington contend that a participative leadership style for decision-making yields higher efficiency and productivity.[8] Viola supports the participative leadership approach as fostering motivation among subordinates.[57] Still other advantages to the participative leadership style include the following:[42]

Subordinates have a closer identity with the organization.

There is less resistance to change.

Personal growth and development of subordinates is encouraged.

A wider range of experiences and ideas is solicited.

It should be noted, however, that implementing participative management in the laboratory is dependent upon factors other than just the manager's desire to involve employees more in decision-making. Snyder and Manuselis[49] studied the leadership and situational factors of 48 laboratory managers affecting participative management. They found that a manager's perceived leadership role, his leadership style, the number of employees for whom he was responsible (span of control), and the size of the institution (situation) were contributed most to a participative management climate.

Participative leadership is a natural style for managers whose assumptions parallel Theory-Y beliefs. Theory Y supports the concept that creativity is widely dispersed among subordinates, and participative leadership calls for input from staff members when making a decision or solving a problem.

Jewett, Esch, and Shrago described an example of participative leadership in which information to solve a problem was gathered at a variety of levels.[26] In their article, Jewett and colleagues were asked to study the feasibility of consolidating the laboratory systems of two hospitals. The information-gathering tool employed was the "nominal group problem-solving technique," a structured type of brainstorming. The principle of the technique is that everyone has a unique perspective on his work and associated problems. Everyone involved with the laboratory operation was included in the data-gathering step as part of the decision-making process: administrators, laboratory users (doctors, nurses, ward clerks), laboratory supervisors, and laboratory staff. These general subdivisions were further broken down into groups of ten individuals each to probe for information. Everyone was asked to describe both the current and *desired* situation following a series of steps. Group discussion was either solicited or limited, whichever posed the least potential threat to the author of the perspective. All perspectives were recorded in such a way that they were visually available throughout the time of discussion. Table 6-2 lists sample ideas of the current situation statements classified by operation or organization. When one looks at the table, the value of gathering differing perspectives during the decision-making process is clear. This represents just one technique proven successful in participative leadership.

Individual Temperaments

The group problem-solving technique just described highlights the value of many perspectives contributing to decision-making. In the clinical laboratory, individual differences in terms of temperament (personality) can be either very useful or a sizable problem. To maximize the talent of individuals with different temperaments and minimize the disruption of conflicting temperaments, it is helpful for the laboratory manager to understand his superior's, peers', and employees' natural personality traits.[50]

Some managers would dismiss the value of learning about or even trying to accommodate differences in personality. Some laboratory managers would protest on the grounds that accommodation of personal temperaments diminishes treating everyone equally, while others expect that "professional behavior should equalize the differences that are natural in everyone as an individual. This brief discussion is intended only to introduce the foundation premises in temperament typology and provide enough examples of how this information is helpful to stimulate the reader's further study.[27]

The basis for most temperament assessment tools and personality classifications is Carl Jung's

Psychological Types.[40] Jung's theory of psychological type included three pairs of opposing attitudes or functions: (1) attitude toward life; (2) perception or method of taking in information; and (3) use of judgment to reach a conclusion. Isabel Briggs Myers, author and proponent of the widely used Myers-Briggs Type Indicator (MBTI) assessment tool, added a fourth dimension, "orientation toward life."[39] Each of these continua is graphically displayed in Figure 6-5 with select characteristics of each type. While everyone uses both "ends" of the continua—for example, both sensing and intuition sources—to become aware of things, a natural preference for one kind of perception and one kind of judgment prompts individuals to use and develop more skills with one "set" of processes.

Extroversion/Introversion

Everyone falls somewhere along the continuum between fully extroverted and fully introverted. In general, the extrovert's interest flows mainly to the outer world of actions, objects and people. By contrast, introverts focus more on the inner world of concepts and ideas. Research has documented that clinical laboratorians are predominantly introverts, a finding consistent with their characteristics, noted in Figure 6-5. The astute laboratory manager will note that while the extrovert technologist may not seem to "fit" the norm of the group, he has other gifts that make him valuable. The extrovert is the technologist of choice to plan the holiday season party, tour a group of high school students through the laboratory, and arrange a schedule of speakers for inservices. The extrovert will probably not do as well with a long, tedious technical procedure that requires maximum concentration.

Sensing/Intuition

The perception continuum contrasts two distinct ways an individual becomes aware of something. Those who prefer to perceive the immediate, real practical facts of experience and life are sensing types. Intuitive types prefer to perceive the possibilities, relationships, and meanings of experiences. Again, individuals use both methods of perceiving but are better at one and depend on it more. The sensing person really smells the coffee, sees the writing on the wall, and hears the music. The intuitive grasps for "the big picture" and relies on hunches and insight. A review of the characteristics of these two types (Fig. 6-5) shows some noteworthy strengths of each—the sensing type will most closely follow the procedure manual in doing a lab-

(*Text continues on p 112*)

Table 6-2
Sample Ideas of Problem-solving Groups on the Current Situation

Statement Areas	Supervisors		Administrators		Laboratory Staff		Laboratory Users	
	Sample Ideas	*Percent Ideas in Areas*	*Sample Ideas*	*Percent Ideas in Areas*	*Sample Ideas*	*Percent Ideas In Areas*	*Sample Ideas*	*Percent Ideas in Areas*
Laboratory Operation Reporting	Data-management system overload of test results. Difficult to get access to data.	4%	Inadequate collection reporting system.	4%	Nothing goes on chart to indicate that blood is cross-matched. Untrained clerks calling for reports.	6%	Frequent typographical errors and illegibility. Reports late. High percent outpatient reports don't get to chart. Delayed tissue and autopsy reports. Poor reporting abnormal data back to MD. Results completed but not on charts.	21%
Ordering	Too many tests per patient. Duplication of tests. Too many tets requested for no real purpose.	18		0	Too many unnecessary blood orders. Requisitions not properly filled out or signed. Medical students order blood for doctors.	10	High rates of test per patient.	2

(continued)

Table 6-2 *(Continued)*

Statement Areas	Supervisors		Administrators		Laboratory Staff		Laboratory Users	
	Sample Ideas	Percent Ideas in Areas	Sample Ideas	Percent Ideas in Areas	Sample Ideas	Percent Ideas In Areas	Sample Ideas	Percent Ideas in Areas
Collection of Specimens	Hemolyzed blood not redrawn by technician. No contral receiving point for specimen collection. Specimen containers not stoppered on wards. Too much blood drawn.	18		0	Too many repeated drawings of blood.	4	Large amounts of blood drawn from patients not able to tolerate it.	7
Transportation	No transportation system for taking specimens to the lab after the regular morning pickup.	4		0	Difficulty in transporting cultures. Blood bank takes blood to surgery.	4	Excessive delays.	0
Lab Facility	Clincal lab has no windows. Limited and inefficiently arranged space. No available equipment for stat results. The priority of the lab is high output but not quality.	14	Labs inadequate (space, number of instruments, computerization, number of technologists). Overcrowded facilities.	8	Limited space. No new equipment. Poor heating and cooling system. Labs too far apart. No lockers. No lounge.	11	Space tight, not well designed. Need facilities for manual platelet counts.	11

Staffing	7 — Coverage not sufficient on weekends and holidays.	17 — Lack of fulltime doctorate level directors in many labs. Scarcity of qualified personnel. Personnel excellent but unappreciated.	4 — Personnel shortage.	17 — Have highly qualified pathologist. Poor technologist morale. Short number of technical personnel.
Other	11 — Lost specimens; lost slips. Policy regarding services isn't distributed to users.	21 — Inadequate amount of time for method development. Need to expand the range of services provided. Lack of assessment of quality of service.	22 — No continuing education program. Technicians have too many bookkeeping jobs. New employees lack training. Don't like punching time clock. Must transport files at end of month to isolated area.	16 — Lab accredited. Blood bank accredited. Procedures list for collections of specimens not available.
Organizational Laboratory*	0	12 — Unsatisfactory training program. No continuing education.	14 — Lack of supervision. Poor communication in labs. Too much absenteeism among new employees on weekends.	2 — Inability to communicate with responsible person in lab for specific tests.
Hospital	7 — Merit performance system not used. Good interpersonal relations.	12 — Lack of communication with hospital administration. University has inadequate knowledge to run hospital. No technical school.	6 — Almost impossible to get rid of someone who needs to be fired.	0

(continued)

Table 6-2 (Continued)

Statement Areas	Supervisors		Administrators		Laboratory Staff		Laboratory Users	
	Sample Ideas	Percent Ideas in Areas	Sample Ideas	Percent Ideas in Areas	Sample Ideas	Percent Ideas In Areas	Sample Ideas	Percent Ideas in Areas
Financial	Budget overruns could be controlled.	4%	No control over income generated. Poor identification of financial basis of lab by hospital administration. Inadequate provision for lab directors to determine level of pay for new technicians and technologists with experience.	26%	Low starting salaries and increased pay scale.	6%	Budget for supplies, SVCs, and equipment inadequate	4%
Other	Problem of interhospital data management. Should be an intercom system to all operating rooms from pathology. No actual label on blood tubes from hospital. Good salaries.	13		0	Cumbersome working with personnel office.	13	Proper equipment to collect specimens not on wards. Some lab work done outside on fee basis. Delays, confusion on procedures for tests done outside.	20
	(Total statements—26)		(Total statements—24)		(Total statements—50)		(Total statements—43)	

*Administration, supervision, personnel, communication.

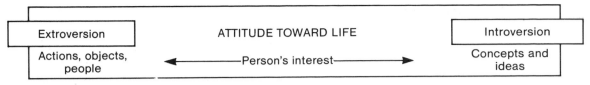

ATTITUDE TOWARD LIFE

Extroversion		Introversion
Actions, objects, people	←—————Person's interest—————→	Concepts and ideas

Extroverts:

Like variety and action.

Tend to be faster; dislike complicated procedures.

Are often good at greeting people.

Are interested in the results of their job, in getting it done, and in how other people do it.

Often don't mind the interruption of answering the telephone.

Often act quickly, sometimes without thinking.

Like to have people around.

Usually communicate freely.

Introverts:

Like quiet for concentration.

Tend to be careful with details; dislike sweeping statements.

Have trouble remembering names and faces.

Tend not to mind working on one project for a long time without interruption.

Are interested in the idea behind their job.

Dislike telephone intrusions and interruptions.

Like to think a lot before they act, sometimes without acting.

Work contentedly alone.

Have some problems communicating.

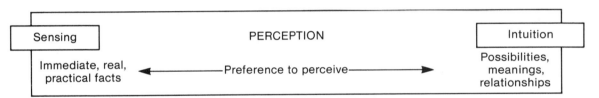

PERCEPTION

Sensing		Intuition
Immediate, real, practical facts	←—————Preference to perceive—————→	Possibilities, meanings, relationships

Sensing Types:

Dislike new problems unless there are standard ways to solve them.

Like an established way of doing things.

Enjoy using skills already learned more than learning new ones.

Work more steadily, with realistic idea of how long it will take.

Usually reach a conclusion step by step.

Are patient with routine details.

Are impatient when details get complicated.

Don't often get inspired, and rarely trust the inspiration when they do.

Seldom make errors of fact.

Tend to be good at precise work.

Intuitive Types:

Like solving new problems.

Dislike doing the same thing over and over again.

Enjoy learning a new skill more than using it.

Work in bursts of energy powered by enthusiasm, with slack periods in between.

Put two and two together quickly.

Are impatient with routine details.

Are patient with complicated situations.

Follow their inspirations, good or bad.

Often get their facts a bit wrong.

Dislike taking time for precision.

(continued)

(Part A)

FIGURE 6-5. Temperament dimensions and select characteristics. (Adapted from Myers IB: Type and Teamwork. Gainesville, FL, Center for Applications of Psychological Type, 1974)

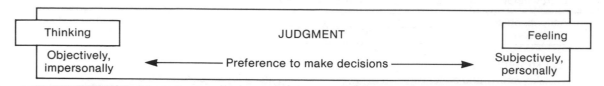

Thinking Types:

Are relatively unemotional and un-
interested in people's feelings.

May hurt people's feelings without
knowing it.

Like analysis and putting things
into logical order. Can get along
without harmony.

Tend to decide impersonally, sometimes ignoring people's wishes.

Need to be treated fairly.

Are able to reprimand people or fire
them when necessary.

Tend to relate well only to other
thinking types.

May seem hard-hearted.

Feeling Types:

Tend to be very aware of other
people and their feelings.

Enjoy pleasing people, even in
unimportant things.

Like harmony. Efficiency may be
badly disturbed by office feuds.

Often let decisions be influenced
by their own or other people's
likes and wishes.

Need occasional praise.

Dislike telling people unpleasant
things.

Relate well to most people.

Tend to be sympathetic.

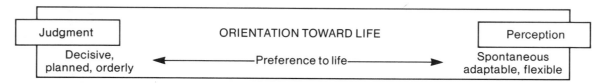

Judging Types:

Best when they can plan their work
and follow the plan.

Like to get things settled and
wrapped up.

May decide things too quickly.

May dislike to interrupt the project
they are on for a more urgent one.

May not notice new things that need
to be done.

Want only the essentials needed to
get on with a job.

Tend to be satisfied once they reach
a judgment on a thing, situation
or person.

Perceptive Types:

Tend to be good at adapting to
changing situations.

Don't mind leaving things open for
alterations.

May have trouble making decisions.

May start too many projects and have
difficulty in finishing them.

Want to know all about a new job.

May postpone unpleasant jobs.

Tend to be curious and welcome new
light on a thing, situation, or
person.

FIGURE 6-5. *(Part B)*

oratory analysis, whereas the intuitive type will be happy to learn how to use a new piece of equipment, for example—and some drawbacks of each —sensing types prefer not to take a research procedure and adopt it for use in the routine laboratory, whereas intuitives may make decisions on a "gut feeling" that is incorrect.

Because of the different preferences for perceiving information, intuitives need sensing types and vice versa. When putting together a committee to work on a problem or oversee the development of a new policy, the laboratory manager can capitalize on the gifts both types would add. For example, intuitives need sensing types to bring up pertinent facts, read the fine print in a union contract, and notice what needs attention most urgently. Sensing types need intuitives to bring up new possibilities, to see how to prepare for the future, and to supply ingenuity on problems.

Thinking/Feeling

This continuum, judgment, is the process of coming to a conclusion about something. The thinking individual prefers to make judgments or decisions objectively and impersonally by considering causes of events and where decisions may lead. By contrast, feeling types arrive at conclusions more subjectively and personally, weighing values of choices and how they matter to others. For the clinical laboratorian, the thinking end of the continuum is an expected and even learned approach based on the scientific method for work. This obviously is not always the stronger of the two approaches when one is dealing with interpersonal relationships as a peer or supervisor. Thinking types are analytical and logical and do not show emotion readily, characteristics that help them do some tasks like disciplining or terminating an employee and hinder them when faced with an employee or colleague who is upset. The feeling individual, in reaching conclusions based on a set of values and standards that take into consideration what matters to himself and others, is more people oriented and tends to be more sympathetic. When faced with interpersonal conflict, the feeling type will be the better listener but will have difficulty taking corrective action by talking to the person at fault in the conflict.

The laboratory manager should consider the strengths of both thinking and feeling types when planning a group activity because the two types are mutually useful. Feeling types need thinkers to hold consistently to a policy, to stand firm against opposition, and to reform what needs reforming. Thinkers need feeling types to persuade and conciliate, to forecast how others will feel, and to arouse enthusiasm.

Judgment/Perception

Opposite ends of the continuum for an individual's approach to life include the judging types, who prefer an orderly, planned, and controlled life, and the perceptive types, who tend to be flexible, adaptable, and spontaneous. Once again, both types have strengths—the judging types will see a project through to completion and be satisfied when a matter is settled, and perceptive types adapt well to changing situations and welcome new insights on a situation—and weaknesses—judging types may reach a decision too quickly or not notice new things that need to be done, and perceptive types may start too many projects and postpone unpleasant jobs.

Readers should have, with this brief introduction, an appreciation of the natural differences in their supervisor, peers, and subordinates. The clinical laboratory work force is composed of "different drums and different drummers." With all the richness of the human personality, no two people are totally alike—a fact that makes individual differences best thought of as "gifts," or individual contributions. Clearly identifiable common threads are woven through each of us, however; and a knowledge of them can be useful in understanding how human behavior affects the accomplishment of work in the clinical laboratory. This knowledge is not to be used for stereotyping individuals on the basis of a few characteristics; rather, the types described here should be viewed as a template. Kindler notes that when managers handle differences well, they can identify underlying concerns, stimulate creative effort, reduce antagonistic feelings, correct misunderstandings, and guide commitment to needed change.[28]

LEADERSHIP AND THE SITUATION

Beyond the investigation of various leadership styles resulting from individual differences and the needs of the followers is the consideration of how the *situation* affects leadership effectiveness. Fleishman concluded that no single leadership style is most effective; rather, leadership effectiveness depends upon the integration between task, power, personality, attitudes, and perceptions.[15] Tannenbaum and Schmidt, whose leadership continuum was considered earlier, maintain that the successful manager is one who consistently and accurately assesses the situational forces determining the most appropriate leadership behavior.[52]

Research on leadership effectiveness in the late 1960s and early 1970s began to focus more on the effect of situational variance on leadership behavior, rather than on "situational determinants."[30]

Situational Leadership Theory and the Tridimensional Model

Hersey and Blanchard have added to the typical four quadrants of the Ohio model two additional situational dimensions. Figure 6-6 contains both a

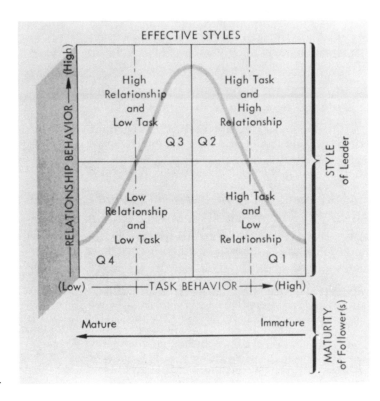

FIGURE 6-6. Situational leadership theory.

maturity of followers continuum and an effectiveness dimension, represented by the shaded, three-dimensional appearance.[23]

The maturity factor is part of Hersey and Blanchard's life-cycle theory. Maturity is considered in relation to a specific task to perform, rather than implying that an individual is mature or immature at all times. For example, a technologist may be very responsible (mature) in completing a particular laboratory procedure and somewhat irresponsible (less mature) in filling out all necessary forms to document preventive maintenance. This may require the

manager to more closely supervise the technologist's report-filing but exercise less supervision over specimen-testing.

The life-cycle theory suggests that as the followers mature, the leader's behavior should change. This is displayed in Figure 6-6 as the line representing a curvilinear design between relationship, tasks, and other variables. The sequence proceeds from (1) high task-low relationship behavior to (2) high task-high relationship behavior to (3) high relationship-low task behavior to (4) low task-low relationship behavior. Consider the development of a new

Table 6-3
Managerial Styles with an Effectiveness Dimension

	Orientation	*Ineffective*	*Effective*	*Leader Behavior*
Q1	High task/low relationship	Autocrat	Benevolent autocrat	Telling
Q2	High task/high relationship	Compromiser	Executive	Selling
Q3	High relationship/low task	Missionary	Developer	Participating
Q4	Low relationship/low task	Deserter	Bureaucrat	Delegating

testing procedure to be added to a clinical laboratory's regimen. Early in the development, when the supervisor and staff technologists are attempting to modify a research design to make it practical for clinical application, the supervisor may need to exercise high task-low relationship behavior. Once the procedure is developed and implemented on-line, the supervisor can progress to Quadrant 2 or 3 leadership behavior characterized by high relationship and low task emphasis.

The effectiveness dimension was first added by Reddin to the task-concern and relationship-concern dimensions.[44] This addition reflects the fact that a variety of leadership styles may either be effective or ineffective, depending on the situation.

With the third effectiveness dimension, eight possible combinations exist, as depicted in Table 6-3. Hersey and Blanchard's contribution to the effectiveness dimension is in the perceptions of followers, supervisors, and associates when these leadership styles are employed. Table 6-4 contrasts some of these perceptions of leader behavior for effective and ineffective styles.

The Contingency Model

Fiedler postulated the first contingency model of leadership supporting the premise that effective group performance is dependent upon the leader's

---

Table 6-4
How the Basic Leader Behavior Styles May Be Seen by Others

Basic Styles	Effective	Ineffective
High task and low relationship	Seen as having well-defined methods for accomplishing goals that are helpful to the followers	Seen as imposing methods on others; sometimes seen as unpleasant and interested only in short-run output.
High task and high relationship	Seen as satisfying the needs of the group for setting goals and organizing work, as well as providing high levels of socio-emotional support	Seen as initiating more structure than is needed by the group and often appears to be insincere in interpersonal relationships
High relationship and low task	Seen as having implicit trust in people and as being primarily concerned with facilitating their goal accomplishment	Seen as primarily interested in harmony; sometimes seen as unwilling to accomplish a task if it risks disrupting a relationship or losing "good person" image
Low relationship and low task	Seen as appropriately delegating to subordinates decisions about how the work should be done and providing little socio-emotional support where little is needed by the group	Seen as providing little structure or socio-emotional support when needed by members of the group

(From Hersey P, Blanchard KH: Management of Organizational Behavior: Utilizing Human Resources, 3rd ed, p 107. Englewood Cliffs, Prentice-Hall, 1977. Used with permission.)

style of interacting with subordinates and the degree of influence and control allotted the leader by the situation.[14] An instrument was designed by Fielder to measure a leader's relationship or task orientation within the parameters of three situational criteria. The measurement tool contains 16 bipolar adjectives (such as efficient-inefficient) that the leader selects to describe an individual he is least able to work with. From this set of instructions, the title of the questionnaire, Least-Preferred Coworker (LPC), is derived. If a leader responds by selecting relatively favorable terms on the LPC, his orientation is toward establishing relationships. If the leader responds in unfavorable terms, he is considered task oriented.

The three situational criteria, or contingency dimensions, include

1. Leader–member relations—how well the leader is liked, respected, and trusted
2. Position power—the amount of influential power the leader has in terms of hiring, firing, discipline, and control of the rewards systems
3. Task structure—the degree to which job assignments of subordinates are specifically defined (structured versus unstructured)

Fiedler reports that the more positive the leader-member relations, the greater the position power. Also, the more highly structured the tasks to be performed, the greater the leader's influence.

Figure 6-7 depicts eight situational conditions (I-VIII) correlated with task-motivated or relations-motivated leadership styles. If a laboratory manager is relations oriented, job performance will be better

for situations characterized in IV through VII. On the other hand, productivity is enhanced by a manager with a task orientation for those situations described in I through III and VIII.

Both the tridimensional model and the contingency model support the premise that effectiveness of leadership style is dependent upon situational variables such as maturity of the followers, relationship between the manager and his subordinates, the manager's power to influence, and the degree to which subordinate's tasks are structured.

DIAGNOSING THE SITUATION

At times it is helpful to have a tool that can be used to diagnose a difficult situation confounding the leadership efforts of the manager. Getzels proposed a theory of administration that considers management as a social process.[19] Within Getzels' model (Fig. 6-8), two dimensions operate simultaneously: an impersonal (normothetic) dimension and a personal (idiopathic dimension). The impersonal dimension consists of the institution with its roles (positions) and expectations (responsibilities) within the roles. The personal dimension consists of the individual selected to fill a position, his personality (knowledge and skills factors) in the role, and motivators required to alleviate needs. Conflict within the system may exist whenever there is a disharmony between the corresponding components of the two dimensions: role and personality. These may exist as an inter- or intrarole conflict, inter- or intrapersonality conflict, or a combination role–personality conflict.

FIGURE 6-7. Fiedler's situational favorableness dimension. (From Fiedler FC: A Theory of Leadership Effectiveness. New York, McGraw–Hill, 1967)

THE SITUATIONAL FAVORABLENESS DIMENSION.

	I	II	III	IV	V	VI	VII	VIII
Leader–member relations	Good				Poor			
Task structure	High		Low		High		Low	
Position power	Strong	Weak	Strong	Weak	Strong	Weak	Strong	Weak
Most appropriate leadership style	T	T	T	R	R	R	R	T

T = Task-motivated; R = Relations-motivated

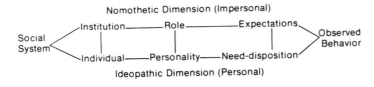

FIGURE 6-8. Getzels' social systems model of administration. (From Mattran KJ: Conflict management, organizational and personnel needs, performance evaluation. In Langerman PD, Smith DH: Managing Adult and Continuing Education Programs and Staff, p 351. Washington, National Association for Public Continuing and Adult Education, 1979. Used with permission of the publisher)

Role Conflict

Interrole conflict occurs when two individuals clash over the boundaries of their job responsibilities, resources available, or "turfdom." An example might be a dispute over the priority for use of a refrigerated centrifuge shared by two technologists. Intrarole conflict usually occurs at the time a position is created if the responsibilities are not clearly or reasonably defined.

Personality Conflict

Rather than referring to the incompatibility of two co-workers, interpersonality conflict refers to a lack of shared attitudes, values, or interests in achieving organizational goals. For example, two technologists may have differing views on whether or not they should be required to perform phlebotomy as part of their daily routine. Intrapersonality conflicts exist when needs–disposition precludes achievement of expectations within a role: the performance of the closet drinker, for example, is affected by his habit.

Role–Personality Conflict

This is probably the most common form of organizational conflict. In this situation, an individual may not be qualified for a particular role (responsibility) or may be overqualified for the position and hence underutilized, or a change in the job requirements or personal preparation may bring about this conflict.

To demonstrate the utility of Getzels' model in diagnosing the situation, consider the following example:

> The laboratory manager of a large microbiology section directs a staff of fifteen technologists who do most of the day-to-day testing for routine cultures and sensitivities. One of the senior technologists has recently completed an advanced degree in microbiology at a nearby university. During the time he was pursuing his studies the laboratory supported his efforts through a 75% tuition-reimbursement policy and the special privilege of being released early from work in the afternoon to attend class.
>
> Since completing the degree, this senior technologist has seemed unhappy at work, arriving late and often leaving early. There has been much bickering between the technologist and fellow staff members, especially with the recent addition of a senior technologist to specifically perform the mycology tests. General staff morale has slumped, it seems, and the manager has had to spend much time arbitrating disputes that most often involve the senior technologist of concern in this study.

This example is not an unusual situation to be faced by the laboratory manager. Using Getzels' model, the situation can be analyzed to identify the root cause of the problem. In this case, the problem stems from a role-personality conflict in which the senior technologist feels he has outgrown his role on the basis of his newly acquired advanced degree. The problem is typical in that people frequently want to take on new responsibility with the completion of an advanced degree; this situation is referred to as "flexing newly credentialized muscles."

In this particular case, the manager was astute enough to diagnose the situation. At a counseling session, the perceived type of conflict was validated. The solution the manager chose to implement included an expansion of the role of the individual. This entailed delegating more responsibility to the senior technologist without expanding the hierarchical structure.

Fell and Richard point out the necessity for laboratory managers to be cognizant of the occurrence of role and personality conflict in their study of factors contributing to occupational stress of medical technologists and technicians.[13] Information gathered through situational diagnosis with Getzels' model should help uncover occupational stressors such as role overload, role conflict, low participation, and role ambiguity, enabling the manager to minimize their effects.

MANAGEMENT BY OBJECTIVES

Management by objectives (MBO) is a managerial process reflective of a leadership style with high consideration for both production and people. The MBO concept was first described by Drucker in 1954, and much research has been conducted on the process since that time.[12,58] MBO is defined as a process whereby an employee and manager jointly define major areas of responsibility within the work setting, identify the commonality of organizational and personal goals, and establish a mutual understanding and acceptance of plans for future activities.[16]

Odiorne clarifies MBO as a set of procedural rules for management.[41] Figure 6-9 graphically displays a map of the MBO cycle. The key features of a typical MBO program include the following:[20]

The laboratory's common goals and the measures of success in meeting these are reaffirmed and considered, respectively.

In light of past goal achievement, any revisions to the organizational structure are made to facilitate achievement.

The supervisor and subordinate meet to discuss and jointly set goals for the subordinate for a specified period of time (*e.g.,* six months). These goals reflect needs of both the organization and the subordinate.

A joint agreement on the goals established and criteria for measuring and evaluating these goals is determined.

At various intermediate times in the evaluation period, the supervisor and subordinate review the progress of the subordinate toward the mutually accepted goals. The supervisor's role is one of support, coaching, and counseling, rather than judging. Goals may be redefined or eliminated if they are no longer appropriate within the organizational context.

A final evaluation at the end of the predetermined period measures the subordinate's achievement based upon results accomplished, not upon activities, mistakes, or organizational requirements.

The performance of the entire laboratory is reassessed.

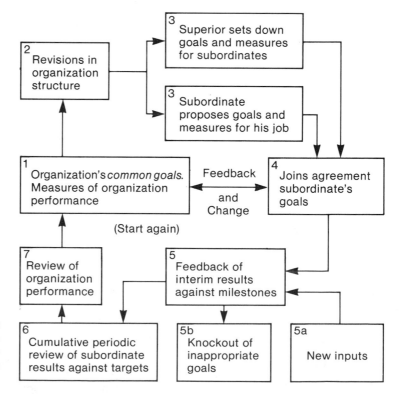

FIGURE 6-9. The cycle of management by objectives. (From Odiorne GS: Management by Objectives. New York, Pitman Corporation, 1972. Reprinted with permission of the publisher)

From this point, the cycle is reinitiated.

A key element in the MBO process is the definition of goals and objectives. *Goals* are general aims or purposes. *Objectives* are specific plans to achieve results through defined tasks within a certain period of time. For example, a goal may be "to increase the provision of appropriate procedures available on the midnight to 8 AM shift." The laboratory manager and hematology supervisor may jointly agree on the following objective:

> To offer reticulocyte counts as a stat procedure during the midnight to 8 AM shift by retraining the technical staff covering these hours such that this procedure will be performed with the same precision exhibited by daytime personnel by November 1, 19—.

Based upon this objective for the supervisor in light of organizational goals, a joint agreement between the supervisor and staff technologist on the midnight to 8 AM shift might be as follows:

> To perform reticulocyte counts routinely on the midnight to 8 AM shift with results not exceeding 5% variance from those obtained by day-shift personnel. This objective is to be reached by October 15, 19—— following two in-service sessions and a structured period of reading and evaluating reticulocyte counts pre- and postanalyses by day-shift technical staff.

From this example, it is obvious that MBO can be implemented at any supervisor–subordinate level. MBO is not a panacea leadership process for involving subordinates in their work. While the advantages generally outweigh the disadvantages, Uris cautions against several counterproductive problems:[56]

Heel-dragging participation. Both the supervisor and the employee must stretch their capabilities, rather than maintain the status quo.

Setting low standards (*objectives*). Some supervisors and subordinates set objectives well within reach, causing the employee to always appear favorable on evaluation and the department to appear full of overachievers.

Quantification. It is critically important that specific criteria be established for measuring achievement of objectives. It is very difficult to define measurable criteria for some objectives, such as the improvement of morale.

Management by objectives is a common sense approach to 9,9 Team management reflective of Theory-Y assumptions.

LEADERSHIP BEHAVIOR IN NEED OF CHANGE

There are some subtle clues that should alert the manager to the need for a change in leadership styles. Leslie surveyed 1000 supervisors and managers from 23 organizations, asking, "What would you say to your boss if there was one thing, if he would do it, that in your opinion would most contribute to the effectiveness of yourself and your work unit?"[54] The following is a rank-ordered list of their responses:

1. Share the company objectives with me.
2. Provide better, more honest communications.
3. Know my problems.
4. Set the objectives. Let me do the job my way.
5. Involve me in the decisions that affect me and my work unit.
6. Eliminate duplication of effort.
7. Back me up in personnel/grievance decisions.
8. Treat managers as if they were human.
9. Get rid of the deadwood.
10. Tell me what is expected of me.

These concerns provide a sound sketch of middle-management concerns when a change in the supervisor's leadership style is needed. Perhaps polling one's own subordinates would enlighten the reader to his own leadership style, and some changes might seem appropriate.

REFERENCES

1. Appley LA: The nature of Management, Film One in a Series. In Supervisory Management Course—Part One. New York, American Management Association, 1968
2. Argyris C: Management and Organizational Development, p 17. New York, McGraw-Hill, 1971
3. Argyris C: Management and Organizational Development: The Path from XA to YB, p 12. New York, McGraw-Hill, 1971
4. Blake RR, Mouton JL: Managerial facades. Adv Manag J, pp 29–36, July 1966
5. Blake RR, Mouton JL: The Managerial Grid. Houston, Gulf Publishing, 1964
6. Blake RR, Mouton JL: The New Managerial Grid. Houston, Gulf Publishing, 1978
7. Burden CA, Dorff PG: Understanding the leadership function: Leaders are not necessarily managers. Lab Med 18:327–329, 1987
8. Cherrington DJ, Cherrington JO: Participation, performance, and appraisal. Bus Horiz 17:40, December 1974
9. Crowley J, Rinker G, Neely AE, Anderson AS: Situational leadership for the laboratory. J Med Technol 3:303–306, 1986
10. Davis K: Human Relations at Work, 3rd ed p 97. New York, McGraw-Hill, 1967
11. Davis K: Human Behavior at Work: Human Relations and Organizational Behavior, 4th ed, pp 120–133. New York, McGraw-Hill, 1972

12. Drucker PF: The Practice of Management. New York, Harper & Row, 1954
13. Fell RD, Richard WC: Health effects on job pressures. Lab World, pp 44–47, July 1980
14. Fiedler FC: A Theory of Leadership Effectiveness. New York, McGraw-Hill, 1967
15. Fleishman EA: Twenty years of consideration and structure. In Fleishman EA, Hunt JG (eds): Current Development in the Study of Leadership, pp 1–37. Carbondale, Southern Illinois University Press, 1973
16. Frank ER: Motivation by objectives—a case study. Res Manag 12:391–400. November 1969
17. French JRP, Raven B: The bases of social power. In Cartwright D, Zander AF (eds): Group Dynamics, 2nd ed, pp 607–623. Evanston, Row Peterson, 1960
18. Fulmer RM: The New Management, p 336. New York, Macmillan, 1974
19. Getzels JW: Administration as a social process. In Halpin AW (ed): Administrative Theory in Education, pp 150–165. Chicago, Midwest Administration Center, 1958
20. Gibson JL, Ivancevich JM, Donnelly JH: Organizations Behavior, Structure, Processes, 3rd ed, pp 30–32, 366–367. Dallas Business Publications, 1979
21. Glassman E: A leadership skills program for scientist/supervisors. Lab Management 20(9):46–49, 1982
22. Halpin AW: The Leadership Behavior of School Superintendents, p 4. Chicago, Midwest Administration Center, University of Chicago, 1959
23. Hersey P, Blanchard KH: Management of Organizational Behavior: Utilizing Human Resources, 3rd ed, p 89. Englewood Cliffs, Prentice-Hall, 1977
24. Jago AG, Vroom VH: Hierarchical level and leadership style. Organizational Behavior and Human Performance 18:131–145, 1977
25. Jennings EE: The anatomy of leadership. Management of Personnel Quarterly (1) (Autumn), 1961
26. Jewett JE, Esch D, Shrago J: Try the team approach to problem solving. MLO 8:63–70, February 1976
27. Kiersey O, Bates M: Please Understand Me: Character and Temperament Types. Del Mar, Prometheus Nemesis Books, 1978
28. Kindler HS: The art of managing differences. Training and Development Journal 37(1):26–32, 1983
29. Knudson HR, Woodworth RT, Bell CH: Management: An Experiential Approach, p 326. New York, McGraw-Hill, 1973
30. Korman AK: "Consideration," "initiating structure," and organizational criteria—a review. Personal Psychology: A Journal of Applied Research XIX, No. 4, pp 349–361, Winter 1966.
31. Lawler EE, Hall DT, Olham GR: Organizational climate: Relationship to organizational structure, process and performance. Organizational Behavior and Human Performance II, 14:139–155, 1974.
32. Leavitt T: The managerial merry-go-round. Harvard Bus Rev, p 131, July–August, 1974
33. Likert R: Management styles and the human component. Management Review 66:23ff, 1977
34. Likert R: New Patterns of Management, pp 113–115. New York, McGraw-Hill, 1961
35. McDonnell J: Participative Management: Can its acceptance be predicted? Human Resource Management 15(2): p 2–4, Summer 1976
36. McGregor D: Leadership and Motivation. Boston, MIT Press, 1966
37. Mitchell TR, Larson JR, Green SG: Leader behavior, situational moderators, and group performance: An attributable analysis. Organizational Behavior and Human Performance 18:254–268, 1977
38. Murnighan JK, Leung TK: The effects of leadership involvement and the importance of the task on subordinates' performance. Organizational Behavior and Human Performance 17:299–310, 1976
39. Myers IB: Type and Teamwork. Gainesville, Center for Applications of Psychological Type, 1974
40. O'Brien RT: Using Jung more (and etching him in stone less). Training 22(5):53–66, 1985
41. Odiorne GS: MBO: A backward glance. Business Horizons 21:14–24, 1978
42. O'Donovan TR: Can the 'participative' approach to management help the decision makers? Hospital Management 112:16, July 1971
43. Rakich JS, Longest BB, O'Donovan TR: Managing Health Care Organizations. Philadelphia, WB Saunders, 1977
44. Reddin WJ: The 3-D management style theory. Train Devel J 30(4):8–17, April 1976
45. Reichman W, Levy M: Personal power enchancement: A way to execute success. Management Review 66:28–34, 1977
46. Schwartz D: Introduction to Management: Principles, Practices and Processes, pp 507–508. New York, Harcourt Brace Jovanovich, 1980
47. Scott WG, Mitchell TR, Birnvarum PH: Organization Theory: A Structural and Behavioral Analysis, 4th ed. Homewood, Richard D. Irwin, 1981
48. SInger HA: Human values and leadership: A ten-year study of administraters in large organizations. Hum Organ 35(1): 83–87, 1976
49. Snyder JR. Manuselis G: Factors affecting participative management in the clinical laboratory. J Med Technol 2:532–536, 1985
50. Steger J, Manners G, Zimmer T: Following the leader: How to link management style to subordinate personalities. Management Review 71(10):22–51, 1982
51. Stogdill RM, Coons AC (eds): Leader Behavior: Its Description and Measurement. Research Monograph No. 88. Columbus, Bureau of Business Research, The Ohio State University, 1975
52. Tannenbaum R, Schmidt WH: How to choose a leadership pattern. Harvard Bus Rev pp 162–180, May–June 1973
53. Taylor JK: Participative management lifts lab productivity. MLO 18(4):46–50, 1986
54. This LE: A Guide to Effective Management: Practical Applications from Behavioral Science, pp 96–97, 108–11. Reading, Addison-Wesley, 1974
55. Townsend R: Up the Organization, pp 33, 86. Greenwich Fawcett Publications, 1970
56. Uris A: The Executive Deskbook. New York, Van Nostrand, Reinhold, 1970
57. Viola RH: Be a manager and a motivator. MLO, pp 131–136, September–October 1974
58. Weihrich H: Management by objectives: Does it really work? Bus Rev 28:(4)27–31, 1976

ANNOTATED BIBLIOGRAPHY

Barron RA: Behavior in Organizations: Understanding and Managing the Human Side of Work, 2nd ed. Boston, Allyn and Bacon, 1986

While this text does not address employees specifically working in the clinical laboratory, readers will find the following chapters of particular interest: Chapter 5, "Work Related Attitudes: Job Satisfaction, Organizational Commitment, and Prejudice"; Chapter 6, "Personality: The Nature and Impact of Individual Differences"; Chapter 7, "Stress at Work. Its Causes, Impact, and Management"; and Chapter 8, "Group Dynamics": "Understanding Groups at Work."

Blake RR, Mouton JS: The New Managerial Grid. Houston, Gulf Publishing Company, 1978

This resource is, in essence, a second edition to the author's classic text on the Managerial Grid published in 1964. Additional research and insights are included to support the validity of the Grid organization development and its application to leadership styles and group effectiveness.

Blalock HM, Wilken PH: Intergroup Processes: A Micro-Macro Perspective. New York, The Free Press, 1979

This reference addresses relationships and theories of complex social processes. Readers who wish to investigate the implications of social power on leadership style and effectiveness will find this source useful.

Fielder FE, Chemers MM, Mahar L: Improving Leadership Effectiveness: The Leader Match Concept (rev). New York, John Wiley & Sons, 1977

This self-teaching guide first supplies a basic review of leadership philosophy and theory. The majority of the text provides a straight forward approach for the reader to rate himself or herself on a number of style factors relevant to situational variables. The discussion of comparative thinking and actions is enlightening.

Gibson JL, Ivancevich JM, Donnelly JH: Organizations: Behavior, Structure, Processes, 3rd ed. Dallas, Business Publications, 1979

This text integrates the leadership activity of managers with other managerial functions and the organization setting. Chapter 8 specifically deals with trait and personal-behavioral approaches to leadership, while Chapter 9 focuses on situational approaches. Chapter 19 also relates to leadership effectiveness in a discussion on organizational climate.

Hersey P, Blanchard KH: Management of Organizational Behavior: Utilizing Human Resources, 3rd ed. Englewood Cliffs, Prentice-Hall, 1977

The emphasis of these two authors is on leadership styles appropriate for situational differences. This is reflected throughout this text addressing behavior within organizations. Of particular interest is the Leader Effectiveness and Adaptability Description (LEAD) instrument, which measures supervisor's perception of leadership style, style range (flexibility), and style adaptability (effectiveness). After completing the LEAD questionnaire in Chapter 1, the reader is provided with leadership theory and self-analysis in subsequent chapters.

Hollander EP: Leadership Dynamics: A Practical Guide to Effective Relationships. New York, The Free Press, 1978

This single resource provides an exhausting look at leadership styles and group effectiveness. Chapter 2 contrasts several ways of approaching leadership for study. Both the parameters of leadership effectiveness discussed in Chapter 6 and the summation of leadership dynamics in Chapter 8 are excellent readings.

Ivancevich JM, Matteson MT: Organizational Behavior and Management. Plano, Business Publications, 1987

This resource integrates various components of organizational behavior and management following a diagnostic model. Of particular note, this text includes diagnostic exercises, group exercises and cases. Readers will find Part II, "The Individual in the Organization," and Part III, "Interpersonal Influence and the Group Behavior," of particular interest.

Keirsey D, Bates M: Please Understand Me: Character and Temperament Types. Del Mar, Prometheus Nemesis Books, 1978

This resource includes a temperament assessment questionnaire for self-assessment of one's specific temperament type. The foundation for temperament types is described in Chapter 2, and the lengthy appendix provides interesting insight into the 16 different temperament types. Readers will also be interested in Chapter 5, entitled "Temperament in Leading."

Maude B: Leadership in Management. London, Business Books Ltd, 1978

This resource is easily read and focuses largely on pragmatic applications of leadership based on manager's experiences and insights. Of particular note is the author's discussion of integrating personal and organizational goals throughout the book as he describes effective leadership for a variety of different roles.

seven

Employee-Involvement Work Groups

Dietrich L. Schaupp
Barbara L. Parsons

During the past decade, change has swept through the medical profession and exposed the laboratory manager to a wide variety of methods and programs to enhance management effectiveness. Some of these programs offer specific, short-term approaches, while others promote the benefits of long-term change.

Quality assurance programs, cost-containment programs, morale-enhancement efforts, and productivity-improvement programs are just a few approaches currently facing the laboratory manager. Although each method promises long-term laboratory improvement, after adoption and implementation these programs often fall short of their promises for productivity and human resources. Some of these programs have achieved spectacular results; however, the majority have proved to be lackluster, sometimes destructive, and often costly during and after implementation.

Recent management thought extols the benefits of participatory group approaches for the health-care sector. Although participative management techniques have been on the management horizon for some time, only recently have they been actively prescribed for medical fields.

Three of the more popular approaches are quality circles (QCs), and quality of work life (QWL) programs, and autonomous work groups. From an employee-involvement perspective, these three approaches are similar, but they differ in one respect: QCs and autonomous work groups usually operate in a non-union setting, whereas QWL programs function in a union environment.

This discussion explores the feasibility of these three approaches in a laboratory environment. Furthermore, it explains the background, function, and brief supervisory overview required to establish these approaches.

WHY EMPLOYEE INVOLVEMENT?

Although employee involvement approaches are not foreign to the United States, they have recently received considerable exposure as a Japanese import, with Japanese success in competitive manufacturing strengthening the image. Management practitioners can no longer dismiss Japanese products as mere copies of American products and techniques, nor can they afford any longer to ignore the Japanese competitive threat: Japanese manufacturers and their products clearly seem to be more competitive than their American counterparts in the manufacturing sector.

It has been suggested that Japanese performance and productivity can be linked directly to the

Japanese management style. Although the relationship is somewhat oversimplified, it is true that the Japanese have been strong advocates and practitioners of employee-involvement groups. Americans generally have been lukewarm to the idea. Americans have a long history of one-to-one management where the superior–subordinate interaction is the basic management unit. Furthermore, cultural differences between Japan and the United States are reflected in their respective management styles because most managers practice what is culturally "natural" to them. The Japanese style reflects a collective society, whereas American techniques express the virtues of individualism. Finally, American managers often do not really understand or know what employee involvement is. Our discussion addresses this issue.

When advocating employee-involvement approaches for American medical services, we assume that they are transplantable from the manufacturing sector and will readily take root. Overwhelming evidence exists that employee-involvement approaches are feasible in American manufacturing, but fewer data are available in the service sector, even though some evidence strongly implies that employee involvement is workable and should be considered.

Put simply, employee involvement means utilizing employee groups to increase performance, quality, and productivity. Its roots lie in the American human-relations approaches so popular after World War II. Although it addressed worker satisfaction and group interaction, the human-relations approach stressed the employee's need for recognition and job security, as well as a sense of belonging and importance.

An outgrowth of the human-relations approach emphasized the developmental aspect of human needs. It sought employee participation based on the premise that it would satisfy needs associated with personal development. This human-resources approach stressed employee self-control, self-direction, creativity, and innovation. It strove to create an environment that allowed employees to contribute to organizational goals and experience direct control of their work environment. Through an attitude of "ownership" or "control," employee productivity and performance were expected to increase.

The employee ownership/control argument is also the basis of the employee involvement approaches presented in this discussion. However, the techniques presented here stress group involvement as opposed to individual participation. Although there are participative schemes that involve employees on an individual basis, such as manage-

ment by objectives, the major emphasis in QCs, QWL programs, and autonomous work groups is that they utilize the group to achieve organizational goals. Furthermore, groups that practice high-involvement approaches tend to make knowledge necessary to manage these activities. The first approach to be examined is the QCs movement that has recently attracted the attention of the health-care providers.

QUALITY CIRCLES APPROACH

As with most new management approaches, experts lack data regarding the effectiveness of the QC approach in the United States. There is significant evidence, however, to suggest that it has become one of the most adopted human-resource activities in recent years. Although problem-solving groups have been in existence in the United States since the 1930s, QCs have had phenomenal growth recently. In a 1982 survey conducted by the New York Stock Exchange, 65% of companies with over 25,000 employees used some form of QC program. Obviously, the trend is well established. And it is now being adopted by service-oriented organizations.

Why the popularity? The Japanese competitive threat—and success with employee-involvement programs—certainly is one answer. Also, American managers are aware of employee needs and desires to participate in achieving organizational goals and recognize QCs as one way to satisfy these needs. Quality circles also do not significantly alter the traditional managerial power structure, so they are less threatening than other employee-involvement programs. Furthermore, the QC approach portends significant quality outputs and productivity increases.

A quality circle in its most basic form, is a group of employees meeting to solve problems related to their immediate work environment. Although this basic model differs from one organization to another, the major characteristics are discussed here:[3]

1. *It is a people-building philosophy*: Quality circle programs will work only if there is a sincere desire on the part of management to help their employees grow and develop through QCs. We would advise any company whose only goals are selfish gains for management not to bother to try QCs. It would be seen just for what it would be—another attempt at employee manipulation.
2. *It is voluntary*: This is the second most important element of the program and one

that seems difficult for management to accept. This is the visible proof to the member employees that quality circles are for their benefit—they are completely free to take or not take advantage of them.

3. *Everyone participates*: Quality circles are a participative program; therefore, the leader must see that the quiet, more introverted person also has a chance to say what is on his mind.

4. *Members help others to develop*: Because all members will not be equally skilled in understanding and participating, it is important that all the members help in everyone's development. It is not only the leader's job to see that this happens: every member must see to the development and growth of the others.

5. *Projects are circle efforts, not individual efforts*: A QC is a group, a team effort. Everything a circle does should be done as a team. The projects chosen should be of interest and value to all of the members. The circle as a whole should receive recognition for any achievements it has accomplished.

6. *Training is provided to workers and management*: It is not enough to turn the workers loose to find answers to their problems in an unstructured manner. They need to know effective techniques for doing this, or they will become frustrated with their ineptitude. Management must also receive training in the role they are to play—one of support, not domination.

7. *Creativity is encouraged:* A nonthreatening environment for ideas must be created. People will not risk suggesting a half-developed idea if they feel they may be ridiculed or rejected. From seemingly wild ideas often come practical solutions.

8. *Projects are related to members' work*: The projects that circles undertake need to have something to do with their work—not the work of others or non-work-related subjects. Members are experts at what they do, but not at what other people do.

9. *Management has to be supportive*: Unless someone in management is willing to give QCs some time, some advice, and some commitment in the beginning, they will not have the encouragement they need to grow and mature.

10. *Quality and improvement consciousness develop*: All of the above will be useless unless the steps result in an awareness on the part of members that they must be thinking always of procedures to improve quality and reduce errors.

11. *Reduction of the "we" and "they" mentality*: Each of us strives to make his or her job more creative and meaningful. Quality circles, when used correctly, help a company to reduce the "we and they" mentality of the employees. Since everyone (labor and management) is encouraged to participate in problem-solving, the feeling develops that the employees are all in it together and that it is up to each of them to try to produce products of the best quality.

Additional characteristics of QCs include a strong emphasis on training and development of individual members who usually are trained in group processes and problem-solving techniques. Information-sharing during the problem-solving phase usually is directly concerned with the problem being investigated. In most cases, management shares little information about operations, plans, or long-range objectives of the organization. Likewise, members do not receive direct monetary awards or benefit from cost savings; instead, symbolic rewards such as special recognition, hats, patches, and T-shirts are common rewards for their suggestions.

Leadership of the QC is usually not representative of management. A "facilitator" steers the QC during the start-up phase, until a team leader, usually a supervisor, is selected from the members. Most QCs have little or no authority over budgetary matters or organizational resources. They are structured to make recommendations; therefore, they are less threatening to management than other forms of employee involvement.

Often, QCs are mandated by top management. That is, an executive thinks using QCs is a good idea, and the idea is implemented.

Expectations

With these characteristics, what can one expect from QCs? In broad terms, one can expect better communication with management and with other working units, improved quality, and, to a lesser degree, greater productivity and group awareness, which result in a harmonious team-building atmosphere. For example, in a recent survey of hospitals using QCs, the following reasons were given as the initial attractions to the QC approach[2]:

- to improve the quality of patient care
- to increase productivity

- to increase morale and improve employee attitudes
- to refocus problem-solving activity
- to change or improve communication
- to support quality assurance activities
- to assist in recruitment and retention
- to identify the participative methodology for adoption
- to avoid unionization
- to decrease cost
- to increase employee involvement
- to improve the quality of work life
- to increase job satisfaction

Organizational Structure

Participative management is the basic premise underlying the QC concept. This implies employee involvement and an organizational structure that facilitates this process. Quality circles will not work if management opposes the idea or if the structural changes threaten administration. Because problems are to be solved by individuals directly involved, the structure of QCs must reflect this. The QC program overlays or parallels the existing hierarchical structure.

For an understanding of how this structure (Fig. 7-1) operates in a hospital or laboratory, an explanation of each structural component is necessary.

Steering Committee

The steering committee functions as a board of directors. It establishes policies on implementation and administration of the program. It also sets program objectives and resources and, in general, provides guidance and direction for the program. The steering committee selects a facilitator and meets regularly with him. The committee also attends management presentations. It is important that representatives of the major organizational functions be on the committee. If a union exists, representation should be solicited.

Facilitator

The facilitator is a key element in the success or failure of the program. This individual must have excellent human-relations skills. Ultimately, he conducts the training of team leaders and/or members. The background of this individual should reflect extensive organizational experience, and he should be trusted by both management and nonmanagement. Because the facilitator works closely with the steering committee, he should have the ability to communicate with a wide variety of individuals regardless of background or organizational status. Likewise, a facilitator should have administrative experience or interests, because he is responsible for the operation of the program. This implies recordkeeping, directing, evaluating, and other regular duties and responsibilities associated with implementing a project.

Teams

The teams are the backbone of the QC concept. After all, it is a team concept where the team identifies and solves its own problems. Team members are volunteers from a similar work area or department and usually number from 8 to 15 individuals. Rarely are all members of a work area involved; the supervisor or manager usually is not a member. Supervisors have been appointed team leaders, but the general feeling is that management should not determine membership, nor take a leadership position unless selected by the team's members. Experience indicates that a management-selected team with

FIGURE 7-1. Quality circle structure.

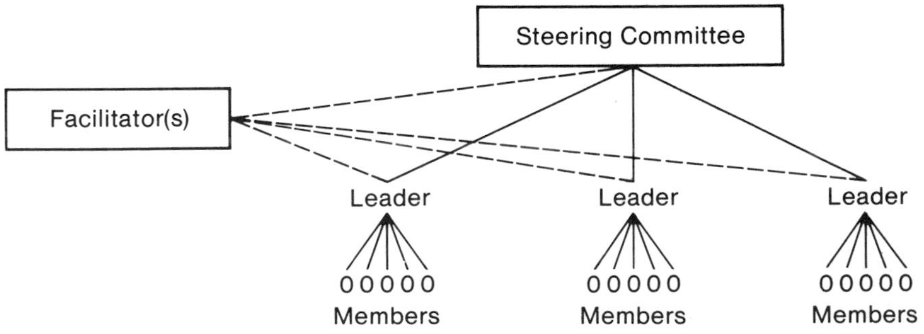

management-endorsed leadership resembles a "management" process that will solve "management" problems the way "management" wants them solved. From an employee viewpoint, this often is interpreted as another management technique to increase productivity at the workers' expense.

Initially, enthusiasm for the program results in oversubscribing. More employees want to be involved than the program can realistically handle. However, as the QC program matures, some circles cease to function and new ones emerge, so that everyone eventually has an opportunity to participate.

Team Leader

Because success hinges so dramatically on the group dynamics of a QC, the facilitator initially leads and helps the circle to establish itself. The facilitator trains the group in intragroup dynamics, in problem-solving, and in making presentations to the steering committee or management. After the QC is established, a team leader is selected from the team, and the facilitator becomes a liaison, linking the team to other teams and the steering committee. The leader is not in a traditional hierarchical power relationship with members. Rather, the role of the leader is to promote the team process, work closely with the facilitator, teach circle members QC techniques, and see that the goals of the team are accomplished.

A QC program does not compete with the existing administrative hierarchy. It parallels it but has no budget and can only make recommendations or suggestions. Therefore, the QC concept cannot work if it is not enthusiastically endorsed by upper and middle management.

Should We Introduce Quality Circles?

Before implementing a QC program, management first must determine whether this is the most desirable approach. It is difficult to suppress the program once QCs have been initiated. Circle members and nonmembers may interpret attempts at suppression as a form of administrative manipulation. Administration also should be aware that although the QCs have no budgetary responsibilities, the process does take time and is costly. The cost factor cannot be ignored, because QC teams meet on hospital or laboratory time (most teams meet 1 or 2 hours a week). Management should ponder the following points before implementing a QC program:

- Is the existing managerial style compatible with a participatory management philosophy that resembles the QC approach?
- Are the board of directors, top management, and middle management knowledgeable about the QC concept?
- What is the organizational history of previous programs (*e.g.,* management by objectives, cost containment, quality assurance, and hospitality training)?
- Is the organization willing to commit resources over the long-term tenure of the program?
- What is the organizational climate associated with employee morale, commitment, and flexibility regarding new programs?
- Will existing union(s) accept QCs?

This list is not exhaustive, and other factors may be more pertinent to the reader's situation. These factors do, however, highlight specific concerns that should be considered before hastily embarking on a QC program. For example, most hospital QC programs have been implemented by someone on the board of directors who was familiar with the concept. In some cases, the board members actually introduced and encouraged management to implement the program.[2]

Implementation

Once a decision to implement a QC program has been made, it must be carefully orchestrated. In Japan, the introduction of QCs was compatible with a culture stressing collective decision-making; in the United States, this is not the case. Some American organizations receive orders to implement QCs from top management. They are encouraged, cajoled, or sometimes even pointedly told to implement the program. Often the QC program is introduced into the American organization with the hope that it will influence the organizational culture and indirectly change the quality of work life. In fact, it takes on the trappings of an organizational development effort with all the claims of success that often are difficult to substantiate even after a period of several years. The claims of QCs are achievable, but it is a slow and arduous journey that demands planning and a culture receptive to implementation. For example, a QC program is not a panacea that will immediately erase a long history of strained management–employee relations. It can build new relationships that foster mutual problem-solving and trust between participants. For successful implementation, consider the following suggestions:

- Contain initial enthusiasm; be patient and let it evolve.
- Allocate sufficient resources to train; start with the board of directors and top administration and work downward.
- Provide an environment for open, honest, and positive communication.
- Reassure, train, and encourage middle management with regard to the merits of a quality circle program.
- Allocate sufficient financial resources.
- Publicize the program and its benefits.
- Keep the program voluntary.
- Plan for scheduling problems and solve them.
- Management expeditiously implements the acceptable recommendations of the circles.

In general, conditions for successfully sustaining a QC program hinge on organizational commitment and environment. In most cases, this means that the organization must make substantial efforts to educate organizational members about the QC concept. This implies that participants must have access to information that in the past was considered confidential—for example, information dealing with quality, cost, and output are essential. Furthermore, the organizational climate must support a cooperative atmosphere that encourages open communication, sharing of information, and a genuine feeling of cooperative problem-solving. Because some consultants would assert that this atmosphere is an end-result variable, the chicken-or-the-egg dilemma is an appropriate analogy: Without these conditions at the outset, implementation of the program is difficult; yet these conditions are the philosophic heart of a program, and that assures operation of the Pygmalion effect on the environment. In any case, management must support these conditions if the program is to succeed. These conditions reduce resistance to the program and allow implementation to proceed, usually in a sequential fashion, as in the displayed list opposite.

Training

Integral to a QC program is training. Enthusiasm alone will not do it. Because the QC concept relies on cooperative problem-solving, a major emphasis of any program is on the behavioral and technical skills associated with group dynamics. This includes interpersonal skills, group problem-solving, group leadership skills, and QC techniques. Quality circle

---

Sequential Implementation of a Quality Circles Program

- Disseminate QC material
  ▼
- Research similar situation using QC
  ▼
- Discuss with impacted parties, all levels of management, union, and employees
- Get outside help consultant
  ▼
- Establish steering committee
  ▼
- Identify baseline data points
  ▼
- Select facilitator
  ▼
- Develop implementation plan and secure approval
  ▼
- Develop or purchase training materials
  ▼
- Publicize program
  ▼
- Train management, staff, and circle leaders
  ▼
- Start several pilot circles
  ▼
- Train participants
  ▼
- Shepherd pilot circle(s) to assure successful outcomes
  ▼
- Review and circulate pilot circles
  ▼
- Expand program and evaluate

---

techniques may include instruction in how to collect data, select and utilize sampling techniques, draw histograms and scatter diagrams, understand Pareto analysis and stratification theory, develop cause and effect diagrams, and construct control graphs. They also include training in making presentations to top management and fundamentals of conducting meetings and keeping minutes.

Pitfalls and Conclusions

The chief advantages of QCs are obvious. If implemented correctly, QC techniques can create major changes in employee attitudes and increase productivity and quality. However, they also can be costly, they require constant management vigilance, and they can deteriorate into a program identified more with management than with employees. In union situations, a QC program can be criticized as having co-opted the union, reducing employees' influence over their work situation. A possible solution is a modified approach to employee involvement, QWL programs.

THE QUALITY OF WORK LIFE APPROACH

The second major employee involvement approach is the QWL program. Although traditionally identified with manufacturing in the United States, QWL has been adopted by some service sectors in recent years. Its adoption and adaptation to a health-care environment seems feasible, and it is for that reason that this approach is presented here.

The primary difference between QWL programs and QC programs is the inclusion of the union as an active participant. Quality circle programs can function in a union environment and often have the endorsement and encouragement of the union. However, QCs do not significantly change or otherwise affect the traditional hierarchical structure and therefore never address the limited degree of involvement or power-sharing between management and labor, one of the major shortcomings of QCs. On the other hand, QWL programs attempt to increase employee prerogatives and feelings of empowerment through active union involvement.

The QWL movement is broader than that of QC. It has a greater impact on work life in general because it legitimizes its efforts through union participation. Quality of work life programs attempt to improve product quality or service, improve union–management relationships, and increase employee involvement. Most QWL programs have a structure similar to that of QC approaches, relying on problem-solving groups. However, the presence of a union introduces an extra dimension in traditional management problem-solving methods. Ordinarily, the traditionally adversarial collective bargaining relationship holds certain issues sacrosanct. Therefore, both union and management decide at the outset of QWL implementation which issues are untouchable. Usually, both sides agree that the collective bargaining contract remains in place, and management usually allows certain issues that traditionally were within the province of management to be addressed by the problem-solving teams. Gener-

ally, then, a QWL approach permits organizational problems to be divided into three groups, the three-legged stool of collective bargaining, management authority, and joint problem-solving (Fig. 7-2).

Objectives

As depicted by the three-legged stool analogy, such an arrangement tends to categorize questions into collective bargaining (union) problems, management problems, or joint problems, representing each constituency's objectives. In reality, the objectives overlap, for the same people involved in the collective bargaining process also participate in the joint problem-solving (QWL) process. Each has entered the process with an objective, to reduce the adversarial relationship existing among the parties, to gain popular support, to increase influence in changing the work environment, or to increase productivity or quality performance. Usually the broad objectives of the process are written as a mutual contract.

Memorandum of Agreement

Because the QWL process will change the traditional way of deciding and implementing change in the organization, the union and management negotiate an agreement that defines the objectives and boundaries of the process. Such an agreement may include the following items:

- Participation is voluntary.
- Objectives are to improve the quality of work life (that may range from a better work environment for employees to greater performance in quality and productivity).
- Collective bargaining issues will not be addressed.
- Employee attitudes and morale will improve.
- Jobs will be secured (through no layoffs) because of increased productivity or quality.
- Both sides will have the right to withdraw from the agreement.

Organizational Structure

The organizational structure resembles that of QC programs. Like QCs, the QWL structure parallels and complements the traditional hierarchical structure. Steering committees are established, facilitators or coordinators are selected and trained, and

Organizational Problems

Collective bargaining	Management authority	Joint problem solving

Win/Lose Outcome	Act/React Outcome	Win/Win Outcome

Problems	Problems	Problems
Contract items	Capital investment	Quality
Wages	Quality control	Production
Grievances	Affirmative action	Alcohol/drugs
Overtime	Engineering	Work methods
Seniority		Layoffs

FIGURE 7-2.   The three-legged stool.

work teams are established. Although the QWL program's structure superficially resembles a QC program, the fundamental difference is *power*. The authority of a QWL program to implement suggestions and to influence outcomes is dramatically enhanced through the participation and legitimization of the union. The union is represented on the steering committee and in the role of the facilitator. The union comprises 50% of the steering committee membership and has equal representation in the position of facilitator; usually, one facilitator is selected by the union and one by management. Because union officers frequently are members of the steering committee and facilitators are highly visible personalities with well-developed human-relations skills and generally accepted by all parties involved, the participants have a greater stake in assuring the implementation of problem-solving suggestions. This mutual interaction of the union and management results in greater awareness of problems facing the organization and may lead to mutual trust as the process expands and is established throughout the organization. Work-team attitudes should progress from the adversarial win/lose atmosphere to a cooperative outlook that fosters win/win solutions (Fig. 7-3).

Implementation and Training

The implementation process relies heavily on training. In fact, the intervention strategy most clearly identified with the QWL process is training, which takes two forms: (1) awareness training, which highlights the conceptual background and the need for the program; and (2) training in interpersonal relations and problem-solving skills, focusing on the QWL team. Training, by outside consultants and by the coordinators, provides the structure that allows the change process to take place. The awareness phase facilitates unfreezing of traditional attitudes. Team training for interpersonal-relations and problem-solving skills encourages experimentation with the QWL concept. The positive outcomes experienced by work teams reinforces new attitudes about the process and the two collaborating parties, management and the union.

Examination of the training sequence and the progressive sequential implementation of the QWL process suggests three distinct, yet interrelated training packages are appropriate (Fig. 7-4). Initially, management and labor must be brought together, preferably off-site, to familiarize themselves with the concept and to attempt to create cohesion

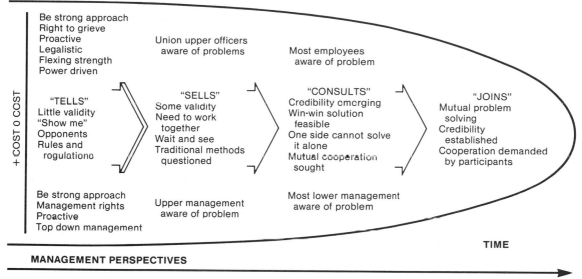

UNION PERSPECTIVE

FIGURE 7-3. Attitudinal evolution of quality of work life (QWL) teams. (From Schaupp D, Elkin R: A model of communicating employee responsibility through labor-management participation teams in an organization in financial difficulty. In Chimezie AB, Osigweh Y [eds]: Communicating Employee Responsibilities and Rights, p 183. New York, Quorum Books, 1987)

between the two parties. The result of this meeting is a joint mission statement of commitment to the concept. Once the mission statement (memorandum of agreement) is completed, the parties select a steering committee with equal representation from both sides. Training is designed to help the steering committee set policy and function as a board of directors for the program. Usually the steering committee is composed of members who represent the leadership of the company and the union, so that the need for training in policy formulation and implementation is minimized. Both groups are already familiar with that process. However, they usually are unfamiliar with joint problem-solving techniques, and this becomes a major element of their training. At this stage, coordinators are usually selected, who attend the steering committee training. Finally, after the pilot teams have been identified, they are trained in group problem-solving skills.

The role of the consultant is very much in evidence during the start-up phase of the program. The initial awareness session and training of the steering committee are usually conducted by an outside con-

sultant. Experience suggests that the two coordinators should conduct the initial QWL training in conjunction with the consultant. This "train the trainers" exercise is a significant factor in arresting any fears the coordinators might have regarding their impending role as trainers. Once pilot groups are in place, the coordinators monitor and evaluate their progress. Initial problems are selected that are relatively easy and solvable, to help ensure initial positive outcomes. Thus encouraged, the pilot groups provide internal endorsement of the process and function as catalysts for further implementation.

Training Content and Mechanics

A salient objective of QWL teams is to bring decision making about work-related problems directly to the laboratory or worksite. Because this decision-making style is probably unfamiliar to most participants, training must include acceptance of the concept, the skills necessary to conduct joint problem-solving, and the techniques required to implement the problem's solution. Changing old behav-

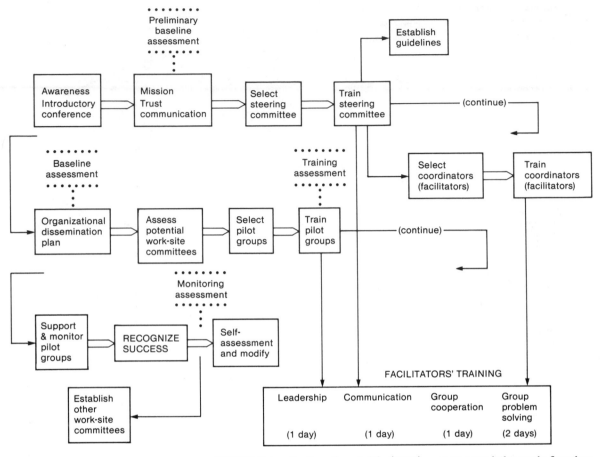

FIGURE 7-4. Quality of work life (QWL) commitment/pilot study flowchart.

iors and habits is difficult for most adult learners who are not accustomed to a classroom. Therefore, training attempts to integrate the QWL work-team concept with these broad guidelines:

- Examples must be job-specific.
- Conceptual ideas must be "discovered" by the participants to enhance ownership by the trainees.
- A lecture teaching format is minimized, and group activities are utilized wherever possible.
- Role playing, group involvement, and group discovery are emphasized.
- Skills are taught by utilizing an on-the-job training format.
- Off-site training is to be encouraged wherever possible.

With these training prescriptions, the process can be introduced with positive results. The training material is designed to minimize note taking by trainees and is structured to present the essential idea, yet allow for note taking should additional information evolve out of group discussion and/or "lecturettes." The objective is to create a feeling of ownership with the information that is discovered through the training process.

Pitfalls and Conclusions

Experience has shown that the sudden euphoria created by initial implementation success results in "backsliding" to more traditional attitudes about institutional training. Management especially tends to question the expected duration of training. Because most hospitals and institutions conduct training on organizational time, the cost can become problematic. The question often asked by administration is, "Can this process be reduced to 3 days or 2?" To accelerate the process, training often is much reduced in length and intensity over time—in some instances by almost 50% in the first 6 months of implementation.

Management is aware of the "opportunity cost" associated with training and unfortunately sometimes is seduced by actions suggesting short-term cost containment at the expense of long-term survival. On the basis of our experience, training still seems to be relegated to specific job-related skills training that stresses "how" instead of "why" things happen as they do in an organization.

Initial success also breeds complacency. Both parties sometimes lose sight of the fact that the QWL process, to be fully implemented in an organization with 700 employees, may take a minimum of 2 years. Both sides desire immediate improvement based on their own time agenda and criteria. Experience has shown that the organization will have a greater chance for success if it retains an outside consultant who intervenes periodically to provide guidance and encouragement.

Overall, the feeling seems to be that the very least to be expected is significant improvement in communication through sharing of information. Some units experienced significant cost reductions, increase in morale, and noticeable changes in behavior, suggesting that collaboration occurs in a win/win atmosphere that benefits both sides for long- and short-term survival.

AUTONOMOUS WORK TEAMS

The third and final high-involvement team approach results in problem-solving groups that have significantly greater influence over their work environment than permitted by either QC or QWL programs. Although varied levels and degrees of employee prerogatives exist in the management of problem-solving teams, this approach stresses a philosophy that goes beyond a human resources viewpoint presently practiced by participation-oriented organizations.

Autonomous work groups or teams, as a management approach, strive to push knowledge, power, information, and extrinsic rewards to the lowest level of the organization. It is believed that this will increase productivity, employee commitment, and satisfaction. It is assumed that people can

be trusted to make important decisions about their work, that their skills in making these decisions can be developed, and that greater organizational effectiveness will result.

Although most laboratory managers would agree with—and even identify with—these assumptions, autonomous work groups formalize them through an organizational structure that complements its philosophic base. At present, the authors know of no formal study or organization that has implemented this approach in the health-care sector. However, it appears to be a powerful alternative to present-day management practices. Autonomous work groups seem a natural extension of group problem-solving approaches already used in an informal manner in laboratory settings. Variations of this model are used throughout the United States in manufacturing and service industries, with generally impressive results. Unfortunately, little has been written about their use, and even less is known about them in the health-care environment.

As described by Edward E. Lawler III,[1] autonomous work groups are a radical departure from traditional management hierarchies but still fit philosophically with laboratory managers who practice participative management. This method is egalitarian in the sense that it attempts to give important decision-making powers to the individuals directly associated with a task. This means giving as much control as possible to individual work teams that determine almost all boundaries and objectives associated with the task.

A major tenet of this approach is that the team should have some voice in the selection of members, the arrangement of work flow, the establishment of standards for evaluation, and the supervision of quality control and productivity. As much as possible is delegated to the work teams. The teams are entrusted with responsibility to accomplish the activity or group of activities. This means that the teams are responsible for production goals, quality, purchasing, control of absenteeism, and job rotation. Although the limits and goals may change from team to team, responsibility for getting the job done rests with each team.

Structural Considerations

Because a philosophic underpinning of this approach is that work should be satisfying, challenging, and motivating, team members are cross-trained for all jobs under its authority. The thinking behind cross-training is that it allows mixing interesting jobs with routine ones and thus creates greater job flexibility. It instills responsibility not only for a specific job, but also for more broadly defined undertakings.

The work team concept is further reinforced by a compensation structure that is skill-based. Although all employees start at the base level of pay (for newly established units), they progress to higher levels of pay on the basis of skills acquired through cross-training. In some teams, for example, team members set standards for appraisal and actually evaluate their co-workers. Usually, all participants are salaried, and the team concept is strongly encouraged. For work teams to function properly, individuals require the knowledge of more than one job.

Management

What happens to management? Management survives in a modified form. The management hierarchy is flattened as much as possible. In some organizations, work teams report directly to the unit or divisional manager. In other situations, the first-line supervisor is eliminated and a key individual is selected by the team to maintain relationships with other, lateral units or functional groups. Naturally, the work area and the tasks themselves ultimately determine the limitations of the team's managerial prerogatives.

Management personnel develop a strongly egalitarian philosophy that extends beyond decision-making and the work task. In many of the newer organizations utilizing a team approach, egalitarian principles are reflected in the physical facilities, dress, parking, organizational benefits, and dining facilities. Individual managers are encouraged to think in terms of organizational effectiveness and less as functional heads.

Likewise, the staff often is greatly reduced. Because autonomous groups take on many of the duties of traditional staff members such as scheduling, purchasing, and inventory control, their function often is absorbed by the team. Not all staff roles are eliminated, but many become consultants to and trainers of teams, rather than decision-makers. Increased training is encouraged, not only cross-training to master job-related activities, but also training to aid in self-development and career planning. Off-the-job training also is encouraged and supported.

Although there is no exemplary model that addresses all dimensions and problems encountered by autonomous work teams, the preceding description depicts what is happening in the United States.

A more definitive model must be fleshed out at a later date, because there is as yet no perfect plan.

Pitfalls and Conclusions

As with most innovative approaches, potential problems and pitfalls are abundant in autonomous teams. A major problem often occurs with employee expectations: How much participation can be allowed? When does participation turn into permissiveness? What happens to individuals who do not fit into the team concept? What role should key individuals accept as pseudo-supervisors? Because the team concept relies heavily on team participation and an understanding of group dynamics, how does an organization handle personnel unable or unwilling to learn interpersonal skills? These questions have not been answered; yet all the evidence suggests that organizations that have begun autonomous work teams also have expanded the program to include other teams. A shortcoming in this area of management research is the scarcity of data surrounding the whole process. Preliminary data suggest that productivity gains have been quite remarkable with the use of this approach, and the scarcity of data can be interpreted as an endorsement of the team structure. Most work team organizations, it is speculated, want to retain their own competitive edge and therefore are reluctant to share their successes at this time.

CONCLUSIONS AND SUMMARY

The overwhelming trend in management in the United States indicates a wholesale adaptation of some form of employee-involvement work groups. Although the health-care industry has only recently experimented with QC programs, QWL and autonomous work group approaches seem compatible with health-care goals and existing managerial structures. Considering the industry's recent cost-containment emphasis and the general shift to a more competitive environment for clients and services, the health-care industry should seriously consider these approaches to enhance organizational effectiveness and long-run survival.

Depending on existing organizational parameters, managerial philosophy, and employee managerial relationships, one of the three approaches is feasible (Fig. 7-5). Regardless of which approach is selected, enhanced employee satisfaction and morale are the universal outcomes. Increased produc-

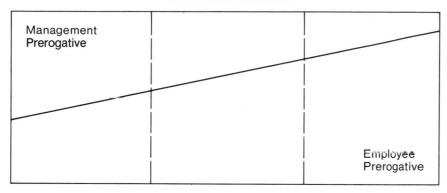

FIGURE 7-5. Employee involvement work groups. (Adapted from Lawler EE III: High-Involvement Management. San Francisco, Jossey-Bass, 1986)

tivity, better quality control, lower absenteeism, and lower turnover often accompany improved satisfaction and morale. The degree to which management is willing to empower its employees with managing their work environment determines which approach is selected. The techniques are available. It is up to management to utilize them for mutual employee–management gain.

REFERENCES

1. Lawler EE III: High Involvement Management. San Francisco, Jossey-Bass, 1986
2. Orlikoff JE: Quality Circles in the Health Care Setting, pp 41–42. Chicago, American Hospital Association, 1982
3. Rieker WS: Tapping the creative power of the work force. In Quality Control Circles. W. S. Rieker, Inc., 1978. In Ingle S. Quality Circles Master Guide, pp 4–5. Englewood Cliffs, Prentice-Hall, 1982

ANNOTATED BIBLIOGRAPHY

Barra R: Putting Quality Circles to Work. New York, McGraw-Hill, 1983
    Very practical, very basic. Excellent first source for getting acquainted.
Goldberg AM, Pegels CC: Quality Circles in Health Care. Rockville, Aspen, 1984
    Excellent quality circle source for health-care settings. Generally basic and to the point.
Ingle S: Quality Circles Master Guide. Englewood Cliffs, Prentice-Hall, 1982
    Industrial orientation, but excellent "how to" approach for actually implementing a quality circles program.
Kregoski R, Scott B: Quality Circles. Chicago, Dartnell Corp, 1982
    Excellent source for training materials. Basic, practical approach that leads you by the hand through the quality circles implementation process.
Lawler EE III: High-Involvement Management. San Francisco, Jossey-Bass, 1986
    Excellent source for up-to-date analysis and research findings on high-involvement groups. Probably best single reference source, although not a "cookbook" or "how to" manual.

eight

Authority and Delegation

Arthur L. Larsen
Arden E. Larsen

SOURCES OF AUTHORITY

If you are a supervisor who is never ill, never takes a vacation, is available to handle laboratory problems 24 hours a day, and is an expert in all areas of the clinical laboratory, this chapter is not for you. Delegation is an activity from which you would derive no benefit. On the other hand, if you are a supervisor with twice as much work to do as time available, this chapter may provide you with some valuable help.

Before we can address the subject of delegation, we have to consider the source that enables us to delegate, namely authority. We all accept the fact of authority blindly. Our parents had authority over us when we were children; our teachers had authority over us in school. Certainly, our boss holds authority over us. But where does this authority come from, and how extensive is it?

In an organization, there is an ultimate source of authority. Not even the chief executive of a company is the final source of authority, because he is usually answerable to a board of directors and a group of stockholders. In most instances, the real source of authority is probably the person or group who makes an activity financially feasible.

If monetary support is the foundation of authority, one can see that every supervisor in an organizational hierarchy has only limited authority, and that authority is exerted over a limited number of subordinates. In the medical laboratory, authority is also curtailed by government regulations, hospital poli-cies, certifying and accrediting agencies, and some-times union rules. However, a supervisor can dele-gate his authority to those below him.

TYPES OF AUTHORITY

Authority can take many guises, depending on the leadership style of the supervisor. Some of the more common ways of exercising authority are despotic-ally, in which a supervisor is autocratic and does not consult his subordinates; paternally, in which the supervisor treats the subordinates with kindness but little respect; and collaterally, in which authority is shared between superior and subordinates both ver-tically and horizontally.

An example of how these types of authority might be exercised is shown in the following exam-ple: A scheduling problem over Christmas holidays arises. An autocratic supervisor arbitrarily assigns technologists to cover the emergency; a paternalis-tic supervisor simply assumes the extra workload himself; and a collateral supervisor discusses the problem with the technologists involved, and some reasonable solution is achieved.

All three supervisors accomplished the goal of laboratory coverage; all exercised their authority. However, the degree of long-term success in each instance is probably not equal. The third supervisor accomplished the organizational goals while at-tempting to achieve a satisfactory realization of his own personal goals and those of his subordinates.

DELEGATION

Delegation can be defined as the transfer of authority to another person to accomplish a specific finite goal under carefully defined conditions. Delegation is actually an entrusting of authority to another person, usually a subordinate whose position in the organization would not ordinarily allow him to possess that degree of authority. The authority delegated has clearly demarcated limits and is applicable to a specifically circumscribed area.

Reasons for Delegation

Delegation can accomplish a specific aim more efficiently, make a manager's job easier, and help him to achieve full realization of the potential of his authority. If the laboratory is expected to be represented at the Tissue and Transfusion Committee meeting, the blood bank technologist can address the current problems more efficiently than a chief technologist who is not involved in the day-to-day details of interacting with surgery, the emergency room, and the nursing staff with regard to transfusion policies. Personnel with appropriate expertise should be asked to accomplish the delegated task. In cases like this, delegation is common sense.

Another reason for delegation is to free the laboratory manager from specific details in order to permit the coordination of the efforts of subordinates to whom authority has been delegated. For instance, when the clinical laboratory orders and reports, each major area has its own set of problems. How can microbiology delay a report for 48 hours until the culture can be read out? How can the computer handle a type-and-hold order for the blood bank? How can the computer alert the chemistry laboratory to collect a timed specimen? If it is the responsibility of the administrative technologist to see that the laboratory becomes computerized, he can accomplish that goal by delegating to the head of each section the responsibility and the authority to work out the problems relative to his section. The administrative technologist then coordinates all efforts, dovetailing suggestions and integrating common policies for the total laboratory. If he spends his time tackling the details specific to each section, the laboratory will never become computerized. So another important reason for delegation is to give a manager the time and opportunity to coordinate smaller segments of a large project.

In terms of long-range benefits, the most important reason for delegation is *personnel development.* Supervisors don't just happen. They must be nurtured in an appropriate environment, and future supervisors come from current subordinates who are allowed to grow and develop. Properly encouraged, subordinates are ready and able to step into supervisory roles when such positions became available. Subordinates to whom authority for specific activities has been delegated are also more satisfied employees, because they have input into the overall work organization and they develop an enhanced self-image. With the concept of personnel development in mind, it is evident that not only unchallenging or unrewarding tasks should be delegated. Subordinates deserve the opportunity to become involved in exciting developmental activities and not merely in drudgery and details.

How to Delegate

If delegation is to make managers more productive and efficient, they should begin by analyzing their activities in order to see what aspects of their jobs can and should be delegated. Breaking down their jobs into components enables them to envision which of their subordinates can presently handle which parts of the job and to decide which employees could be trained to assume those responsibilities.

Routine details that recur frequently in the job can easily be delegated, as can minor decisions that must be made on daily matters. Those job details that take the most time, such as meetings, filling out reports, keeping inventory, filing quality control data, making out schedules, and so forth, can often be at least partially delegated. Similarly, those parts of the job that the manager feels least qualified to handle from the standpoint of technical skills should be delegated.

Unfortunately, delegating responsibility is not as easy as saying, "Here, you do it." There are certain ground rules and refinements that must be followed.

First, a manager should have in mind a broad outline of the overall job he expects to accomplish, both through his own efforts and the efforts of those to whom he has delegated responsibility. For example, he intends to develop a quality control program for the laboratory. Included in this program will be internal and external check samples, daily statistical analysis of precision and accuracy, checks of purity of reagents, development of an assayed serum pool, records of instrument maintenance and function checks, and so on. The overall objective is to develop a quality control program, and the manager has firmly fixed in his mind what components of the program are required and what degree of excellence these components are expected to reach. However, it is not necessary to explain in detail the overall program to the person who has the responsibility for checking the calibration of automatic pipettes. The pipette-checker needs to know only that part of the program specifically relating to his responsibility. In this instance he is delegated the responsibility to check pipettes within stated limits of accuracy. He is told the frequency with which the checking is to be done and the records that must be kept. He also is given the authority to retire from use any pipette that does not meet the predetermined criteria.

To reiterate, then, the manager has an overall outline, but the delegate is given a specific goal with specific restrictions.

In delegating, the manager must establish with his designee the resources available to accomplish the goal desired. What equipment is available? What personnel? How much money? How much time may he take from his routine duties to accomplish the special job delegated? These conditions must be clearly delineated at the outset.

Any delegated job must carry with it a time reference. A reasonable period for the accomplishment of the task must be estimated and a deadline set. This deadline may have to be revised as unforeseen circumstances occur, but at least it is a goal. A manager who delegates many specific tasks might

like to develop a standard form (Table 8-1) of which both he and the delegate should have a copy. If the manager prefers a less formal approach, he should note on his calendar the appropriate deadline so that he can check on the progress of the project when that day approaches.

How does a manager choose his delegates? The fortunate supervisor has a number of potential delegates from whom to select, and a good supervisor knows his people well enough to be able to select the best one for a given job. The supervisor should be able to evaluate the strengths and weaknesses of potential designees, both in terms of technical competence and personality traits. However, the supervisor must avoid the unconscious habit of always selecting the same employee for a delegated job. Sometimes the brightest, most eager person seems the logical choice, but other employees may become jealous and lose motivation if delegation is not equitably distributed. For example, when a teaching position became available in the chemistry section of a large hospital laboratory, the person with the most experience as a chemist was not the one best qualified to teach. The wise supervisor delegated the teaching responsibility to a technologist who enjoyed working with students and who had a real talent for explaining theory and principles of tests, even though that technologist was not the quickest technical worker.

Whenever possible, the person selected as a

Table 8-1
Suggested Form for Monitoring Delegated Tasks

Date	Assignment	Assigned to	Special Conditions	Progress Report Due	Final Report Due
Aug. 15	Evaluate antiglobulin reagent from at least three suppliers. Consider titer, storage stability, sensitivity, shipping efficiency of manufacturer, ease of use and cost. Recommend the product that best fulfills criteria.	J. Brown	Cost not to exceed $50.	Oct. 1	Nov. 1

delegate should be asked if he is willing to accept that responsibility. Delegation grudgingly accepted usually leads to mediocre performance. If it is not possible to offer the delegate an option, then he should be told why he has been chosen to carry out the delegated job and why he cannot be offered the choice of acceptance or rejection of the assignment. For example, in one hospital, illness left the serology department without a supervisor for several months. However, the supervisor was expected to return upon recovery; so the position was not filled with a replacement. The Director of Laboratories delegated the responsibility of the serology department to the supervisor of the immunology section in the interim. Delegation to the immunology supervisor was the only logical solution to the problem, and no other option was available. The immunology supervisor recognized the situation and accepted the delegated assignment.

As employees handle delegation, they can be entrusted with larger and larger degrees of responsibility. Employees are developed by being given delegation in easy stages. A good manager evaluates how well an employee performs a delegated job and keeps that performance in mind for subsequent delegation.

Delegation as a Contract

A contract implies an agreement, and that is exactly what the manager and delegate must do: agree. They must agree upon a mutually understood goal and an end-point of the project. Both parties must have the same understanding of the end-result of the delegated responsibility. For example, a director of laboratories expects his administrative technologist to develop a system for inventory control. His understanding of an efficient, workable system in terms of adequacy of stocking for contingencies, most economical purchasing policies, minimum reagent outdating, and optimal reagent quality must not contradict the technologist's understanding of ease of reordering, space for stocking, and convenience of dispensing. The end-point of the inventory control program must be mutually agreed upon at the outset of the contract and looked at from the points of view of both parties.

Once a general agreement of the end-result has been achieved, the manager should ask the delegate to present in writing an initial plan for accomplishing the goal. This plan may be tentative and subject to revision, but it should provide a framework from which to work. If the plan is approved in essence, the delegate should be given the freedom to de-velop the detail. If the manager has fundamental reservations about parts of the plan, he should indicate clearly what parts of the plan are unacceptable and why and ask for contingency plans. This will prevent difficulties from developing later.

Definite intervals for review of the plan as it progresses should be set and mutually revised as necessary. The delegate should be given the freedom to develop details; his ideas may prove to be quite innovative. However, at the outset of the project, the limits of his authority must be set in terms of time, money, personnel, and resources.

If the project that has been delegated involves several sections, departments, or personnel areas, clearly establish at the beginning the appropriate channels of reporting. For example, the nursing staff has asked the laboratory to participate in their in-service education program by instructing new staff in specimen collection. This responsibility is delegated to the head of the phlebotomy service. At the time of delegation, the priorities should be established for approval of the instructional program developed by the phlebotomy supervisor. Must the manager approve the content first? Must the director of nurses be consulted, and before or after the manager's approval? Does the hospital's personnel department need to be involved for inclusion of in-service education information in employee files?

Having given the delegate freedom to develop the plan to accomplish the goal does not mean that the manager automatically abrogates responsibility for the project. He must be available for consultation when the delegate hits a snag outside the limits of his authority. In certain details he may need approval before he can proceed further, or he may wish an opinion on the advisability of several available options. Availability, however, should also imply preparedness, and a poorly thought-out answer to a question posed in the hallway may be a disservice to both manager and delegate. If consultation is necessary, an appointment at a mutually convenient time for discussion will generate the best results.

Keeping in mind that personnel development is one of the key reasons for delegation, the good manager will allow his delegate to make errors and learn from them. Often the supervisor can foresee that a projected action will not accomplish the desired goal, but he will wisely say nothing and allow the delegate to learn by results. Whenever the good of the organization is not jeopardized by such an attitude, and when the time and effort expended are in proportion to the benefits of the lesson learned, the delegate should be allowed to pursue a course of trial and error.

Once a delegated job has been accomplished, the good manager needs to follow through with his delegate. This includes giving credit to the delegate in person or publicly when indicated. It also includes the courtesy of explaining to the delegate his contribution to the overall achievement of a larger organizational goal. Realistically, employees also look forward to tangible rewards for a job well done.

Barriers to Effective Delegation

Once a delegation contract has been entered into, the manager must be able to "let go." He must allow the person to whom the contract was delegated to perform the assignment in the way he judges best. A manager cannot oversee, second-guess, nag, or change the course of action at every step. Once he has delegated a task, the manager must allow his delegate freedom to accomplish the objective. Otherwise, the whole premise of delegation is thwarted.

On the other hand, the manager has to make appropriate and reasonably quick decisions on material brought to him for review by the delegate. The delegate may not be able to proceed until a managerial decision is made, and delay can cause the entire project to be held up. The manager should understand this role in the encouragement of continued progress of the project. However, the manager must be wary of falling into the trap of eventually carrying through the entire project owing to the delegate's relying too heavily on the manager's judgments and decisions along the way.

To delegate an assignment effectively, the manager must be consistent in what he expects, when he expects it, and how well he expects it to be completed. His assessment of the priority of an assignment is conveyed to his delegate, and if the delegate senses the assignment to be a relatively low-priority item, the assignment usually is not completed promptly or well.

The manager must always follow through. He must never allow an assignment to fade away without a formal review of its status. He may dissolve the delegation contract if he desires, but he must not let the delegate think he has ignored or forgotten the assignment. Such an apparent (or real) attitude defeats the success of all future delegation to that individual.

Another barrier to successful future delegation is the failure of the manager to give credit to the delegate for a job well done. An expression of appreciation is in order to the delegate personally, and his contributions should be recognized publicly whenever appropriate. No one wants to work hard and well without recognition.

Another barrier to effective delegation is the selection of a delegate who is not appropriate for the job. Here the manager must decide which of the delegation objectives is most important: getting the job done or developing personnel. Depending on the priority of the delegated assignment, the manager has several choices: he can relieve the delegate of his assignment, he can work with the delegate to accomplish the goal, he can temporarily suspend the importance of the task's being accomplished, or he can give the delegate exceptional latitude to muddle through. Whichever course of action is chosen, it should be a careful decision, so that maximum achievement can be salvaged from an imperfect situation.

Special Problems of Delegation in the Clinical Laboratory

In order for a clinical laboratory to operate efficiently, a large and varied number of employees is necessary, each with his own authority and responsibility and each with a special talent, training, or expertise. The medical director of the laboratory delegates authority for the performance of laboratory tests to his supervisors and technologists, but the responsibility for the validity of those laboratory tests remains his. The medical director can delegate authority to his technologists to perform those duties for which they are qualified, but he cannot delegate to them authority to make medical decisions. For example, the blood bank supervisor is highly competent in erythrocyte antigen typing, antibody identification, and interpretation of the results of a crossmatch, but he does not have the authority to make a medical decision about whether a patient should receive a particular unit of blood. At times the lines of authority in a medical–technical situation are not clear, and there should be written guidelines in the laboratory policy manual outlining the division of authority. For instance, at what critical limits should a pathologist be notified to confer with the physician, as opposed to the technologist's transmitting the information to a floor nurse? Which emergency specimens must be reviewed by a pathologist and which by a technical supervisor? When can an apparently erroneous order by a physician be administratively changed and when must a change be approved by him?

Similarly, many hospital laboratories have clerical–receptionist staffs to accept orders and report laboratory tests. Lines of authority must be clearly understood between procedures that are merely clerical and those that have a bearing on the testing itself, such as scheduling timed specimens, handling stat orders, correcting reports, or advising on specimen collection and handling.

ANNOTATED BIBLIOGRAPHY

Clarke JR: Executive Power: How to Use it Effectively. Englewood Cliffs, Prentice–Hall, 1979
This source teaches recognition of power and explains how and why it works. It gives advice on team development and development of individual potential. It also shows how to increase productivity through subordinates by choosing good designees and lists rules for delegation and obstacles to effective delegation.
Laird DA, Laird EC: The Techniques of Delegating: How to Get Things Done Through Others. New York, McGraw–Hill, 1957
A practical text on the art of delegating, the book discusses when to delegate, how to delegate, how to choose the correct person, what not to delegate. Chapter 10 is especially helpful in analyzing aspects of a manager's job that can be delegated.
McConker DD: No-Nonsense Delegation. New York, American Management Association, 1974
This practical textbook discusses reasons for delegation, the roles of the delegator and delegatee, sources of authority, and evaluation of the effectiveness of delegation.
Sanzotta D: The Manager's Guide to Interpersonal Relations. New York, American Management Association, 1979
This source discusses legitimate authority and obedience, stresses knowing strengths and weaknesses of personnel, and using this knowledge for improving group relations; describes effectiveness of persuasion and influence in getting things done through others; and helps manager toward self-development as well as other-development.

nine

Conducting Effective Meetings

Janie Brown Crane

Within organizational settings meetings are essential to effective communication. Individuals must get together in order to function. They must share information, plan, solve problems, criticize, praise, make new decisions, and find out what went wrong with the old ones. The laboratory manager or supervisor who can conduct an effective meeting to further the objectives of the organization will be one step closer to becoming truly effective in his management and supervision

MEETING PURPOSES

A *meeting* can be defined as that which occurs when three or more persons get together with a leader to accomplish an objective. Meetings can be held for various reasons and with an equal variety of objectives. The departmental or staff meeting takes place when the chief calls his subordinates together to give them information, to solve a problem, to get information, to exchange ideas, or for a combination of these. The committee or task force, composed of a chairperson and members, meets to accomplish an objective. Training meetings are held for a leader to teach knowledge, skills, attitudes, or a combination of these to a group of students.

More than eleven million meetings are held every day in the United States. It is estimated that middle managers spend 35% of their time in meetings, while the figure for top managers is 50%. Seven to fifteen percent of personnel budgets is

spent on meetings, not including preparation time or training programs.

As one can see from these statistics, the meetings should play a significant role in attaining the organizational objectives as set forth. However, many persons will voice the opinion that group meetings are held too frequently, that they take too much time, and that they do not achieve results. In fact, on one survey of 50 hospital administrators, meetings were listed by 34 persons as timewasters and were ranked fourth overall in a list of the biggest time-wasters. (Meetings were listed right after telephone interruptions, drop-in visitors, and ineffective delegation![2])

To avoid these negative attitudes, the laboratory manager or supervisor would be wise to ask, "Is this meeting really necessary?" before proceeding to schedule one. Since laboratory meetings are usually held for the common purposes of information-giving, information-getting, problem-solving, attitude-creating, or instruction, one should first examine other communication alternatives. The dissemination of information to employees can be done in memo form. If the manager needs to gather information from employees, a questionnaire can be distributed to be returned to the manager, or information from individual employees can be solicited. For problem-solving, the manager can again present the problem in memo form and request written suggestions and opinions from individuals. Attitude-creating communication would be more difficult in the written form, but a well-worded explanation or "pep talk" on paper is possible. Instructional communication could be accomplished through individual study followed by written examination, with practical training given on an individual student basis.

By no means is it expected that an organization could do without meetings. However, alternatives to meetings are practical under many circumstances. If the manager employs appropriate alternative methods as feasible, meetings could be held less often. Those meetings that are held should be purposeful and necessary for objective accomplishment.

Meeting alternatives would not be wise choices whenever group face-to-face interaction is desired. If memos for information giving or getting require further explanation or the objectives cannot be easily understood, then a meeting should be held. Likewise, group interaction is often necessary for problem-solving. This is especially true if members of the group, perhaps representative employees, can help to solve the problem or are needed to carry out the solution. If the manager must sell an idea, a policy, or a decision that has already been made, then an attitude-creating meeting may be the most beneficial communication form. Instructional meetings have the obvious advantage of uniformity, which individual instruction would lack. Group interaction also can save the manager time because he will have to present the material and answer questions about it only once.

After the manager has answered yes to the question, Is this meeting really necessary? he can then proceed to ensure that it is a successful, effective one. By allowing an opportunity for interaction, meetings can build group cohesiveness and improve manager–employee relations while accomplishing the objectives.

PLANNING

The first and probably the most important step toward conducting effective meetings is planning. It is estimated that 50% of a meeting's effectiveness comes from the mental preparation of the person who wants to have the meeting and the physical preparations he makes.[3]

The manager must realize that there is a vast difference between simply *scheduling* a meeting and *planning* for that meeting. His role in planning includes establishing the objectives, selecting the participants, distributing the agenda, making the physical arrangements, and considering of the psychologic forces at wok in him and the participants.

It has been said that the better one understands that which he is trying to accomplish, the greater one's chances are of accomplishing it. Therefore, objectives should be clearly defined. "To look at overtime in the lab" should be rejected in favor of "To find a method of reducing overtime in the lab," if indeed it must be reduced. If the manager is holding an information-giving or information-getting meeting, he should state clearly that which he expects to be understood by the participants or received from them. "To have all participants understand the new dress code" would be better than "To explain the new dress code." Likewise, "To discuss possible causes of employee turnover" would not promote as much thought as "To have each participant contribute at least three possible causes of employee turnover for discussion." Whatever type of meeting the manager decides to hold, he should stay with his original objective. If participants are led to believe that they are making problem-solving decisions when actually the manager intends only to gather information to make his own independent decision, the participants will soon learn that the manager does not mean what he says and will become disillusioned with future meetings held by that manager.

Once the meeting objective(s) has been established, the manager must give careful consideration to who should attend, since often there is a direct connection between the participants in a meeting and the content and quality of decisions that come from it. If possible, all persons who must ultimately approve, accept, or implement a decision should be involved from the beginning in making that decision. Naturally, if the manager is holding a staff or departmental meeting, then all of the designated representatives should be asked to attend. However, when calling a meeting for a specific reason, the manager should hand-pick those whom he feels can accomplish the objective. There are several resource individuals who should be included. The person with all the facts is necessary. The idea man who can stimulate thinking and promote discussion is valuable, while the compromiser who is good at keeping the meeting on an even keel is an asset. Of course, the person who can approve the project because of his informal power should be included, as well as a key person who could be a barrier to the project. Representatives who could help sell the decision or project to others should also be included.

It is best if the manager can avoid surprise meetings. When possible, a 48-hour notice to the participants of when and where the meeting will be held, how long it will last, and why it is being held should be given. The distribution of the meeting's agenda at the time of notice will also improve meeting success. It must be noted here that objectives and agenda are not one and the same. Objectives are what is to be accomplished. The agenda consists of individual items to be discussed in consideration of the objectives. "Employee sick leave" would be the entry on the agenda with the objective clarified as "To find a method to reduce sick leave by 4 days/year/employee." The agenda items included at any one meeting should be related if possible and limited to fit into the designated time frame. When distributing the tentative agenda in advance, the manager may find it helpful to ask for comments or additions before the meeting and to request participants to think about the problem(s) beforehand. The meeting will be better if the participants as well as the manager are prepared.

The physical preparations for a meeting should receive more attention than is usually given to them. If participants are unhappy about the chosen time, if the room and the seating arrangements are uncomfortable, if the leader, chairman, or instructor cannot be easily seen or heard, then the meeting is off to a bad start with a dwindling chance of success. Making the physical preparations is just as much the manager's responsibility as establishing objectives. He can decide on the basic physical plan and delegate the footwork to someone else if there are many details to be handled.

The meeting should be scheduled at a time and place convenient for the participants. The manager may be free at 8:30 AM, but this may be a busy time for supervisors and others responsible for getting out the morning work. Therefore, the meeting should be held at a time when the participants are most likely to be relatively free of immediate obligations and can devote their full attention to the matters at hand. Also, the meeting place should be readily accessible. If it must be conducted at a place unfamiliar to the participants, the exact location and directions to get there should be provided.

Despite what many managers may think, the meeting room itself can be a critical factor. The room selected should fit the participants and be conducive to the type of meeting being held. The room should not be cramped, nor should it be too large. Unfortunately, within the laboratory there may be only one or two choices of meeting places. For a special meeting the manager may find it worthwhile to obtain a more desirable room outside the laboratory or to rearrange one of the usual meeting places to make it more suitable. Movable partitions or blackboards can be used to reduce the feeling of a too-large room, and chairs can be rearranged and tables removed from a too-small room. For an information-giving or instructional meeting, chairs should be arranged so that all participants can easily see and hear the leader. A semicircle or U-shaped arrangement with the leader seated or standing at the edge of the open area is appropriate for information-getting and problem-solving meetings. (This also allows participants to see notes as they are written on the board by the recorder, as will be discussed later.)

The meeting room should be adequately ventilated for avoiding stuffiness and lingering cigarette smoke. If ventilation is not possible and the meeting will run longer than an hour, short breaks should be permitted. Breaks during long meetings allow participants to get some fresh air and give them a chance to collect their thoughts before the next phase of the meeting. Lighting should be adequate for seeing visual aids and note-taking. A dark room may put people to sleep or at least hamper their ability to contribute and understand the material. The area should not be noisy. Extraneous conversations or noise from outside the room would definitely be distracting.

Visual aids may be beneficial to objective accomplishment. It has been noted that people retain about 10% of what is heard and 20% of what is seen, but about 50% of what is both heard and seen.[1] The manager must remember, however, that aids are merely carrier devices for presenting ideas more effectively, and he should not rely on them exclusively for making important points. If he employs a visual aid, it should convey only one idea so that participants can keep their focus on the topic under discussion and not on the aid itself.

Just prior to meeting time, the manager or his designee should check to make sure the physical preparations are complete. Electrical outlets for projectors and microphones should be tested, and lighting and seating arrangements should be checked. If needed, chalk for use at the blackboard, marking pens and paper for the recorder, and handouts should be ready. A meeting that is delayed or hampered because of the physical factors is likely to produce less than optimum results.

Finally, after the manager has completed his mental preparation and has made all of the physical arrangements, he should examine his psychologic forces that will influence the progress and outcome of the meeting. This may be the most difficult aspect of planning, but a necessary one, especially for problem-solving and attitude-creating meetings. If the manager is aware of and has given consideration to the hidden agendas at work in himself and the participants, his chances of conducting the meeting effectively will improve. The psychologic forces that determine a person's behavior deserve more attention than can be given here; however, they will be briefly discussed to help the manager understand the attitudes displayed and the positions expressed at a meeting.

An individual's hidden agendas are composed of his external and internal pressures (Fig. 9-1). Pressure is not used here in the negative sense, but as a feeling that has an impact on the group and its ideas. External pressures may be groups to which one is affiliated, such as unions, social organizations, or political groups; past commitments made that have an effect on current behavior; personal life forces; and forces that exist because of the person's relationship with the organization. Internal pressures are generated by the individual's own goals and aspirations. An example of these hidden agendas at work would be the different reactions of two participants to the problem of excessive overtime in the laboratory. One person might defend overtime on the basis of its necessity to provide proper patient service, when subconsciously he is concerned about his personal loss of income needed to support his family. On the other hand, another person might express beliefs that schedules and shifts could be rearranged to reduce overtime, when actually his concern is to protect his next-in-line position as a manager.

There is little the manager can do to control these hidden agendas in himself and in the meeting's participants. However, knowledge of the participants and awareness of the forces behind them will help the manager evaluate contributions made at meetings. Recognizing that everyone in the organization is influenced by a hidden agenda permits the manager to look beyond surface expressions or actions and to attempt to determine the motivations underlying them.

CONDUCTING THE MEETING

The manager should insist on prompt attendance and start the meeting on time. A delay in starting penalizes those who arrive on time and rewards latecomers. If staff meetings are known to start late, participants will soon stop coming on time, and more time will be wasted waiting for everyone to assemble. Interruptions other than extreme emergencies should not be allowed. If someone outside of the meeting can screen calls and take messages, the meeting will run more smoothly. When participants must come and go, it is distracting to others, and they must catch up on the discussion upon their return, usually by whispering with a neighbor.

Participants should arrive at the meeting with the initial attitude of enthusiasm. This eagerness should have been generated by the manager during the planning phase when he notified participants

FIGURE 9-1. Hidden agendas—factors influencing a participant's contribution in a meeting.

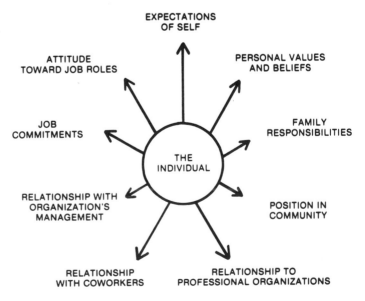

of the meeting and its purpose, but it will wain unless the manager is able to maintain it. His leadership style, which will be discussed separately, and his ability to maintain control of the meeting once he has involved the participants are important in keeping interest and enthusiasm.

The technique of conducting an effective meeting is essentially a technique of communication. In reference to this point, Benjamin Franklin is purported to have said, "If you state an opinion dogmatically, which is in direct opposition to my thought, and you imply no room for negotiation, then I must conclude in order to protect my own self-esteem that you are wrong, and I will immediately undertake to prove you wrong. On the other hand, if you state your opinion as a hypothesis, with evidence of a willingness to discuss and explore, I will like as not undertake to prove you correct."

The wise manager will keep this in mind not only for himself, but also for participant interaction. He should make each person feel that his ideas are welcome, that he is given credit for them, and even more importantly, that an occasional useless idea will not bring disgrace. The more opportunity participants have to incorporate their ideas and suggestions in a decision, the greater is their emotional ownership in it and the harder they will work to make it succeed.

As the manager begins the meeting, he should clearly define the objective(s) and the method the group should undertake for its accomplishment. It is extremely important here that he distinguished between *process,* how the problem is solved, and *content,* the problem and its solution. Once this is clearly established, the responsibility is still his to see that the meeting stays on track.

If he is looking for information or problem-solving, he must elicit free and creative suggestions from the participants. To do so, he should withhold criticism or comment, which might inhibit imaginative suggestions. He must also keep control of participant interaction to protect individuals from attack by others. If participants feel inhibited or that their ideas will be ridiculed, they will be less likely to contribute. When seeking information and involvement, it is better to use "overhead" questions so a volunteer can answer. The asking of direct questions should be used sparingly for avoiding embarrassment if the participant does not know the answer. The manager should not dominate the meeting or allow one participant to dominate the discussion, because other participants will become resentful. Wandering from the agenda should not be allowed. The manager should expect and demand adherence to it. He should also be aware of

and resist hidden agenda ploys. Socializing and allowing interruptions will cause the meeting to get off track. Unnecessary prolonging of a meeting causes participants to lose interest and hence should be avoided.

Although it is the manager's responsibility to stimulate and balance the discussion, this does not mean that he must discourage healthy differences of opinion. A certain degree of conflict can play a constructive and positive role in fostering creativity and innovation. Some friction between participants creates an atmosphere conducive to the generation of fresh ideas. A conflict-free group may be static and operate at considerably less than capacity.

The manager's aim in reaching the objective should be to obtain a win/win solution through consensus. If it becomes apparent to the group that consensus cannot be reached despite meaningful discussion, then a decision made by the manager will be accepted more readily. At the meeting's conclusion, the manager should restate the objectives, summarize the accomplishments, thank participants for their contribution, and give assignments and announcements if appropriate. It is important that the participants should leave feeling glad that they attended. They will be more likely to accept and react positively to the decisions made if they felt the meeting was worthwhile.

FOLLOW-UP

The manager's job in conducting a meeting does not end when the meeting itself is concluded. He must now provide a record of what happened, follow-up on decisions made, and evaluate the meeting so he can upgrade future ones.

A summary or minutes should be distributed if the manager wants the participants to have a record of decisions made and assignments given, if he needs to communicate with those who did not attend, or if the participants want a summary for their files or a clarification of what happened. The summary should state concisely what the decisions were, the assignments and deadlines made, and any unfinished business to be taken up at another meeting. It should be distributed within one day of the meeting while it is still fresh in the participants' minds.

The manager must follow-up to ensure that the decisions made are carried through. He should set deadlines for their implementation. Oftentimes decisions that involve policy changes or major operational changes will require another meeting to determine the implementation method, if time and resources did not permit that at the meeting where the decision was made. If assignments to individuals were made, he should request progress reports at set intervals to ensure timely implementation of decisions.

An evaluation of the meeting should be performed. The real importance of a meeting must be judged by the results obtained from it; therefore, a meeting that produces no results fails and probably should not have been held in the first place. Opinions differ as to what constitutes a "productive" meeting. One set of criteria by which to judge the meeting would be to ask, Were the objectives accomplished? Were they accomplished in minimum time? and Are the participants satisfied? If the objectives were not accomplished, the manager must investigate why. The information he obtains may help him to plan and improve the next meeting and better the chances of achieving objective accomplishment. If the meeting exceeded the established time limit, the manager must evaluate the process of the meeting. Maybe there were too many items on the agenda, or perhaps his ability to maintain control needs improvement. It is more difficult to judge the impact and significance of dissatisfied participants. The manager must try to assess why they were dissatisfied. Meetings that leave participants unhappy or frustrated about the decisions made might cause them not to attend future meetings, to decide the manager is ineffective, thereby affecting future relationships, or to carry negative attitudes and low morale back to their jobs. If in evaluating the meeting, the manager cannot say that the meeting accomplished its objectives in minimum time with satisfied participants, he should seriously review all phases of planning and conducting a meeting so that the same problems will not recur. Table 9-1 summarizes the most common hurdles the manager must overcome to turn nonproductive meetings into productive ones.

Table 9-1
Causes and Solutions to Nonproductive Meetings

Causes	Solutions
Before the meeting	
Lack of purpose	Hold meetings only when there is a definable, managerial purpose to be served in doing so.

Table 9-1 (continued)

Causes	Solutions
Participants do not want to come or are unprepared	Create enthusiasm—distribute agenda when giving notice; explain benefits of attendance; set convenient time and place in comfortable surroundings.
Lack of planning	Allow for and schedule appropriate planning.
Wrong participants	Include only those who are needed.
Not starting on time	Start on time
During the meeting	
Objectives unclear	Clarify objectives early in the meeting.
Participants disinterested, confused	Create enthusiasm—use understandable language; clarify as necessary.
Socializing, interruptions	Do not allow interruptions.
Wandering from agenda	Keep discussion under control.
Indecision	Keep objectives in mind and work toward them.
Too much time spent on each subject, meeting runs too long	Set realistic time limits; keep meeting moving.
No summary	Summarize so participants are clear about what is to happen.
After the meeting	
No minutes	Record and distribute minutes within one day.
Failure to follow up	Make assignments and check up on implementation.
Participants unhappy	Determine causes of dissatisfaction and correct for future meetings.
No meeting evaluation	Evaluate meeting to improve future ones.

AVOIDING NONPRODUCTIVE MEETINGS

Many of the solutions to causes of nonproductive meetings are straightforward and can be handled by the manager with practice once he recognizes their importance. Planning for the meeting is time-consuming but can be accomplished efficiently if the manager takes all of the planning factors into account. After the meeting, the manager should be able to follow through by distributing minutes and establishing a method for implementation of any decisions made. However, as is the case for managers of almost any group or organization, laboratory supervisors will probably find actually conducting the meeting to be their downfall. Conducting an effective meeting is easier said than done. For practical purposes, the concern here will be the problem-solving meeting, the one most likely to cause frustration in laboratory operations and employee relations.

Usually when a staff or special meeting is held, one or more entries on the agenda deals with a problem. Topics such as vacation coverage, physician overuse of stat requests, and technologists call-in policies are common examples. The typical way the problem is handled goes something like this:

Manager: As everyone knows, Sam *(the only night-shift tech)* is quitting at the end of the month. It will take at least six weeks to hire and orient a new tech. How do you propose we cover during the interim?

Supervisor 1: Maybe a tech from each dayshift section could rotate onto nights for a week at a time.

Supervisor 2: There's no way I can have someone from my section rotate onto nights. I'll be short-staffed because of vacations all summer as it is.

Evening Supervisor: *(getting off track)* I think we ought to hire two nightshift techs so we don't keep running into this problem every time someone on second or third shift quits.

At this typical meeting, potentially good ideas are immediately judged, found to be faulty in some way, and then dismissed. The person who contributed an idea feels that he has been personally attacked and is more likely to tear down another idea if it is suggested by the person who attacked his idea. The meeting can easily get off-track, good solutions can be ignored, and the meeting may end with the manager saying he will have to think about it. Participants leave not knowing what will happen,

and the final solution to the problem may be less than satisfactory to all concerned.

To avoid these problems and conduct an effective meeting, the manager should consider the New Interaction Method as described by Doyle and Straus.[1] It is a method by which several persons play roles that aid in separating the meeting process from its content, thus keeping the discussion focused on the objective. With this method, a facilitator is appointed who is neutral and nonevaluating. It is his job to make sure that participants use the most effective methods to accomplish their task in the shortest time. He helps the group decide on how they will solve the problem and then sees to it that they stay on track. It is also the facilitator's job to protect participants from being attacked by others. The group will need a short-term memory so everyone will record the same events in the same way. The recorder does this by writing the group memory on the blackboard or on large sheets of paper that are then posted on the wall in everyone's view. It is the manager/chairperson and participants' responsibility to make sure that the facilitator does not manipulate the group and that the recorder's record is kept accurately. The manager/chairperson should keep the group focused on the agenda, set realistic time limits, and be aware of the organizational constraints when it comes to making final decisions.

If this method is used, the meeting described earlier might go like this:

Manager: As everyone knows, Sam *(the only night-shift tech)* is quitting at the end of the month. It will take at least six weeks to hire and orient a new tech. We need to discuss how to cover during the interim. Facilitator, how do we begin?

Facilitator: We could try kicking out some ideas for the recorder to write down. After we have a list of ten, we could mix and match them and come up with a workable solution. Does everyone agree? *(Heads nod in agreement.)* OK, then, let's try to come up with the ten ideas in five minutes. Remember, no evaluation until the recorder has all ten down. Ready? Who's first?

Supervisor 1: Maybe a tech from each dayshift section could rotate onto nights for a week at a time *(Recorder busily writes down this idea.)*

Supervisor 2: *(jumping in)* There's no way I can have someone from my section rotate onto nights. I'll be short-staffed because of vacations all summer as it is.

Facilitator: Wait a minute, Number 2, you may have a valid point, but we'll discuss the feasibility of each idea after we have them all listed. Who's next?

Evening Supervisor: Overtime might be a possibility. Some techs on second shift have expressed interest in it.

Facilitator: OK. Anyone else? We need eight more ideas.

After the ten ideas are amassed, the feasibility of each idea is discussed. The manager inputs advice if a possible solution could not be contained within the budget, within legal limits, and so forth. Because the ideas are recorded first and discussed later, participants forget who suggested what idea, and rejection of an idea is not taken personally. Because they are all on visual display, ideas can be combined until a workable solution is found.

If during the meeting the facilitator or recorder wants to contribute as a participant, he can request of the manager to step out of his role temporarily, say what he has to say, and then go back to his role. Or, if available, the manager can have individuals not involved in the problem-solving play the roles of facilitator and recorder.

At the conclusion of the meeting, the manager summarizes the decisions and states what will happen next. He then proceeds as discussed earlier.

Portions of this imaginary meeting express another idea useful to the manager for problem-solving. Even if he does not choose to use the New Interaction Method in its entirety, brainstorming is a useful tool. *Brainstorming* is a technique of problem-solving in which a group of people gather together and contribute ideas spontaneously, hoping to find together the solution they could not find alone. Quantity of ideas is important, freewheeling is encouraged, and "piggybacking" (building on someone else's idea) is welcomed. Evaluation and judgment are reserved until all ideas are amassed.

In reality, brainstorming is difficult to practice. Because people are taught to immediately evaluate an idea, they hold back if they do not think their contribution will be accepted or if they feel they might be ridiculed. The manager may be able to overcome resistance to the brainstorming approach by having the group practice with an imaginary problem. He must be aware and keep participants aware that brainstorming does not solve the problem; it is only one step in the process.

EFFECTIVE LEADERSHIP

Most laboratory managers and supervisors are unschooled in communications. They have spent many years concentrating on the subject matter of their profession and have not had the time or opportunity to devote to developing communication skills. Also, many managers and supervisors have reached their present positions because of their technical abilities or their rapport with fellow workers and their supervisors. A person who can function well at the technical and production aspects of a job does not necessarily possess the attributes necessary to handle the managerial duties of his supervisory position. Suddenly, upon promotion or transfer from a staff technical position to a managerial/supervisory role, the individual is faced with problems and situations requiring good communication skills. It is no wonder that laboratory meetings held to give or get information, to solve problems, to give instruction, or to sell decisions already made may be less than effective.

Meeting success rests heavily upon effective leadership. In all meeting types, the leader (manager) has the same responsibility and accountability to conduct a productive meeting. He must be able to get things done through people. To do so he must adapt his leadership style to fit the type of meeting, which means he may need to change or modify it to make the meeting as fruitful as possible. To provide information, an autocratic-type style is necessary for presenting and explaining directives without receiving any feedback. When collecting information, the manager will need to share the leadership to increase participation and stimulate the group so that he can gather as much data as possible. For decision-making, the leadership is again shared because each participant's ideas are important to the final decision. Decision-selling is a combination of the above-mentioned characteristics: autocratic with regard to the decision but shared leadership with regard to carrying out the decision. Meetings held for problem-solving also involve shared leadership to use all resources available.

Another option for the manager to consider in leadership styles is to temporarily step down and allow someone else to chair the meeting if he has a stake in the decision. The conflict of running the meeting and having a personal stake in the outcome can lower participation and cause the process to control the content.

There are several basic "do's" and "don'ts" to effective meeting leadership. Some have been discussed already but merit reiteration. The Boy Scout motto, "Be Prepared," is of prime importance. Without proper planning there is no point in having the meeting. The manager should not bluff if he does not know the subject. Adequate research beforehand should alleviate this problem. Dominating the meeting discussion or allowing one participant to dominate will intimidate other participants, who will then be less likely to contribute. The manager should never appear to resent questions or comments or criticize individuals publicly. The impact of that type of behavior is evident. When giving technical information or holding a discussion with participants who do not know the background material, the manager must be sure to use language that is understandable. Maintaining tact while thwarting off-track discussions and side conversations will be beneficial to meeting progress. Finally, steering the participants to come to some positive conclusion so that they leave the meeting feeling that something has been accomplished is most important.

The more skillful one becomes at conducting meetings, the more critical one becomes of the meetings he attends. Therefore, the manager will find that effective leadership characteristics will be beneficial when he attends meetings as a participant. He should know why he was asked to participate and be prepared to the extent that he can. He should arrive on time, stay on the subject under discussion, and remain open to the ideas of others. The manager should be able to identify with the leader's role and therefore not cause problems for him. On the contrary, he should be able to help the leader maintain control of the meeting by using his own leadership skills. As a listener, taking notes during the meeting will force him to keep his mind on the topic, and he will be able to contribute more fully as a participant.

REFERENCES

1. Doyle M, Straus D: How to Make Meetings Work, The New Interaction Method, pp 4, 264. Ridgefield, Wyden Books, 1976
2. Kirkpatrick DL: How to Plan and Conduct Productive Business Meetings, p 29. Chicago, Dartnell Corporation, 1976
3. Lewis PV: Organizational Communications: The Essence of Effective Management, p 187. Columbus, Grid Inc, 1975

ANNOTATED BIBLIOGRAPHY

Auger BY: How to Run Better Business Meetings. Minnesota Mining and Manufacturing Company, 1972
> A very good source for basic reading on meetings. Focuses on the different meeting types and the factors influencing meeting quality.

Casella C: Training Exercises to Improve Interpersonal Relations in Health Care Organizations. Greenvale, Panel Publishers, 1977
> Chapter 1 deals with the individual in the group. A useful source for understanding why group members differ.

Doyle M, Straus D: How to Make Meetings Work, The New Interaction Method. Ridgefield, Wyden Books, 1976
> A very good approach to conducting effective meetings. Concepts require practice but are worthwhile. Designed mainly for task-oriented meetings of 3–30 persons.

Kast FE, Rosenzweig JE: Organization and Management: A Systems Approach. McGraw-Hill Series in Management. New York, McGraw-Hill, 1974
> Part Five, "The Psychosocial System," deals with communication and conflict in committees. A useful source for understanding communication patterns within the group.

Kirkpatrick DL: How to Plan and Conduct Productive Business Meetings. Chicago, Dartnell Corporation, 1976
> An excellent source for learning about the meeting process. The text goes into detail on almost every aspect of the meeting. Very good for managers and supervisors at all levels.

Knudson HR, Woodworth RT, Bell CH: Management: An Experiential Approach. New York, McGraw-Hill, 1973
> Exercise 5, "Invisible Committees," provides understandable information on the psychological forces at work in every individual. Useful in all management practices.

Lewis PV: Organizational Communications: The Essence of Effective Management. Columbus, Grid Inc, 1975
> Chapter 11 contains a concise overview of group meetings and a manager's conference checklist. Provides the basics for planning the meeting.

ten

Management of Conflict and Change

Dietrich L. Schaupp
Barbara L. Parsons

Recently a sage remarked that the only truism about change is that it is constant. The same could be said about conflict. Both change and conflict have consumed the minds of some of the world's great thinkers; yet a casual survey of writings on management indicates that much more remains to be said.

Contemporary writing on both change and conflict suggests that the process is still not totally understood. This chapter provides a general discussion of what recent writers think about change and conflict and how this information might be used in the workplace.

At the outset we make several assumptions:

1. Change and conflict are inevitable in normal organizational behavior.
2. Responsibility for initiating change and maintaining an acceptable level of conflict lies with the laboratory manager.
3. The laboratory manager works toward the goals of the organization.

We will look at change and conflict from management's perspective.

CHANGE AND CONFLICT ARE NATURAL

The assumption that change and conflict are inevitable suggests that they are a natural outgrowth of the managerial process. Regardless of hierarchical level or specialty, a manager must perform the basic functions of planning, organizing, staffing, directing, and controlling. He is expected to manage these functions and at the same time meet the organization's demands.

It is impossible to manage these functions without introducing change into the work environment. Change inevitably elicits some form of opposition, either from subordinates or from others directly or indirectly involved with the goals or objectives of the organization.

The novice manager often feels that the problems he faces are unique to his setting and situation. Although human relationships and the working environment do interact to create totally individual situations, the underlying causes and solutions to these problems are often very similar.

Once the manager realizes that change and conflict are a natural phenomenon in the management process, he can facilitate change and control

153

conflict with minimal disruption and opposition. The effective manager will integrate the needs and desires of subordinates with the goals and aims of the organization.

THE LABORATORY AS AN ORGANIZATIONAL ENTITY

The medical laboratory exists to provide a service. In general, its staff performs a variety of anatomic and pathologic services that range from routine medical procedures to highly complex research. Whatever its specific responsibilities, the laboratory provides a valuable diagnostic function in the health-care process.

Because the laboratory is an essential element of modern diagnostic and therapeutic hospital services, it is usually an important subunit of the hospital's organizational structure. A hospital is composed of a triad: the governing board (also called the board of trustees, board of directors, board of councillors, or some other variation), the administrator, and the medical staff. Authority is organized along two lines: administrative and professional.

The governing board provides overall objectives and legal responsibility for the institution, but it is removed from direct participation in hospital operation. Administrative authority extends from the governing board through the administrator to the various department heads. Department heads include the controller, housekeeping manager,

laundry manager, engineer, purchasing agent, and so on.

The administrator relinquishes authority for patient treatment to the medical staff. Functions associated with the medical staff include nursing service, pharmacy, pathology, social service, medical records, and food service.

The administrative side of a hospital deals with day-to-day survival of the institution, and the professional side deals with patient care and treatment. This is a simplified view of a hospital, and the structure may vary depending on size and objective, but even this superficial overview makes it readily apparent that the administration of a hospital is difficult and complex.

As Figure 10-1 illustrates, the hospital laboratory is only one subfunction of the organized medical staff. It functions in harmony and competition with the other subunits in the organization while concentrating on its own objectives. It is usually subordinated to pathology, and its organization chart may resemble the one shown in Chapter 2, Figure 2-9. A medical laboratory may also be a separate entity that provides diagnostic services to medical institutions and physicians. In this instance, the laboratory is unencumbered by the multiple demands of the health-care process usually associated with hospitals. When it is a separate business, the laboratory has great autonomy and operates under the profit orientation of its owners. Whether part of a hospital or a separate financial entity, the medical

FIGURE 10-1. Typical hospital organization chart.

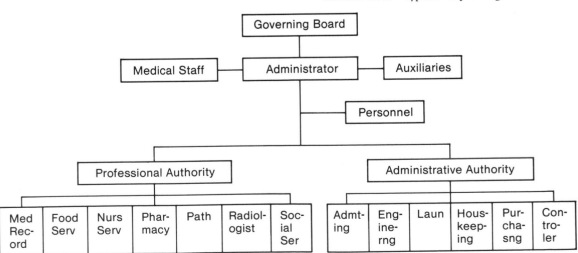

laboratory is subject to change and conflict that will ensure its survival or demise.

Forces for Change

No laboratory functions in a vacuum. The laboratory must seek sustenance in the form of clients, scarce financial resources, personnel, and equipment to complete its mission. In order to survive, it must be aware of its environment. A chief characteristic of that environment, and of all modern society, is change. The laboratory manager must possess the ability to recognize change and act accordingly.

Twenty years ago, few would have imagined that court rulings regarding medical malpractice suits would precipitate the onslaught of demand for laboratory services. A laboratory's external world is highly volatile. In general, any manager must acknowledge four broad areas of change:

1. The increasing trend for advanced education and training, coupled with employee aspirations for more interesting work and advancement
2. The accelerating demand for employee loyalty to the organization relative to the societal changes occurring in the market place
3. The problem of unionization and employees' demands for more rewards—financial and psychological—from their work environment
4. The challenge of increased revenue production coupled with cost containment and high quality standards

A closer look at the four areas of change reveals that factors affecting change also occur within the organization. For example, most middle managers are acutely attuned to personnel shifts that might affect their ability to manage their work groups. These changes may be drastic or subtle. In any case, the manager is aware that these forces exist and that he must deal with or diffuse them.

Most managers, after studying their internal and external environments, are able to distinguish between those changes that will impede or enhance their ability to manage their own work unit. However, the ability to distinguish between the changes that are superficial or negligible and those that might have a major impact comes only with experience and knowledge of the process of change.

TRYING TO UNDERSTAND CHANGE AND CONFLICT

Faced with forces for change, the supervisor is caught in something of a dilemma. On one hand, based on his knowledge of the work environment, the manager realizes that there are compelling reasons for change. On the other hand, he realizes that organizations and the people in them tend to perform most efficiently under stable and predictable conditions. If the manager changes the work environment too much, he risks unexpected and detrimental outcomes. If he does not react to the demands of change, he may jeopardize the very survival of his laboratory.

The laboratory manager must also function as a problem-finder. He must not only react to change, but he must also identify and plan for change. He must realize that a planned program for change allows greater control of and flexibility for the laboratory. To achieve both control and flexibility, he must initiate change and function as an agent of change.

Change forces are not often of equal intensity or attractiveness; moreover, they are not always intense enough to be recognized nor attractive enough to prompt action. However, feeling compelled to make changes that are unwarranted is as dangerous as failing to recognize the need for change. Too much change may be as dangerous as too little.

A clearer understanding of change and conflict is possible with a motivational explanation. In the individual motivation process, needs create drives that lead to the accomplishment of goals. A need or deficiency is created where there is some form of psychologic or physical imbalance. The need then manifests itself in some form of action or direction which is directed toward a goal that satisfies the initial imbalance. Although we recognize that such an explanation is clearly simplistic, it does serve as a basic explanation of behavioral change.

Carrying the motivational model a step further, we find an explanation for conflict. Conflict occurs when something or someone erects a barrier that does not allow attainment of the goal (Fig. 10-2). The barrier creates frustrations that may lead to a variety of defense mechanisms.

Conflict, then, occurs when an individual encounters some form of opposition in his motivational cycle. The barrier may be physical (outward)

FIGURE 10-2. A simple model of frustration.

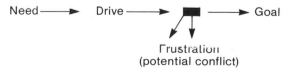

or psychologic (inward). These frustrations are not necessarily negative from an organizational standpoint. For example, a manager who is rejected for promotion may not react defensively, but may be spurred on to greater and better performance in order to achieve a denied objective.

So far we have implied that the individual process of change begins in the motivational cycle and is somehow linked with conflict. The cause–effect relationship between change and conflict is not that simple, however; and most evidence today suggests that we still do not clearly understand this relationship.

The practicing manager is bombarded every day with a multitude of factors that he must evaluate before making a decision. We do not clearly understand how a manager weighs his decision concerning strategy for action because individual values and perceptions vary. We will assume, however, that whatever course of action he pursues will take into consideration the long- and short-run survival of his work unit or laboratory. Therefore, we will assume that the change/conflict process within an organization or organizational subunit will be influenced, and to a certain degree managed, by the individual most responsible for its direction: the manager (Fig. 10-3).

Quite simply, the association between change and conflict generates some action or reaction that will ultimately change the human, technologic, or structural elements of the work unit to ensure its survival. However, the underlying managerial questions still remain: When should I change? How should I go about it? How does the change process work? To help the manager answer these questions, Edgar H. Schein offers the following observations[10]:

1. Any change process involves not only learning something new but unlearning something that is already present and possibly well integrated in the personality and social relationships of the individual.
2. No change will occur unless there is motivation to change, and if such motivation to change is not already present, the induction of that motivation is often the most difficult part of the change process.
3. Organizational changes such as new structures, processes, reward systems, and so on occur only through individual changes by key members of the organization.
4. Most adult change involves attitudes, values, and self-images. The unlearning of present responses in these areas is initially and inherently painful and threatening.
5. Change is a multistage behavior modification cycle that is complex and requires a systematic approach.

The Change Sequence

In order to manipulate change, the manager must understand the sequence of change. There is nothing so frustrating to a manager as to examine his action in retrospect and conclude that he should have pursued a different course of action. It is easy to analyze actions in retrospect, but it is quite difficult to decide what should be done when confronted with external and internal forces for change. Understanding how far he has progressed through the change sequence can help the manager make that initial decision. Figure 10-4 shows one interpretation of this process.

The key to surviving in an organization is how well one reads the forces for change, not necessarily how actively one pursues change. Many managers are successful without being preoccupied with the change process. Also, many effective managers exert minimal influence on the functioning of their units, while others constantly initiate new programs and implement new procedures. To suggest that one style is correct and the other wrong would be foolhardy. Each may reflect the forces demanding change in their respective working units. Some units function effectively in a very turbulent environment, while others function better in a calm and stable environment.

FIGURE 10-3. Change/conflict survival model. (Adapted from Robbins SP: The Administrative Process, p. 343. Englewood Cliffs, Prentice-Hall, 1980)

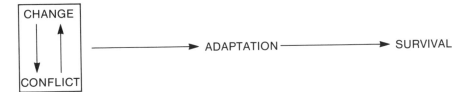

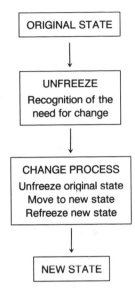

ORIGINAL STATE

↓

UNFREEZE
Recognition of the
need for change

↓

CHANGE PROCESS
Unfreeze original state
Move to new state
Refreeze new state

↓

NEW STATE

FIGURE 10-4. The change sequence.

Complacency can also be a problem. After initial attempts to improve his unit's efficiency, a manager eventually realizes that organizational barriers affect his ability to improve productivity and employee morale. Coupled with an organizational philosophy that discourages change, the manager often becomes complacent about the operation of his work unit and lapses into a management style that encourages the status quo.

The manager must possess curiosity, discontent, open-mindedness, and self-respect to be able to recognize the need for change.[1] He must understand and recognize the attitudes that are most conducive to change. The manager should question himself about how something can be done more effectively or why something happens. He should be dissatisfied with complacency or the "tried and true" method and seek ways to improve the functioning of his unit.

The manager should be open to suggestions from sources other than his own experience and intellect. True open-mindedness is the realization that good ideas and suggestions also reside among subordinates. An effective change agent fosters communication from all levels of the hierarchy.

Ultimately, the manager must have a genuine respect for his own abilities. Many managers ignore changes that evoke initial resistance when implemented. It is easier to submit to the status quo than initiate a procedure that might elicit short-run resist-

ance. The successful manager overcomes the pressures to maintain the status quo.

Having concluded that change is necessary, the manager must decide what type of change strategy should be used. The objective of the change process is the survival of the organization. Many recent change methods advocate a participatory approach which involves both the management hierarchy and subordinates. This approach facilitates ownership and acceptance of the change process by the participating parties. Many organizational-development, sensitivity-training, and management-development programs reflect this philosophy. Many other change techniques exist and will be discussed later in this chapter.

The Change Process

The change process is a difficult one. Trying to change individual human behavior is very hard. Changing the behavior of an entire work group is even more difficult, but it begins with changes in individuals. For individuals to internalize and accept change, a three-step sequence must occur: the individual must *reject* the old pattern or behavior, *move* to the new one, and ultimately *accept* the new behavior.

The first stage can be characterized as unfreezing the existing status quo. This step forces a person to unlearn or alter his way of thinking. He must be made aware of why his behavior may be ineffective, unproductive, or outmoded. This stage reduces the forces for resistance, and the person experiences doubt about his way of thinking. For example, medical technologists might be given information about a new testing procedure that promises high productivity. To overcome resistance to change, the technologist must be convinced that this procedure is superior to the existing one and that using the new procedure benefits him. In other words, he must be provided information by the manager to combat any resistance.

After a person rejects old behaviors, the must be persuaded to adopt new behavior. This starts the second step, the period of change or transition. At this stage, individuals should be willing to give the new procedure a try.

Through identification and internalization mechanisms, the manager can move individuals toward acceptance of new behavior. For example, the manager might reveal that the new procedure is used by other, very prestigious laboratories (identification) and suggest that his technologists try it to see how they like it (internalization). In this stage, the manager can facilitate the process by providing genuine two-way communication with the subordinates. For example, he can provide information and guidance regarding the new procedure, but the employees should be encouraged to make suggestions and contribute to the change process. This might mean modification or reformulation of the procedure to meet the demands of the employees. The manager must also be malleable about the new procedure—after all, the objective of the process is the acceptance of the new procedure.

The third step is sometimes identified as the refreezing stage: the individual internalizes the new behavior, and it becomes part of his daily life. In our example, the technologists have accepted the new procedure. Reinforcement occurs through their own perceptions of its advantages and through information supplied by the manager about increased productivity, greater reliability, lower cost, and so on. It is important in this stage that the change is not extinguished. The environment must remain rewarding to the individuals who have adopted the change; if the environment does not continue to be rewarding, it is possible that old behaviors will resurface. People tend to repeat behavior that is rewarding.

Diagnosing Resistance

Understanding the change process does not guarantee acceptance of change. In some instances, the most improbable changes initiated by management are embraced cheerfully by work units. Yet in other instances, change programs have been initiated with disastrous results. Often, the very programs that management thought would be accepted with enthusiasm fail badly. Why does one change strategy succeed, and others, with seemingly meritorious objectives, fail?

The answer may lie in change strategy selection and available information about possible resistance to the change. The manager must think through possible implications for the work unit before he implements any change that affects it. A manager must assess the change process in light of potential overt and covert resistance. Furthermore, he must consider the ramifications of the change itself.

Often, a change strategy is adopted because it seems to work somewhere else; however, what is feasible in one work unit does not guarantee success in another. The manager who bases change on his own environment has a greater chance for success. One way to increase the probability of success is to be aware of factors that might cause resistance to change. Although one could compile numerous

factors, the obvious ones appear to be insecurity, social and economic costs, union intervention, and the reduction of autonomy.

INSECURITY. Change inherently creates feelings of uncertainty and anxiety. Humans are creatures of habit. The person who has ample experience with and knowledge of one job procedure often exhibits inflexibility regarding a job change. It is quite logical that someone who has achieved status and recognition in a position would be threatened by a change in which the outcome is uncertain. An employee may feel threatened if he believes that changes may cause him to lose face or be inconvenienced. Many employees are "organization-wise." They think that management transforms "harmless changes" into more work, inconvenience, or loss of status. A good laboratory manager should never allow a technologist to equate change with insecurity. The field of laboratory medicine is dynamic; every professional who practices in one of the paramedical fields must be continually exposed to change and made to feel comfortable with it.

SOCIAL AND ECONOMIC COSTS. Change may also demand social and economic costs. As employees orient themselves to their work environments, they establish elaborate social relationships with their co-workers and superiors. Cliques and informal work groups emerge. A sense of security, identity, and belonging exists with membership in a group. If change of one form or another threatens this relationship, workers will resist that change. For example, the introduction of a new testing procedure is often resisted by the persons who are most familiar with the weakness of the old method. Yet these people will attack the new procedure for a variety of reasons. The real reason, however, may be that the new procedure means different working hours, destruction of the existing work group, or the possibility of having to report to someone else. These negative responses are mere symptoms of the underlying social threat to the individual or the work group.

Likewise, the economic costs associated with change should be confronted. Individuals are extremely sensitive to anything that affects their income, especially if the income is a reflection of status or recognition. Economic costs may include replacement of an employee by more efficient technology or rejection of a new work schedule because it entails higher parking costs.

THE UNION. The relationship between union and management is the pivotal issue in the introduction of change. If both sides trust each other and there is harmonious cooperation, resistance to change is significantly reduced. The degree of resistance is often determined by past experiences, and it is critical that the manager understand the political dimensions of the union hierarchy. He cannot and should not expect to win approval of every proposal of plan of action that he presents to the union. Neither should a proposal be submitted only once if there is some possibility of finding a way to effect change that satisfies both sets of needs.

REDUCTION OF AUTONOMY. An increase in control or accountability will usually be resisted by a technologist. No one likes to be evaluated if the evaluation takes the form of closer supervision or the reduction of discretionary decision-making. Employees often interpret closer control as a lack of trust by management.

Likewise, if a work-related task that requires some form of judgment and skill is redesigned as a routine, repetitive task, the laboratory manager should expect resistance. This is especially true for tasks that have been assigned high status and prestige.

A Framework For Analysis— Diagnosis and Implementation

Before implementing a change process, a manager must have a clear understanding of what he wants to accomplish. Hersey and Blanchard indicate that the manager must have or be able to obtain the necessary skills to diagnose and implement the change process.[3] The success of a change process hinges on diagnosis and implementation skills.

In Hersey and Blanchard's model, diagnosis is the critical first step of any successful change process. The manager evaluates what is *likely* to happen if change does not occur, what *ideally* should happen, and what forces of resistance could block the actual from becoming the ideal. If there is a discrepancy between the actual and the ideal, the question, "Should I change something?" is answered—"Yes."

In reality, the answer may not be so simple. Hersey and Blanchard point out, for example, that the diagnostic phase is essentially an evaluation stage. The manager must correctly read the organizational and human variables that may impede or encourage the change process. For example, conflict in a work group may not be a problem if it does not impede group efforts to achieve the ideal or planned goals. Conflict might actually promote attainment of organizational goals through healthy competition. Only when it interferes with ideal

goals does conflict become a problem. Naturally, if harmonious intragroup relations are a goal, conflict then becomes a problem. This approach forces the manager to think through what he wants to accomplish before he haphazardly introduces some change process.

The second step of the Hersey and Blanchard analysis is implementation. In this step, the laboratory manager uses the data from the first step and translates it into a systematic change process or strategem. The manager examines alternative solutions to the problem and then assigns appropriate stratgems that will effect the change.

Hersey and Blanchard's approach can be condensed into six questions the manager should ask himself when contemplating change:

1. What do I want to accomplish?
2. Should I change anything based on what I want to accomplish?
3. Is there a problem(s), and what are its parameters?
4. What possible solutions are available to me?
5. Which solution or strategy is the most appropriate?
6. How can I monitor and evaluate the change?

These questions force the manager to think through the whole change process systematically. They provide structure and direction to the thought processes associated with organizational change. All too often a manager takes corrective action without systematically diagnosing and analyzing the organizational and human changes that it might precipitate.

Leavitt categorizes organizational change approaches into structural, technologic, or people-oriented approaches.[5] The structural approach facilitates change through the formal rules, procedures, and guidelines of the organization. The technologic approach stresses the work flow, as exemplified by job descriptions and physical layout. People approaches favor training programs and appraisal techniques to change attitudes, motivational levels, and behavioral skills. Leavitt's views the three approaches as interrelated: one does not change without affecting the other two.

Whatever viewpoint a manager chooses to follow, he must be an excellent diagnostician. The management prerogatives he possesses must be tempered by the realization that few of his managerial actions are isolated. However, a manager who considers too many variables and sees too many forces of constraint and resistance can render himself ineffective. Caution is important, but the manager serving as an agent of change quickly realizes that the change process is not for the fainthearted.

Some General Statements about Change Efforts

We have stressed that understanding the change process facilitates control of the process and lessens the chance that the manager will be overwhelmed by it. Also, we have strongly implied that the managerial role is probably the most effective and realistic change vehicle in the laboratory. Although third-party (consulting) relationships are effective, most situations must be resolved within limited time and financial frameworks. The role of an outside consultant is often not realistic or feasible. Therefore, we offer guidelines that might help the manager facilitate change.

Realize that mutual trust tends to facilitate change. If there are harmonious, trusting relations between the manager and his subordinates, the chance for successful change implementation is greatly enhanced. If, on the other hand, the organizational climate resembles that of an armed camp, a manager can expect resistance. Simply put, trust facilitates change, and lack of trust breeds resistance.

Create a climate that encourages and reinforces open, honest communication and supportive behavior. Also, acquire adequate resources to implement change; and most importantly, be creative and adaptive. Naturally, it is helpful if all believe in the organization's goals and culture.

Only make changes that are necessary. Change is very threatening and should be used with discretion. Employees may interpret frequently changed directives and goals as a lack of planning instead of judicious reaction to external and internal forces for change. Furthermore, constant change turns a stable work environment into one plagued by turbulence and uncertainty. Employees accustomed to a stable, predictable environment often resent changes introduced by management. Frequently changed work patterns or objectives can diminish commitment to organizational goals.

Do not be afraid to try something on a tentative basis. Nothing should be written in stone. Although some change processes must be very structured and inflexible, there are others that should be tried on an evaluative basis. Not everything can be planned, nor will every result be anticipated. This is extremely important

from the subordinate's viewpoint. Most employees are more willing to try something on a tentative basis than to be forced to make a change with little opportunity for modification. Resistance can often be overcome if employees know in advance that it is possible to negotiate changes.

Try to include employee participation in the planning stages of change. People tend to be very supportive of change processes in which they are involved. A note of caution: it is foolhardy to include persons in decision-making who have neither the maturity nor the skill to make the decision. To do so establishes a dangerous precedent that the manager may not be able to satisfy in future decision-making.

Be careful of upsetting established customs and traditions. Changes often appear revolutionary when viewed by the informal work group. The manager must be careful that change does not occur so quickly and intensely that insurmountable opposition to the change results. Sometimes a slower, evolutionary approach is just as effective, especially if the change attacks long-standing ways of doing things and threatens established interpersonal relationships and alliances.

Be aware of a "wallet mentality." If a change affects people's pocketbooks negatively, they tend to resist it. Technologic changes are resisted because employees perceive that the change will demand more of them in less time. They fear that such change will jeopardize their job security or overtime. The manager should anticipate these fears and attempt to assure employees that they will maintain their present levels of income.

Try to provide as much information about the change as possible. Although it is not always possible, try to implement changes with knowledge as the base of support. Most people want to know why a change needs to take place. Once the reasons are explained to them, most resistance evaporates. Some managers feel that the organizational merits of the change are sufficient to convince employees to adopt the change. Often, managers forget that selling the change to subordinates is necessary. Managers who hold that attitude often find themselves blocked because employees perceive organizational merits in a completely different way than the manager. Withholding information can be especially troublesome when dealing with unions. It is probably wiser to share information regarding anticipated changes with the union than to surprise it. If the union can be brought into or identified with the change process, the process will tend to defuse this source of resistance.

Selection of a Change Stratagem — A Continuum

The selection of a change strategy depends on the diagnosis of the problem and the indicated remedy. The manager today is presented with a wide variety of procedures and must choose the one most feasible for what he wants to accomplish. The critical point, however, is the validity of the original analysis of the intended change. Selecting the correct change technique greatly facilitates the success of the change.

Numerous tactics and procedures are available to the manager; these methods represent a variety of philosophic orientations regarding the selection of a change process. To better understand how a manager can choose the best technique, it might be wise to examine two extreme orientations-to-change stratagems. One tries to overwhelm resistance, and the other tries to dissipate any resistance.

A strategy that tries to overwhelm resistance usually relies on hierarchical authority or power to impose the change. It is directive in nature and allows little input from the people who will be affected by the change, which is clearly planned and affects the total group or organization.

In this instance, change is often swift and complete. Opposition might be anticipated, but the manager's power to impose the directive is greater than the power of the forces resisting it. Naturally, the change may sustain itself if hierarchical powers or efforts diminish or disappear.

Often, the manager imposes some change that he realizes will be unpopular; but he tries to convince his subordinates that if they try the change, they will see that it was the right move. An example of this was the Federal government's imposition of civil rights laws on a population that strongly resisted it. The feasibility of such an approach is strongly tied to the manager's past record and power to effect such changes, the time he has available to impose the change, and the general preference of the subordinates regarding implementation style.

When the Civil Rights Act was passed, the population was aware that the federal government had the power to implement such legislation and had done so in the past. The Federal government settled on a time frame and chose a style legitimized by the Federal system. Such an approach is certainly feasible in the workplace.

At the other end of the continuum is the "bottom up" or participatory approach. In this approach, the manager uses tactics designed to win over the opposition. Such an approach is used where acceptance of the change is important. Subordinates are brought into the decision-making process and are strongly encouraged to contribute to diagnosis, analysis, and implementation of the change. Such an approach usually requires more time and, by the very nature of its style, is less specifically planned than a directive approach. Employees are less threatened and tend to become part of the change process. This generates commitment, motivation, and a sense of achievement among most participants.

Because the change is not forced on the employees, it tends to have a much longer staying power than a hierarchically imposed change. The objective is the evolution of a behavioral change, not the imposition of one. Again, the organizational climate and the manager's prevailing style are critical variables. A well-liked manager who projects a certain amount of personal power tends to have greater success with this approach than one who is not trusted and uses an authoritarian approach to problem-solving.

Depending on the actual environment of the change process, either approach is feasible. Selection of the appropriate approach is clearly dependent on how well the manager has diagnosed the change problem. Both strategies can be superimposed on a continuum developed by Kotter and Schlesinger.[4] They have investigated methods for dealing with resistance to change and have identified four situational variables that should be considered before choosing a change strategy. Their strategic continuum, adapted to our needs, and the situational factors are shown in Figure 10-5.

Kotter and Schlesinger point out that change efforts based on inconsistent strategies invariably run into problems. A quickly implemented change that is not well-thought-out or planned tends to run into unanticipated problems. Likewise, a rapidly implemented change strategy that involves a large number of people usually stalls in its own inertia and takes on fewer participative characteristics over time. According to Kotter and Schlesinger, successful change efforts are located on the strategic continuum in relation to their four situational variables:[4]

1. The type and degree of anticipated resistance. The greater the degree of resistance anticipated, the more the initiator will move to the right in selecting a strategy to win over or minimize the resistance.

Strategic continuum	
OVERWHELM	WIN OVER
Fast	Slower
Clearly planned	Not clearly planned at the beginning
Little involvement of others	Lots of involvement of others
Attempt to overcome any resistance	Attempt to minimize any resistance
Key situational variables	
The amount and type of resistance that is anticipated	
The position of the initiators vis-a-vis the resistors (in terms of power, trust, and so forth)	
The locus of relevant data for designing the change, and of needed energy for implementing it	
The stakes involved (e.g., the presence or lack of presence of a crisis, the consequences of resistance and lack of change)	

FIGURE 10-5. Change continuum and situational variables affecting choice of strategy. (Adapted from Koiter J, Schlesinger LA: Choosing strategies for change. Harvard Bus Rev 57:111, March 1979)

2. The amount of power and trust the manager is given. The less power he has, the more the manager is forced to select a strategy to the left of the continuum; conversely, the greater his personal power, the more he can afford to move to the right.

3. Data and energy needed to implement and design the change process. If the manager requires commitment and data from individuals who might resist the change, it behooves him to involve them in the design of the change effort. Likewise, if he has the power and information to overwhelm any resistance, then a strategy on the left side of the continuum is feasible.

4. The stakes involved. If a short-run crisis exists and the survival of the firm is in jeopardy, then a move to the left on the continuum is warranted. Likewise, if radical action is not called for and the problem involves many people, a win-over strategy from the right side of the continuum is reasonable.

The Kotter and Schlesinger strategems are listed below and summarized in Table 10-1. Each

strategem has been illustrated in a manner that will identify the appropriate context for its utilization.

Education and Communication. This approach is feasible when inaccurate or inadequate information creates resistance to change. It is especially appropriate when the manager needs to create commitment among the people who resist change because of misinformation or lack of information about the change. Although such a strategy appears simple, it can be time-consuming if a large number of people are involved. It will have a greater chance of success if the "teacher" and the "pupil" trust one another. The assumption here is that communication and logic will prevail.

Participation and Involvement. Bringing subordinates into planning or implementation of change is an excellent method when the manager does not possess the expertise or knowledge to implement the change himself and the resisters have significant power to impede his efforts. As discussed before, participation often generates commitment by the participants to the change process. This approach can also re-

Table 10-1

Strategies for Dealing with Resistance to Change

Approach	Applicable Situations	Advantages	Drawbacks
Education plus communication	Where there is a lack of information or inaccurate information and analysis	Once persuaded, people will often help with the implementation of the change	Can be very time-consuming if many people are involved
Participation plus involvement	Where the initiators do not have all the information they need to design the change, and where others have considerable power to resist	People who participate will be committed to implementing change, and any relevant information they have will be integrated into the change plan	Can be very time-consuming if participants design an inappropriate change
Facilitation plus support	Where people are resisting because of adjustment problems	No other approach works as well with adjustment problems	Can be time-consuming, expensive, and still fail
Negotiation plus agreement	Where someone or some group will clearly lose out in a change, and where that group has considerable power to resist	Sometimes it is a relatively easy way to avoid major resistance	Can be too expensive in many cases if it alerts others to negotiate for compliance
Manipulation plus co-optation	Where other tactics will not work or are too expensive	It can be relatively quick and inexpensive solution to resistance problems	Can lead to future problems if people feel manipulated
Explicit plus implicit coercion	Where speed is essential, and the change initiators possess considerable power	It is speedy and can overcome any kind of resistance	Can be risky if it leaves people angry at the initiators

sult in time-consuming compromises that do not fit the organizational needs. It must be handled carefully because once a decision has been made by the group, it is difficult for the manager to push it aside.

Facilitation and Support. This works best with problems that deal with adjustment to the change process. It helps people adjust to change by facilitating their reaction to the change and by being supportive as the change occurs. It tries to reduce anxieties and fears by providing time for reflection, educational training, or additional counseling. This approach is time-consuming and expensive and requires a certain amount of patience of the part of the manager. It tries to smooth the disruption by allowing time for coping with change. Like the others, however, it is not always successful.

Negotiation and Agreement. This strategy is feasible when someone has to lose or give up something and that person possesses a significant amount of power to resist the change. Under these conditions the manager might barter or offer something to gain compliance and avoid major resistance or create commitment. This sometimes is an easy way to get compliance, but it can become expensive. If individuals or groups understand that the manager is willing to negotiate, they are likely to comply only when something is offered in return. It can establish a dangerous precedent.

Manipulation and Co-optation. When all other methods do not work or are too expensive, the manager may resort to covert change tactics. The manager manipulates the situation in order to evoke compliance. He may selectively release important information or orchestrate events that endorse his change efforts. Another kind of manipulation is co-optation. The manager might ask a key individual to participate in the design of the change process. This creates the appearance of endorsement or identification, rather than participation. Either of these tactics can be inexpensive and quick, but also very dangerous. If people perceive that they are being manipulated, the manager runs the risk of having all his actions perceived as covert attempts to influence. If discovered, he destroys his trust and may create doubt about his motives when changes occur in the future.

Explicit and Implicit Coercion. If speed is essential and the manager has considerable power, he might resort to coercion. Fear can be used to gain compliance, as can direct or implied force. A manager sometimes uses this approach when other techniques and methods have failed. It is effective if the manager can overwhelm his resistance, but it can be risky. Most people strongly resist such tactics. If a manager is going to attack resistance by force or fear, he must know he can win. If he loses, the defeated manager will have a long way to go to regain power.

What are the implications of this for the laboratory director? A variety of change methods are available to the manager, although much of the literature today tends to advocate and endorse a participative approach to change. We tend to agree with this trend. As suggested in the discussion of developments in the next decade, the work force will be highly educated, mobile, and specialized. For this reason alone, a manager should consider strategies located on the right side of the continuum. In general, people do not want to be ordered about and directed; this invariably generates resistance and resentment. The immediate and long-run effects are better served if, where possible, the chosen strategy involves the people affected by the change. People like to feel that they have some control of their work environment. Likewise, a win-over philosophy tends to build bridges of trust between people.

Conflict and Conflict Management

No matter how carefully a manager chooses his strategy, conflict still occurs during the change process. We previously implied that functions associated with the management process invariably lead to conflict. This conflict is rooted in the individual's motivational need–drive–goal cycle: when someone or something erects a barrier that blocks or opposes goal attainment, frustration results. This encourages the individual's development of defense mechanisms, and these mechanisms may be a cause of conflict.

Conflict has been defined as "any kind of opposition or antagonistic interaction between two or more parties."[7] Conflict also has a conceptual basis. If conflict is perceived, conflict exists; if it is not perceived, it does not exist. This means that conflict can be latent or overt, accurate or inaccurate. The point is that conflict is a matter of individual perception.

This perspective can be expanded to include conflict situations between individuals, groups, and organizations, or any combination thereof. It is not difficult to imagine that incompatible interests and goals among different parties can result in some form of conflict. Thus, conflict can occur internally or externally.

The managerial role requires not only an understanding of conflict but also an ability to control and direct it. Because the manager must live with conflict, he must also be able to manage it. To manage it, however, requires understanding the conditions that foster conflict in an organization.

Sources of Conflict

What conditions nourish and breed conflict in an organization? The formal organization attempts to specify in advance the nature of human relationships in that organization. No matter how carefully planned and executed work-oriented behavior might be, the very existence of a formal organization seems to assure conflict. Individuals want to control their own work environments, and this need for self-determination is often a basis for work-related conflict. Let us examine several of the more common underlying causes for organizational conflict.

SCARCE RESOURCES. Most organizations have a common resource base from which resources are reallocated to the various units and subunits of the organizations. Everyone wants the biggest part of the resource pie. The scarce resource could be anything: time, equipment, money, employees, or other items. Because each unit sees its mission as the most important or most critical, its members sometimes resort to extreme measures to secure the scarce resource. When this happens, conflict usually occurs. Often individuals or groups will present biased or exaggerated evidence to ensure the "proper" allocation of resources.

VALUES. The health-care field attracts highly competent, specialized individuals. Each employee in a hospital brings with him many years of training and his own perception of what professional behavior should be. Because a hospital is a complex organization staffed by many diverse professionals, it is easy to understand why professional value orientations may differ. A nurse may need immediate results from tests performed by medical technologists, but she may be unaware that the technologists also have other, more critical, work to perform. The two groups often misunderstand one another's duties and responsibilities and the work pressures associated with them. Furthermore, the nurse functions in a line relationship, the medical technologist in a staff role. Unfortunately, each group often misinterprets the actions of the other, and neither seems to understand the hierarchical limitations and relationships regarding their respective responsibilities and authority.

AMBIGUOUS ORGANIZATION. Organizational conflicts often result because of undefined or overlapping duties and responsibilities. Organizations usually try to prevent this by developing job descriptions and organization charts that clearly define the roles of separate groups and individuals. Because of the dynamic nature of most organizations and the less formal daily interactions that develop, overlapping duties and responsibilities do exist. This results in political behavior such as bickering and complaining about one party's jurisdictional responsibility to another. When the manager observes such behavior and cannot attribute credit or blame to one party over the other, more definitive jurisdictional responsibilities may be needed.

DEPENDENCE. Conflict often occurs when one party is dependent on another. For example, during a flu epidemic a physician will order certain tests for a patient, and these tests will be sent to the laboratory for analysis. After a period of time the physician might urge the nurse to contact the laboratory about the test results. The laboratory is now besieged with extra work because of the epidemic and reschedules the work flow accordingly. A misunderstanding may result based on the laboratory's perception of the doctor's impatience, the nurse's numerous telephone calls for the test results, and the hospital manager's strict inflexibility with overtime pay.

COMMUNICATION. Communication barriers are often the cause of conflict. The most obvious example occurs when two parties use such specialized jargon that communication ceases. Physicians often explain diagnosis to patients in such technical language that patients are too intimidated to admit a lack of comprehension. When this happens, communication ceases. It is important to express the information clearly and in a way the intended audience will understand.

INTERPERSONAL CONFLICT. A common conflict in organizations is the clash of incompatible personalities. Although a manager might try to segregate the individuals, educate them about their perceptions of one another, and preach tolerance and understanding, the fact is simply that some personalities affect each other the wrong way. There are interpersonal conflict situations that are so one-sided that the other party does not know conflict exists. Some people become highly dissatisfied when their roles are compared with the role of another person, for example, when someone is promoted or receives an increase in pay not granted to co-workers. The organization may unwittingly foster such dissatisfaction by encouraging excessive competition for promotion or merit increases.

Different Viewpoints On Conflict

Managers hold three different viewpoints about conflict.[8] Some managers see conflict as primarily destructive, signaling a breakdown in the management process. Others tend to look at conflict as natural and inevitable and will learn to live with it. Finally, there are those who view conflict as an essential variable in the continued survival of the organization. They feel that the laboratory manager who admits that resolving conflict and clarifying misunderstanding consumes much of his time may be functioning very effectively in his role as manager.

TRADITIONAL VIEWPOINT. The classical management theorists look upon conflict as the malfunctioning of the management process. If the manager had planned, organized, or controlled his work unit better, conflict would not occur. If conflict does occur, it is an indication that the manager is not correctly performing his job. It also assumes that conflict is dangerous and should be resolved by management as soon as possible. The management of conflict means that better planning has to be initiated, that the hierarchical structure should be used to resolve conflict, and that conflict should be avoided when possible. Under this approach the causes of conflict are analyzed and resolved by removing the cause of conflict. This is a classical management approach to handling conflict, and it still is prevalent in many organizations.

BEHAVIORAL VIEWPOINT. The behavioral viewpoint holds that harmony and tranquility do not necessarily mean high productivity. This perspective has it that conflict is not all bad and that there actually are some constructive aspects of conflict. All organizations are recognized to have built-in conflict situations, and it is assumed that the manager's duty and responsibility is to accept and manage it. This viewpoint warns the manager, however, that making or allowing too many waves could result in outcomes detrimental to the organization.

INTERACTIONIST VIEWPOINT. With this viewpoint it is argued that there might not be enough conflict in organizations.[7] Although the negative and destructive aspects of conflict are recognized, it is also believed that organizations sometimes need conflict as a stimulus for adaptation and survival. The manager is not only concerned with reducing and resolving conflict but also with stimulating it.

With this viewpoint, conflict may be functional or dysfunctional. If it furthers the goals of the organization, it is functional; if it hinders organizational performance, it is dysfunctional. Simply put, it states that organizations need to be responsive to their internal and external environments in order to survive. If a manager becomes too complacent or snuffs out the forces that facilitate change, there is great danger that the organization will lack the adaptability necessary to survive in today's highly competitive world. Furthermore, it views conflict as an integral part of the change process.

A reexamination of our initial model on conflict and change shows that we agree with this viewpoint. While his model displays conflict as the determinant for change, it is our belief that there isn't enough empirical evidence for us to state that conflict causes change. They are, however, closely interrelated, and this relationship is the catalyst for organizational adaptation and ultimately organizational survival.

We believe that the interactionist viewpoint is a realistic one. It not only incorporates much of the thinking from the other two viewpoints, but it allows growth and change to occur and makes the manager directly accountable for this process. It is inconceivable to us that a formal organization will not encounter conflict if it is responsive to its internal and external environments. It also appears realistic that adaptation and survival of the organization requires the subordination of individual interest to that of the organization. This means that the stimulation of conflict initiated by the manager may disturb some employees.

We are cautious, however, of endorsing behavior that stimulates conflict. Once conflict is introduced into the work setting, it is our belief that control and management of the "conflict" is often difficult to control and contain.

THE JAPANESE VIEWPOINT. It seems to be fashionable to adapt or adopt Japanese management styles to an American setting. Some well-managed American firms have adopted a Japanese orientation to conflict, which seems to correspond to many of our own viewpoints on conflict and change. The Japanese approach to conflict holds that conflict is inevitable in organizations, but uncontrolled conflict is considered intolerable. Conceptually, a Zen approach to management stresses harmony and tranquility. The Japanese believe that harmonious relationships are the underpinnings of effective management. This does not mean that competition should be avoided, only that conflict should be avoided. Conflict and change should be managed through approaches that stress cooperation through participative intervention techniques.

Participative intervention techniques such as quality circles, task groups, labor–management committees, and productivity programs all resemble a "bottom up" form of management. The individual as a member of a group is asked to participate in a change process or problem-solving situation that solicits commitment, creativity, and acceptance. The emerging viewpoint among many well-managed organizations is the importance of organizational harmony for successful implementation of change and the management of conflict.

Conflict Diagnosis and Coping Techniques

Much of what has already been said in our discussion about the diagnosis and implementation of various change processes also holds true for conflict techniques. Selection of an appropriate technique to deal with conflict depends on an accurate analysis of the conflict situation in the first place.

Conflict does not usually appear overnight. It often festers without the knowledge of the recipient party. Furthermore, conflict usually passes through several progressive stages before it manifests itself to others:[6]

1. Latent conflict. At this stage the basic conditions for potential conflict exist but have not yet been recognized.
2. Perceived conflict. The cause of the conflict is recognized by one or both of the participants.
3. Felt conflict. Tension is beginning to build between the participants, although no real struggle has yet begun.
4. Manifest conflict. The struggle is under way, and the behavior of the participants makes the existence of the conflict apparent to others who are not directly involved.
5. Conflict aftermath. The conflict has been ended by resolution or suppression. This establishes new conditions that will lead either to more effective cooperation or to a new conflict that may be more severe than the first.

The parties may be at different stages of the conflict cycle, which complicates management of conflict. For example, one person may be manifest-ing conflict behavior while the other is still trying to figure out what is happening.

The manager must have a keen sensitivity to and understanding of his work environment to deal effectively with conflict. He must not only be alert to potential conflict situations and know how to handle them, but must also know when to encourage conflict.

Knowing how to prevent conflict situations means understanding the underlying causes of conflict. A laboratory manager must be able to diagnose potential problems and structure situations to prevent them. People generally disagree over facts (perception of the present situation or problem), goals (how each party would like things to be), methods (the best way to achieve the goal), and values (the qualities and beliefs each thinks is important); the manager must be able to deal with these disagreements.[11]

For example, teaming two individuals with divergent viewpoints as to what constitutes a fair day's work creates a potential conflict situation. It should not come as a surprise that disagreements will occur between the two. A manager must be alert to these potential disagreements and carefully think through his managerial actions.

No matter how carefully the manager has analyzed a situation, open disagreement between parties can occur. The manager must ask himself what causes the conflict. Was each party exposed to a different informational base? Has the same information been perceived differently by the opposing parties because of past experience? Or have the parties been put in a situation or role that forces them to take opposing positions?[11] The answers to these questions define the parameters of the conflict situation. Only after the manager has attempted to clarify the parameters can he effectively influence the opposing parties to select the appropriate mode of conflict resolution or reduction.

It is generally understood that it is easier to resolve differences caused by misunderstanding or lack of information than differences caused by opposing values. Likewise, there are appropriate conflict resolution modes that are more effective with one type of conflict problem than with others. Table 10-2 presents some of the more common conflict resolution techniques and briefly describes their strengths and weaknesses. Selection of the appropriate technique depends on the resources available to the manager, the stage of the conflict cycle, the consequence of doing nothing, the timing of the intervention, the power of the hierarchy, and the manager's own leadership style.

(*Text continues on p 170*)

Table 10-2
Conflict Resolution Techniques

Technique	Brief Definition	Strengths	Weaknesses
Problem-solving (also known as confrontations or collaboration)	To seek resolution through face-to-face confrontation of the conflicting parties. Parties seek mutual problem definition, assessment, and solution.	Effective with conflicts stemming from semantic misunderstandings. Brings doubts and misperceptions to surface.	Can be time-consuming. Inappropriate for most non-communicative conflicts, especially those based on different value systems.
Superordinate goals	Common goals that two or more conflicting parties each desire and cannot be reached without cooperation of those involved. Goals must be highly valued, unattainable without the help of all parties involved in the conflict, and commonly sought.	When used cumulatively and reinforced, develops "peace-making" potential, emphasizing interdependency and cooperation.	Difficult to devise.
Expansion of resources	To make more of the scarce resource available.	Allows each conflicting party to be victorious.	Resources rarely expandable.
Avoidance	Includes withdrawal and suppression.	Easy to do. Natural reaction to conflict.	No effective resolution. Conflict not eliminated. Temporary.
Smoothing	To play down differences while emphasizing common interests.	Points of commonality stressed. Cooperative efforts are reinforced.	Differences not confronted and remain under the surface. Temporary.

(continued)

Table 10-2 (Continued)

Technique	Brief Definition	Strengths	Weaknesses
Compromise	To require each party to give up something of value. Includes external or third-party interventions, negotiation, and voting.	No clear loser. Consistent with democratic values.	No clear winner. Power-oriented —influenced heavily by relative strength of parties. Temporary.
Authoritative command	Solution imposed from a superior holding formal positional authority.	Very effective in organizations because members recognize and accept authority of superiors.	Cause of conflict not treated. Does not necessarily bring agreement. Temporary.
Altering the human variable	To change the attitudes and behavior of one or more of the conflicting parties. Includes use of education, sensitivity, and awareness training, and human-relations training.	Results can be substantial and permanent. Has potential to alleviate the source of conflict.	Most difficult to achieve. Slow and costly.
Altering structural variables	To change structural variables. Includes transferring and exchanging group members, creating coordinating positions, developing an appeals system, and expanding the group or organization's boundaries.	Can be permanent. Usually within the authority of a manager.	Often expensive. Forces organization to be designed for specific individuals and thus requires continual adjustment as people join or leave the organization.

Often the manager must exercise his leadership function in the role of supportive facilitator or counselor. Here his function is not to resolve the conflict himself but to bring the opposing parties together and let them resolve the conflict. He acts more as a referee than a judge. He interferes only to explain and define the variables, issues, and boundaries of the conflict. Likewise, he makes the parties understand that it is their responsibility to resolve the conflict, not his.

This requires a certain amount of skill on the part of the manager because this type of conflict management usually results in some form of verbal confrontation. Some commonsense rules, however, help the manager maintain a facilitating role[9]:

- Review past actions and clarify the issues before the confrontation begins.
- Communicate freely; do not hold back grievances.
- Do not surprise the opponent with a confrontation for which he is not prepared.
- Do not attack the opponent's sensitive spots that have nothing to do with the issues of the conflict.
- Keep to specific issues; do not argue aimlessly.
- Maintain the intensity of the confrontation but ensure that all participants say all that they want to say. If the basic issues have been resolved at this point, agree on what steps will be taken next toward reaching a solution.

The manager must provide a constructive climate for the confrontation and prevent it from deteriorating into a destructive, name-calling feud. He can, for example, allow for a cooling-off period if one of the sessions becomes too heated. Likewise, he may reveal new information about the situation. However, his most important objective should be to keep the resolution session going and on track. Many managers are uncomfortable in the role of facilitator because they feel a strong sense of accountability and responsibility for the outcome. These managers feel that they would have functioned more effectively had they resolved the problem in the first place. However, allowing the participants to resolve their own problem forces them to think through the problem and the parameters and consequences associated with it. Once a solution has been resolved they are more committed to it than to one imposed by the manager.

ENCOURAGING CONFLICT. So far we have been concerned with the prevention and resolution of conflict, but there are instances where the encouragement of conflict makes good management sense. Conflict is an essential component of the adaptation and survival of the firm. Furthermore, some evidence suggests that conflict spurs greater productivity and that decision-making characteristics are enhanced by it. Likewise, many practicing managers realize that stress and conflict are sometimes the only feasible solutions to lackadaisical and complacent attitudes. In fact, conflict is the basis of competitive techniques found among work groups who require self-motivation.

The question remains, however, of when to initiate conflict stimulation. Although there is no specific criterion for determining when conflict should be introduced into the work environment, Robbins has compiled a list of ten questions that are appropriate for managers to ask themselves:[7]

1. Are you surrounded by "yes men"?
2. Are subordinates afraid to admit ignorance and uncertainties to you?
3. Is there so much concentration by decision-makers on reaching a compromise that they may lose sight of values, long-term objectives, or the company welfare?
4. Do managers believe that it is in their best interest to maintain the impression of peace and cooperation in their unit, regardless of the price?
5. Is there an excessive concern by decision-makers in not hurting the feelings of others?
6. Do managers believe that popularity is more important for obtaining organizational rewards than competence and high performance?
7. Are managers unduly enamored with obtaining consensus for their decisions?
8. Do employees show unusually high resistance to change?
9. Is there a lack of new ideas forthcoming?
10. Is there an unusually low level of employee turnover?

According to Robbins, a positive answer to one or more of the questions suggests a possible need for conflict stimulation.

Likewise, Robbins has identified three broad categories for stimulating conflict among individuals and groups. These stimulation techniques include the following:[7]

Manipulate communication channel
   Deviate messages from traditional channels
   Repress information

Transmit too much information

Transmit ambiguous or threatening information

Alter the organization's structure (redefine jobs, alter tasks, etc.)

Increase a unit's size

Increase specialization and standardization

Add, delete, or transfer organizational members

Increase interdependence between units

Alter personal behavior factors

Change personality characteristics of leader

Create role conflict

Develop role incongruence

Manipulation of the communication channel, for example, allows the manager to control information for functional purposes. Holding back information not only enhances the power of the manager but also increases hostility among the work group. Lack of information regarding merit increases or transfers may create stress situations that result in greater productivity. Likewise, a strategically planted piece of information can often create uneasiness and lay the groundwork for a major policy change. It is an excellent strategy for testing the new policy. Although the use of such techniques may appear unethical to some managers, more seasoned managers already consciously or subconsciously use such tactics. It is not really a matter of what kind of manipulation is used but one of degree.

Changing structural variables can increase hostility. For example, increasing the size of an organizational unit can generate conflict by strengthening bureaucratic tendencies. Transferring several task-oriented individuals into a work group recognized as complacent can also create conflict.

Finally, the manager can alter personal behavior factors. The classic example of such a tactic is to put an authoritarian, dogmatic, and inflexible individual into a leadership role with a flexible, compatible work group. Likewise, changing the status or altering the privileges of an individual or group can cause dissatisfaction. Even such simple steps as revoking parking privileges or invoking a uniform dress code can generate discord.

It should be obvious that using these tactics can be dangerous. To do so involves gamemanship and shows disregard for individual sensitivities and feelings. Many managers resort to such tactics anyway, for they realize that a manager cannot satisfy the needs of all employees all the time. Often individ-

ual aspirations and needs must be sacrificed for the survival of the unit or organization. This does not mean that a manager should be callous to the needs of his subordinates, but that he should be aware that he represents and serves two constituencies: his subordinates and his organization. A manager electing to serve only one is usually ineffective.

Some General Statements About Conflict

The logical approach to conflict management is a contingency one. Whether a manager stimulates or resolves conflict is a matter of the variables surrounding the conflict situation. It is doubtful that only one method of conflict resolution can be expected to resolve the problem. There appears to be no universal cure all when it comes to conflict-resolution techniques. The selected technique must conform to and be compatible with the parameters and variables identified in the diagnostic stage of the analysis. A manager does not mirror his perceived expertise with that mode, rather than what is appropriate for the situation. We tend to repeat behavior with which we are comfortable, but that action is not sufficient for all situations.

Much of the literature today, especially that found in textbooks, tends to advocate a humanistic approach to conflict management. The increased collaboration as a change objective. In itself, this approach is admirable. Most managers, however, do not have the time and resources to deal with it effectively. Furthermore, many of them may be afraid of it, and probably with some justification.

Recent research indicates that a participation approach is not as feasible in large systems as it is in small ones and that power equalization may be necessary for collaboration to occur. Furthermore, interdependency between conflicting parties may better facilitate the problem-solving approach. Likewise, in situations of great conflict, unconditional collaboration may be naive.[12]

Problem-solving techniques require some very basic assumptions in order to be successful. The conflicting parties must desire a mutually acceptable solution. Couple this with trust in the other party, a belief that cooperation is better than competition, the idea that opposing opinions are not only healthy but legitimate, and the basic conditions for successful confrontation and problem-solving are met.[2] The objectives of such an approach certainly are noble, although the conditions that facilitate its success are somewhat more difficult to come by. The point is that collaborative problem-solving is just one tool available to the manager in resolving conflict.

The manager is always confronted with the problem of choosing a conflict-handling mode that is compatible with his desired outcome. Regardless of the technique selected, someone often has to pay the price with regard to satisfaction, personal and organizational resources, and influence. There are costs and benefits associated with each technique; they should be considered before a choice is made.

A note of caution should be interjected for managers contemplating stimulating conflict. The danger associated with the various stimulating techniques is found in the nature of the conflict itself. Although the objective of the conflict may be to increase the effectiveness and efficiency of the organization, the costs to the organization may be substantial. The danger is that the manager may lose control of the situation. The manager must be careful that he does not ignite a flame that could consume him in the process of conflict stimulation.

Because of time constraints, because of a crisis situation, or because other techniques have failed, a manager may resort to a hierarchical, authoritative solution. If a manager uses his positional power to impose a resolution, the participants may feel that his actions are arbitrary, personal, and discriminatory. The manager who opts for such a solution should have the support of higher level management.

A FINAL NOTE

Change and conflict are intertwined, and an understanding of the two concepts is essential for good management. The degree of effectiveness a manager achieves in handling these two concepts depends to a great extent on how effectively he diagnoses the conditions and parameters surrounding them. The ultimate framework for analysis will be each manager's individual value system.

We believe that the desire of most employees for greater involvement in their work environments strongly endorses a participative approach to management of both conflict and change. Participative approaches are not only more effective but will invariably reap high standards of quality and efficiency.

Our faith in participation is based on the premises that the size of most laboratories is well suited for participative schemes, that most laboratories are either "relatively" autonomous subunits within a larger system or independent "stand alone" units, and that a harmonious climate in laboratory fosters

efficiency and effectiveness more than any other approach to change and conflict. Coupled with the increased educational and professional expertise in today's laboratories, we feel that employee involvement techniques are worth considering.

However, the manager is faced with a variety of other options concerning conflict and change management. Should he sacrifice self-interest over the collective good, or individual expectations over organizational ones? Should he stress the rational, the efficient, or the humane solution?

Acknowledging these dilemmas does not make the selection of the appropriate change process or conflict resolution any easier. However, the reader now has the ability to ask questions that will orient him to the process of choice. Ultimately, the answers must come from within the manager himself. With the techniques and stratagems presented here, the flexible manager now possesses a repertoire of skills to help him find those answers.

REFERENCES

1. Bennet AC: Improving the Effectiveness of Hospital Management, pp 162–166. New York, Preston Publishing Co, 1972
2. Filley AA: Interpersonal Conflict Resolution, pp 60–69. Glenview, Scott, Foresman and Co, 1975
3. Hersey P, Blanchard KH: Management of Organizational Behavior: Utilizing Human Resources, 3rd ed, pp 273–284. Englewood Cliffs, Prentice-Hall, 1977
4. Kotter J, Schlesinger LA: Choosing strategies for change. Harvard Bus Rev 57:112–113, 1979
5. Leavitt HJ: New Perspectives in Organization Research. New York, John Wiley and Sons, 1964
6. Pondy LR: Organizational conflict: Concepts and models. Administrative Science Quarterly 12:296–320, 1967
7. Robbins SP: Conflict management and conflict resolution are not synonymous terms. California Management Review 21(2):67–75, 1978
8. Robbins SP: Organizational Behavior, pp 287–289. Englewood Cliffs, Prentice-Hall, 1979
9. Rue LW, Byars LL: Management: Theory and Application, p 252. Homewood, Richard B. Irwin, 1977
10. Schein EH: Organizational Psychology, 3rd ed, pp 243–244. Englewood Cliffs, Prentice-Hall, 1980
11. Schmidt WH: Conflict: A powerful process for (good or bad) change. Management Review 63:5–8, 1974
12. Thomas KW: Conflict and collaborative ethic. California Management Review 21(2):58–59, 1978

ANNOTATED BIBLIOGRAPHY

DuBrin AJ: Contemporary Applied Management. Plano, Business Publications, 1985
   An excellent summary of current management concepts and techniques. It presents practical behavioral science oriented techniques for managers and professionals.
Filley AC: Interpersonal Conflict and Resolution. Glenview, Scott Foresman & Co, 1975

This book addresses the problem of interpersonal conflict and presents techniques and methods for conflict resolution and management. It is a good supplement for workshops on understanding and handling personal conflict.

Harvard Business Review. Boston, Graduate School of Business Administration, Harvard University (bi-monthly publication)

Although it has a general orientation, this journal often presents articles of interest to the health professional, such as articles that have wide applicability for laboratory management.

Hersey P, Blanchard KH: Management of Organizational Behavior: Utilizing Human Resources. Englewood Cliffs, Prentice-Hall, 1988

This is a general text on management emphasizing a behavioral approach. Although not specifically targeted for laboratory administration, it provides an excellent overview of current management thinking and should be an invaluable guide for the health professional who has not had formal management training.

Lippitt GL: Visualizing Change: Model Building and the Change Process. La Jolla, University Associates, 1973

This is a model-oriented text dealing with change. Although conceptual in orientation, it provides a broad discussion of change and includes an excellent bibliography.

Robbins SP: Managing Organizational Conflict: A Nontraditional Approach. Englewood Cliffs, Prentice-Hall, 1974

This book discusses conflict from an organizational perspective. It is essential reading for practitioners who view the survival of the organization as paramount. It provides an excellent explanation of constructive conflict from a management orientation.

Vecchio RP: Organizational Behavior. Chicago, Dryden Press, 1988

A board survey of behavioral concepts applicable to managers in general. Although targeted for college audiences, it is an excellent source book for laboratory managers.

part three

Processes in Personnel Administration

eleven

Interviewing and Employee Selection

John R. Snyder
Stephen L. Wilson
Linda L. Otis

The most important resource of any manager is his personnel.[34,38] The clinical laboratory is no different. Laboratory medicine is a labor-intensive service, as evidenced by the percentage of budget allocated to salaries. For this reason, a good deal of time and effort should be devoted to planning for an effective and efficient staff. This chapter covers personnel administration aspects of recruitment, interviewing, selection, transfer, and promotion in the clinical laboratory.

Turnover of personnel in the laboratory was a problem which plagued many institutions a decade ago. Karni, Studer, and Carter reported annual job turnover among clinical laboratory personnel in a large Midwestern city for the years 1970, 1975, and 1980 to be 20%, 19%, and 15%, respectively.[14] It is evident that diagnosis related groups (DRGs) have played a major role in reducing turnover by limiting the opportunities for relocation. In a 1987 survey of 200 laboratories, 85% had experienced a 3–7% decrease in full-time equivalent positions.[41] Beyond reduced staffing levels, hiring practices are changing somewhat in response to prospective payment, including a trend toward hiring more generalists. Anticipated increases in the numbers of technician-level workers replacing technologists in clinical laboratories have not materialized as predicted. Perhaps the slim pay differential between the two levels of technical personnel, usually only $1500 to $4000 per year, does not merit hiring staff with fewer problem-solving and disease-correlation skills. Other aspects of personnel have also been affected by DRGs: "The tight economic climate has forced laboratory managers to demand more work from fewer workers, and in many cases it has resulted in smaller salary increases, salary caps, reduced benefits, and postponement of work-place improvements."[41]

In addition, the seasonal peaks and valleys in laboratory volume often complicate the staffing picture, which in turn is reflected in recruiting, interviewing, and selection activities. A supervisor must plan in advance for the usual attrition (normal resignations and retirements). Erratic ups and downs in staffing volume, expedient hiring, and substantial overtime are all indicators that a problem may exist either in the selection process or in the work setting.[40] Retraining and constant orientation of new personnel is costly, in terms of both operational efficiency and quality of results.[29]

RECRUITMENT

The group of applicants from which a manager may select is variable. A laboratory supervisor cannot assume that the right employee will come along just when needed. Many rural and some metropolitan areas experience shortages of qualified laboratory personnel on a rather continual basis. Declining enrollments in today's clinical laboratory sciences educational programs may herald more severe laboratory manpower shortages for some institutions. Therefore, it behooves laboratory administrators to recruit in advance of staff vacancies and follow up all requests for information concerning the availability of current and future positions.

Recruitment of laboratory personnel relies primarily on newspaper and professional journal advertising. As competition for certified practitioners has heightened, some institutions have prepared enticement packets describing promotional opportunities, personnel benefits, and community educational/recreational advantages. Still others have prepared elaborate slide/tape recruitment programs that can be taken to professional meetings and college campuses.[7] Professional recruitment agencies are an expensive option, although their efforts usually are successful in securing applicants. Perhaps the most rewarding recruitment of bench-level staff is the result of efforts directed at the professional educational programs. Some institutions encourage potential employers to meet with their students through a placement option. Regardless of the tactic employed, the need for recruitment activities as part of the interviewing and selection process is becoming more evident.

A strong laboratory staff is the result of years of perceptive hiring.[37,39] The long-term health of the department is not assured if the employees are too similar in experience, age, job development, and promotability. Often it appears less costly and more efficient to recruit from within an institution's own educational program, but beware the phenomenon of in-breeding. Too many of one institution's graduates over too long a period of time may be detrimental. The introduction of new perspectives is always healthy. The infusion of new blood keeps the laboratory system from growing stagnant, repetitious, and overly reliant on internal judgment. Optimally, there should be a mix of newcomers and oldtimers, since too many hard-driving, overly ambitious outsiders can be almost as destructive as too many long-term "old fogies."

LEGAL ASPECTS OF INTERVIEWING AND EMPLOYEE SELECTION

During recent years a variety of Federal and State laws have been enacted to insure equal employment opportunities for all individuals.[13] The provisions of these laws apply to daily employer decisions of recruiting, hiring, promotion, training, and termination.[32] Moreover, these regulations extend to selection procedures.[35] Devices used to select an employee for employment, such as written tests, seniority systems, interviews, and application forms, are subject to scrutiny under these laws.[15,30] A brief summary of the major regulations that apply to employee selection follows.

Title VII

Title VII of the Civil Rights Act enacted by the Congress of the United States in 1964 is the major legislative effort to guarantee equality to all persons. The act was amended by the Equal Opportunity Act of 1972 and the Pregnancy Discrimination Act of 1978. Title VII forbids employers of more than fifteen persons from limiting, classifying, or segregating employees in such a way that would deprive any person of employment opportunities or adversely affect his status as an employee on the basis of that individual's race, color, religion, sex, or national origin.

Although Title VII is often associated with women and minorities, several other groups have been included by subsequent legislation. These are the handicapped (Rehabilitation Act of 1973 and the Equal Employment Opportunity for Handicapped Individuals Act of 1980), veterans of the Vietnam conflict (Vietnam Veterans Readjustment Act), and persons between the ages of 40 and 70 (Age Discrimination Employment Act of 1967).[16,17]

The original emphasis in Title VII was on protection of the individual from discrimination in employment. The act also emphasized opportunity, based on the equal-treatment test. Nevertheless, it is clear that certain minorities still suffer from discrimination. The unemployment rate for blacks continues to be twice that for whites;[33] women employed full-time have a median annual income less than men.[11] Because of these inequities, a movement to redefine discrimination in terms of outcomes, rather than opportunities, began. This movement emphasized the statistical *effects* of employment practices on minority groups, rather than the violation of individual rights.[20,23]

Affirmative Action

Affirmative action programs are based on the effects of discrimination. President Johnson, in 1965, instituted an executive order (E.O. 11246) calling for equal opportunities to be applied to all aspects of the personnel process. These orders applied to all contractors working for the Federal government. This action greatly improved on the affirmative action orders of the Kennedy administration (E.O. 10925, 1961), which were at best symbolic. However, it was not until 1968 that goals and timetables became a part of these programs. In a later executive order, President Nixon clarified the meaning of affirmative action (E.O. 11749, 1969). Additionally, he added provisions assuring that recruitment efforts would be extended to all sources of job candidates by requiring employers to make use of the present skills of employees, as well as to provide programs to upgrade their skills, and to participate in school and government efforts to improve community conditions affecting the employees. These executive orders were part of an effort to equalize the percentages of minorities in federal or federal contract employment and apply only to government employees; they are distinct from the provisions of Title VII.

A variety of State and Federal laws determine who must adopt affirmative action programs. Any employer holding federal contracts or subcontracts totaling more than $2500 must have affirmative action programs for the handicapped; if the contracts total more than $10,000, the employer must have a program including women, blacks, Hispanics, Asians, American Indians, and Vietnam veterans. Since Federal research grants are considered to be contracts, almost all university-affiliated hospitals are bound by these orders. Many States have similar regulations. Employers who have been found by the courts to have discriminated in the past (under Title VII) may be required to institute affirmative action programs.

Affirmative action is a plan for positive steps that an employer will take to ensure equal opportunity. It cannot be viewed as a standardized program that must be accomplished in the same way at all times by all employers.[10] There are three basic elements in an affirmative action program.[43]

1. The employer's current work force is analyzed to determine whether the percentages of minorities employed are similar to the percentages available in the labor pool who possess the basic job-related qualifications. When substantial disparities are found, an analysis is made of the selection process that is operating to exclude the minority individual.
2. A statement of hiring and promotion goals and a timetable for correcting deficiencies is established.
3. A plan for attaining the goals and a system for regularly monitoring the effectiveness of the affirmative action program is implemented.

There are several criticisms of affirmative action. Some see it as a quota system that imposes unfair burdens on white males and leads to reverse discrimination. However, the goals of affirmative action programs are clearly defined and distinct from rigid, inflexible requirements or quotas. In fact, quotas are specifically prohibited, as illustrated in the Supreme Court's decision in *Bakke* v. *The University of California at Davis* (1978) and *Weber* v. *Kaiser Aluminum* (1979). Goals are simply statements by the employer that the number of minority individuals employed will reach the level that would be achieved by drawing from the labor pool without bias.

Other critics contend that affirmative action programs lead to lower standards, implying that the relative qualifications of candidates will be ignored at the expense of mandatory percentages, resulting in preferential selection. Preferential selection in actuality occurs only in the infrequent situation of equally qualified candidates where a minority candidate is given preference; or when, in the process of ranking, positive credit is given for minority status. A recent ruling by the Supreme Court in *Johnson* v. *Transportation Agency, Santa Clara, California* (1987) has further emphasized that employers who voluntarily set hiring and promotion goals to improve representation of women and members of minority groups where a "manifest imbalance" exists have some protection against claims of discrimination by nonminority men. In this case, a male employee charged "reverse discrimination" when a woman with slightly less qualification was promoted to the job he was seeking. Although it is too early to ascertain the total impact of this ruling, it should not be construed as a quota system. Rather, institutions are able to modify their affirmative action plans to allow consideration of sex and race where a "manifest imbalance" exists.

By focused recruiting and employee development, larger numbers of well-qualified minorities can be brought into the labor market, resulting in a larger, more diverse pool of talent. Additionally, as equal opportunity goals are reached, the number of reverse discrimination conflicts will decrease.

Because affirmative action has been in existence a relatively short time, it is still too early too assess the full potential of these programs in terms of measurable practices such as changes in outreach, interviewing, skill-upgrading programs, promotion reviews, and employee selection and the effect they will have on the goal of achieving full integration.

Discrimination is deeply ingrained in our society. Fry recently published a study that predicts affirmative action programs will not achieve full integration for minorities until the year 2013.[8] The future success of affirmative action programs will not depend on formal programs, but rather on our society's commitment to end discrimination and improve the status of disadvantaged groups.

The Equal Employment Opportunity Commission

The effectiveness of Title VII and affirmative action programs depend largely on employers' willingness to comply with the law. When employers do not comply, the Equal Employment Opportunity Commission (EEOC) and the courts determine what constitutes violation of the law and set the penalties for noncompliance. The EEOC was formed in 1965 as the enforcing arm of the Civil Rights Act. It is a compliance agency whose investigative powers are evoked by the charges of discrimination filed by an aggrieved person or EEOC commissioner. The State governments have similar agencies commonly referred to as fair employment practices commissions to regulate similar State statutes. Affirmative action programs, being executive orders, are under the jurisdiction of the Departments of Justice and Labor (Office of Federal Contract Compliance [OFCCP]) and the Civil Service Commission (CSC).

The EEOC has identified three aspects of discrimination:

1. Disparate treatment
2. Disparate impact
3. Perpetuation of past discrimination

Disparate treatment is the most easily understood type of discrimination. The employer simply treats some people less favorably than others because of age, race, color, religion, sex, marital status, or national origin. Disparity in treatment includes failure to recruit, hire, transfer, or promote minority group members on an equal basis with white persons. Usually it must be proved that disparate treatment is a

matter of practice and that the differences are "racially premised." Statistical evidence showing a difference in treatment is "relevant only to prove that the employer regularly made discriminatory decisions, not to support the contention that a work force is racially unbalanced.

The disparate-impact doctrine is designed to prevent unintentional discrimination resulting from apparently neutral practices. A case of discrimination can be proved by showing that an employment practice has a disparate effect between white males and any protected group. If disparate effect is shown, employers must prove that such practices result from business necessity or are unrelated to the employment status of the employee allegedly discriminated against.[26]

Perpetuation of past discrimination is sometimes built into an employer's hiring and promotion practices, especially when he uses a merit or seniority system for promotion or selection. These procedures exclude minorities because past discrimination has resulted in their lacking the necessary skills, education, training, or job attitude. The objective of Title VII is to remove barriers that have operated in the past to exclude minorities. This is usually accomplished by the modification of seniority systems and by the recruitment of minorities into training and continuing education programs that influence selection for promotion.

Many employers are finding that the issue of discrimination is far from academic. There are hundreds of cases in the Federal courts, and many of the court decisions have cost employers a great deal of money. In one case, Standard Oil Company of California agreed to a $2 million settlement as restitution for laying off 160 older employees during a reduction in force.* An employer who fails to comply with EEOC guidelines can be subject to judgments under Title VII calling for significant back-pay awards; if the employer is a Federal government contractor, he can be barred from receiving any additional government contracts. Under Title VII the employee has the right to bring a civil suit against the discriminating employer. However, the employee must give notice to the EEOC that he intends to bring suit 60 days before he files. During this period the EEOC usually conducts an investigation of the alleged discrimination and attempts a reconciliation between the employer and the employee. In cases where there is strong evidence of discrimination, the EEOC will actually bring suit against the employer. If the EEOC does not bring suit, the employee still has the right to bring his

*Business Week, p 91, February 24, 1975.

civil suit. The employee may seek both legal and equitable remedies, usually wages lost because of the discrimination. The employee may even recover damages for pain and suffering, or the employee may ask for retroactive seniority as restitution for past discrimination.

Additional Legal Considerations in Hiring

Several recent legal actions have had a considerable impact on how prospective employers must assess applicants. House Rule 4154, amending the Age Discrimination in Employment Act (ADEA), extends protection under the Act to workers in the private sector and to most State and local government employees beyond the age of 70. The amendments eliminate mandatory retirement for workers over age 70. The new amendments also require that employers cannot discriminate against any individual over 40 in terms of paid benefits or continued employment. Although this law became effective January 1, 1987, there is a 7-year exemption for implementation of these amendments for State and local government employers when dealing with public safety employees such as police, firepersons, prison guards, and tenured college professors. This has caused some consternation on the part of employers who feel they will have less power to determine the composition of their work force. They fear the potential for discrimination suits brought by an older worker can be an increasing problem for which they are ill prepared. Also, there is some concern that a "gray-haired work force" will, potentially, create morale problems for other workers.[18] These concerns can be minimized by creative use of retirement plans. In summary, age cannot be a discriminating factor in the hiring process, and potential applicants must be assessed on the basis of individual merit.

On June 1, 1987, the Immigration Reform and Control Act (IRCA) of 1986 took effect. This legislation prohibits employers from knowingly hiring or continuing to employ illegal aliens. Personnel departments in institutions will most likely handle the responsibility of checking potential employees' identity documents such as a driver's license with photograph and work eligibility records such as a social security card or certificate of United States citizenship.

THE APPLICATION FORM

In the process of interviewing candidates for employment, the employer gathers preliminary information about the applicant's potential for success in a given position by use of an application form. Because the application is often used as a screening tool to eliminate at an early stage unqualified individuals from consideration for employment, and because eventual hiring decisions are made on the basis of answers given on the application, it must conform to Title VII of the Civil Rights Act: Questions appearing on the form must be established to be related to legitimate occupational qualifications. Further, it must not have a disparate impact on minorities by the use of qualifying factors that disproportionately screen out protected groups in favor of white male applicants. With the exception of questions pertaining to an individual's arrest record, Title VII does not specifically forbid the inclusion of non-job-related items. However, when the employer is charged with discrimination, the burden of proof (of the business necessity of the question) rests with the employer. In a study published by *Fortune* magazine on May 8, 1978, it was found that some 99% of the employers studied included at least one inappropriate question on their application form; 38% included more than ten inappropriate items.

The investment of time and effort in preparing an application that is unbiased will be rewarding both in terms of obtaining suitable employees and in terms of avoiding charges of discrimination and consequent costly legal proceedings. A good method to use in designing such an application is to make up a worksheet containing the information needed about an applicant before a decision to hire is made and the information needed for recording purposes after the applicant is hired.[36] This list will vary for each job description. Accordingly, specific applications must be tailored for specific jobs. Then list the reasons the information is needed. This will help determine whether the information is indeed job-related. Using this information, prepare an application with the following points in mind:

1. Do the questions conform to Title VII of the Civil Rights Act, EEOC guidelines (*guidelines on the Employment Selection Process,* a publication available from local offices of the EEOC)?
2. Do the questions relate specifically to the job that the applicant is seeking? Can it be proved to be a bona fide occupational qualification or an absolute business necessity?
3. Do the questions violate the applicant's right to privacy?
4. Will the questions disqualify a disproportionate number of minorities or

protected group members? Are there any valid studies that indicate that these items are valid predictors of occupational success?

It is probably best to discard any question if there is even a remote possibility that it cannot be justified by these criteria. In some cases, merely rewording an inappropriate question will make it acceptable. Table 11-1 identifies acceptable and unacceptable inquires.[13] Questions may be established as an occupational qualification by conducting research to validate the item as a predictor of success for a specific position. Also, such research can be used to substantiate that the item does not have a disparate impact on any protected group. Some information that you may need for the record or statistical purposes and that cannot be asked on the application can be obtained after hiring. Such information includes photographs for identification purposes, age, sex, race, marital status, and so forth.

It is a good idea to include on the application a blanket statement indicating that you are an equal employment opportunity/affirmative action employer and are not interested in receiving information that may be construed to be discriminatory in nature. The application should include a statement signed and dated by the prospective employee indicating that he has not falsified any information on the application. This is necessary in the event you wish to terminate the employee for such reasons. If you intend to check references, you will need the applicant's signed permission for this also.

As a final check for the validity of your application you may want to submit it to the local offices of the EEOC for their advice and approval. An application example is shown in Figure 11-1.

The application is often your first contact with prospective employees. For this reason it should, in addition to gathering vital information, make a positive statement about the employer. Because it is a vital part of the employee selection process, the use of the most appropriate application will be to the employer's best interest.

REFERENCE CHECKS

Reference checks are important because how a prospective employee has performed in the past is a good predictor of how he will perform in the future. However, the nature of information that can be obtained from a former employer has been rigidly limited by various State and Federal regulations designed to protect the applicant.

The major restriction is the applicant's written permission to contact the persons he has listed as references. Any inquiry as to the person's previous salary, scholastic aptitude, or work habits violates his right to privacy. Information supplied concerning the applicant's lifestyle may indicate race, national origin, or other protected-group status and thus may be discriminatory in nature and violate the applicant's civil rights under Title VII. Moreover, any previous employer or supervisor who gives deleterious information is subject to charges of slander by the applicant.

The purpose of the reference check, then, is to validate the applicant's employment record. This can be best accomplished through a telephone call or personal visit. Obviously, it is important to validate the information supplied to you by the applicant (dates of employment, position) with the employer's record. Any discrepancies found do not speak in the applicant's favor.

Other information can be gleaned from the employment record. An individual who has a record of short stays with employers may indicate a lack of stability, which should be assessed further in an interview. The advancements in job position or attendance of training programs or participation in continuing education by the applicant suggest positive qualities that can be further evaluated in the interview.

Although reference checks are a limited source of information concerning a prospective employee, they remain a vital part of the selection process. In the clinical laboratory, an individual's credentials are critically important for assuring the quality of laboratory results. One of this chapter's authors recalls an incident in which a chemistry supervisor was hired on the basis of his self-stated academic preparation equivalent to a doctoral degree. The individual at the time appeared to be a godsend in the middle of a crisis following several evening-shift resignations. Months later, after the manpower shortage had been alleviated, technical problems arising in the laboratory prompted the chief technologist to check a reference or two on the new chemistry supervisor. The resulting information revealed academic preparation perhaps equivalent to the baccalaureate level but without the degree. Reference checks, therefore, as evidenced by this example, play an important role in the interviewing and selection process if quality is to be maintained.

CONDUCTING THE INTERVIEW

An interview is essentially a conversation between two people which permits a give-and-take exchange
(*Text continues on p 190*)

Table 11-1
Eliminating Discrimination from Preemployment Inquiries

Category	Acceptable Inquiries	Unacceptable Inquiries
Age	Valid if necessary to secure proof of age to comply with child labor laws. Valid in age-based occupations requiring strenuous manual labor. Valid in professions where the age-related degenerative process could affect job performance and safety because of impaired reflexes.	Inadvisable to ask applicant's age for any reason other than to ensure compliance with child labor laws. Law generally forbids discrimination against individuals 40–70 years of age.
Arrests	None.	Questions concerning arrests and *not* convictions may be viewed as discriminatory because in some geographic areas certain racial minorities have a higher percentage of arrests than Caucasians. Rejection for employment on this basis could thus have an untoward effect on these minorities.
Convictions	Permissible in security-sensitive positions. Inquiries concerning convictions for theft or embezzlement would be considered acceptable when hiring a laboratory purchasing agent.	Questions concerning convictions unrelated to job requirements and responsibilities.
Credit	None, unless job related.	Inquiries about personal finances to ascertain an applicant's level of affluence. This may be viewed as discriminatory because the nonminority population is perceived to be more affluent.
Education and experience	Questions to determine if an applicant has the specific education or training required for a particular job. Permissible when experience is critical to successful job performance, as in requiring a minimum amount of flight time for commercial pilots.	General inquiries about high school or college degrees, unless you can prove the educational degree in question is needed to perform the job. Questions about specific institutions attended may be regarded as discriminatory, since some schools have predominantly racial or religious minority student bodies. Asking for dates of attendance could be interpreted as an indirect means of getting at an applicant's age.
Emergency notification	Name and address of person to be notified in case of an emergency.	Name and address of relative to be notified in case of an emergency. Asking for information about an applicant's relatives could be viewed as an indirect attempt to learn national origin, especially in the case of a married woman with an ethnic maiden name.

(continued)

Table 11-1 (Continued)

Category	Acceptable Inquiries	Unacceptable Inquiries
Family status	Permissible if relevant to job performance. Valid inquiries concern any commitments that might prevent the applicant from meeting such professional responsibilities as travel, late hours, or weekend work. The questions, however, must be asked of *both* men and women.	Questions designed to ascertain the applicant's parental or marital status, spouse's profession, number and age of children, or child care arrangements. Any questions asked of only one sex.
Handicaps	Questions to find out if an applicant has any specific physical or mental handicaps that would interfere with the ability to perform a particular job. Permissible in jobs requiring rapid reflexes, high degree of speed, strength, coordination, dexterity, or endurance if these standards are shown to be reasonably necessary for job performance.	Inquiries of a general nature, such as: "Do you have any handicaps?" These questions might cause an applicant to reveal handicaps that are not related to the ability to perform a specific job.
Marital status	None, unless job related.	Any questions about whether the applicant is single, engaged, married, separated, divorced, or widowed, unless it is job related.
Military service	Inquiries pertinent to education or training gained in the United States Armed Services if applicable to job requirements and responsibilities.	Asking the type, condition, and date of discharge. Inquiries concerning foreign military experience. Questions to determine the applicant's whereabouts during 1914–1918, 1941–1945, 1950–1953, and 1964–1975. Any questions concerning general military experience.
National origin	Questions concerning the applicant's ability to read, write, or speak English or any foreign language when required for a specific position.	Asking about an applicant's place of birth, native tongue, language spoken at home, or length and status of residency in the United States.
Organizations	Inquiries about memberships in job-related professional organizations, societies, or associations.	Questions about memberships in specific organizations to ascertain an applicant's nationality, color, creed, religion, sex, marital status, political affiliation, or social or economic class. Some private clubs have historically banned certain minorities and religious groups; membership in others is limited to certain minorities and religious groups.

(continued)

Table 11-1 (Continued)

Category	Acceptable Inquiries	Unacceptable Inquiries
Photograph	May be requested for identification purposes *after* the applicant becomes an employee.	Requiring an applicant to supply a photograph with the application. Such prescreening is discriminatory.
Physical data	Valid only if the information pertains to a *bona fide* occupational qualification. When questioning an applicant about height or weight, be prepared to prove that a specific size is necessary for job performance.	Any question concerning height, weight, or other physical characteristics that are not job related.
Pregnancy	None.	Asking anything about the applicant's medical history related to pregnancy. The EEOC has ruled that refusing to employ a woman solely because she is pregnant amounts to sex discrimination.
Race or color	None.	Any question on a form about the color of the applicant's skin, eyes, or hair. Any inquiry concerning race or color.
References	Names of persons willing to provide professional references. Valid when solicited in good faith, given appropriate consideration, and not used to accomplish a discriminatory result.	Inflexible policy of rejecting applicants solely on the basis of adverse reports from previous employers, as these references could be shaded by the employer's own prejudices. Inadvisable to request the name of the applicant's pastor or religious leader.
Relatives	Questions about relatives, other than the applicant's spouse, already employed by the organization.	Inquiries designed to encourage employees to recruit their friends and relatives when minorities are underrepresented in the current work force. Additionally, you must be able to prove good business reasons for not hiring the spouse of current employees, because women often suffer disproportionately under this policy.
Religious preference	None.	Questions concerning an applicant's religious holidays observed.
Sex	None.	Any question asked.

(From Ivey TR: Keeping the employment interview legal. MLO 13(11):109–110, 1981.

Reprinted with permission from Medical Economics Company, Inc., Oradell, New Jersey.)

FILE #_ _ _ _ _ _ _ _ _ _

THE UNIVERSITY OF NEBRASKA MEDICAL CENTER
42ND AND DEWEY AVENUE
OMAHA, NEBRASKA 68105

COLLEGE OF MEDICINE
  SCHOOL OF ALLIED HEALTH PROFESSIONS
COLLEGE OF NURSING
COLLEGE OF PHARMACY
COLLEGE OF DENTISTRY
UNIVERSITY HOSPITAL AND CLINICS
EPPLEY INSTITUTE FOR RESEARCH IN
  CANCER AND ALLIED DISEASES
C. LOUIS MEYER CHILDREN'S
  REHABILITATION INSTITUTE

AN EQUAL OPPORTUNITY EMPLOYER M/F/H

APPLICATION FOR EMPLOYMENT

1. CURRENT INFORMATION

Name (Type or Print as on Social Security Card) _____
                                     Last   First   Middle

Social Security Number _____ _____ _____
                                 Application Date _____
                                         Month Day Year

Position(s) applied for (1) _____ (2) _____ (3) _____

This application is for Full Time ☐ Part Time ☐ Permanent ☐ Temporary (normally, 3 months or less) ☐

Date available for work _____ _____ _____
                  Month Day Year   Minimum salary acceptable $ _____

Present Mailing Address _____
                      Street & No. or RFD   City   State   Zip Code

Permanent Mailing Address _____
                      Street & No. or RFD   City   State   Zip Code

Telephone Home _____ Business _____ If none, where can you be reached by telephone? _____

Driver's License Number (If Applicable) _____

Citizenship U.S.☐ If not U.S. Visa Type _____ Date Granted _____ ____ _____ Immigrant No _____
                                             Month Day Year

Military Service Are you a veteran? No ☐ Yes ☐ Dates of Military Service From _____ _____ To _____ _____
                                                  Month Year   Month Year

In case of emergency notify _____ Telephone Number _____

* The Age Discrimination in Employment Act of 1967 as amended prohibits discrimination of age with respect to individuals who are at least 40 but less than 70 years of age. Federal law prohibits employing persons 16 and 17 years old in certain high-risk positions.

Are you between the ages of 16 - 70? Yes _____ No _____

2. EDUCATIONAL & TRAINING RECORD

Give your complete educational history below. For any position requiring special education, transcripts of all college education may be requested for employment.

Elementary or High School	Name of School	City & State	Circle Highest Grade Completed 1 2 3 4 5 6 7 8 9 10 11 12 G.E.D.	Graduate: ☐Yes ☐No	Graduation Date or Last Year Attended

College	Name of School	City & State	Circle Highest Grade Attended: 1 2 3 4 5	Graduate? ☐Yes ☐No	Graduation Date or Last Year Attended:
Major		Minor	Degree(s)		

College	Name of School	City & State	Circle Highest Grade Attended: 1 2 3 4 5	Graduate? ☐Yes ☐No	Graduation Date or Last Year Attended:
Major		Minor	Degree(s)		

College	Name of School	City & State	Circle Highest Grade Attended: 1 2 3 4 5	Graduate? ☐Yes ☐No	Graduation Date or Last Year Attended:
Major		Minor	Degree(s)		

Graduate School	Name of School	City & State	Graduate? ☐Yes ☐No	Graduation Date	No. of Credits Earned	Major	Degree(s)

Other Courses Completed	Name & Addresses of Schools			
Courses		Date Completed	Certificate or Diploma	

Rev. 6/79

Side 1

FIGURE 11-1. Four-sided general application form. (Reprinted with permission of the Chancellor, University of Nebraska Medical Center)

APPLICANT LOG

The University of Nebraska Medical Center is an Equal Opportunity/Affirmative Action Employer. The Federal Government requires us to collect and be able to produce data pertaining to each applicant's ethnic background, citizenship and sex, as well as any handicap. Please complete the following Applicant Log information, which will be removed from the application, retained in the Human Resource Department and not forwarded to any employing department. In keeping with the University's status as an Equal Opportunity/Affirmative Action Employer, this information will not be used in making any decision affecting employment or any personnel action following employment.

The following information is needed for voluntary or affirmative action efforts. We invite you to furnish the information on a voluntary basis; however, your refusal to provide it WILL NOT subject you to any adverse treatment. This information will be kept confidential.

PLEASE ENTER INFORMATION REQUESTED ABOVE THE HEAVY LINE

Today's Date	Name (Print or Type as on Social Security Card)	Sex	Date of Birth	Are you a Vietnam Era Veteran? (Vietnam Era begins August 4, 1954)
Mo Day Yr	(Last) (First) (Middle) SS #	☐ Female ☐ Male	Mo. Day Yr.	☐ No ☐ Yes

ETHNIC BACKGROUND

☐ **W** White (not of Hispanic origin): Persons having origins in any of the original peoples of Europe, North Africa, or the Middle East.

☐ **B** Black (not of Hispanic origin): All persons having origins in any of the black racial groups of Africa.

☐ **H** Hispanic: All persons of Mexican, Puerto Rican, Cuban, Central or South American, or other Spanish culture or origin, regardless of race.

☐ **AI** American Indian or Alaskan Native: All persons having origins in any of the original peoples of North America, and who maintain cultural identification through tribal affiliation or community recognition.

☐ **AA** Asian or Pacific Islanders: All persons having origins in any of the original peoples of the Far East, Southeast Asia, the Indian Subcontinent, or the Pacific Islands. For example, China, Japan, Korea, the Phillipine Islands, and Samoa.

CITIZENSHIP

☐ Resident foreign national [Alien who has been admitted for permanent residence (must have Alien Registration Card, Form 1-151)]

☐ Non-resident foreign national (Alien admitted temporarily for specific purposes and periods of time)

☐ U.S. Citizen

PHYSICAL OR MENTAL HANDICAP (IF ANY)

☐ Blind

☐ Deaf

☐ Communicative

☐ Orthopedic

☐ Other (specify) _____

Position(s) Applied For:

1. _____
2. _____
3. _____

This application is in response to (please specify):

☐ Newspaper _____   ☐ Walk In

☐ Telephone Job Listing (541-4446) _____   ☐ Other (please specify) _____

☐ Nebraska Job Service _____

Side 2

FIGURE 11-1. (Continued)

3. CURRENT PROFESSIONAL REGISTRATION

States license in: _____ Current Registration Number: _____

If not licensed in **Nebraska, have you applied?** Yes _____ No _____

Membership in professional and honorary organizations: _____

_____

_____

4. SKILLS

(Please list any skills and abilities you wish considered. Include skills with equipment or machines you operate, special computer knowledge, laboratory techniques, and the like.

_____

_____

_____

_____

_____

_____

5. GENERAL INFORMATION

a. Are you employed? No ☐ Yes ☐ If *Yes*, may we inquire of your employer regarding your experience and qualifications? No ☐ Yes ☐

b. Have you filed an Application for Staff Employment with the University within the last two years? No ☐ Yes ☐

c. Will you accept employment requiring night shift or weekend work? No ☐ Yes ☐

d. Are you, or have you ever been, employed by the State of Nebraska or at the University? No ☐ Yes ☐ If *Yes,* where? Give places and dates.

_____

_____

_____

_____

*e. Are you related by blood or marriage to any person now employed by the University of Nebraska Medical Center? No ☐ Yes ☐ If *Yes*, give name, relationship, and department.

_____

_____

**f. Have you ever been convicted of any offense (other than a minor traffic violation with a fine of $50 or less)? No ☐ Yes ☐ If *Yes*, please explain.

_____

_____

* to avoid conflict of interest or violation of the UNMC Nepotism policy only.

** conviction of a crime does not necessarily exclude a candidate from employment.

6. NURSING ONLY

1. What areas of clinical service do you prefer? (Peds, Surgery, etc.)

   1. _____ 2. _____ 3. _____

2. What shift (tour of duty) do you prefer? Please check appropriate block.

   ☐ Any   ☐ Rotation   ☐ Permanent Evenings   ☐ Permanent Nights

3. If preferred shift not available, will you accept another shift?   ☐ Yes   ☐ No

   If yes, please check appropriate box: ☐ Rotation   ☐ Permanent Evenings   ☐ Permanent Nights

FIGURE 11-1. (Continued)

7. EMPLOYMENT RECORD (List your present or most recent employer *FIRST*. Include U.S. Armed Forces experiences. *Account for all time during the past 10 years* including periods of unemployment. Include any unpaid work experience.)

Firm _____ Address_____

City_____ State_____ Phone _____

Job Title_____

Nature of Duties (Explain fully) _____

	Employed	
From: Mo. Yr.	To: Mo. Yr.	
	Salary	
Start		End

Reason for Leaving_____

Immediate Supervisor _____

Firm _____ Address_____

City_____ State_____ Phone _____

Job Title_____

Nature of Duties (Explain fully) _____

	Employed	
From: Mo. Yr.	To: Mo. Yr.	
	Salary	
Start		End

Reason for Leaving_____

Immediate Supervisor _____

Firm ___

City

HIRING AGREEMENT

I certify that the information contained in this application is true to the best of my knowledge and belief. I understand that any willful omission of facts or misrepresentation is cause for denial of employment and or dismissal as applicable.

I grant permission for the authorities of the University of Nebraska Medical Center and Hospital to investigate my work references and release said agency from any and all liability resulting from such investigation. Upon my termination, I authorize the release of reference information on my work.

I agree to submit to a pre-employment physical and recognize employment is contingent upon successfully meeting Hospital physical requirements.

I further agree that if I've been convicted of a crime, the authorities of the University of Nebraska Medical Center and Hospital may obtain the details of my conviction to determine it's relationship to the position I'm applying for as a condition of my employment.

_____   _____

Signature   Date

Side 4

FIGURE 11-1.   (Continued)

of information and ideas. Even though the interview process has not been shown to be particularly reliable, it is still the primary process by which employment decisions are made.[18] An employment interview should have structure and purpose (e.g., to gather information, give directions, or motivate). The preemployment interview serves two basic functions. First, it provides the opportunity for the employer to get to know the applicant. The applicant's qualifications for the job, his background, and previous employment records are analyzed and discussed. Subjective information concerning maturity, personal appearance, attitudes, potential, and other pertinent areas is gathered. Second, the interview gives the applicant essential information about the nature of the job, hours, benefits, continuing education and training programs, and opportunities for advancement. Further, it serves to create an early feeling of mutual understanding between the employer and the applicant. A good initial relationship not only gives a positive impression to the most valuable prospective employee but also is the basis for a lasting rapport between management and the employee.

The major advantage of the interview is that it is more flexible than written statements. It is particularly useful because it allows the interviewer to probe for more information than is on the written application.[12,22] The interview process has five separate but overlapping stages: (1) warm-up, (2) getting the applicant to talk, (3) drawing-out, (4) information, and (5) forming an opinion.[21]

The *warm-up* stage allows the interviewer to put the applicant at ease and to begin to develop a rapport in a relaxed atmosphere for the interview. This is important because most applicants are somewhat apprehensive. At this point, it is helpful to initiate a constructive atmosphere through a few general social remarks or similar interactions. The interviewer should create an atmosphere of sincere and genuine interest, recognizing the applicant as worthy of attention. An applicant who is at ease is far more likely to provide candid self-expression and an accurate assessment of attitudes, feelings, and ideas.

In the second stage, the interviewer must *get the applicant talking*. The interviewer must make the purpose of the interview clear quickly, explaining its function in terms that can be readily understood. The interviewer must have formulated goals and purposes for the interview, primarily from a review of the completed application and other pertinent information that has been gathered about the applicant. A good first question is extremely important to trigger the applicant's flow of conversation.

This question should be one with which the applicant will probably be comfortable. For instance, asking an open-ended question, "I see that you have worked as a chief technologist at Memorial Hospital for the last three years. Can you tell me what you enjoy most about your job?" This allows the applicant to set the pace of the conversation.

In the *drawing-out* stage, the applicant is encouraged to further describe his background, qualifications, and other attributes he believes support his candidacy. During this stage, the interviewer should use various questioning techniques to learn as much as possible about the applicant. This is a critical time for the interviewer to assess as accurately as possible whether the applicant has appropriate knowledge, skills, and attitudes for the position. Information that is missed at this stage is likely not able to be retrieved later on. Some critical interviewing techniques are reviewed later in this chapter.

In the *information* stage, the interviewer presents a picture of the institution and the specific job for which the applicant has applied. At this point, also, the applicant may ask any questions about his perceived role. Through this interaction, potential problems can be expressed or fears presented that can affect the job. Also, the interviewer is able to get some sense of the applicant's real interest in the position, aspirations, and future goals.

The last stage of the interview is when an *opinion is formed*. This is usually done after the applicant has left the office and when constructive note-taking can take place. Generally, it may be appropriate to take a few notes during the interview; however, major observations and analyses should be delayed until after the applicant has left. The interviewer must assess the applicant's qualifications against the requirements and conditions that have been identified for the position.

Interviewing Basics

A few basic planning techniques can help the manager conduct an effective interview.[5,9,19]

INTERVIEW PREPARATION. The interviewer should take ample time to plan the process by carefully reviewing the job description. The interview should be scheduled so that there is ample time to conduct a quality, interactive process with the applicant and to ensure that there is a sense that ample time was spent with the applicant.

ANALYSIS OF THE RESUME. Careful review of the resume for analyzing the applicant's experience and abilities is extremely important before the interview. The resume detail is the applicant's chronologic work record and other data useful in determining whether the candidate seems appropriate for the position. Through careful analysis, questions can be formulated for the interview. A review of the resume should determine, for instance, the chronologic record of the person's employment, educational qualifications, service to the profession, community activities, and other information that profiles the applicant. The reviewer can also pinpoint potential areas of concern such as lapses in the work record, numerous job changes, lack of advancement, and other data to be investigated during the questioning portion of the interview.

INTERVIEW ENVIRONMENT. The interview process is a complex task involving screening and evaluation of much verbal data from the applicant; thus, a quiet atmosphere with minimal distractions is advantageous. Also, the interviewee will feel more comfortable in a setting that is private, free from phone calls or interruptions from staff. It is also important for the interviewer to create an environment without bias that may distort perceptions.

STRUCTURED INTERVIEW. It is important that in any interview the interviewer proceed in an organized fashion, generally proceeding in reverse chronologic order from the applicant's current position and covering prior work and educational preparation. All of this information will give the applicant an opportunity to demonstrate qualifications for the position, as well as identify such items as career progress, job stability, overall motivation, and salary history.

COMMUNICATION SKILLS. The communication during the interview process should be as simple and nonthreatening as possible. The interview itself is designed to determine the match between the applicant's experience and training with the duties and responsibilities of the position. The questions posed by the interviewer should not be complex. An understanding of some basic questioning techniques enables the interviewer to be more precise in the data-gathering process. Types of questions typically used in the interview process include:

Leading Questions. This type of question tends to lead the applicant to a predetermined answer. These have really no place in the interview and should be avoided. If they are used, the amount of information obtained is minimal, and the answer only tends to confirm what is implied in the question. For example:

"You obviously don't like working at Metropolitan Hospital, do you?"

"You really haven't had much experience related to this position, have you?"

"You seem to have had some problems at your last job, hadn't you?"

Open-Ended Questions. Questions that are open-ended cannot be answered with a yes or no. They require more explanation and provide the interviewee an opportunity to offer unsolicited information or clarify comments. While such questions allow the interviewee to control a portion of the interview, they also create an environment in which the interviewer is able to glean a great deal of information. Some examples:

"You've heard the description of the job, could you now tell me how you think you fit into it?"

"If you were to take this position, how would it fit into your future ambitions?"

"Can you tell me your reasons for leaving your last job?"

"As you can see, the job of senior medical technologist at this hospital has some problems attached to it; how do you think you would help solve these problems and make the laboratory more productive?"

Direct Questions. These questions can be answered with a "yes," "no," or one-word answer. The best use of these questions is when you want to gain specific information, rather than a general explanation. The questions should be quick and to the point, and are most effective when followed by an open-ended question. Some examples:

"What is your current salary? What salary considerations do you feel are important in the position for which you are applying?"

"Having seen the laboratory, are you still interested in this position? What do you think you can do to make the laboratory more productive?"

Probing Questions. Probing questions are designed to delve more deeply into the interviewee's answers. There are a number of different situations in which probing questions are appropriate. For instance, in response to a short incomplete answer, the interviewer may wish to delve more deeply to gain more specific information. For instance:

First Question: "Have you gone to any continuing education programs, recently?"

Applicant response: "A few."

Probing Question: "Can you describe these programs for me?"

Some probing questions may be used where there is need for further clarification or to explain a response that was unclear or did not make sense in the context of the question. For instance:

First Question: "What do you think you would enjoy most about being the supervisor of the laboratory section?"

Applicant Response: "The job looks really challenging."

Probing Question: "What would you enjoy about the challenge?"

Sometimes a probing question will be channeled more directly to focus on a perceived feeling or attitude that has been identified by the interviewer. Thinking that it is important to amplify on it, the interviewer may wish to probe more deeply in an attempt to ascertain the true frame of reference of the interviewee. For instance:

First Question: "What particularly appeals to you about the technologist position for which you are applying?"

Applicant Response: "It seems like the kind of position in which I could work independently from others without any of the usual hassles with the other technologists."

Probing Question: "What kinds of hassles have you experienced when working closely with others?"

Hypothetical Questions. These questions provide the interviewer excellent insight into the problem-solving thought processes of the applicant. Good hypothetical questions will pose a potential problem and ask the interviewee to propose a solution. These provide an opportunity for the applicant to demonstrate insight, experience, and innovation. Some examples might be:

"If this laboratory is going to maintain its present level of activity, some entrepreneural ventures are going to have to be pursued. Do you have any ideas as to how we might be able to expand our services or scope of testing offered?"

"The job you are applying for requires a lot of interaction with hospital management who have so far been insensitive to problems that cost-containment measures have caused us. Do you have any ideas about how we might be able to help them better understand the laboratory operation?"

Effective use of questioning techniques is an interviewer skill that maximizes the gathering of information about the applicant.[12] The development of questioning techniques takes concentrated practice; however, over time, the interviewer should be able to develop the interviewing process to the point that a considerable amount of critical information is gained during a relatively short interview period.

INTERVIEW TERMINATION AND FOLLOW-UP. The interviewer establishes the conclusion of the interview when he decides that all the relevant information is gathered and the purpose of the interview has been achieved. The interviewer should summarize the major points and tie up loose ends brought out at the interview. As at the beginning, casual social comments are an appropriate way to wind down the interview. Often, the last words of the interviewer are remembered longest. In particular, the interviewer should express an appreciation for the opportunity to talk to the applicant. It is appropriate in closing to give the applicant some idea of how the interviewer has assessed the applicant's qualities. It is also appropriate for the interviewer to indicate how he will be communicating with him after the interviewing process has been completed. The applicant should be provided with a realistic date by which he can expect to hear from the employer. On the other hand, if the candidate appears to be unsatisfactory, the interviewer should clearly indicate that the applicant may not be matched with the job.

Misunderstandings can lead to charges of discrimination. At the conclusion of the interview, the interviewer must ensure adequate follow-up by consolidating results, updating employment records, and other routine procedures such as contacting the personnel department. Some information gathered in the interview may not be as easy to quantify. Writing up notes taken during the interview serves to clarify impressions or ideas and to emphasize the applicant's strong or weak points.

Limitations of Interviewing

Anyone with supervisory responsibilities eventually becomes involved in the interviewing process. Successful interviewing is a challenge; however, interviewing skills can be mastered by simple training, exposure, and practice. Although much of the success of the interview is based on the skills and discipline of the interviewer, there are some limitations inherent in all interviews.

First, it is important to emphasize that there are certain questions that may not be asked during an interview. These are the same as those prohibited on the application form (see Table 11-1). For instance, race and color are never acceptable standards for hiring, and no questions should be asked that relate to these areas. Although recent court rulings indicate that institutions may hire on the basis of sex or race where there are clear inequities, it is never appropriate to focus upon such areas as part of the interview. Questions related to sex are always to be avoided. For instance, questions related to marriage (Are you married? Do you have any children?) or spousal relationships (Where does your husband work?) are inappropriate and should be avoided. It is discriminatory to ask a woman about who will take care of her children. If the position requires the ability of the applicant to work extended hours during peak periods of time, a question may be asked such as, "At certain times of the year, we have especially heavy workloads, and overtime may be required. Is there anything that would prevent you from performing this part of the job satisfactorily?" Questions related to national original, religion, age, and arrest or conviction records are all inappropriate as well.

The second limitation of interviewing is that the reliability of the interview is markedly lower when the interview is unplanned, aimlessly directed, and vague. In this situation, the interviewer is likely to rate the applicants inconsistently: the same applicant might receive different ratings in two interviews with the same interviewer. A thorough knowledge of the job description, a firm set of qualifications, including standards for each level within a position, and a systematic plan for assessing each applicant increase the interviewer's reliability.

Team interviewing is another method that increases reliability. Often, individual interviewers do not rate applicants similarly; pooled judgments more successfully assess the applicant. It is a good idea to have as a member of the interviewing team a person who has current information on the job vacancies, wages, and benefits (e.g., laboratory manager, personnel representative). An interviewer's lack of knowledge in this area may discourage valuable applicants. The interviewing team should also include individuals with the necessary technical skills to accurately assess the applicant (e.g., bench

technologist, technical supervisor). Team interviewing can be accomplished in a conference or by progressive interviews.

The third limitation of the interviewing process consists in the degree to which the interviewer intervenes in the interviewing process. When the interviewer dominates the conversation, useful information cannot be gathered. When the interviewer fails to listen or give mental attention to what is being said, important information will be missed, and the value of the interview will be limited. The interviewer should encourage the applicant to speak freely. He should not only listen but also attempt to comprehend the speaker's intent. The interviewer should avoid interrogating the applicant by overuse of statements beginning with "what," "when," "where," and "why." Placing the applicant in a stressful situation will limit information exchange as well as as frighten valuable applicants away.

A fourth limitation of interviewing is created by the interviewer through attitudes, biases, and prejudices that influence the appraisal of the applicant. These are responses over which the interviewer has little control and which can never be totally eliminated. A good interviewer, being aware of these weaknesses, can discount them in his assessment of the applicants. One common interviewer bias is called the "halo effect." The halo effect occurs when a single characteristic of the applicant dominates the interviewer's judgment in other areas. For instance, the fact that an applicant may have graduated from the interviewer's college may dominate the interview and may overshadow the applicant's limited job experience. The halo effect can also take a negative form. For instance, an applicant's appearance or dress (having a beard, wearing jeans) may create an initial negative impression about the applicant that will unfairly bias the overall assessment.

Another interviewer problem is the lack of flexibility. The interviewer who asks the same questions and in the same order with no variance cannot accurately evaluate the applicant's responses. Optimum information can be exchanged only through thoughtful, individualized probing.

Finally, the interview is often limited by the interviewer's decision to hire too early in the interview process. Immediate decisions based upon such preliminary information as personal appearance and general manner, rather than experience and training, can cause job-related problems later.

In summary, the interview process is a complex task requiring effective communication skills; careful attention to constructing a planned, organized interview; appropriate use of questioning techniques; and a genuine desire to select the best qualified applicant on the basis of the candidate's knowledge, skills, and attitudes under fair and open competition.

THE SELECTION PROCESS

Once the interviews are completed, the supervisor is faced with sorting out the information gathered and making a selection. This decision will affect many facets of the supervisor's realm of influence and responsibility. A common pitfall in the selection process is the assumption that the personal judgment of the hiring laboratory manager is sufficient to determine an applicant's qualifications. Some managers attempt to make a selection based on *body chemistry*—a feeling of whether a person is right for the job. Be aware that reliance on personal feelings has caused the downfall of many individual laboratory supervisors.

Input should be solicited from all those involved in the interviewing process; this will increase the value of the selection decision. The final decision of which applicant to hire, however, must be the responsibility of the immediate supervisor. Unfortunately, there is no single formula one can apply to screen out those not well-suited for a position and select the most-qualified applicant. One of the most successful approaches is to list the qualifications necessary for the vacant position (based on specific tasks and the job description) with a corresponding semiquantitative evaluation. One category of qualifications may address the academic preparation and work experience relevant to the position. For example, if the job description calls for major responsibilities in the repair and preventative maintenance of particular instrumentation, qualification items may include the following:

Has the applicant attended any manufacturer's workshops for this particular instrument?

Does the applicant have any experience in working with the particular instruments?

Or perhaps the job description calls for evaluation and implementation of new procedures:

Has the applicant evaluated procedures in the past?

How has the applicant responded to an open-ended question dealing with the appropriate approach for determining the impact of an interfering substance?

For nearly all applicants, regardless of the specific job description, a category dealing with individual work characteristics and interpersonal relations skills would be appropriate.[4]

How closely supervised does the applicant need to be? Is he able to plan and organize his own work?

Is the applicant able to make sound decisions?

What is the applicant's predicted ability to get along with even the most troublesome fellow laboratorian in the department?

Semiquantitation of these qualifications can be accomplished by establishing a numerical scale (perhaps 1–10) for each item.[25] This will force critical evaluation of those components essential for a given position and assist in ranking the applicants. One inherent problem with this approach is the weighting of the characteristics. Avoid selecting someone whose extremely high ratings on academic preparation and work experience shadow some problems recorded as low ratings in the area of interpersonal relations. Particularly noteworthy is guarding against hiring a career-entry staff member on the basis of his academic performance. A study by Firestone, Lehmann, and Leiken found that characteristics other than academic ability are more important predictors of the professional success of medical technologists.[6]

Finally, a manager should not be afraid to hire someone perceived as being more capable than he is. The success of many administrators is largely dependent upon their ability to draw together a group of highly skilled individuals and to unify their expertise to create an exceptional team.

TRANSFER AND PROMOTION

When vacancies occur in staff and supervisory positions, transfers and promotions may be viable alternatives to outside recruitment and selection[35] The clinical laboratory would seem to provide substantial breadth for transfer. It may appear to technologists that transferring from one department to another in the clinical laboratory as a lateral move is an excellent option based on their current generalist education. Unfortunately, technologic advances in the laboratory make such transferring a less than optimal situation if the laboratory is departmentalized. If a laboratorian has not worked within the department to which he wishes to transfer, a considerable amount of retraining will be necessary.

At times, employees will request transfers to different departments or different specialties within a department. The transfer in this manner plays a vital role in providing an alternative for the individual who finds himself in a situation with no upward mobility. A staff technologist may request a transfer in order to get around a blockage in his career ladder aspirations or as a means of seeking greater challenge in technical responsibilities.

Transfers are a managerial tactic used at times to cope with incompatibilities between a given position and the employee holding it. A transfer may effectively resolve a problem situation in which an employee is not capable of performing the required tasks or has developed personal friction in dealing with his supervisor or peers. Frequent remedial transfers from department to department when conflict arises among the staff are not advised. This results in a glossing over of serious problems. Rather than postpone the resolution of these problems with a transfer, the problem needs to be identified and handled directly.

Promotion to a supervisory position or selection of a supervisor from outside warrants special consideration. Few technologists are adequately prepared to assume managerial roles solely on the basis of career-entry education. Yet such responsibilities are often expected soon after completion of the entry-level degree. A recent study by Peddecord and Taylor of the education, training, and experience of supervisory personnel in interstate laboratories found most supervisors to be prepared at the baccalaureate level and having more than 10 years of experience.[27] Historically, technologists have been promoted on the strength of their technical expertise and tenure in the laboratory, and less emphasis has been placed on their managerial skills.

Promotion from within may be an ideal approach for filling supervisory positions that have been vacated. The techniques described earlier concerning interviewing and selection would still apply. Laboratory administrators should encourage the maintenance of good individual evaluation records to identify achievers with growth potential. A wise manager will maintain an ongoing, informed grooming process for possible candidates for future promotion. This is best accomplished by delegating some supervisory responsibilities and counseling the potential leader when appropriate. Some institutions maintain rather elaborate *career-ladder tracks* for employee improvement in preparation for promotion opportunities of the future.

The use of career ladders can be an effective means of developing a more productive staff.[2,24]

Such staff development plans offer employers an opportunity to realize professional advancement and job satisfaction without changing institutions. Other job enrichment opportunities such as participatory decision-making and contact with other patient service representatives help prepare staff technologists for promotion.[3,31,42]

Of significant importance is the degree of support and assistance provided the newly promoted individual. Despite the fact that the new position probably carries increased responsibilities, management must not make the promotion a "sink or swim" transition.

While the benefits of promotion to both the individual and the organization are obvious, the process is not without problems. The mere existence of the promotion policy creates what is perhaps the most difficult situation—the employee who is unlikely to be promoted. The laboratory supervisor has the responsibility of not only watching out for and developing potential staff for promotion but also helping those not promotable to accept their fate. An individual unsuitable for promotion must not be allowed to take for granted that he is in line for various promotions on the basis of longevity. After several occasions of being passed over, a problem is likely to develop that might result in serious charges of favoritism. The most effective tactic to use in dealing with the employee unlikely for promotion is a one-to-one discussion about the responsibilities of the new position long before a decision is made. The supervisor should attempt to point out the incongruities between the employee's abilities and the requirements of the new position. Perhaps guidance can be provided to help the employee supplement his background or improve his performance in order to prepare himself for eventual promotion.

Another promotion-related problem is the employee who does not want to be promoted. Laboratory administrators are frustrated from time to time by the employee with excellent potential who lacks the desire for advancement. This person has reached the limit of either his ambition or perceived ability. Most often, refusal of promotion by laboratory personnel hinges on the employee not wishing to take on additional responsibility or problems associated with the new position. This should not be held against the employee. A discussion of the benefits to both the organization and promotable employee may assist in convincing him to try the new responsibilities. If the employee still declines the promotion, administration must look elsewhere.

Promoting an employee always involves a degree of risk. The new position undoubtedly has responsibilities for which the candidate has not had the opportunity to display competence. Most people have observed a leader who was promoted beyond the level of his competence. So widespread is this phenomenon, in fact, that it has achieved the distinction of being termed the *Peter Principle:* "In a hierarchy every employee tends to rise to his level of incompetence."[28] The effect of this phenomenon on the staff is likewise interesting: "Employees in a hierarchy do not really object to incompetence (*Peter's Paradox*). They merely gossip about incompetence to mask their envy of employees who have Pull."[28] The promotion of an individual may yield an incompetent at a key level in the organizational hierarchy. Therefore, the promotion process must be undertaken with great care.

REFERENCES

1. Boe GP: Picking a winner: A guide to effective employment interviews. MLO 14(6):97–102, 1982
2. Crane VS, Jefferson K: Clinical career ladders: Doing more with less. Health Care Supervisor 5(3):1–11, 1987
3. Crystal JC, Deems RS: Redesigning jobs. Training and Development Journal 37(2):44–46, 1983
4. Douglass GR, Wood JM: Interpersonal value profiles as indicators for the selection of clinical laboratory workers. J Med Technol 3:409–416, 1986
5. Famularo JJ (eds.): Handbook of Human Resources Administration. New York, McGraw-Hill, 1986
6. Firestone DT, Lehmann CA, Leiken AM: Predictors of career advancement for laboratory professionals. Lab Med 17:759–762, 1986
7. Fruend M, Somers P: Ethics in college recruiting: Views from the front lines. Personnel Administration 24(4):30–33, 1979
8. Fry FL: The end of affirmative action. Business Horizons 25(1):34–40, 1980
9. Galassi JP, Galassi MD: Preparing individuals for job interviews: Suggestions from more than 60 years of research. Personnel Guidance Journal 57(4):188–192, 1978
10. Goodman J: Indirect discrimination and the employer's right to select. Pub Per Mgt 12(2):38–41, 1980
11. Hoffman NM, Martin BG: Affirmative action: What does it really mean? MLO 11:49–57, May 1979
12. Hopkins JT: The top twelve questions for employment agency interviews. Personnel J 58(5):379–381, 1980
13. Iry TR: Keeping the employment interview legal. MLO 13(11):97–115, 1981
14. Karni KR, Studer WM, Carter SJ: A study of job turnover among clinical laboratory personnel. Am J Med Technol 48:49–59, 1982
15. Kraft JD: Adverse impact determination in federal examinations. Pub Per Mgt 7(6):362–367, 1978
16. Lehr RI: Employer duties to accomodate handicapped employees. Labor Law Journal 31(3), 1980
17. Linenberger P, Keaveny TJ: Age discrimination in employment: A guide for employers. Personnel Administration 24(7):87–98, 1979
18. Makin P, Robertson I: Selecting the best selection techniques. Personnel Management. November: 38–42, 1986
19. McConnell CR: The Effective Health Care Supervisor. Rockville, Aspen Systems, 1982
20. McQuire JP: The use of statistics in Title VII cases. Labor Law Journal 30(6):361–370, 1979
21. Metzger N: Personnel Administration in the Health Services Industry. Jamaica, Spectrum Publications, 1979
22. Micheals DT: Seven questions that will improve your managerial hiring decisions. Personnel Journal 59(3):199–224, 1980
23. Miller EC: An EEO examination of employment applications. Personnel Administration 25(3):63–81, 1980
24. Miller K: How rotation can help boost productivity. MLO 19(1):53–58, 1987
25. Morris FJ, Fernandez ZC: Bayesian analysis: An objective approach to hiring. MLO 15(11):63–70, 1983
26. Norwood JM: But I can't work on Saturdays. Personnel Administration 25(1):25–30, 1980
27. Peddecord KM, Taylor RN: Education, training, and experience of supervisory personnel in interstate laboratories. J Med Technol 2:114–118, 1985
28. Peter LJ, Hull R: The Peter Principle. New York, William Morrow, 1969
29. Pigors P, Meyers C: Personnal Administration: A Point of View and a Method. New York, McGraw-Hill, 1977
30. Portwood JD, Koziara KS: In search of equal employment opportunity: New interpretations of Title VII. Labor Law Journal, 30(6):353–359, 1979
31. Rosland FA: A study of job enrichment perferences among medical technologists. J Med Technol 2:127–130, 1985
32. Sawyer S, Whatley AA: Sexual harassment: A form of sex discrimination. Personnel Administration 25(1):36–44, 1980
33. Sherman M: Equal employment opportunity: Legal issues and societal consequences. Pub Per Mgt 7(2):127–137, 1978
34. Sikula AF: Personnel Administration and Human Resources Management. New York, John Wiley and Sons, 1976
35. Simon WA: A practical approach to uniform selection guidelines. Personnel Administration 24(11):75–80, 1979
36. Smith RE: Successful People Management: How to Get and Keep Good Empoyees. Toronto, Macmillan, 1978
37. Stockard JG: Rethinking people management: A new look at the human resources function. New York, AMACOM, 1980
38. Strauss G, Sayles LR: Personnel: The Human Problems of Management, 3rd ed. Englewood Cliffs, Prentice-Hall, 1972
39. Sweet D: The Modern Employment Function. Reading, Addison–Wesley Publishing Co, 1973
40. Terry GR: Supervision. Homewood, Richard D. Irwin, 1978
41. Tune L: DRGs three years later: Lab staffing trends mixed. Clin Chem News 13(6):1–2, 1987
42. Umiker WO: Job enrichment: Whose responsibility is it? MLO 14(11):58–64, 1982
43. Zahsin EM: Affirmative action, preferential selection, and federal employment. Pub Per Mgt 7(6):378–393, 1978

ANNOTATED BIBLIOGRAPHY

Dann JD, Stephens EC: Management of Personnel: Manpower Management and Organizational Behavior. New York, McGraw-Hill, 1972

Part 2 of this reference, entitled "The Employment of Manpower," provides a concise look at determining the demand for manpower, recruitment, selection, and testing and interviewing.

Famularo JJ (ed): Handbook of Human Resources Administration. New York, McGraw-Hill, 1986

>This comprehensive book covers all aspects of personnel management with current information. Part 4 has several chapters devoted to recruitment, selection, and placement of personnel.

Flippo EB: Principles of Personnel Management, 4th ed. New York, McGraw-Hill, 1976

>Part 3 of this book discusses job analysis, recruitment and hiring, and tests and interviews. Part 4 describes development of personnel, covering such topics as training and education, advancement, and performance appraisal. Part 5 addresses the compensation issues of personnel management.

Halper HR, Foster HS (eds). Laboratory Regulation Manual. Rockville, Aspen Publications (updated annually)

>Part 10 of Volume III addresses laws concerning clinical laboratory employees. Also of interest might be Part 12 of the same volume dealing with malpractice. The three-volume set serves as an efficient, complete, and authoritative resource.

Lewis PV: Organizational Communication: The Essence of Effective Management. Columbus, Grid Inc, 1975

>This reference is especially useful for considering the communication process in the interview setting. Chapter 11 addresses communication strategies appropriate for planning and conducting both preemployment and counseling interviews.

Metzger N: Personnel Administration in the Health Services Industry. Jamaica, Spectrum Publications, 1979

>This book is an excellent administrative overview for personnel management. Chapter 4 has a comprehensive description of the recruitment, screening, and selection process.

McConnell CR: The Effective Health Care Supervisor. Rockville, Aspen Systems, 1982

>This book provides a fine description of supervision in the health services industry. Chapter 8, entitled, "Interviewing: The Hazardous Hiring Process," provides excellent information on conducting the interview.

Pigors P, Myers CA: Personnel Administration: A Point of View and a Method, 7th ed. New York, McGraw-Hill, 1973

>Readers will find this a thought-provoking examination of the ramifications of employee selection and developing human resources with a personnel policy system. The authors provide 19 case illustrations from their experiences, which aid the reader in understanding theoretical concepts.

Strauss G, Sayles LR: Personnel: The Human Problems of Management, 3rd ed. Englewood Cliffs, Prentice-Hall, 1972

>Part 5 of this resource deals with manpower and employee development. Chapters 19, 20, and 21 address recruitment and selection, technical training, and minority employment. Readers may also find Chapter 11, entitled "Interviewing: The Fine Art of Listening," to be helpful.

twelve

Staffing and Scheduling of Laboratory Personnel

Bettina G. Martin
Anthony S. Kurec

People don't dislike work . . . help them to understand mutual objectives and they'll drive themselves to unbelievable excellence.

Tom Peters

In the evolution of medical laboratory practice, social, economic, scientific, and technologic forces are demanding the serious attention of all concerned with human resource management.

Responses of laboratory management to these forces are affecting profoundly the recruitment, education, and careers of laboratory personnel. In most clinical laboratories employee salaries account for 60%–80% of the total operating budget. To assure sustainment and improvement in quality of laboratory service for patient care as new staffing patterns develop, all individuals engaged in laboratory medicine seek wisdom in finding new alternatives. These alternatives come from careful review, evaluation, and planning for future directions and action.

Only with efficient staffing and scheduling can management make the best use of personnel, supplies, instrumentation, and facilities in a prompt and cost-effective manner.

STAFF PLANNING

By definition, *to staff* is to provide a group of workers for the purpose of securing united and cohesive performance. Specifically, staffing of a clinical laboratory is then a two-step process. The initial step is to set up a table of organization denoting laboratory structure and chain of command. It is of utmost importance to clearly define what the *function* of the laboratory is and how it fits into the overall organization—whether a tertiary-care hospital, an extended-care facility, or one catering to a particular type of patient, *i.e.*, elderly, pediatric, ethnic, and so forth. Once the mission and purpose of the laboratory have been determined, decisions in efficient utilization of personnel and equipment can be made with accuracy. After thought is given to the need for present and future numbers of positions, a comparison can be made between predicted demand and supply. Differences can then be assessed and finally a plan formulated to recruit, train, and meet suitable staffing needs.

The establishment of employee positions is best accomplished by using *laboratory organization charts* that outline the structure of the laboratory. These charts should include physical plans and work-flow diagrams. Procedure lists, classified as to proposed methodologies, time specifications, and instrumentation, are also requisites for setting forth employee positions. These data are necessary for projecting the number as well as classes (levels) of employees required to operate the laboratory properly. Essentially, this involves knowing what type of service a particular laboratory is to provide and establishing employee positions to ensure that service can be provided adequately. Before it is possible to forecast the number of staff required, information has to be collected about existing staff, i.e., numbers recruited, length of employment, how many qualified (certified/licensed), and percentage of turnover and reasons for it. This type of information, once gathered and reviewed, can be very useful in forecasting future needs.

The second step in staffing consists of the actual selection and development of personnel to fill positions. *Selection* is a process of matching people with available jobs. Staffing begins with recruitment and includes interviews, reference checks, selection, employee orientation, training, and subsequent performance appraisal. Readers are encouraged to review Chapter 11, "Interviewing and Employee Selection," which addresses this step of the staffing process in detail.

Staff utilization, *i.e., scheduling,* is defined as the planning of work assignments for a certain time period. Initially, this involves determining the number and types of positions needed and secondly, assigning employees from the necessary job categories to appropriate positions. Work assignments can be made on a very short-term basis, hourly or daily, or on a more long-term basis, such as weekly or monthly. What really is important is how people are utilized to obtain maximum efficiency and productivity. Ongoing data acquisition and analysis of actual workload are useful in setting productivity levels for the laboratory.

RESPONSIBILITY AND IMPORTANCE OF SCHEDULING AND STAFFING

In the laboratory arena, service is the product and people the major resource. Great emphasis must be placed on those who make decisions and take action. The size and complexity of the laboratory organization will determine who is assigned responsibility for staffing and scheduling. Staffing is usually the responsibility of the laboratory director, manager, or administrator. Supervisors, whether section supervisors in the larger laboratory or the chief technologist in the smaller organization, may be responsible for the scheduling of those employees directly assigned to them. In some laboratories these individuals work as a team.

Staffing and scheduling should not be static parameters in management. Staffing must be adaptable and scheduling flexible for quality to be maintained. On a day-to-day basis the laboratory must respond quickly and effectively to changes in instrumentation, workload, test priorities, cost analysis, and regulatory demands. Therefore, staffing and scheduling are important, forceful activities that require the good manager/supervisor to use management techniques that include frequent review and modification as necessary for optimal effectiveness.

The implementation of prospective reimbursement of hospitals by diagnosis-related groups (DRGs) has resulted in added burdens for hospital laboratory management and has clearly forced the need for improved information on staffing costs and productivity. Third-party insurers and compulsory rate review agencies are demanding more accurate laboratory activity data.

HISTORIC CHANGES IN STAFFING AND SCHEDULING

The clinical laboratory has been refining its labor productivity measurement system since 1960. While not perfect, the College of American Pathologists (CAP) work-load recording system is by far the most widely used. Refer to Chapter 29 for more information regarding work-load analysis. With many advances in medicine and innumerable innovations in medical technology, the clinical laboratory has also undergone extensive change in the last decade. Increased utilization of clinical laboratory testing has been a product of this dynamic medical era. Never before have so many laboratory services been available and so extensively used and scrutinized. There have been several factors contributing to these changes.

Physicians have influenced to a great extent the type of procedures and service priorities the laboratory offers. With attempts to reduce health-care costs, efforts have also been made to decrease patient *length of stay* (LOS) in the hospital. Physicians continue to demand increased availability of laboratory tests, along with decreased turn-around time (TAT). Procedures previously offered once or twice a week are often now required on a daily basis. *More, faster, at a lower cost, with fewer staff,* and *high quality* are the new guidelines, which are indeed challenging. Increased consumer knowledge has led to increased utilization of all physician-support services. The patient of the mid-1980s became more knowledgeable and continues to take a more active role in monitoring health-care services. The fear of medicolegal action has led the physician to use more extensive testing to rule out potential incorrect diagnosis and treatment. With the advent of *physician review organizations* (PROs), it becomes essential for all phases of laboratory testing to be monitored carefully by appropriately trained and credentialed laboratory professionals.

Another factor that has led to increased utilization of the clinical laboratory is the introduction of new methodology and "high-tech" instrumentation, including computers. Both have made feasible many assays not previously practical owing to cost or the large volume of specimen required. Initially, there was a trend toward organ profiling, presurgical battery testing, and patient service packages, all designed to aid the physician in providing a standard, comprehensive patient-care plan. Single assay techniques were replaced with instruments capable of performing multiple assays on a single specimen. However, third-party payors continue to demand justification for tests performed when not ordered by the physician, which has reduced or eliminated profiles in some institutions. Microsampling instruments have now made most laboratory tests available for use with pediatric and neonatal patients.

Surviving clinical laboratories nationwide have grown, and some have diversified. The resulting and extensive modifications in staffing and scheduling are further defined in terms of quantity, quality, and category. In response to increased work loads, some laboratories have increased production, test menus, and number of employees, as well as extended hours of operation. Still others have reduced work loads and staff alike. Aggressive marketing has become a common practice for laboratories on the upward move. Increased work load is not the only cause for the longer workday or workweek. Physician demand for increased availability of laboratory test results and the trend toward preadmission testing, as well as an overall trend toward patient management on an outpatient basis, have required adjustments in hours of service.

In general, the traditional 40-hour workweek, "9 to 5," is no longer practical. In a hospital setting, the laboratory must provide 24-hour-a-day, 7-day-a-week service. Some smaller hospitals still provide 24-hour service on a *stat basis* only. In some instances, on-call scheduling has been replaced by a more structured, full-compliment staffing on day, evening, and night shifts. As a result, modifications in staffing and scheduling have occurred and are not reflected by quantity alone. Increased automation and highly technical assays often require advanced-level specialization of employees. Specialization contributes to proper operation and maintenance of complex instruments and affords better quality assurance. The need for high-level quality employees has increased with the growth of services in laboratory medicine. This has also resulted in the formation of new and additional categories of employment in the health-care organization.

CRITERIA-BASED JOB DESCRIPTION

Once function of the laboratory has been established, the next priority involves establishing employee positions within the laboratory structure and filling those positions with the appropriate qualified technical and nontechnical personnel. To accomplish this, we recommend the *criteria-based job description*, based on definitions set forth by the Board of Registry of the American Society of Clinical Pathologists (ASCP). The criteria-based job description defines positions in terms of technical, administrative, and teaching responsibilities (Table 12-1). Several examples with different format styles are provided for review on the following pages.

Staffing policies depend upon volume of work to be handled for specific hours each day of operation. This includes the number of shifts scheduled the proposed availability of laboratory services on all shifts, including weekends and holidays, the test menu offered, and the methods used to provide service. Factors to be considered are the ratio of routine to stat specimens and manual versus automated procedures. Laboratories without critical-care areas, as well as those receiving less than 5% stat requests, have fewer rapid turn-around difficulties and generally require fewer employees. In some institutions governmental and regulating agencies' accreditation may insist that certain staffing requirements be met. Teaching hospitals have further staffing obligations in order to provide academic and research activities.

Nontechnical Service Duties

In addition to actual diagnostic duties in laboratory testing, many nondiagnostic activities involved in daily operation of the laboratory must be considered when staffing. Phlebotomy, reagent and specimen preparation, reporting, charting, telephone calls, filing, and billing all consume much personnel time in the workday and must be considered in planning the work flow. Positions such as phlebotomist, safety officer, medium and reagents preparation technician, glassware worker, receptionist, secretary, word processor, laboratory aide, and computer entry clerk all have vital roles in maintaining a smooth and efficient operating laboratory.

Table 12-1
Criteria-Based Job Description

	Technician	Technologist	Specialist
Knowledge	Has working knowledge of routine tests.	Understands the technical aspects of tests and their underlying scientific principles; knows biologic factors associated with lab testing; is familiar with other lab services.	Knowledge of advanced scientific principles within the specialty area; applies that to the technical, procedural, and research aspects of laboratory testing; knows the organization of the other health care areas.
Technical skills	Performs routine tests and instrument maintenance; understands the basics of quality control.	Performs routine and more complicated tests; implements and monitors quality control; introduces and evaluates new procedures and instruments.	Performs all tests within the specialty area; is able to maintain and troubleshoot equipment; researches, develops, implements, and evaluates new and existing methods, instrumentation, and quality control.
Judgment and decision-making	Recognizes common technical problems and is able to correct them.	Uses independent judgment of technical and procedural problems; participates and delegates in decision-making regarding quality control, instrument selection, preventive maintenance, safety, and reagent purchases.	Implements and delegates decisions in laboratory operations; anticipates and shows independent judgment in problem-solving and other unique situations; participates in policy-making decisions.
Communication	Reports laboratory results, normal ranges and specimen requirements.	Generates technical or general information for medical and nonmedical personnel.	Communicates with other health-care personnel on the applications and validity of laboratory data, laboratory policies and operations, and detailed information about specialty areas.
Supervision and management	None.	Uses basic management practices; establishes technical and administrative procedures; supervises technicians, aides, clerical personnel.	Performs and directs administrative functions over laboratory personnel.
Teaching and training responsibilities	Demonstrates learned skills.	Teaches and evaluates basic theory, technical skills, and application of tests.	Plans, implements, and evaluates educational programs.

(Adapted from Board of Resistry, American Society of Clinical Pathologists: Professional levels definitions. Lab Med 13:312, 1982)

The *job description* matches the employee with the kind of work to be performed, level of responsibility to be assumed, and job requirements to be met. The job description is an essential management tool in the staffing process. In addition to serving as a training and evaluation guide, it contributes to establishment of employee incentives. The most basic job description should include (1) job title, (2) job duties, (3) work aids, (4) qualifications, and (5) job relationships. The job description may also include a category such as worker traits. This would include limitations such as physical demands and working conditions unique to the position.

Job duties include responsibilities and objectives—what the employee does and how he accomplishes his duties. *Work aids* consist of necessary equipment, including computers, tools, and machines the employee uses in job performance. Necessary education, training, or experience required for the job are included in *qualifications. Job relationships* involve workers to be supervised by the employee and the titles of those exercising supervision over the employee.

Technical Service Duties

The criteria-based job description uses the ASCP Board of Registry definitions as a foundation and adds to it specific duties as deem necessary by laboratory and hospital administration, as well as the various accrediting services. These criteria consist of three levels, *technician, technologist,* and *specialist,* and reflect abilities and skills that should be present at entry level, in addition to being hierarchical, in that each advanced level includes the skills of the preceding. Furthermore, each of these levels is applicable to medical technology, cytotechnology, histology, and computer science. As a laboratory becomes larger and more sophisticated, a "division of labor" may become necessary. In addition to the laboratory manager, supervisors, technologists, technicians, and ancillary support personnel, other administrative personnel within the laboratory structure may be justifiable in promoting a smooth operation. These positions may include an equipment inventory coordinator to maintain inventory on all major equipment; equipment repair specialist for repair and maintenance of equipment; business manager with responsibility for laboratory marketing, advertising, negotiating with reference laboratories, billing, and so forth; computer specialist; purchasing agent; educational coordinator; quality control/assurance coordinator, and so on. Not all

---

> **Example**
>
> ### JOB DESCRIPTION — PHLEBOTOMIST
>
> **Title**
>
> Phlebotomist
>
> **Duties**
>
> The phlebotomist receives the physician's request and collects blood specimens from patients, properly identifying the patient and promptly drawing and correctly labeling the specimens.
>
> He accurately performs venipunctures, heelsticks, and fingersticks, ensuring proper specimens for testing as well as ensuring patient safety. He distributes the specimens to the proper laboratory area as soon as possible.
>
> The phlebotomist also stocks phlebotomy rooms and trays.
>
> **Work Aids**
>
> Blood collection equipment
>
> **Qualifications**
>
> High school diploma or equivalent; phlebotomy experience preferred
>
> **Job Relationships**
>
> Workers supervised — none
> Supervised by medical technologist, phlebotomy supervisor

---

laboratories have a need for all of the above, and combinations are encouraged where applicable.

Job descriptions should not remain static; rather, the laboratory manager should periodically review each employee to ensure that each position is current and accurate. Changes in technology, equipment, administration policies, state and federal laws, and accreditation procedures should be appropriately incorporated into the job description. Reviewing job descriptions with the Personnel Department and with employees may generate motivation not originally considered. A well-developed and current job description ensures smooth operations and can often prevent potential administrative or legal problems. Furthermore, the job description sets guidelines for each individual and may be useful in evaluating personnel, as well as aiding in projecting future staffing needs.

Phlebotomists are employees specifically trained in obtaining blood samples and are essential

(*Text continues on p 207*)

Example

JOB DESCRIPTION — MEDICAL TECHNOLOGIST – GENERALIST

I. Qualifications

Bachelor's degree in medical technology or equivalent education plus certification by American Society of Clinical Pathologists (ASCP) or equivalent required. Previous experience in a clinical laboratory preferred.

II. Schedule

Monday through Friday, 8 hour daily shift. Holidays, evening/nights and weekends on rotation.

III. Duties

A. Technologist performs clinical testing in laboratory areas including blood bank/histocompatibility, immunology, microbiology, hematology, virology, microscopy, cytogenetics, and chemistry.

B. The technologist obtains or receives laboratory specimens, including blood, urine, and body fluids, and performs and interprets clinical laboratory tests, obtaining data for use in the diagnosis and treatment of disease; performs a variety of standardized procedures, both manual and automated, using established standards and controls in order to ensure correct data.

C. The technologist understands the principles of and competently performs a variety of techniques, including spectrophotometry, microscopy, fluorometry, titrimitry, immunology, chromatography, toxicology, and gravimetric analysis; performs quality control and preventive maintenance; and correctly performs analysis and interprets results obtained as far as accuracy, acceptability, and critical limits.

D. The technologist works independently, organizing work to meet established deadlines and records and files all data obtained.

IV. Administrative

A. Report directly to Laboratory Manager/Assistant Manager and section supervisor. Secondary source to be consulted: Laboratory Director.

B. Prepare documentation as necessary for:

1. Patient demographic data and other information.
2. Incident reports concerning patients, equipment or staff.
3. Quality control/Quality assurance.
4. Accreditation procedures (State, Federal, ASCP, CAP, JCAHCO, etc.).

C. Be able to contribute to and perform quality control in chemistry, hematology, microbiology, virology, microscopy, immunology, blood bank/histocompatibility, and cytogenetics.

D. Be able to maintain and perform preventive maintenance in chemistry, hematology, microbiology, virology, microscopy, immunology, blood bank/histocompatibility, and cytogenetics.

E. Be involved in decision-making processes of the laboratory as requested.

F. Supervise other technicians, aides, support staff as assigned.

G. Attend, participate, and evaluate continuing and in-service education programs.

H. Be aware of, contribute to, and observe laboratory safety at all times.

I. Maintain strict patient confidentiality at all times.

J. Work as a team player during all assignments.

V. Technical Responsibilities

A. Perform emergency and routine testing accurately for chemistry, hematology, microbiology, virology, microscopy, immunology, blood bank/histocompatibility and cytogenetics.

B. Perform other testing as time permits with accuracy, efficiency and cost-effective methods.

C. Telephone "panic-value" results promptly and document them immediately.

D. Perform phlebotomies as needed, including both venipuncture and microsampling on adults and children.

(continued)

Example

JOB DESCRIPTION — MEDICAL TECHNOLOGIST – GENERALIST (*Continued*)

E. Correctly prepare reagents and test samples.
F. Be able to set up (start-up) instruments in all areas of rotation.
G. Be able to enter and retrieve patient data accurately, utilizing the laboratory computer system if applicable.
H. Become familiar with troubleshooting techniques for the major instruments in each laboratory section.

I. Be familiar with the billing process of patient testing, including audit procedures.
J. Participate in the development, evaluation, and implementation of new methods and equipment if requested.

VI. Work Aids
A. Include cell counters, chemistry analyzers, centrifuge, microscope, spectrophotometer, automated coagulators, computers, calculators, etc.
B. Include the safe use and handling of toxic and biohazardous substances.

For Personnel File:
Reviewed with new employee_____by_____
                                                    Date   Title

Signed by_____
                                  New employee

Example — More Specific

JOB DESCRIPTION — SUPERVISOR OF CLINICAL CHEMISTRY

I. Qualification
Must be registered Medical Technologist (M.S. preferred, B.S. required) with at least 6 years' laboratory experience, including a minimum of 3 years in Clinical Chemistry.

II. Authority
A. Act and report to no one as long as consistent with the policies of the Clinical Chemistry Laboratory, the Department, and the Hospital.
B. Act as long as consistent with the policies of Clinical Chemistry Laboratory, the Department, and the Hospital, but inform the Director of Clinical Chemistry.
C. Act only after consultation with specific approval from the Director of Clinical Chemistry.

III. Duties
A. Planning
1. Space needs and space utilization within the area of supervision. (Authority III)*
2. Annual requirements, for budgetary purposes, of capital equipment, supplies, wages, and salaries. (Authority II)*
3. Programs for instruction and evaluation of new personnel and students and cross-training of personnel in all sections of Clinical Chemistry. (Authority II)
4. Organize work-flow pattern for Clinical Chemistry. (Authority III)
5. Develop and maintain an organization plan showing the number, types, and duties of personnel in all sections of Clinical Chemistry. (Authority I)†
6. Evaluate and finalize position descriptions for personnel within the incumbent's direct authority. (Authority III)*
7. Maintain adequate personnel files on each individual under the incumbent's direct authority to include attendance records, evaluation records, and documentation relevant to employee performance. (Authority I)
8. Organize and update programs on quality control of laboratory tests,

(continued)

Example — More Specific

**JOB DESCRIPTION — SUPERVISOR OF
CLINICAL CHEMISTRY (Continued)**

preventive maintenance of
instruments, and safety in the
laboratory. (Authority III)

9. Evaluate and implement new
procedures and instruments and
update existing methodologies.
(Authority III)

10. Review, update, and write
laboratory technical procedures
and instrument preventive
maintenance procedures.
(Authority III)

11. Maintain good communications
within all divisions of Clinical
Pathology, and meet personnel
needs within the areas of the
incumbent's authority. (Authority
I)

12. Review present functions of areas
of the incumbent's direct
authority, and revise and optimize
functions to better meet the goals
and objectives of the Department.

B. Controlling

1. Monitor the time records of
personnel within the incumbent's
area of authority. Institute
corrections when necessary
(Authority I)†

2. Monitor the rotation of personnel
to all sections of Clinical
Chemistry. Monitor straight
overtime needed to fill staffing
needs. (Authority I)†

3. Monitor for accuracy and
acceptable turn-around time of all
testing done in all sections of
Clinical Chemistry. (Authority I)

4. Monitor preventative maintenance
schedules on all laboratory
equipment. (Authority I)

5. Schedule and conduct regular
meetings of personnel within the
incumbent's area of direct
authority for purposes of
information and general
communication. (Authority II)

6. Monitor the timely handling of all
proficiency-testing surveys within
all sections of Clinical Chemistry.
(Authority I)

C. Decision-Making

1. Conduct performance evaluation
for personnel within the
incumbent's area of direct
authority. (Authority III)*

2. Hiring of personnel within
incumbent's area of direct
authority. (Authority III)*

3. Additions to the table of
organization or personnel roster
in the incumbent's area of direct
authority. (Authority III)*

4. Initiate requests and conduct
follow-ups on orders for
equipment and medical supplies
for the incumbent's area of direct
authority:

Capital Equipment (Authority III)*

Supplies up to $100 per order
(Authority I)*

Supplies above $100 per order
(Authority III)*

Renewals of orders for reagents
and expendables (Authority III)*

Maintenance contracts (Authority
III)*

5. Recommend personnel for the
participation of continuing
education programs and
workshops on a local level that
involve no special funds and
absence of no longer than one
day. (Authority II)*

6. Recommend personnel for the
participation of continuing
education programs and
workshops involving special funds
and absence of more than one
day. (Authority III)*

D. Other Duties

1. Perform clinical tests at work
station(s) where help is required,
i.e., scheduled rotation, heavy
workload, instrument breakdown,
or personnel shortage.

(continued)

Example—More Specific

JOB DESCRIPTION—SUPERVISOR OF CLINICAL CHEMISTRY (Continued)

IV. Working Relationship

  Report to: Director of Clinical Chemistry

  Also to: Director of Clinical Pathology
      Laboratory Manager

Has reporting to him/her:

  All Assistant Supervisors of Clinical Chemistry
  All technologists, technicians, and technical assistants in Clinical Chemistry, work study students

*Act only after consultation with specific approval from the Laboratory Manager.
†Inform the Pathology Laboratory Manager.

additions to the laboratory work force. With increased ambulatory workload has come the need for increased phlebotomy. It has become increasingly difficult and expensive for technologists to free themselves to obtain a blood specimen.

The number of laboratory requests for newborn and pediatric patient specimens have increased markedly because of advances in neonatology and the increased availability of micromethods and instrumentation. Obtaining blood from newborns and pediatric patients requires special training in technique as well as patient management. In general, the time required to obtain a heelstick, fingerstick, or venipuncture specimen from the younger patient is greater than time required for adult phlebotomy. A second factor to consider is the number of phlebotomists needed to manage a pediatric patient during phlebotomy. Phlebotomists, when adequately trained, can and should relieve technologists of primary phlebotomy responsibilities. This is especially important if, during certain shifts or on certain days, such as weekends and holidays, the technical work load permits the scheduling of fewer technologists while phlebotomy requirements remain constant. It is not cost-efficient to schedule more technologists than are needed to perform diagnostic work in order to have personnel available for phlebotomy.

A second area of the clinical laboratory that has expanded greatly is specimen-receiving and sample preparation. Increases in work load in this area are due to a greater volume of laboratory tests performed. Personnel time increases are reflected by more time spent processing specimens for mailing to reference laboratories. Some use a group of employees designated as specimen processors. These employees have been trained to receive as well as process laboratory specimens. They are responsible for evaluating specimens for adequate volume, proper anticoagulant, proper collection time, and specimen suitability. Duties also include measuring

and recording urine volumes as well as properly distributing specimens to various sections in the laboratory.

With the increasing amount of paperwork and the computer entries involved in the day-to-day operation, new positions have emerged with titles ranging from data entry to computer/operator clerk. In the computerized laboratory, data entry clerks are responsible for entering specimens received, and printing and distributing computer work lists, and a select few enter laboratory results into the computer. In the noncomputerized laboratory, the record clerk is responsible for maintaining work lists for distribution to work areas and transferring results from work lists to reporting forms with subsequent distribution for charting.

SCHEDULING FOR EFFICIENT SERVICE

The major goal of the clinical laboratory should be to provide high-quality, cost-effective, timely, and efficient service. Factors to consider when scheduling staff include the following:

1. *Laboratory hours.* Hours of operation dictate the number of shifts to be scheduled.
2. *Procedures offered and days of the week procedures are performed.* This takes into account time requirements for all procedures as well as high-volume versus low-volume workdays, and determines the number and type of employees needed at a given time.
3. *Ratio of stats to routine work.* These data can help predict work flow. Generally, stats interrupt work flow of batch routine procedures, decreasing laboratory efficiency. Where a high percentage of stats exist, in order to meet established priorities and deadlines, more employees may have to be scheduled per shift.

4. *Workload trends.* It is the exceptional laboratory that maintains a constant workload hour to hour or day to day. Most laboratories have hourly, daily, and even monthly fluctuations resulting in volume peaks and valleys. However, when work-load trends can be predicted, more cost-effective and efficient scheduling is possible. Regretfully, the alternative generally used is overscheduling, with resulting decreased employee productivity and decreased cost-efficiency.

5. *Personnel benefits.* On a nationwide average, each day 10% or more of the work force is absent. Some of these absences can be predicted and controlled—for example, vacation, business leave, and compensatory time. Other absences, owing to illness or other personal reasons, are neither predictable nor controllable. Overstaffing may result when predictable absences are not effectively managed or controlled or when employees take excessive advantage of sick and personal leaves. Monitoring of both is strongly encouraged.

6. *Physical design.* With the many changes occurring in the clinical laboratory with regard to instrumentation and work-load fluctuation, the old physical design of the laboratory is difficult to maintain and should be modified as necessary to ensure optimal work flow. Where this is not done, there is often an increase in number of employees needed to overcome deficits in physical design alone. For example, if the outpatient facility is located a great distance from the hospital phlebotomy area, the laboratory is forced to maintain two phlebotomy teams as well as two reception areas, requiring extra staffing, scheduling, equipment, and supervision.

STAFFING AND SCHEDULING GUIDES

There are several data-gathering systems that can be useful guides when staffing and scheduling. These include work-load recording, performance or work-flow charts, a productivity monitoring system, and projected work load.

Work-load recording involves counting the number of tests performed for a given time period and then calculating a number for the employees performing tests and the number of employees assigned to various laboratory areas and shifts. Data obtained can reflect the cost-efficiency of a test as well as staffing and scheduling efficiency in a given area, on a given shift, or throughout the laboratory.

Busy and slow work-flow periods can be identified by this system. Alternate staffing and scheduling might improve the efficiency in terms of employee productivity and operating costs. Modified procedures and instrumentation changes might improve work flow and productivity. A work-load recording system is described in detail in Chapter 29.

A second system guide for staffing and scheduling is the *performance chart, or work-flow diagram.* This chart records the present system of operation with regard to activities and work flow. All steps necessary for reaching the desired end-point are presented. The most simple form of performance chart is a listing of all steps in sequence:

1. Obtain physician order.
2. Draw blood.
3. Receive specimen.
4. Process and aliquot specimen.
5. Perform analysis.
6. Record data.
7. Report result.
8. Bill patient.
9. File data.

A diagram might better show the interaction of laboratory areas and employee job duties. Work-flow Diagram—Plan A (Fig. 12-1) is an example of a large, complex laboratory organization. Work-flow Diagram—Plan B (Fig. 12-2) represents the smaller laboratory operation. The performance chart can be prepared in much more detail, reflecting which employee is performing a given step in the system as well as time required. In this way, any lags in the process, duplication of duties, or under- or overutilization of personnel can be readily documented and the system revised as needed. Revision might involve reassigning duties or procedures or establishing new test priorities and work flow.

The third data system is the *productivity monitoring system,* which allows, in some cases, enhanced managerial responsibilities. This system involves the determination of variable work-load factors (determining standard unit values), developing fixed time standards (work load as a function of "calender time"), establishing target utilization (accounts for constraints or inefficiencies not controllable by the laboratory manager or supervisor), establishing a fixed reporting period (biweekly, monthly, and so forth), collecting data (work-load volume), and a report format that collates all the information within the reporting period(s) in a manner that is quick and efficacious.

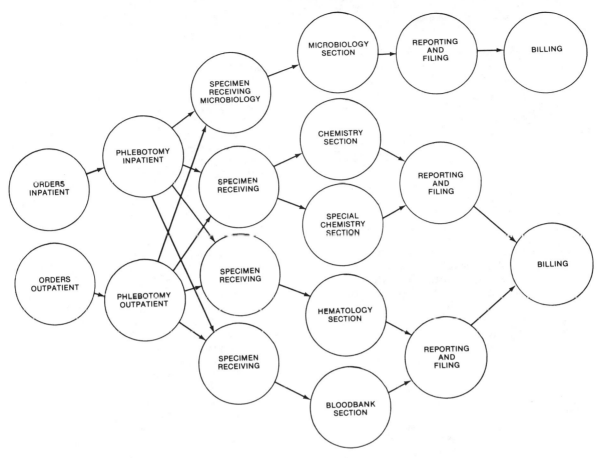

FIGURE 12-1. Laboratory work flow—Plan A.

FIGURE 12-2. Laboratory work flow—Plan B.

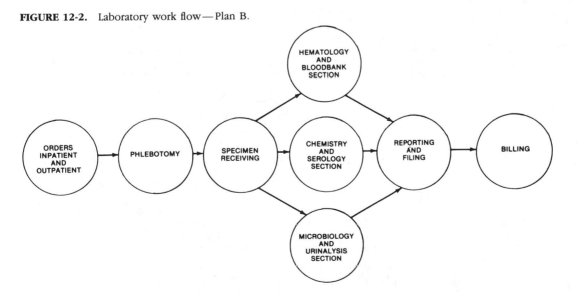

A fourth data system is the *projected workload.* Any planned changes in laboratory operating hours, test priorities, or days on which tests are to be performed can affect work load. The introduction of new procedures, new instrumentation, or alternations of inpatient or outpatient numbers may also alter work load. In any of these instances, there may be a need for revised scheduling. It is best for management to anticipate these changes and allow adequate time for changes to occur. In some instances, the use of mathematical models may be useful in predicting daily and weekly work-load variations. Staffing assessment can then be made, and a productivity monitoring system can be constructed; thus, utilization of laboratory personnel can be maximized in an efficient and cost-effective fashion.

One of the simplest methods for evaluation of a current staffing and scheduling system is to ask the following questions: Is the turnaround time for most tests adequate? Is the laboratory meeting established priorities and deadlines? Is there negative feedback from supervisors and employees? If the turnaround time is not adequate, the problem might be in scheduling. It might be a matter of not having enough laboratory personnel available at appropriate times or perhaps having an improper category of employees available. One should also consider lack of motivation and morale problems if applicable. If staffing and scheduling is adequate, a reassessment of methodologies, instrumentation, human resources, or work assignments might be necessary.

Efficient scheduling also involves maintaining continuity and communication between shifts and on weekends and holidays. If current schedules do not provide for smooth transitions between shifts, staggered arrival and departure for selected staff should be considered. If the increase in volume of tests on Monday or on the day after holidays becomes so great that normal work flow suffers, staffing should be adjusted with more of the appropriate employees scheduled as needed.

AVAILABLE RESOURCES

One of the major human resources available, yet often not managed properly, is support (ancillary) personnel: phlebotomists, laboratory workers, clerks, data entry operators, volunteers, receptionists, and secretaries. Scheduling efficiency and technical performance are greatly increased when these employees are supervised and managed properly. They should relieve more highly paid technical personnel of many time-consuming, nontechnical tasks. Part-time employees can be utilized during peak work-load periods and are very beneficial in the clerical, data entry, and phlebotomy areas. Volunteers are also useful in well-defined, nontechnical functions.

While absences cannot always be predicted or controlled in the case of vacation or compensation time, the supervisor can limit and control time taken. Supervisors should encourage employees to take compensation time during slack periods when possible. The supervisor can set limits as far as the number of employees taking time off on a given day and should encourage employees to take vacation year-round, instead of only in summer months. Many junior and senior staff like winter vacations.

In the laboratory that must provide 24-hour service, weekend and holiday scheduling is necessary. Part-time employees can be used in these time slots, or regular employees can work for compensatory time off or for overtime. It is most cost-efficient to ask employees to take compensatory time for overtime worked because these hours are usually paid at a higher rate. Remember, however, that fair practice labor laws prohibit forcing the employee to take compensatory time instead of pay if he worked beyond the 40-hour week.

Some laboratories still use an on-call system for coverage during nontraditional hours. If full-time night service is available, then routine maintenance, quality control, and routine testing can be done as time permits, which eases the work load for the day shift and eliminates the need for on-call service. This system should be evaluated closely, because there is a point at which the volume of work necessitates a scheduled shift instead of on-call, becoming more cost-efficient with a more rapid turnaround.

A valuable and important resource available to management is the *rotating generalist staff.* Unanticipated and temporary decreases in the work force and increases in work load can be responded to quickly and adequately with the least interruption in service when generalists are available on a rotation basis within the various job classifications. Such flexibility is one of the most decisive factors in effective scheduling and can boost productivity while saving overtime dollars. There continues to be controversy surrounding rotational versus nonrotational staff. In the smaller laboratory, necessity or opportunity for specialization is not present. In the larger laboratory, however, the trend has been for specialization of employees, ranging from receptionist to advanced, highly skilled medical technologist. The decision for rotational or nonrotational scheduling must be based on the needs of the individual laboratory. Recognizing advantages and disadvantages of both systems, management must evaluate and rate the need for flexibility in scheduling and for cost-efficiency versus benefits derived from the expertise and continuity of specialized employees.

INNOVATIVE APPROACHES IN SCHEDULING

One problem that can be encountered with a change in shifts is a lack of continuity, or interruption in service. Utilizing staggered work shifts (Fig. 12-3) may offer better work flow and keep open communication lines between shifts when an employee's work hours overlap two standard shifts. For instance, in staggered shifts, a technologist working from noon to 8 PM is available for lunch coverage for day-shift technologists and dinner coverage for evening-shift technologists. A technologist involved in this shift-sharing provides a strong degree of continuity between shifts and functions as a mediator between the shifts involved. Increased utilization of employees is possible if they are hired and trained to work two of the three shifts, either day/evening or evening/night. The increased flexibility obtained with this oscillating shift schedule allows for better coverage during emergencies, vacations, and extended maternity leave.

There was an attempt in the mid 1970s to increase workday hours and to decrease the workweek, but this idea has not gained acceptance in most laboratories. It may be possible for certain laboratories to make more effective use of their employees by scheduling 10-hour days and 4-day workweeks (Fig. 12-4), but such a practice should be evaluated very carefully before put into use. One should consider the possible decrease in overtime and the work force in relation to the possible decrease in productivity of employees required to work 10-hour days. Some employees complain that such a workday is physically tiring and not conducive to personal lifestyle.

Another alternative, schedules of 7 days on/10 hours per day/7 days off have the advantage of decreased overtime and better weekend coverage and shift transition. The disadvantages include a straight 7 days of 10-hour shifts and the necessity for extremely flexible, well-motivated, and healthy technologists. Absenteeism in either of the above-mentioned categories can cause serious staffing and productivity problems.

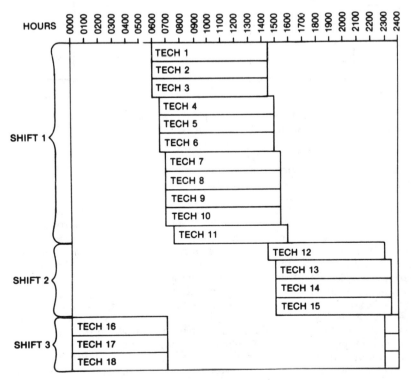

FIGURE 12-3. Staggered shifts. Shifts 1 and 2 are assigned to the chemistry section in 8½-hour shifts with a half-hour lunch period. Shift 3 technologists work all areas of the laboratory, with all three technologists working 8-hour shifts with a starting time of 2300 hours. Staggered starting times enable 1-hour overlap between Shift 3 and Shift 1, allowing Shift 1 technologists time for worklist preparation and blood collection. Overlapping hours between 1430 and 1600 allow good work flow from Shift 1 to Shift 2, when the work load is characteristically high. The half-hour overlap between Shift 2 and Shift 3 is usually sufficient for the work flow at that hour; however if work flow is high, Shift 3 may be assigned a starting time of 2230 with half-hour lunch period.

		SUNDAY	MONDAY	TUESDAY	WEDNESDAY	THURSDAY	FRIDAY	SATURDAY
WEEK I	TECH 1		WORK	WORK	WORK			WORK
	2	WORK	WORK			WORK	WORK	
	3	WORK	WORK				WORK	WORK
	4		WORK	WORK	WORK	WORK		
	5			WORK	WORK	WORK	WORK	
	6			WORK	WORK	WORK	WORK	
WEEK II	TECH 1	WORK	WORK			WORK	WORK	
	2			WORK	WORK	WORK	WORK	
	3			WORK	WORK	WORK	WORK	WORK
	4	WORK	WORK				WORK	
	5		WORK	WORK	WORK	WORK		WORK
	6		WORK	WORK	WORK			
WEEK III	TECH 1			WORK	WORK	WORK	WORK	
	2		WORK	WORK	WORK			WORK
	3		WORK	WORK	WORK	WORK		
	4			WORK	WORK	WORK	WORK	
	5	WORK	WORK				WORK	WORK
	6	WORK	WORK			WORK	WORK	
WEEK IV	TECH 1			REPEAT AS ABOVE OR				
	2			REASSIGN LINES AND REPEAT				
	3							
	4							
	5							
	6							

FIGURE 12-4. Schedule for the 10-hour day, 4-day workweek. This schedule is for a microbiology section, day shift, with a staff of six technologists.

An example of a clinical laboratory schedule making use of some of these innovative techniques can be seen in Figure 12-5.

Most hospital laboratories have experienced the problem of increased stat or rush orders at 7AM. Either the patient is going to surgery, or the physician needs results to evaluate patient data before morning rounds. One possible solution would be an early morning shift responsible for work ordered from critical intensive care areas, including the neonatal unit, as well as laboratory work needed for patients immediately prior to surgery. Because the shift begins 1 or 2 hours before the regular day shift begins, laboratory results are available to the physician earlier. If this cannot be done, request that blood from all such units be delivered to the labora-tory before 3 AM and guarantee results back on the unit by 6:30 AM. The third shift performs this work as part of the routine. There is greater efficiency in the laboratory with either of the above because the day shift is not overwhelmed with stats from these areas while trying to perform start-up and routine early morning laboratory work. This also eliminates the need to overstaff the night shift in order to handle any rush of laboratory requests from these areas just before day shift begins.

Some laboratories with a large volume of stat requests consider it advantageous to set up a stat laboratory as a separate area within the laboratory, with its own staff of employees. It is true that interruptions in routine work flow each time a stat specimen is received are eliminated, but one must weigh

		WEEK 1 S	M	T	W	Th	F	Sa	WEEK 2 S	M	T	W	Th	F	Sa
TECHNOLOGIST (SHIFT 1)	1		C	C	C	C	C	C	C	C	C	C			
	2	C	C	C	C					C	C	C	C	C	
	3					C	C	C	C	C	C	C	C	C	
	4	C	C	C	C					C	C	C	C	C	
	5		C	C	C	C	C	C	C	C	C	C			
	6						C	C	C	C	C	C	C	C	C
	7	C	C	C	C	C	C						C	C	C
	8	C	C	C	C	C	C	C				C	C	C	
	9	M	M				M	M							
	10		M	M	M	M									
	11			M	M	M	M								
	12	H	H	H			H	H							
	13	H	H	H	H			H							
	14		H	H	H	H	H								
	15	BB			H	H	H	BB							
	16		BB	BB	BB	BB	BB								
	17		BB	BB	BB	BB	BB								
	18	12→2030					H								
RECEPTIONIST/ CLERK	1		R	R	R	R	R								
	2	R	R	R	R			R							
	3						R	R							
PHLEBOTOMIST	1		P	P	P	P	P								
	2	P	P	P	P			P							
	3	P				P									
	4						P	P							
TECHNOLOGIST (SHIFT 2)	19		C	C	C	C	C								
	20	C	C	C	C	C									
	21	H	H				H	H	H						
	22	C	H	H	H	H									
	23			H	H	BB	BB	BB							
	24	BB	BB	BB	BB			C							
RECEPTIONIST/ CLERK	4		R	R	R	R	R								
	5	R						R							
PHLEBOTOMIST	5		P	P	P	P	P								
	6						P	P							
TECHNOLOGIST (SHIFT 3)	25		W	W	W	W	W	W	W						
	26	W								W	W	W	W	W	W
	27		W	W	W	W	W			W	W	W	W	W	
CLERK/ PHLEBOTOMIST	7		P	P	P	P	P								
	8						P	P							

FIGURE 12-5. An example of a clinical laboratory schedule that makes use of innovative scheduling techniques. Technologists 1–11 on Shift 1 are on a 10-days-on/4-days-off schedule with lines assigned on a rotating basis each week. Technologists 12–17 are on a rotating weekend schedule. Technologist 18, part-time, is used in shift-sharing, assigned to the 1200–2030 shift in the blood bank each Sunday. This eliminates the need for additional technologists on both Shift 1 and Shift 2 by providing blood bank coverage during the high work-load periods, primarily preop crossmatches. Part-time employees, used on weekends or during the week, include the receptionist/clerks, the phlebotomists, and the phlebotomist/clerk. Technologists 25 and 26, Shift 3, are on a 7-days-on/7-days-off schedule. They are assigned to a 10-hour shift Monday through Sunday every other week. Two week, 70-hour-schedule pay can be adjusted to 80-hour pay by use of shift differential or by assigning an additional day during the off week.

the disadvantages of duplicative costs for staffing and instrumentation. Modern instrumentation also affords performance of random emergency testing without disruption of work flow.

In previous years, most laboratories used evening and night shifts only for presurgical or stat requests. In recent (1987) situations, staff on these shifts have been performing routine and emergency laboratory procedures during these hours as some hospital services have extended their hours (i.e.,

in/out surgery, CAT scans, etc.). Laboratory service has increased, with benefits to both physician and patient. Laboratory results are made available for review by the physician more promptly, with the goal of possible earlier discharge of the patient. This becomes especially efficacious in light of current DRG concepts. In addition, the laboratory becomes more productive by utilization of most laboratory equipment 24 hours a day, rather than only during one shift.

One major potential problem facing management in the 1990s will be recruitment of qualified applicants. At present there is a decrease in medical technology school enrollment, a shifting of available educational funds, and a transition of qualified technologists seeking new career opportunities at higher pay in industry and management.

Many promising applicants are not hired because they seek part-time employment or are not able to work standard shift hours. *Job sharing* is the policy of allowing two or more employees to occupy one position within a particular job category. This alternative for experienced professionals offers great value to both the laboratory and the employee and should be encouraged. Another alternative is flex-time, which enables employees to perform their job duties during hours when they are best able to work. In some situations, set work hours are not absolutely necessary for a given employee position. Job duties such as reagent preparation, water testing, pipet-checking, inventory control, and so forth, are not usually restricted to a given shift or time. However, job descriptions must clearly define all responsibilities, rules, and regulations.

Many times, medical technologists who have left the work force for a period of time are reluctant to resume careers. They do not find it easy to return to the clinical laboratory because of the many changes that have occurred while they were away. In addition, some want to work on a part-time basis only. These technologists are a great resource and should not be overlooked as potential contributing employees. Reentry into the profession should be encouraged by offering free retraining programs, with subsequent employment opportunities as they become available on either a full-time or part-time basis.

In summary, the reader should keep in mind that selection and placement of employees are continuous processes. The selection process and other human-resource functions are essential for effective management.

BIBLIOGRAPHY

Allen LA: Professional Management: New Concepts and Proven Practices. Maidenhead, Berkshire, England, McGraw-Hill, 1973

Board of Registry, American Society of Clinical Pathologists: The Three Levels of Certification. In Rolen HB (ed): Study Guide for Clinical Laboratory Certification Examinations. Chicago, American Society of Clinical Pathologists Press, 1986

Board of Registry, American Society of Clinical Pathologists: Professional Levels Definitions. Lab Med 13:312, 1982

Chruden HJ, Sherman AW Jr: Managing Human Resources. Cincinnati, South-Western Publishing Co., 1984

Dorsey DB: Personnel management. Clin Lab Med 3:453, 1983

Fitzgibbon RJ: Legal Guidelines for the Clinical Laboratory. Oradell, Medical Economics Co., 1981

Holloway LA: Laboratory productivity: Assessing productivity in the laboratory. Hospitals 56:92, 1982

Johnson AP: Staff management. In Organization and Management of Hospital Laboratories, 98. London, Butterworths, 1969

Koenig AS: Laboratory planning and design. Clin Lab Med 3:485, 1983

Kurec AS: Management Tech Sample, Criteria Based Job Description. American Society of Clinical Pathologists, In press

Longest BB: Management Practices for the Health Professions. Reston, Reston Publishing Co, 1976

Martin BG: How to improve your hiring techniques. MLO, May–June:126, 1973

Martin BG: Reflections: Know and appreciate part-time technologists. MLO March:31, 1976

Martin BG: Reflections: Let's put more effort into human relations. MLO September:141, 1976

Martin BG: Reflections: The need for technical specialists. MLO January:20, 1977

Martin BG: Developing supervisors for tomorrow. Lab Med January:32, 1979

Martin BG: Reflections: What makes an employee tick. MLO July:64, 1979

Martin BG: Reflections: How not to attract top employees. MLO May:137, 1980

Martin BG: Reflections: Secretaries are indispensable team members. MLO January:119, 1981

Martin BG: Participative management: Let's turn the myth into reality. MLO July:113, 1982

Martin BG: Preparing for the potential personnel shortage: Or will there be one? MLO February:80, 1983

Martin BG: New goals; new roles; changing directions in the clinical laboratory. MLO July:77, 1984

Martin BG: Cost containment: Strategies and responsibilities of the laboratory manager. Clin Lab Med 5:697, 1985

Martin BG: Change and change makers. Lab Med January:49–51, 1986

Miller K: How rotation can help boost productivity. MLO 19:52, 1987

National Conference on Education and Career Development: Manpower for the Medical Laboratory, p 4. Washington, DC, US Government Printing Office, 1967

Newell JE: The people in laboratories. In Laboratory Management, p 7. Boston, Little, Brown, 1972

Nopper P: Personnel management. In Lundberg GD (ed): Managing the Patient-Focused Laboratory, p 155. Oradell, Medical Economics, 1975

Olsen KE, Durej RJ: A laboratory productivity monitoring system. Am J Med Technol 47:631, 1981

Pang CY, Swint JM: Forecasting staffing needs for productivity management in hospital laboratories. J Med Syst 9:365, 1985

Reed LB: Assessing productivity and staffing through workload recording. MLO, September 1979

Rubenstein NM: Handbook of Clinical Laboratory Management. Rockville, Aspen, 1986

Shuffstall RM, Hemmaplardh B: Organizing and staffing the hospital laboratory. In The Hospital Laboratory. Modern Concepts of Management, Operations and Finance, p 29. St. Louis, CV Mosby, 1979

Strauss G, Sayles LR: Personnel: The Human Problems of Management. Englewood Cliffs, Prentice-Hall, 1972

Taylor HW: A study of factors affecting laboratory workload. Clin Biochem 11:179, 1978

United States Department of Labor, Manpower Administration: Job Descriptions and Organizational Analysis for Hospitals and Related Health Services. Washington, DC, US Government Printing Office, 1971

Wertman M: Job classification. In Lundberg GD (ed): Managing the Patient-Focused Laboratory, p 139. Oradell, Medical Economics, 1975

Widman J: Using Matrixes to Simplify Scheduling. MLO, August 1980

thirteen

Standards and Appraisal of Laboratory Performance

Jana Wilson Wolfgang
Louis M. Brigando

Appraisal of performance is part of any human endeavor. During performance of a task and at its completion a person will ask himself, "Did I do well?" Similarly, when people pool their efforts under a common leader, the leader must ask whether each person has done his share of the task and whether each performance met the leader's expectations.

In the clinical laboratory, as in other organizations, performance appraisal plays an essential role in effective management. Appraisal may be formal or informal, or both. It may serve as a vehicle of communication, as a basis of promotion or salary decisions, or as a means employed by managers to change their subordinates' behavior.

The need for planned, thoughtful appraisals is as great in the laboratory as in nonlaboratory settings. Sometimes, however, this aspect of management is neglected in the face of high staff turnover and the special time constraints of the clinical laboratory. On the other hand, the clinical laboratory is uniquely able to deal with the issues associated with performance appraisal. Measurement and its applications are intrinsic to the very processes associated with the laboratory. Issues of reliability and validity are no less critical to the success of a performance appraisal than they are to clinical laboratory testing.

In the following pages, we will define some terms associated with performance appraisals and present purposes for which they may be used. We will then attempt to distill the essentials of effective appraisal and give examples of the different formats a laboratory manager might consider when planning for this important task.

PERFORMANCE APPRAISALS — DEFINITION AND PURPOSES

Among the terms applied to periodic assessment of an employee's job performance are employee rating, performance evaluation, merit review, and performance appraisal. The selection of one term over another is usually arbitrary.

Despite the profusion of terms, *performance appraisal* may be defined concisely as a planned, formal, and periodic management activity in which subordinates' on-the-job behavior is evaluated for some self-serving purpose. Although the elements of planning, formality, and periodicity are important, the key to this definition is purpose. In order to function effectively, a performance appraisal should reflect and serve the purpose for which it was designed.

Some possible purposes for performance appraisals are as follows:

217

Salary decisions

Promotion decisions

Behavior modification

Determination of level of competence

Determination of need for training

Communication (obtaining feedback from subordinate)

Evaluation of progress toward or achievement of job objectives

Discussion of interface between subordinate's and organization's goals and how each can be achieved

The most commonly cited reason for evaluating a subordinate is to make salary and promotion decisions.[3,5,9,10,13] In practice, this does not always require direct communication with the subordinate; a manager can, and often does, make such a decision unilaterally. The detrimental effects of such a non-participatory action are probably known to many readers from personal experience. The subordinate feels left out of the decision-making process and is often dissatisfied with the results.

Another purpose for performance appraisals is to attempt to change a subordinate's behavior. Whether a manager wishes to motivate a subordinate who is performing adequately or to bring a below-average performer to an acceptable level, the manager may try to use the performance appraisal to accomplish this goal. If further training is needed to attain an acceptable level of performance, such training would be specified during the course of the evaluation. Attempts to change behavior ordinarily involve face-to-face communication with the subordinate and a more complex performance appraisal system than salary decisions require.

When the primary purpose of a performance appraisal is communication, personal contact between manager and subordinate is essential. The performance appraisal becomes a forum for interactive discussion of the subordinate's responsibilities and how they have been met. Progress toward goals that had been agreed upon at the beginning of the period can be examined in light of the actual demands and constraints of the period. Finally, new goals can be set for the future, with the understanding that less formal discussions may take place in the interim before the next performance appraisal.

The various purposes for performance appraisals are not mutually exclusive. However, the purpose or purposes must be clear, both in design and execution, in order for an evaluation system to function well.

ESSENTIALS OF MEANINGFUL PERFORMANCE APPRAISALS

No matter what the purpose or format of an appraisal, there are a few critical elements without which an appraisal system will not function. These include standards and criteria of performance, communication of these standards and criteria to the subordinate, sufficient frequency of appraisal, and clear communication of appraisal results.

Standards and Criteria

A *standard* might be defined as a measure to which like objects are expected to conform, while a *criterion* is a standard used in forming judgments. For example, a standard for glass cuvettes in the chemistry laboratory might consist of a given internal diameter, such that the cuvette fits into the spectrophotometer. Whether or not the cuvette will go into the spectrophotometer is easily decided; a yes or no answer is possible. In contrast, how readily the cuvette can be removed from the instrument might be a criterion for judging whether the cuvettes are good, bad, or indifferent. To some extent, this is a matter of judgment.

In order to evaluate performance of a task, both standards and criteria for that performance must exist. This may seem self-evident, but standards and criteria are not always clear. For instance, a new pathologist may be given the responsibility of evaluating the chief technologist without being told what the chief technologist is expected to do. Should the pathologist judge according to the standards of a previous hospital environment? How does the pathologist know what the job of chief technologist entails here? On the other hand, if the job standards are known, by what criteria should this individual's performance be measured? A good performance in one laboratory might be considered fair somewhere else or excellent at a third institution.

Sources of Standards

Performance standards must be specified for performance to be evaluated meaningfully. One possible source of standards is the job description. Depending on the detail included, this may serve as a general guideline or give a clear understanding of the responsibilities that accompany a given job.

In general, however, job descriptions are short and not very specific. A more exacting set of standards may be derived from a job analysis. In this process, someone who is currently fulfilling the responsibilities of a job writes down or reports all the different tasks the job includes. Each task may then be broken down into its component skills (task analysis). For example, in the case of a bench-level technologist, a job analysis might show that the technologist runs anticoagulated blood specimens through an automated cell-counting instrument, performs manual differential counts, screens urine specimens using chemical strips, and examines urine sediments. Each of these tasks demands a large number of component skills (*e.g.,* use, care, and basic trouble-shooting of microscopes and cell counters, recognition of abnormal cells or casts, and so forth), which could be further subdivided. At the conclusion of the job analysis, a list of tasks and required skills may serve as a set of standards for performance of the job.

A third possible source of standards is mutual consent to specified goals, as found in management by objectives (MBO). In this case, the subordinate and manager agree upon certain tasks that the subordinate is to perform during the evaluation period. Provided that these standards are clear to both parties, they often provide very useful performance standards.

Performance criteria are more difficult to specify than performance standards. As implied in the definition, criteria serve as the basis of judgment; they allow performance to be characterized as good, poor, or average. An ideal set of performance criteria would allow ten different supervisors from ten clinical laboratories to independently produce exactly the same performance appraisal for one hematology technologist. This is a very difficult goal to reach in any situation where individual judgment is involved.

Performance criteria require clear definitions of what constitutes poor, fair, and excellent performance. If the definition is left to the individual, performance appraisals will be inconsistent from rater to rater, and from the same rater at different times. Some reproducibility can be attained through rater training, where managers are taught to use a certain performance appraisal format. However, the validity of a rating system may be increased by providing criteria that are based on observable behaviors.[6] If a criterion gives the rater a clear choice among alternatives A, B, and C, with minimal judgment involved, that criterion is more likely to contribute to a successful performance appraisal.

Communication of Standards and Criteria

Once performance standards and criteria have been specified, the subordinate to be evaluated by them must be aware of them. Again, this seems obvious, but many laboratory employees have had occasion to ask, "How did I know I was supposed to check the refrigerators every day?" or "Why does my supervisor think my technical skills are average instead of good?" Standards and criteria may be communicated during the initial job orientation session by the manager or personnel department, during the subordinate's first meeting with the manager, or by means of a written document, such as a detailed job description along with the performance appraisal form.

Frequency of Evaluation

The frequency with which performance appraisals should take place depends on the purpose they are intended to serve, as well as the efficiency of other means of communication. The most common interval for appraisal is every 12 months; this is usually adequate for salary and promotion decisions. However, formal review of progress toward goals might be required at more frequent intervals, depending on the nature of the job, the subordinate's ability to work independently, and his supervisor's management style. Certainly, if a manager wants to change a subordinate's behavior, regularly scheduled communications must supplement the more formal medium of the performance appraisal.

Communication of Results

A final vital element in effective performance appraisals is communication of the results to the subordinate. These results must be clear and indicate that the purpose of the performance appraisal was fulfilled. Ordinarily, the appraisal will indicate areas for improvement to the subordinate. If these goals are explicit and detailed, they can serve as guides for improvement and as additional criteria against which performance can be measured.

DESIGNING PERFORMANCE APPRAISALS

The structure of a performance appraisal may generally be divided into two areas, the written component and the interview. These areas should complement and reinforce one another in achieving the purpose for which the performance appraisal was designed. Accordingly, a number of possible formats should be considered during the design process.

Performance Appraisals: The Written Component

Barrett has presented an excellent, detailed discussion of designing written performance ratings.[2] As he points out, an employee's on-the-job behavior may be classified and rated in three areas: personality, performance, and product. Evaluation of these areas may involve any of a variety of formats (Table 13-1). In the following discussion, the three most common formats will be described first, followed by less common performance evaluation methods.

Graphic Scales

The most common method for performance evaluations is probably the use of the *graphic rating scale* (Fig. 13-1). In graphic scales, a quality or characteristic is rated by choosing a point along a horizontal

FIGURE 13-1. Examples of graphic rating scales. (Modified from Snyder JR, Wilson JC: J Allied Health 9:125–131, 1980 and Lynch BL: Am J Med Tech 43(1):54–63, 1977)

INSTRUCTIONS: Evaluate the technologist's technical proficiency using the following key: 1 = unsatisfactory, 2 = fair, 3 = average, 4 = superior, 5 = outstanding.

		Rating
I.	Technical manipulative ability — dexterity	1 — 2 — 3 — 4 — 5
II.	Ability to follow written procedures and protocols	1 — 2 — 3 — 4 — 5
III.	Adaptability — capable of learning new tasks	1 — 2 — 3 — 4 — 5
IV.	Competency with automated analysis	1 — 2 — 3 — 4 — 5

INSTRUCTIONS: Place an X along the continuum at a point which best represents the technologist's behavior.

Skills and competency in performance of tests

A. Test performance

| Consistently performs tests with precision and accuracy | May occasionally repeat some mistakes but is improving | Performs work mechanically with little attention to quality | Exhibits poor sterile technique |

B. Care of equipment

| Makes adjustments and repairs when appropriate | Operates functioning instruments skillfully but will not attempt repairs that should be within his ability | Handles equipment roughly or carelessly | Cannot operate functioning instruments |

Table 13-1
Written Performance Evaluation Formats

Common evaluation methods

Graphic scale
Checklist
Narrative

Less common methods

Ranking
    Rank order
    Paired comparison
    Man-to-man comparison
    Forced distribution
Forced choice
Free-form
    Critical incidents

axis. The scale may be discrete (1—2—3—4—5; A—B—C—D—F; excellent—good—fair—poor —unacceptable); or it may be continuous:

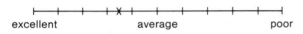

excellent	average	poor

There is usually an uneven number of points on the scale so that a middle or average can be selected; however, an even number is occasionally used.

Barrett offers a practical set of guidelines for constructing rating scales:[2]

Express one, and only one, thought in a scale.

Use words the rater understands.

Have raters rate what they observe, not what they infer.

Eliminate double negatives.

Express thoughts simply and clearly.

Keep statements internally consistent.

Avoid universals.

Stick to the present.

Avoid vague concepts (*e.g.,* honesty).

Perhaps the most important of these guidelines is to "have raters rate what they observe, not what they infer." Most of the other guidelines help the manager state the behavior being evaluated in an unambiguous manner. Barrett also suggests using between five and nine rating steps to allow the rater to differentiate similar but distinct performances.[2]

An example of a special type of graphic-rating scale is shown in the lower portion of Figure 13-1.

This is called a *behaviorally anchored rating scale.* It is based on "critical incidents," or actual examples of how people behaved in a given situation. Such critical incidents are gathered and placed along a continuum by groups of judges from the same populations as the raters who will use the rating scale.[1] The technique has been successfully applied to medical technology student evaluation.[6] However, development of behaviorally anchored rating scales requires conscientious input from a group of prospective judges. This may not be practical in some management situations.

Checklist

After graphic rating scales, a second common evaluation method is use of the *checklist*. A list of adjectives or descriptive phrases is presented along with instructions for checking those that apply or for circling a prescribed number. According to Barrett, this format is very easy to use but rarely distinguishes average from good or poor performers.[2] A checklist rating form might look like this:

INSTRUCTIONS. Circle at least three of the adjectives given below which best describe the technologist's outstanding personal characteristics. The qualities may be desirable and/or undesirable.

aggressive	flexible	observant
articulate	imaginative	open-minded
careful	immature	punctual
careless	impulsive	push
casual	inarticulate	resourceful
cautious	indifferent	responsible
discriminating	inflexible	self-assured
eager	inquisitive	sloppy
efficient	lazy	tenacious
energetic	loud	vigorous
enthusiastic	mature	witty
erratic	meticulous	
excitable	neat	

Narrative

In combination with other rating methods, the free-written rating or *narrative* is a third common vehicle. The rater may be given explicit directions for writing the narrative or may simply be asked to comment on the adequacy of the subordinate's performance. While easy to construct, this rating method has the dual disadvantages of difficulty in comparing subordinates' ratings and subjective bias.[2] An example of a narrative evaluation form follows.

INSTRUCTIONS. Please give other information that will assist in appraising the technologist. Comment on exceptionally outstanding performance or unsatisfactory ratings, as well as qualities not covered elsewhere. Do not include comments that are only a restatement of the various ratings; specific illustrations are always more helpful than remarks of a general nature. Be concise.

TECHNICAL SKILLS
INTERPERSONAL SKILLS
DEPENDABILITY
ORGANIZATION
OTHER

Ranking

A less common evaluation method is termed *ranking.* Ranking methods have proven neither reliable nor valid experimentally,[2] but they are still used. A group of subordinates who perform similar duties may be *rank-ordered,* or assigned a rank in the group according to their overall performance. Alternatively, subordinates may be compared two at a time (*paired comparison*). In this rating method, ranking occurs on the basis of the number of times a given subordinate is deemed the better performer of a pair. In the very similar *man-to-man comparison,* subordinates are ranked as average, below average, above average, or outstanding on the basis of comparison with *only* those of their peers who are currently performing similar tasks. Last, the *forced distribution* method of ranking subordinates assumes a predetermined distribution of performance. For instance, a rater might be compelled to designate 67% of a group of subordinates as average, with the remaining 33% evenly distributed between above and below average. These four ranking methods share the requirement that subordinates be performing closely similar tasks. They also share the characteristic of subjectivity, since subordinates are usually ranked on the basis of the composite, ill-defined overall performance, rather than on a comparison of performance with present standards.

Forced-Choice Rating

Another less commonly used rating method is the *forced choice,* which relies on the idea that a rater

will choose the most applicable of several unrelated descriptions of performance.[2] The choices are purposefully made difficult with the intent of improving the reliability of the rating. We have not encountered this rating method among the written performance evaluations we have reviewed.

Free-Form

Free-form evaluation methods are in wide use as adjuncts to other methods, as noted in the discussion of narratives, but they are rarely used as the only evaluation method. One variation of this format not mentioned previously is the *critical incident* performance evaluation. During the evaluation period, the rater observes the subordinate and makes written notations of exceptional performance, whether good or bad. For example, if a technologist assumes the responsibilities of the supervisor during the supervisor's absence, the laboratory manager might write that the technologist performed creditably during that period. If the same technologist had a loud argument with the nursing supervisor the following week, this, too, would be noted. These critical incidents and others would be summarized in the written performance evaluation. Among the problems with this rating method is the lack of reference to the day-to-day, noncritical performance that makes up the greatest portion of any person's on-the-job behavior.

Whatever the format used in a written appraisal, it must be recognized that individual managers will be using it to evaluate individual subordinates' behavior. It is important that the rater understand the purpose the appraisal was designed to serve. The appraisal must be flexible enough to allow its use to be adapted to the rater's own management style. Finally, the standards and criteria that underlie the appraisal must allow an objective evaluation of the subordinate.

The Performance Appraisal Interview

For many managers, the interview is the most difficult aspect of the performance appraisal. Some managers avoid the appraisal interview altogether, saying they do not have time or that they have nothing to discuss with the subordinate. Unfortunately, this avoidance of personal interaction denies both the manager and the subordinate a unique opportunity for review, discussion, and planning.

Planning The Interview

The purpose of the appraisal interview is to discuss, modify, or reinforce the written performance appraisal. Therefore, it is important for the manager to plan for the interview carefully. The standards and criteria for the subordinate's job should be close at hand; any written records of performance should be reviewed immediately before the interview. The interview should be scheduled well in advance, so that both the subordinate and manager will be prepared. In addition, the interview should be held privately, with no interruptions, so that both can speak freely and without distractions.

Once the interview begins, the interpersonal communication skills of the manager become important. Even when a good relationship exists and a manager and subordinate communicate frequently, the formality of the performance appraisal is likely to make the subordinate (and manager!) nervous.

Interview Methods

A number of interview methods have been proposed.[4,7,10,11] Maier, for instance, suggests three basic approaches: the "tell-and-sell" method, the "tell-and-listen" method, and the problem-solving method.[7] In the tell and sell, the manager tells the subordinate the results of the appraisal and tries to talk him into improving on-the-job behavior. This method is advocated for new, young, or timid employees. In the tell-and-listen method, the subordinate has a chance to respond to the manager's observations before returning control of the interview to the manager. In the last method, which is recommended for experienced and mature employees, the subordinate and manager discuss the appraisal as equals. Deficiencies in job performance are considered problems to be solved through joint effort.

Lefton and colleagues have related these ideas to modern management theory and added the important requirement of the follow-up interview.[4] According to these authors, the performance appraisal is simply the most structured type of feedback along a continuum that also includes ordinary feedback, coaching, and counseling.

Scanlon has recommended a results-oriented performance review emphasizing mutual agreement on standards, criteria, current performance levels, and goals.[10] In this type of appraisal, the interview becomes a planning session where both manager and subordinate participate in goal determination.

Although interview methods vary, it has been demonstrated that involving the subordinate in his own appraisal yields improvement in performance. If the manager regards the appraisal interview as an occasion for discussion, preceded by planning and followed up according to a specific timetable, it is most likely to satisfy the needs of both the manager and the subordinate.

Selection or Design of a Performance Appraisal System

Often, performance appraisal systems are already in place when a manager assumes responsibility in a new setting. However, a manager may sometimes have the opportunity to consciously select an appraisal system, or at least decide how the existing system will be applied. When selecting or designing a written performance evaluation, a manager must consider four factors: (1) the purpose of the appraisal; (2) the work environment itself; (3) the self-directedness and verbal and analytical skills of the subordinates to be evaluated; and (4) the manager's preferred management style and verbal and analytical skills. Selection of one or more of the written appraisal formats will depend on these factors. For instance, in a busy medical center laboratory, it might not be practical to depend on narrative evaluation alone because of the time and writing skills required. A set of graphic scales, filled out by the shift supervisor and the technologist before the appraisal interview, might be an adequate basis for discussion and planning.

With attention to the principles and techniques of performance appraisal as reviewed in this chapter, it is possible for managers in the clinical laboratory to design or apply appraisal systems to improve their own special working environments. An example of a management performance appraisal form to prompt the reader's thoughts or creativity is provided on pages 224–225.

PERFORMANCE APPRAISALS IN THE CONTEXT OF PERFORMANCE MANAGEMENT

Performance appraisals do not occur in a vacuum; they are part of the ongoing and variable process of performance management. In the clinical laboratory, this concept seems virtually unknown. Technical personnel are often promoted on the basis of their technical expertise, not on the basis of managerial skill. Eligibility for positions at higher levels of laboratory management seems to depend on academic or medical degrees, with little regard for the administrative and interpersonal demands of the posts.

The job of any manager is to ensure that the goals of the organization are reached through the people on whom the organization depends. The broad goals of clinical laboratories include accurate and timely laboratory analyses, service to the patient, and service to the physician, with the overriding concern being the welfare of the patient. The people who collect and prepare the specimens and

(*Text continues on p 230*)

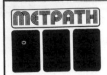

MANAGEMENT PERFORMANCE APPRAISAL

Employee Name:		Title:		I.D. No.	
Department:	**Location:**		**Time with Company:**	**Date of Previous Appraisal:**	
				Time in Present Pos.:	
Appraiser's Name:	**Title:**		**Appraisal Period:** From / / To / /	**Date of this Appraisal:** / /	

PURPOSE:

This form is intended to help the process of manager/employee performance evaluation and planning. To be effective the employee should receive clear feedback about how he or she is doing so that realistic plans may be made for employee development and growth.

EVALUATION CRITERIA:

The objective of the following pages is to reflect and document what has actually been accomplished during the entire review period. Results achieved are to be evaluated against the job description, the work standards which flow from it and previously agreed to goals.

Base your judgements on the entire period covered and not on isolated incidents alone. Be objective. Rate each factor separately. Try not to allow judgement on one factor to influence judgement on other factors.

PROCEDURES:

The manager and the employee review the objectives which were set at or close to the beginning of the work year, comparing the employee's achievement against standards set. This is a two-way conversation with first the employee presenting results achieved and then the manager providing input and his/her evaluation of results.

Immediately after this discussion, the manager completes the Performance Appraisal form and signs it. The manager and the employee discuss the appraisal and the employee signs the form and provides his or her comments.

The manager then forwards the appraisal to the next level of management for review and signature.

Both the manager and the employee keep a copy of the appraisal. The manager forwards the original to Personnel for the employee's permanent file.

Side 1

(Courtesy of MetPath Inc., Teterboro, New Jersey)

SECTION I - EVALUATION OF OBJECTIVES AND ACTION PLANS

Completion of this section is optional at the discretion of the manager and the employee. For this section to be used as part of the performance evaluation, performance objectives must have been established at or close to the beginning of the performance year. If this section is inappropriate or if you choose not to use it, you may begin the performance appraisal with Section II.

OBJECTIVES/ACTION PLANS ACHIEVED:

List the primary objectives established for this performance year and their measures in order of importance. (Should not generally exceed four.)	Describe the employee's performance in achieving objectives. Highlight significant results, goals achieved, not achieved.

Describe Affirmative Action goals, if appropriate.

Describe the developmental goals you established for your subordinates.

Describe any specific accomplishments which support the overall organizational goals but which are not necessarily a normal part of your job responsibilities.

OBJECTIVES NOT ACHIEVED:

For objectives not achieved, what are the probable causes and relevant circumstances?

1H - 713 6/81

Side 2

SECTION II - OTHER JOB PERFORMANCE FACTORS

Importance Scale: (1) Minimally or least important   (2) Important part of this assignment   (3) Critical or a most important aspect

On the preceding page you focused on **achievement** of **results.** On the next two pages, you will now focus on the **processes by which** the employee attained or missed goals; i.e., having seen what he/she did, you now need to see how he/she did it. To facilitate this processs, you will be asked to read each performance factor and select the value which best represents **how** the employee performed with reference to that factor.

Read each performance factor and definition carefully; determining the importance of that factor to the job being appraised and enter the appropriate value into the performance Rating box. Consider the effectiveness of the person being appraised, basing your evaluation on the TYPICAL LEVEL of PERFORMANCE during the entire review cycle. Check the <u>one</u> box which best describes the employee's performance with regard to each factor. If you have not had an opportunity to observe the employee's performance with regard to the specific factor, leave blank and indicate that in the comments section. Use the Comments space to give specific examples most typical of this person's performance.

Organizational Job Performance Factors	Importance Enter Rating	Effectiveness Check One

1. Planning: Planning goals and allocating resources to meet them.

—Identifying programs and actions, including contingency plans, necessary to obtain objectives.

—Monitoring progress toward objectives and adjusting them as needed.

—Allocating and scheduling resources.

Below Expectations   Achieves Expectations   Above Expectations

Comments:

2. Organizing: Completing activities in a timely and thorough manner.

—Managing time effectively by following the priorities set in advance of taking action.

—Using systematic planning and follow-up to avoid crises.

—Maintaining appropriate records and documentation for future reference.

Below Expectations   Achieves Expectations   Above Expectations

Comments:

3. Oral Communications: Communicating effectively one-on-one and in groups.

—Presenting ideas in a clear and concise fashion.

—Sharing information needed by others within the organization to achieve their objectives.

—Actively listening to others and giving appropriate feedback.

Below Expectations   Achieves Expectations   Above Expectations

Comments:

4. Written Communications: Communicating effectively, thoroughly and accurately in writing.

—Writing well-organized, concise proposals, reports and memos.

—Preparing accurate, complete reports.

—Writing letters and internal memos which convey courtesy and sensitivity to the receiver.

Below Expectations   Achieves Expectations   Above Expectations

Comments:

5. Problem Solving: Recognizing and analyzing problems effectively.

—Asking the critical questions to obtain accurate problem definition.

—Accurately analyzing data to determine cause.

—Identifying potential problems for preventive action.

Below Expectations   Achieves Expectations   Above Expectations

Comments:

Organizational Job Performance Factors	Importance Enter Rating	Effectiveness Check One		
		Below Expectations	Achieves Expectations	Above Expectations

6. Decision Making: Selecting viable alternatives in a timely manner.

—Selecting viable alternative actions when faced with an opportunity or obstacle.

—Assessing strengths and weaknesses of various proposals through objective analysis of the facts.

—Balancing practical and theoretical alternatives.

Comments:

7. Know-How: Keeping abreast of changes and innovations.

—Keeping informed of the latest developments in the area of specialty

—Performing the function of resource aid for others.

—Responding accurately to complex questions within area of expertise.

Comments:

8. Innovation and Creativity: Developing ideas which increase quality/quantity of services through innovative and/or creative processes.

—Developing new approaches to business concerns.

—Anticipating significant changes or trends and capitalizing on them.

—Assimilating and using new information to modify or adapt existing processes to increase its effectiveness.

Comments:

9. Delegating: Assigning responsibilities that challenge the ability of subordinates.

—Establishing appropriate work assignments to assure optimum utilization of human and material resources.

—Providing the support necessary to assist in completion of responsibilities.

—Assigning responsibilities, not just tasks.

Comments:

10. Development of Subordinates: Providing structure and support for the personal and organizational growth of subordinates.

—Preparing and following through on subordinates development plans.

—Conducting work planning, progress reviews and performance appraisals regularly with each employee.

—Providing advice and counsel to guide subordinates along ethical and professional concerns.

Comments:

11. Organizational Commitment: Acceptance of organizational goals, policies and practices.

—Maintaining high ethical standards in business interactions.

—Offering management constructive criticism of decisions and policies put forth.

—Operating in synchronization with the overall organizational goals and objectives.

Comments:

Side 4

Overall Performance Summary

Review both Section I objectives and action plans and the other performance factors in Section II to decide on the overall performance evaluation earned. Summarizing all preceding performance information, this employee is rated as:

☐ **(Unsatisfactory) Performance Clearly Below Expectations.** Consistently unable to maintain required objectives. Nature of skills or ability is such that improvement is unlikely. Employee is clearly not qualified for this position. (Usually 0-1% of employee population)

☐ **(Needs Improvement) Performance Marginally Below Expectations.** Adequately performs the majority of objectives but does not do so consistently. Needs to improve skills to fully qualify for position. However, with improvement in designated areas, employee should be able to meet expectations with a reasonable time frame. (Usually 10% of employee population)

☐ **(Good) Performance Fully Meets Expectations.** Usually meets the majority of goals or job requirements. May occasionally exceed in some objectives or fall short in some, but on balance, the goals and job responsibilities are competently performed. (Usually 60% of employee population)

☐ **(Excellent) Above Expectations.** Has consistently exceeded the goals and job responsibilities, with overall performance clearly better than most individuals at this level. (Usually 20% of employee population)

☐ **(Clearly Outstanding) Far Exceeds Expectations.** Has far exceeded job responsibilities and has made significant contributions to the organization above and beyond the requirements of the job. Is consistently successful in meeting difficult challenges and initiating improvements. (Usually 10% of employee population)

SECTION III - DEVELOPMENT PLAN

This section enables the planning of performance improvements based upon the performance evaluation discussion and the employee's interests and aspirations.

Summary of Strengths and Improvement Areas (Comment upon two significant strengths and at least one area where improvement can occur.)

Performance Effectiveness Plan

After considering the performance objectives and measures not accomplished by the employee, describe the work experiences, special assignments, educational activities or training you and the employee plan to increase effectiveness the present job.

Areas for Improvement	Activities Planned	Date

Performance Development Plan

If the employee's performance indicates he/she probably has the capability for developing beyond present level of work, describe the work experiences, educational activities or training you and the employee plan for the next 12-18 months.

Appraiser's Review and Signature:

Name	Signature	Date

Employee's Review and Signature:

Name	Signature	Date

Employee's Comments

Managerial Review and Signature:

Name	Signature	Date

perform the analyses achieve or do not achieve these goals. However, the effort requires teamwork and leadership, which are the responsibility of the laboratory's managers.

Performance management in the clinical laboratory may be perceived as an iterative process involving planning, monitoring, and discussion (Fig. 13-2). Performance appraisal is an integral part of this process. In this model, the management process begins with a discussion of the subordinate's responsibilities and goals. When performance standards are clearly defined, the framework is already built; the discussion can fill in the gaps.

For an example, let us consider a hematology technologist for whom a job description was derived earlier. To enter the cycle of the performance management process, let us say that the supervisor of the hematology laboratory undertakes a job analysis with the technologist's help and writes a set of performance standards. The supervisor and the technologist then sit down together and discuss how the standards apply and whether additional

ones should be added. Criteria for good performance are discussed and agreed upon. Finally, the technologist's personal goals—perhaps learning a new technique or attending more professional meetings—are examined and related to the requirements of the job. At the end of this meeting, both the technologist and the supervisor leave with a clear understanding and a *written summary* of what the technologist is supposed to do.

The second part of the performance management process is performance monitoring. It is the responsibility of the manager to make sure that the subordinate is carrying out his duties. The subordinate's work experience and previous performance will govern how closely he must be observed; a technician with 2 years' experience and an excellent quality-control record might be left to work independently until a question or problem arises, whereas a new phlebotomist might require close supervision and instruction during the first few weeks of work. If a performance problem surfaces, the manager should discuss it with the subordinate

FIGURE 13-2. Clinical laboratory performance management process.

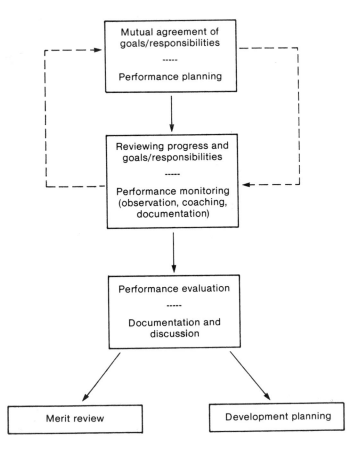

as soon as possible so that they may work together to correct it. Such instances should be recorded to facilitate performance appraisal.

When the time arrives for a performance appraisal, the stage is already set. The manager and subordinate can evaluate the subordinate's performance by comparing it with the standards, criteria, and goals agreed upon at the beginning of the period. The documentation of performance maintained during the monitoring period can aid in the appraisal. From this session, new goals can be established. In addition, the appraisal results can be considered when a salary review is undertaken.

The potential benefits of this approach to managing performance in the clinical laboratory are clear. They may be summarized in terms that are frequently used within the laboratory setting:

A systematic performance management process is *sensitive* to the needs, strengths, and weaknesses of employees and the organization. With this sensitivity, the clinical laboratory manager can expect early detection of problems and opportunities that otherwise might go unnoticed. Early detection allows corrective action or better use of underutilized abilities.

At the same time, the performance management process is *specific:* Misinformation is avoided by frequent interactions and thorough monitoring. Because misunderstanding of the strengths, needs, or problems of employees leads to errors in decision-making, the process increases the effectiveness of the manager.

This model asks that the same rigorous requirements for reliability and validity be applied to the management of people as the clinical laboratory professional applies to the management of test procedures. This is no small undertaking; performance attributes are not nearly as objective or quantifiable as laboratory test results. However, with continuing research and development in the measurement and evaluation of work performance, this approach of the clinical laboratory manager to performance appraisal can serve as an example of successful performance management for other professional disciplines.

REFERENCES

1. Anastasi A: Psychological Testing. New York, Macmillan, 1976
2. Barrett R: Performance Rating, pp 33, 46, 47, 52, 54. Chicago, Scientific Research Association, 1966
3. Fulmer RM: Supervision: Principles of Professional Management. Beverly Hills, Glencoe Press, 1976
4. Lefton RE, Buzzota VR, Sherberg M, Karraker DL: Effective Motivation Through Performance Appraisal. New York, John Wiley and Sons, 1977
5. Lundberg GD: Managing the Patient-Focused Laboratory. Oradell, Medical Economics, 1975
6. Lynch BL: A behaviorally anchored rating scale for the evaluation of student performance. Am J Med Technol 43:54–63, 1977
7. Maier NRF: The Appraisal Interview: Three Basic Approaches. La Jolla, University Association, 1976
8. Meyer HH, Kay E, French JRP: Split roles in performance appraisal. Harvard Bus Rev 43:123–129, 1965
9. Newell JE: Laboratory Management. Boston, Little, Brown, 1972
10. Scanlon BK: Management 18: A Short Course for Managers. New York, John Wiley and Sons, 1974
11. Smith HP, Brouwer PJ. Performance Appraisal and Human Development. Reading, Addison-Wesley, 1977
12. Snyder JR, Wilson JC: Evaluation of student performance in the clinical setting using the process skills approach. J Allied Health 9:125–131, 1980
13. Wilcox KR et al.: Laboratory management. In Inhorn SL (ed): Quality Assurances Practices for Health Laboratories. Washington, DC, American Public Health Association, 1978

ANNOTATED BIBLIOGRAPHY

Anastasi A: Psychological Testing, 4th ed. New York, Macmillan, 1976

A well-indexed reference text on principles and practice of psychologic testing; addresses issues of validity and reliability of testing, applicable to the development of written performance evaluation.

Barrett RS: Performance Rating. Chicago, Science Research Associates, 1968

An excellent text on a difficult subject. Clearly written and readable, it defines terms, supports conclusions with research and examples, and is eminently reasonable.

Lefton RE, Buzzotta VR, Sherberg M, Karraker DL: Effective Motivation through Performance Appraisal. New York, John Wiley and Sons, 1977

This book provides an in-depth discussion of performance appraisals from the perspective of modern management theory. A good how-to reference for planning and carrying out performance appraisal interviews.

Lynch BL: A behaviorally anchored rating scale for the evaluation of student performance. Am J Med Technol 43(1):54–63, 1977

A careful, detailed report of the development of a specific student evaluation tool; an important reference for medical technology educators.

Scanlan BK: Management 18: A Short Course for Managers. In Wiley Professional Development Programs, Business Administration Series, New York, John Wiley and Sons, 1974

This self-instructional text on all aspects of management is very well organized, concise and readable. It summarizes management theory and offers examples of practice.

fourteen

Educational Responsibilities of Managers and Supervisors

Richard L. Moore II
John R. Snyder

At one time or another, most technicians, technologists, and pathologists are called upon to be teachers.[16] Similar to the case made for technical experts to become managers in Chapter 1, these laboratorians are seldom prepared for their teaching role. Teaching responsibilities include a range of activities, from clinical education, in which the manager is asked to help train and supervise medical technology students,[5,11] to orientation of new employees through inservice education[1] and formal continuing education activities for a large peer group.[6]

At one time a manager would have been able to hire a technologist confident in the knowledge that his educational program had provided the necessary skills for a career of service in the laboratory. This, however, is no longer the case — the field of health care and all of its supportive efforts are in a state of constant change. Medical research continues to push the frontiers of knowledge farther and farther. The result has been new medications, new instruments, new procedures, and even new categories of health professionals, such as physician's assistants, clinical pharmacists, nurse practitioners, and patient educators.

This chapter focuses on the need to meet these changes through acceptance of educational programming as an overall responsibility of the institution, of laboratory management, of section supervisors, and of the individual laboratorian as a professional within the field of health care. The chapter is divided into sections reviewing some current issues in continuing education; summarizing activities and goals of preservice education, inservice education, and continuing education; listing the strengths and weaknesses of different teaching methodologies; and developing teaching programs.

It is clear that a professional's preparatory formal training in certificate and degree programs in just that — preparatory. The practicing professional is not able to remain abreast of the developments in the field without additional educational activity. To be sure, the laboratorian himself to a large degree must assume a responsibility for continued learning, but it is surely a responsibility of the supervisor to both stimulate and provide an environment supportive of learning efforts.

An environment for learning includes a variety of support mechanisms. Among the obvious ones are release time to attend formal education programs, tuition and travel support, and recognition of educational achievement through salary increments and promotions. However, there are a number of other ways in which a manager can support and encourage continued learning. These include

Provision for formal reporting to the other staff members whenever anyone returns from a continuing education course

Formation of study clubs or discussion groups similar to the rounds and conferences commonly attended by physicians in which one person reports on a case or subject of interest.

Selection, purchase, and circulation of appropriate journals and newsletters, which provide current relevant information

Provision of funds for staff to select books and reference works for a small laboratory library

Regular rental or free use of audiovisual self-instructional materials, which are available from medical center libraries and biomedical communication centers, regional libraries, pharmaceutical manufacturers, suppliers of laboratory equipment and products, and many of the professional health-related associations

Discussions or informal presentations by other health professionals who are consumers of laboratory services and who can disucss the laboratorian's work in relationship to the diagnosis and management of the patient.

One of the most important steps a manager can take to encourage continued learning is the encouragement of professionalism. If the laboratorian identifies himself as a true professional, then he will tend to include educational activities among personal responsibilities. This feeling of professionalism can be enhanced through providing for participation in the activities of the local, state, and national associations and paying dues and membership fees; by encouraging an understanding of issues confronting the profession and assisting laboratorians in becoming involved in resolving professional issues; and, finally, by assuming a personal role as supervisor to serve as an advocate for the profession throughout the institution.

An academic program that prepares students to become technologists will involve many different laboratory staff members as teachers, tutors, and clinical supervisors. While there are advantages to such a program through creation of a source of new staff members oriented toward the manner in which the laboratory functions (thereby reducing orientation and familiarization activities), there are also added administrative burdens and budgetary considerations. Although a review of the advantages and disadvantages of this involvement is beyond the scope of this text, a review of the required curricular components in the *Essentials of the National Accrediting Agency for Clinical Laboratory Sciences** is recommended.

LIFELONG LEARNING

In accepting a responsibility for continuing the education of the laboratorian, the manager or supervisor joins a rapidly growing movement generally identified by the term *lifelong learning.* The concept is based on the idea that the complexity of today's society, the rapid introduction of new technologies, role changes within the many professions, and the interests and desires of the citizenry for both greater job satisfaction and more meaningful use of leisure time all combine to support learning activities throughout a lifetime, rather than restricting learning to the traditional years of schooling. Continuing professional education identifies the portion of lifelong learning of direct interest to the laboratory supervisor.

Houle speaks to this as he identifies characteristics of professions that can be related to the goals of lifelong education.[8] These he clusters under broad headings:

Conceptual characteristics, by which the profession establishes a commonly agreed-upon function

Performance characteristics, which define the theory and practice of the profession, including mastery of theoretical knowledge, the ability to utilize that knowledge to solve problems, and the ability to use practical knowledge within the profession

Characteristics of self-enhancement through further individual study

Collective identity characteristics, by which a profession is known to be unique

A system of formal training

Systems for credentialing, which assure expertise of those in the profession

Existence of a subculture, which includes traditions and language unique to the profession as well as systems for role definition and recognition

Legal reinforcements, which recognize the activities of the profession with regard to protection of confidences and protection in fulfilling the common functions of the profession

*Adopted by the American Medical Association Council on Medical Education sponsoring the National Accrediting Agency for Clinical Laboratory Services, 1986.

Public acceptance of the field as a profession, which accords a measure of status to its practitioners

A tradition of ethical practice, often formally codified, which sets limits of professional behavior

Penalties available to and enforceable by associations, governments, and agencies that guard against malpractice and incompetence

Relationships with other vocations, which define the role and scope of activity of the professional in relation to allied occupations

Relationships with users of the service established through the pattern of interactions between professionals and consumers

All of these characteristics of a profession apply to medical technology and provide opportunities for development of learning activities and responsibilities for the laboratorian. No profession, including laboratory medicine, is static. Indeed, each of these characteristics merely introduces a complex dynamic aspect of the total field that describes ways in which one profession differs from another.

EDUCATIONAL ISSUES

Apart from the issue of a general societal concern for lifelong learning, there are a number of specific issues related directly to the education and practice of the laboratorian as well as to other professionals in health care. Among these is the utilization of educational activity as a criterion for continued licensure, which has grown substantially since New Mexico first required such a step in 1971. Other states soon followed, and today various authors note a wide range of requirements throughout most states. There is no particular pattern as to which states require continuing education for relicensure and for which professionals it is required. In 1977, Phillips summarized continuing education requirements for a number of professions, finding a range of requirements varying from only four states requiring continuing education for lawyers to 45 states requiring such activity for optometrists.[13] While these figures have no doubt changed, the point of variation among state requirements remains.

The rationale employed in establishing a relicensure requirement for health professionals is a desire to assure professional competence through continued educational activity. While this assurance is a goal of merit, a direct link between continuing education (or preparatory education) and competence in performance has not been established.

Johnston conducted a year-long study of the relationships among demographic factors, continuing education, and current competence as measured by a career-entry generalist certification examination.[9] Her results showed a positive correlation between continuing education preceding the study and test scores and a negative correlation between years since original career-entry certification and test scores. She concludes that continuing education for continued competence needs an accurate assessment of current knowledge and deficiencies, targeted continuing education activities, and evaluation to determine whether deficiencies have been remedied.

The transfer of cognitive knowledge to performance is difficult, even when the knowledge directly relates to the task to be performed. The relationship between knowledge and performance is even more tenuous when learning activities are only peripherally related, which is the case when a laboratorian attends a course away from the work site. Further, Willoughby, Gammon, and Jonas,[17] among others, in studying competence in physicians and other health professionals, note that although factors such as attitude, peer relations, maturity, and integrity are directly related to competent performance, they are not necessarily related to cognitive knowledge.

Among professionals, there is legitimate concern about the effectiveness of required continuing education for maintenance of competence. However, a manager or supervisor may have some additional concerns. First, there is a budgetary ramification if employees are required to undertake educational activities and therefore need educational support as a possible fringe benefit.[7] Second, the atmosphere (and possibly the value) of the learning experience is potentially different when a large portion of a program audience attends by fiat, rather than by choice. Audience size and attitude clearly affect the learning experience for the participant. Fisher and Britt considered these factors from the perspective of a continuing education provider by identifying preferred formats, schedules, and sites at which to offer programs for practitioners in Florida.[6] They found that attendees preferred lectures and workshops, in weekend programs that moved around the state to reduce travel costs to the participants.

A more positive use of continuing education, perhaps, is to reward participation in a way that recognizes individual effort among professionals. This is commonly practiced by professional associations such as the American Medical Association, which developed the Physician's Recognition

Award to encourage physician participation in continuing education. Other groups, such as the American Academy of Family Practice and the American Dietetics Association, require educational activity for maintaining organization membership, certification, or registration.

The Professional Acknowledgement for Continuing Education (PACE) program sponsored by the American Society for Medical Technology is a recognition program for professionals in the medical laboratory field. Voluntary participation in continuing education programs that have been approved by the appropriate PACE committee will earn the designation of PACESETTER for the laboratorian. The certificate awarded serves to recognize the effort of the laboratorian and symbolizes a continuing involvement in the profession.

While participation in the PACE system is voluntary, the supervisor must be aware that programs must be submitted to the review committee *in advance* for approval to be gained. The PACE system recognizes college credit course work, continuing education units (CEUs) awarded to programs submitted for approval, and individual education units (IEUs) for programs that are worthwhile but have not been submitted for approval. IEUs are generally awarded for programs of short duration (less than 3 hours).

One method a supervisor might use to encourage participation would be to note receipt of the PACESETTER certificate by a staff member through public recognition and as a part of salary consideration. From an individual professional's point of view, these systems confer status and recognition among one's peers. However, some problems may occur for the supervisor if the approval system for educational activities is closely controlled. If approved courses, for example, are available only from the association or a school or college, the options available to the manager for development of a total educational program may be somewhat restricted. Most systems place approval priority on live seminars, rather than on in-house activities designed by the manager or a staff committee or on individual self-study activities.

STAFF DEVELOPMENT

Perhaps the most important teaching role of the manager is in the planned educational activity that results from the performance appraisal conference (see Chap. 13). This educational activity is termed *staff development*. Staff development activities are designed both to correct deficiencies in current performance and to provide opportunities for employee growth.[2] Many managers fail to provide growth opportunities for their employees, reinforcing the status quo and generating job dissatisfaction for unchallenged laboratorians.

Educational activities that are targeted for staff development involve the manager in the subordinate's career planning.[4] Some laboratory managers feel that they should not take an active part in helping to develop skills that will prepare employees for jobs beyond those within a given laboratory. If a manager risks helping an employee develop his skills beyond the current job, certainly there exists the possibility of the employee leaving to acquire a better position, perhaps with a promotion. But if the employee is not challenged beyond the routine, the best will leave to find fulfillment elsewhere anyway. This author recalls asking an applicant during a preemployment interview of her career development plans; she said, "I want your job." She was hired—not because her career goals could be soon met in the current position, but because she was ready for growth and very willing to take on educational activities that would make her a more valuable employee than at the time of initial employment. Besides, she welcomed new delegated responsibilities.

Many laboratories are filled with highly qualified bench technologists and have only a few supervisory slots. When considering staff development for clinical laboratorians, beware the trap that the only way to advance is to become a supervisor. Some technologists have no desire to leave their scientific testing role for a position supervising those doing the testing. Unfortunately, too few laboratories have redesigned jobs that allow advancement to positions of "technical specialist," "interdepartmental generalist," or "clinical laboratory practitioner."

Warren has described a staff development program for technologists and technicians who felt their careers had outgrown the growth potential in her laboratory.[15] The program enabled movement along technical career development tracks progressing from Medical Technologist I to Medical Technologist III. Under the program's guidelines: "(1) A technologist must be able to advance without leaving his or her technical area; (2) the medical center and the employee must make a mutual commitment; and (3) the program must eventually be flexible enough to accommodate all levels of interested laboratorians."[15] Progression from MT I to MT III was based on a mixture of additional education, experience in the institution, and specialty certification. New expanded duties were assigned to match the additional education and experience as one progressed in the career path program.

APPROACHES TO EDUCATIONAL ACTIVITIES

There are two areas of educational programming that must be explored by the supervisor. These are preservice education and continuing and inservice education. Both are necessary for an efficient laboratory operation.

Preservice Education

One of management's primary responsibilities to the new employee is preservice education. The technologist's first few weeks in a new work environment often comprise an awkward and uneasy adjustment period. Although the need for additional technical staff generally requires that the new laboratorian function in a technical capacity as soon as possible, the supervisor must ensure that preservice education (or orientation) does not suffer. Too often this critical adjustment period receives too little attention from the responsible superior. Orientation, in fact, is one of management's most overlooked educational tools. A well-planned and structured preservice education program will ensure that the employee understand his responsibilities, limitations, and expectations initially so as not to hinder full development of performance capabilities. The important components of a preservice program are discussed in the following sections.

Job Description

Although the new employee's duties were discussed during the employment interview, the job description should be thoroughly reviewed at the beginning of the orientation period. The new employee will be more likely to ask questions about the duties and responsibilities of the position, giving the supervisor an opportunity to clarify misunderstandings. The supervisor's frank and open discussion of the job description established the foundation for the remainder of the preservice education.

The method of employee evaluation should be related to the job description. A copy of the evaluation form should be reviewed. This discussion about the evaluation and how it reflects the job description will reinforce the specific requirements of the position.

Staff Introduction

An early introduction to the laboratory staff helps develop the effective interpersonal relationships required to build teamwork. Certainly everyone with whom the new employee is to directly interact should be introduced. The size and structure of the laboratory organization will dictate the extent to which staff of other sections should be formally introduced. If the laboratory is small or open in design, all staff may be introduced to foster the "one large family" atmosphere. If, on the other hand, the laboratory has a large staff or is highly departmentalized, the new employee may be introduced only to each section supervisor. In the latter instance, an introduction to everyone at a general staff meeting would be appropriate. The period of individual introductions will include review of the organizational structure and reinforce work relationships for the new employee. In some instances, a personal introduction to the laboratory director may be in order. Attention to this portion of preservice education will enhance the new employee's feelings of belonging in the new environment.

Laboratory Policies and Procedures

Personnel policies and procedures were probably discussed during the initial interview; however, a review of these during the orientation helps to clarify any misunderstandings that might have occurred under the stress of the interview. This responsibility may be retained by the administrative technologist or personnel director or delegated to the section supervisor, depending on who discussed the policies during the interview.

This discussion should include information about the acceptable dress code, appropriate parking areas, security badge requirements, and the mechanism for completing the time sheet or card. Certainly laboratory policy concerning meal times and breaks for the specific work station needs to be addressed, because there is likely to be variation among sections within the laboratory. Coverage of evenings and weekends, call schedules, and vacation and holiday work should be discussed. Economic, educational, and recreational services such as insurance plans, pensions, continuing/inservice education, athletic or social activities, and health services provided by the institution should be included. Particular attention should be given to discipline and grievance procedures. Finally, a discussion of the opportunities for promotion and transfer will encourage the employee in self-improvement and productivity in the new laboratory environment.

Specific Laboratory Section

The first three steps in preservice education are oriented toward nonperformance details of the position. After these are sufficiently covered, the attention of the new employee can be focused on the laboratory role. The location of key manuals, reagents, equipment and supplies, and operational manuals and guidelines for instruments in the section where the laboratorian is to work should be explained. The new employee should know the location of particular documents for recording preventive maintenance checks and plotting quality-control data. Appropriate safety equipment both in and near the section should be identified. Outside the immediate working area, the location of certain general-use facilities should be noted, including the sterile preparation area, storeroom, and photocopy equipment.

Finally, the new employee can begin to feel that he has a niche in the lab when the area reserved for his personal belongings is pointed out to him. Appropriate stress should be placed on the limits of the institution's responsibility for theft of personal property.

Routine Protocols, Analytic Procedures, and Techniques

A discussion of the routine protocol for daily performance of duties follows orientation in the overall organization and the specific duty station. It is important to note tasks that have priority and tasks that can be completed on a more routine basis. If the section rotates certain duties and responsibilities among employees, such as ordering supplies or stocking disposables, this also should be explained.

Frequently, a new employee is not informed of criteria that indicate a diversion from the standard operating procedure. By describing these unusual circumstances and explaining why a special protocol is followed, the supervisor will have anticipated and avoided a future problem.

Time must also be allotted for describing the procedures and techniques that the new laboratorian is expected to perform. Initially, all routine and specialized tests should be at least talked through, since certain in-house modifications of test procedures will differ from the individual's previous experience. It is important to emphasize that the methods and procedures established in the laboratory must be followed explicitly. Of course, suggestions for modifying a procedure or technique should be considered by the supervisor. An amount of time ranging from several days to several weeks usually is required for the new employee to gain sufficient experience to complete all of the procedures and techniques of the section without extra supervision.

One area of preservice education frequently not given sufficient attention is preventive maintenance and troubleshooting problems with the automated equipment the new employee will use. A list of the most commonly occurring problems, noting the cause and outlining a step-by-step approach to resolving each problem, will avoid delays and further orient the employee in unfamiliar equipment. Omission of this important part of orientation inevitably comes back to haunt the supervisor—usually on a weekend or holiday!

Finally, direction regarding the amount of responsibility held in evaluation of quality control and patient data must be given. Approved "panic values" and appropriate actions and the types of test results that require a supervisor's or pathologist's evaluation before a report is issued to the requesting physician should be identified.

Safety Equipment and Procedures

General instructions for the proper use of all laboratory safety equipment is imperative. This may include a demonstration using the fire extinguishers, rolling oneself in a fire blanket, and a discussion on the use of safety showers and eyewashes. The new employee should also be made aware of appropriate actions to take in the event of a job-related accident. If appropriate, a written description of the new laboratorian's role in the institution's fire and disaster plan should be provided.

Documentation

A brief summary memorandum of the aspects covered during the preservice education period will serve to reinforce much of the information and provide the documentation necessary to satisfy requirements of the various laboratory accrediting and regulatory agencies.[3] It will also verify the completion of the supervisor's responsibility for employee orientation.

In summary, a well-planned orientation period will help the new employee adapt more readily to the new work environment of the laboratory. The result should be an open channel of communication between the supervisor and the new employee and avoidance of some of the usual misunderstandings associated with the new-job adjustment period. Despite the supervisor's most elaborate orientation approach, however, it should be recognized that non-scheduled but relevant "orientation" takes place on coffee breaks. Where else can a new employee learn such valuable information as who plans the lab's Christmas party, who usually has extra football tickets, and who will take phone messages?

Inservice and Continuing Education

In developing an appropriate postorientation educational program within the organization, the supervisor must first consider program goals. Lauffer indicates that there are two basic orientations or themes upon which educational activities are based: improving the capabilities of the laboratorian and improving the manner in which the laboratory functions.[10] Generally, the first of these would be called *continuing education* or *staff development*; and the latter would be *inservice education*. In reality, however, the distinctions are neither clear nor particularly important. Although the manager will pursue both goals at various times, there must be an awareness of which effort is being pursued at any point.

Improving the capability of the laboratorian can be accomplished in a variety of ways. Attendance at a seminar offered by a hospital or medical center or enrollment in a course at a local university can contribute to individual growth and development. These activities are commonly classified as continuing education in that they are designed to build upon previous formal educational experiences. Continuing education rarely provides the initial training required for entering the profession; however, educational activities pursued for enhancing progress within the organization or assuming new functions almost always are considered continuing education. For example, a laboratorian who is promoted to shift supervisor and then attends a seminar on techniques of supervision is attempting to develop a new personal role within the field.

Continuing education, when focusing on improving the capabilities of the laboratorian, is a highly individualistic endeavor, even though one would logically assume that a curriculum could be developed through which all laboratorians could constantly remain current. The fallacy in this attractive idea lies in the variability of employment environments and experiences of the individual after graduation from the initial training program. Individual professional experiences and growth are highly variable. In addition, duties for the laboratorian are likely to vary with work locations.

Because needs, activities, goals, and circumstances of individual practitioners within the field of medical technology vary, care must be given to the selection of continuing education activities. Several questions must be addressed by the professional prior to registering for a seminar.[14] First, can areas of personal need be identified so that the technician will be alert to potential educational opportunities? Examples may include future assumption of new duties that might require review of procedures or mastery of a new technique; the laboratory could be preparing to install new equipment that will require additional knowledge; or the institution could be planning to develop a new health-care service area requiring laboratory support, thereby causing a restructuring of duties.

When the educational goal of the supervisor focuses on the manner in which the laboratory functions, however, educational activity will include a large percentage of the laboratory staff and should be conducted locally. In many cases no outside consultant will be required, because the educational activity will center on development and implementation of new procedures and techniques. In other cases the activities might more properly focus on problem-solving steps, such as identification of barriers preventing accomplishment of tasks, motivational sessions that encourage cooperation among staff members, or informational sessions that reiterate policies and procedures. This, then, is the area of inservice education.[1]

A primary concern of the supervisor when focusing on laboratory operation is to ensure that the problem does indeed spring from a lack of training or can be solved through a training activity. A training or educational activity should be held only after it is determined that the lack of performance is not caused by attitudes, lack of motivation, barriers from other departments or personnel, or a lack of resources, such as funding or equipment. Once all of these possible interveners have been examined and discarded, the manager can proceed to the development of an educational activity, taking care that appropriate documentation is prepared for accrediting bodies, such as the Joint Commission on the Accreditation of Hospitals.[3]

Within the laboratory, target audiences of those who will participate will vary with the information to be included in the inservice activity. Certain modifications in a department's analytic procedure would be appropriate only for those responsible for performing that particular analysis and for those affected by a change in the procedure. This may involve two separate groups and require separate meetings. Other changes, such as a modification in a personnel benefit policy, may require a session for all staff members. In the case of a technologist experiencing difficulty troubleshooting a certain instrument, perhaps only one participant would be involved in the instructional activity.

There are several approaches to assist staff members in updating their technical skills within the routine workday. Each of these requires that the supervisor be alert for opportunities to create a learning situation. The College of American Pathology's Check Sample Program is one such example. By involving everyone in the Check Sample process, the routine is supplanted by an unusual case. For the highly departmentalized institution, the Check Sample patient data sheet may provide results from several laboratories to be correlated in defining the intended diagnosis. A subsequent case review is valuable in understanding the pathology behind the Check Sample findings. This same approach can be used by creating a case study when unusual laboratory results are desired.

Teaching Methodologies

Inservice education is usually a responsibility of laboratory supervisors and managers and requires careful planning and implementation to accomplish the stated goals and objectives. The approaches described here are but a few of the variety available to make inservice more effective for larger groups. The only limitation is one's imagination in creating a learning opportunity as part of the employee's workday.

LECTURE AND DISCUSSION SYMPOSIUM. Most people, when asked to teach, fall back on the dominant technique in American education—the lecture. For presenting new information, the lecture undoubtedly is the most efficient. Since inservice topics are usually of immediate application, the effectiveness of the lecture approach can be greatly enhanced by planning to include time for discussion. Two-way communication (discussion) is more accurate and effective than one-way (lecture only). (See Chap. 5.) When an inservice topic has several points of view, perhaps two or more speakers may be invited. This, then, becomes a symposium and will increase the perspective of the participants.

PANEL DISCUSSIONS. A panel generally consists of three or four speakers and a moderator. When presenting a change in laboratory protocol, for example, perhaps a panel of supervisors whose sections are affected should briefly describe the change. A moderator would then direct the interaction among panel members, as well as receive and direct the questions from the inservice participants. As in the symposium, the panel is an ideal format for expressing divergent views. Panel members should be carefully selected with attention given to speaking ability, and they should be assigned generally equal amounts of content to present. The responsibility is placed on the moderator to see that time frames are adhered to and that each panel member is briefed before the session.

PROBLEM-SOLVING SESSION. As noted elsewhere in this text, the commitment to resolution of a problem will be greater if those affected by the problem are involved in solving it. This can become a type of inservice called a *clinic*, in which the speaker is assisted by a panel and the audience in exploring possible solutions to practical problems. When it becomes necessary to modify personnel policies within a department, for example, this approach could be very effective. The speaker becomes the leader relying on the panel for expertise in a judgmental decision area. Even though the content of the discussion may not be totally anticipated, the leader must plan the session to progress through the following stages: (1) defining the problem; (2) stating and ranking the crucial issues; and (3) listing and selecting the best solution.

INTERACTIVE CASE STUDY. Disease correlation with laboratory results and corresponding pathophysiology is best addressed by interactive case study. In this approach, a case is presented in terms of patient history and physical, followed by the laboratory data and a series of questions guiding the audience in discussion of the case. Several professional journals for clinical laboratory personnel include interactive case studies with appropriate answers and references which may be used.

SIMULATION OR ROLE PLAYING. This approach requires the facilitator to create a representation of reality within which the participants interact. Development of interpersonal relationships, such as dealing with uncooperative patients, is ideally suited for this technique. Of all possible approaches, however, role playing is among the most difficult and requires substantial preparation on the part of the role players to be really effective. It may be advantageous to employ a prepared "trigger" film or tape, followed by audience discussion, rather than involve participants in acting out the simulated role.

THE PROCESS OF DEVELOPING EDUCATIONAL ACTIVITIES

The process of planning and carrying out effective teaching follows similar steps whether completed in a formal continuing education program or through the efforts of an individual professional who will offer a short seminar for colleagues within the laboratory. These steps are (1) assessing needs; (2) developing objectives; (3) determining content; (4) establishing the teaching method; (5) conducting the activity (teaching); and (6) evaluating the teaching effort.[5] Evaluation logically leads to a reassessment of needs, making the entire process circular and continuous, because in an environment where staff members are involved in inservice activities, each session should identify teaching areas for the next session.[1]

Assessing Needs

Needs assessment is conducted at three levels—institutional, program, and individual. The essential question at each level is, What shall be taught?

At the institutional or laboratory level, the process is one of identifying topic areas based on the types of work performed within the laboratory. What are the major tests completed for patient admissions? What comprises the top ten laboratory orders from outpatient clinic visits? What are the major services provided for inpatients? This analysis of the most common orders for patient–physician support will provide a listing of areas in which programming should be developed. Assessment of current teaching efforts, audit information, physician requests, and comments for information will help to determine appropriate program development priorities.

At the conclusion of this process of identifying subjects, an assessment of information needed for each subject or program must be completed. The first step would be to list the topics to be taught within an inservice program. The unique aspects of the individual program related to the hospital and laboratory should be considered, and priorities of what must be learned on this topic must be set.

The third, and final, level of assessment is that of the individual laboratorian's educational needs as related to the program topic. This analysis of the individual tailors the instruction as much as possible to the individual and to the staff of the laboratory. All of the possible topics that might be included in one program will not be appropriate to every staff member, and some parts may not be appropriate at all. Time also may not be available to cover all desired topics; so the teaching plan must be sequenced in order to meet areas of greatest deficiency first. A useful strategy often employs an advanced laboratorian as the inservice instructor, thereby creating a tutorial system within the department.

Developing Objectives

The listing of topics that might be taught on any subject provides only a broad guideline. The topics must be refined to summarize actual behaviors that the laboratorian must perform successfully. Some behaviors may be activity-based, such as performing a reticulocyte count; and some may be knowledge-based, such as noting test abnormalities one might expect if a patient were taking a certain medication. Note that the objective is oriented toward the student, that is, the emphasis is on what the student must do rather than on what the teacher will teach.[12] While this may seem to be a subtle distinction, it underlies the philosophy of adult and continuing education.

There are two steps in developing specific objectives for any teaching program. First, a set of standard behaviors for each topic that applies to all students must be listed. These are derived from the topics previously formulated in the needs-assessment phase. For the reticulocyte example used above, an instructor may list the following behaviors: (1) prepare a blood/reticulocyte stain mixture; (2) prepare a smear from this mixture for counting; (3) determine the number of reticulocytes/1000 red cells; and (4) calculate the patient's corrected reticulocyte count.

These activities are then restated as objectives, which contain three elements: the activity or behavior to be performed, the conditions under which the behavior will be performed, and the evaluation criteria that will determine successful performance of the behavior. The acronym ACE serves as a useful reminder of the three elements—activity, condition, evaluation.[12]

The previously mentioned topics could be translated into behavioral objectives:

> The student will combine equal amounts of the patient's whole blood and supravital stain in a white cell pipette such that both blood and stain can be mixed in the bulb; smear the blood/stain mixture on a clean glass slide, spreading cells into a monolayer feather-edge without accumulation on the edge of the slide; count the number of reticulocytes per 1000 red cells on two smears with comparative totals of ±5 cells between smears using a light microscope with an oil immersion objective; and, given the hematocrit, calculate the patient's corrected reticulocyte count within ±3 from the known value.

In each of these objectives the activity to be performed is clear because it is stated in measurable terms; test abnormality expectations will be stated. The condition under which the activity is to be performed is also clear—use of clean slides, use of a light microscope with an oil objective, and calculation from the patient's hematocrit.

The evaluation portion notes the level of competence that must be reached. When unstated it is understood to be 100%. It could also be stated with ranges of correctness, such as ± 5 or 80%. The evaluation criterion provides a signal that teaching has been completed or that additional efforts will be required.

Secondly, the objectives must be sequenced into priority order. The behaviors that are critical would receive the highest priority and be taught to every laboratorian. Less important objectives would be saved for the future or for certain individuals for whom the information is important.

Determining Content

Only the relevant information for the particular objective should be included. While the content should be complete and accurate, the usual tendency to add extra explanatory and background material should be avoided. An overabundance of information that is of marginal importance to the topic may well serve to confuse, rather than to clarify understanding.

Once the objective is identified, gather resources that provide information relevant to the topic. Journal articles, texts, manufacturer's publications, and pamphlets and brochures from health associations are all good sources of information. These resources will help clarify objectives; provide clear, concise descriptions, illustrations, and helpful suggestions, such as lists of forms the laboratorian could use; and identify common problems that have been experienced under similar circumstances.

From this information, the actual content of the session, consisting of an outline of the lesson as well as supplemental notes of drawings, pictures, forms, calendars, and so forth, must be developed. If a particular brochure or article clearly explains one of the teaching points or covers an entire topic, it could be used with little or no modification. In most cases, however, the instructor will want to develop the information to be included using a variety of sources.

Establishing the Teaching Method

The method(s) to be used for actually teaching the material is developed after the content is determined. The methods available may include one-to-one discussion, group meetings, brochures, movies, flipcharts, case studies, slide shows, demonstra-

tions, audio- and videotapes, and charts. Generally, the use of more than one method is recommended, because a variety of approaches complements the teaching effort. For example, the method to be used should be based on factors such as the time and location available for the teaching; complexity of the information; interfering responsibilities of the clinician, which would affect consistent in-person teaching; type of behavior to be learned; and preference and comfort of the clinician in the teaching situation. A review of the teaching approaches stated earlier in this chapter will note the strengths and weaknesses of each approach.

The distinction between student-oriented planning and teacher-oriented planning becomes clear when thinking through the teaching methodology. The instructor who has focused on teacher strategies, that is, *what he will do,* will be less flexible in changing approaches when the student does not progress quickly. The instructor who focuses on *what the student must do,* however, generally is open to attempting a variety of activities to help the student successfully accomplish the goal.

Conducting the Activity (Teaching)

Once the objectives are set, lessons planned, and resources and supplemental materials gathered, attention can be given to the actual implementation of the program. Consideration of several factors by the supervisor will enhance the acceptance of the program by the laboratory staff.

First, the supervisor must ensure a positive attitude toward participation, particularly in inservice activities. In-house activities could be seen as conflicting with "real" job duties if insufficient emphasis has been given to helping the staff understand the need for inservice education. Too many meetings will cause resistance, and too few will reduce acceptance of educational activities as an overall part of the laboratory environment.

Second, activities that are attended by staff members and taught by a senior laboratorian on the staff could develop into a social meeting or a gripe session if the goals are not clearly stated or the seriousness of the activity is underemphasized. The use of a committee in the planning process may increase commitment among staff members, and guest speakers may help to reduce side activity during the teaching session.

Third, the supervisor should give careful thought to personally teaching in the inservice program. For some staff members the acceptance of the supervisor as a supportive teacher, rather than as a "boss," may be difficult, and this may adversely affect his teaching effectiveness. If the supervisor teaches only sessions with subjects such as policies and procedures, however, he may establish an atmosphere of authoritarianism. Establishing a balance may be difficult but must be considered.

Evaluating the Teaching Effort

There are three types of evaluation to employ— student, teacher, and environment. Student evaluation attempts to determine the gains in knowledge resulting from the activity. This evaluation may be formal or informal but must be based upon the objectives developed for the instruction. It is not suggested that a paper and pencil test be used, because tests often cause anxiety in adults and negatively affect performance regardless of the student's knowledge. The test should be as realistic as possible; so actual demonstrations of procedures, case-study discussions, and similar approaches are recommended.

Evaluation of the teacher will help the instructor to improve his approach in the future. Reporting the results to the instructor should be done in a positive, supportive manner.

Evaluation of the teaching environment will reveal distractions and problems, which, if not corrected, may affect the success of future sessions. Statements about interruptions to call technologists back to the laboratory, too much dropping in and out by the supervisor, and the absence of other staff members are all clues for future planning.

REFERENCES

1. Adams CD: Guidelines for in-service programs. Lab Med 16:561–563, 1985
2. Biddle AM: A strategic plan for staff development. MLO 17(1):62–66, 1985
3. Cabonor RP, DeNofa JR: Design and administration of a continuing education policy. Am J Med Technol 47:715–722, 1981
4. Cross L: Career management development—A system that gets results. Training and Development J 37(2):54–63, 1983
5. Ehrmeyer SS, Ehrmeyer GC: A five-step approach to bench teaching. J Med Technol 1:573–577, 1984
6. Fisher F, Britt MS: An assessment of continuing education needs for clinical laboratory personnel. Lab Med 18:110–114, 1987
7. Garcia LS: A cost containment checklist. MLO 17(4):67–73, 1985
8. Houle CO: Continuing Learning in the Professions, pp 34–75. San Francisco, Jossey-Bass, 1980
9. Johnston VF: A study of the relationships among demographic factors, continuing education and continued competence. J Med Technol 2:779–785, 1985
10. Lauffer A: The Practice of Continuing Education in the Human Services, p 16. New York, McGraw-Hill, 1977
11. Morgenstern F: Clinical teaching: On-the-job training or planned method of instruction? Lab Management 16(1):52–54, 1978
12. Objectives. In Development and Evaluation of Audiovisual Instructional Materials. Atlanta, Educational Training and Consultation Branch, National Medical Audiovisual Center, September 1, 1976
13. Phillips LE: The status of mandatory continuing education for the professions. Presented to the National University Extension Association, Division of Continuing Education for the Professions, March 21, 1977
14. Stroul NA, Schuman G: Action planning for workshops. Training and Development J 37(7):41–42, 1983
15. Warren J: Building a career ladder for the upward climb. MLO 15(1):72–82, 1983
16. Warshaw M, Welch JL: Guidelines for teaching in the laboratory setting. MLO 15(6):85–87, 1983
17. Willoughby TL, Gammon LC, Jonas HS: Correlates of clinical performance during medical school. J Med Ed 54:453–459, 1979

ANNOTATED BIBLIOGRAPHY

Dickinson G: Teaching Adults, a Handbook for Instructors. Toronto, New Press, 1973

This book focuses on the educational process and the adult learner. It should be reviewed by individuals who teach adults in continuing education and inservice programs as well as by course planners.

Heroux GAM: Continuing Professional Education—How. Springfield, Illinois Institute for Continuing Professional Education, 1975

This is a general volume which covers basic aspects of identifying curriculum, planning seminars, advertising and administering seminars. It contains sample budgets and forms. This book should be of particular value to individuals responsible for continuing education for associations.

Knowles MS: The Modern Practice of Adult Education. Chicago, Association Press, 1980

This reference focuses on the process of adult education known as andragogy. The first part of the book addresses the special concerns of the adult learner and the role of the adult educator. The second provides a comprehensive discussion for organizing and administering continuing education programs, from needs assessment through budgeting and evaluation. Chapter 11 in the third part provides some examples and aids which help adults learn.

Langerman PD, Smith DH (eds): Managing Adult and Continuing Education Programs and Staff. Washington DC, National Association for Public Continuing and Adult Education, 1979

This resource contains insights from many individuals who have responsibilities in directing continuing education activities. The book is divided into two major sections: managing programs and managing instructional staff.

Lauffer A: Doing Continuing Education and Staff Development. New York, McGraw-Hill 1978

This book provides a general overview of planning educational programs. It is oriented toward development of a total program of education within an organization. It would be valuable to those who desire additional theoretic information about the relationship of continuing education to organizational goals, the identification of resources, and the structuring of overall programs.

fifteen

Labor Relations and the Clinical Laboratory

Walton H. Sharp

BACKGROUND

The term *labor relations* encompasses the interactions between an employer, or institution, and a representative of the employees, normally referred to as a *union,* a *labor organization,* or an *employee association.* Labor relations is a subset of the broader discipline of industrial relations, which is concerned with all aspects of the functioning of labor markets and the employer–employee relationship. The purpose of this chapter is to introduce to the laboratory supervisor the study of labor relations and its integral parts and processes: law, collective bargaining, and contract administration.

There are several reasons for laboratory supervisors to understand more fully the labor relations process. First, some 19 million persons belong to some form of labor organization in the United States. Second, the passage of the 1974 Health Care Amendments to the National Labor Relations Act provided approximately 1.5 million employees of nonprofit voluntary health-care institutions the opportunity to have union representation. Third, it is proposed here that the laboratory supervisor can be more effective as a part of the management team by understanding the dynamics of the labor relations process.

There is not a single encompassing law governing labor relations in the United States. Rather, there are three identifiable legal frameworks: (1) the Civil Service Reform Act, which has jurisdiction over the federal sector; (2) state labor laws, which deal with states and their political subdivisions; and (3) the National Labor Relations Act, which addresses labor relations in the private sector, including profit and nonprofit voluntary health-care institutions (Fig. 15-1).[9] Each of these systems, in turn, must be viewed as dynamic, rather than static, because of changes in the laws themselves, changes in the regulations, decisions of agencies charged with the administration of the laws, and decisions of the federal and state courts.

LABOR LAW AND THE PUBLIC EMPLOYEE

The National Labor Relations Act exempts the federal government and states and their political subdivisions from the coverage of the Act.[10] Employees of health-care institutions operated by units of government are therefore not protected by the National Labor Relations Act. This is also true of most health-care institutions operated by a taxing authority such as a hospital district.

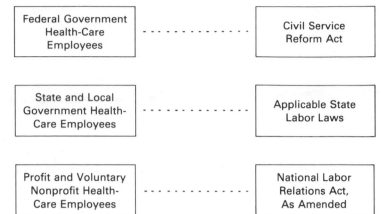

FIGURE 15-1. Appropriate labor law coverage for health-care institutions and employees.

Federal Employees

Employees of the federal government did not have a legal right to engage in collective bargaining until 1962, when President Kennedy issued Executive Order 10988. This executive order contained several major inadequacies. First, recognition of a union was based upon the proportion of employees in a bargaining unit represented by the union. Second, the number of items about which a union could bargain with the agency was limited. Third, the procedures for resolving contractual disputes between labor and management were a part of the statutory framework of the executive order, were cumbersome, and did not provide for a true independent arbiter of the dispute.

In 1970, President Nixon corrected some of these deficiencies in Executive Order 11491. This executive order created a three-member Federal Labor Relations Council to administer the executive order and to take the leadership role in federal-sector labor relations. The authority to determine union eligibility and to determine the bargaining unit to be represented by the union was placed with the Secretary of Labor. The responsibility for settling disputes arising from contract negotiations was granted to a Federal Services Impasses Panel. Additionally, federal employees were prohibited from striking, picketing, or engaging in a work slowdown or any form of work stoppage, which simply continued the established policy of the federal government.

In 1978, the Congress put federal government labor relations into law through the passage of the Civil Service Reform Act.[4] The Act established the Federal Labor Relations Authority (FLRA) as the agency charged with the responsibility for administration of federal-sector labor relations. The FLRA is composed of three members appointed by the President of the United States, not more than two of whom may be members of the same political party. The scope and functions of the FLRA are similar to the scope and functions of the National Labor Relations Board (NLRB), the agency charged with administration of the National Labor Relations Act, which governs labor–management relations of the private economy. The FLRA determines an appropriate employee unit for purposes of collective bargaining, conducts elections for union representation and certifies the results, hears complaints of unfair labor practices, determines whether bargaining is conducted in good faith, and determines whether certain issues are subject to negotiations between the union and the agency of government. The Civil Service Reform Act also provided for a general counsel to the FLRA, who is appointed by the president. The duties of this office are essentially to file, investigate, and prosecute unfair labor-practice charges, making the duties of the office very similar to those of the Office of the General Counsel of the NLRB.

The Civil Service Reform Act also established a Merit Systems Protection Board (MSPB), which is composed of three presidential appointees, no more than two of whom may be from the same political party. The MSPB reviews, upon petition by an employee, an adverse action taken by an agency against an employee of the agency. An adverse action may be defined as discipline that involves a removal, a suspension of more than 14 days, a reduction in grade, a reduction in pay, or a furlough of 30 days or less.

Employee complaints that allege discrimination on the basis of race, color, religion, sex, age, marital status, or political affiliation may be processed through the grievance procedure of the labor–agency contract, through arbitration, and then to either the FLRA or to the Equal Employment Opportunity Commission (EEOC). Cases that allege adverse action and discrimination, termed "mixed cases," may be processed through a negotiated grievance procedure, to arbitration, or to the MSPB, the FLRA, or the EEOC. In the event that the findings and decisions of the EEOC and the MSPB disagree, a special panel is convened to resolve the dispute. Finally, the affected employee may appeal to either a United States district court or a United States court of appeals.

State Employees

After the execution of Executive Order 10988 in the Federal sector, states began to enact legislation that granted the employees of state, county, and municipal agencies the right to unionize and to engage in collective bargaining. To date, 36 states grant public employees such rights, although it should be added that many of these state laws prohibit strikes and limit bargaining issues to those of hours and working conditions. In general, the state laws are not as comprehensive as federal public-sector labor law or the labor laws that govern the private economy

LABOR LAW AND THE PRIVATE-SECTOR EMPLOYEE

The National Labor Relations Act

In 1935, the Congress of the United States passed the National Labor Relations Act, also referred to as the *Wagner Act.* In doing so, Congress exercised its constitutional authority to govern interstate commerce. Prior to 1967, health-care institutions operated for profit were deemed not to be sufficiently engaged in interstate commerce to be subject to the Act's jurisdiction. This was based upon the view of the NLRB that there was not a sufficient flow of patients crossing state lines to receive health care to warrant the inclusion of health-care institutions operated for profit under the Act's jurisdiction. However, in two cases that were heard by the NLRB in 1967, the Board turned its attention to the dollar volume of supplies and equipment that cross state lines to effectuate a new policy that health-care institutions operated for profit would be subject to the Act's coverage.[3] The Board established a dollar-volume jurisdiction yardstick to determine whether the provisions of the Act should be applied to health-

care institutions operated for profit. Hospitals that have annual receipts in excess of $250,000 and nursing homes that have receipts of $100,000 are now subject to the Act's coverage. The Board applied the same yardstick to voluntary nonprofit health-care institutions after the passage of the 1974 Health Care Amendments (discussed later in this chapter) to the National Labor Relations Act.

The Act also established the NLRB as the agency to carry out and oversee the provisions of the Act.[15] As originally established, the board was composed of three members, appointed by the President of the United States, subject to the confirmation of the Senate, who served a specified term of office. The board was also empowered to establish regional and field offices as necessary to carry out the purposes of the Act.

The board has three primary functions: (1) to determine an appropriate bargaining unit when employees seek union representation, (2) to conduct elections for union representation, and (3) to investigate charges of unfair labor practices. These are discussed more fully in the section of this chapter dealing with unions.

Labor-Management Relations Act (Taft–Hartley)

In 1947, Congress amended the National Labor Relations Act and placed additional requirements of labor–management relations into effect with the passage of the Labor–Management Relations Act. Also known as the *Taft–Hartley Act,* the new legislation contained five titles, the first of which amended the National Labor Relations Act. A more detailed discussion of Title I and the amendments follows a brief discussion of Titles II through V.

Title II of the Taft–Hartley Act is concerned with the prevention of work stoppages, especially those that could affect an entire industry and thus threaten the national welfare. In this regard, Congress established the Federal Mediation and Conciliation Service (FMCS) to assist labor and management in resolving impasses in contract negotiations. FMCS is not empowered to make decisions but must use its knowledge and persuasion in attempts to assist labor and management to reach an amicable settlement. Other provisions of Title II outline procedures by which the President of the United States can obtain a federal court injunction when a strike or a threatened strike endangers the national welfare. Under this provision, workers can be compelled to return to work or prohibited from striking for a period of 80 days while attempts are made to settle the dispute between labor and management. Prior to the end of the 80-day period, workers are afforded an opportunity to vote to accept or reject the employer's last offer in a secret-ballot election.

Title III provides that suits to enforce labor–management contracts be brought in a federal district court. This provision is important in the enforcement of grievance–arbitration machinery contained in the majority of union–management contracts.

Title IV established a labor–management commission to study labor–management relations in the United States and to report its findings.

Title V, in Section 502, gives workers a right to refuse to work under abnormally dangerous conditions of employment without such a work stoppage being considered a strike.

It was Title I that made the most substantial changes in the National Labor Relations Act. It increased the size of the NLRB from three to five members and established the Office of the General Counsel of the NLRB. The responsibilities were divided so that the Office of the General Counsel would supervise the regional and field office staffs and the investigation and prosecution of unfair labor practice charges, while the Board itself would adjudicate cases brought before it.

Title I also amended Sections 7 and 8 of the National Labor Relations Act. Section 7 grants employees of employers subject to the Act the right to form, join, or assist in the formation of a labor organization; to bargain through representatives of their own choosing, and to engage in other protected, concerted activities for the purposes of collective bargaining and other mutual aid and protection. Section 8 of the National Labor Relations Act outlines a series of employer unfair labor practices which are violative of employee rights. Among these are:

Interfering, restraining or coercing employees in the exercise of their rights guaranteed in Section 7

Dominating or interfering with the formation or administration of a labor organization

Discriminating against employees in hiring or promotions because of membership in a labor organization

Discharging or otherwise discriminating against an employee because the employee filed an unfair labor practice charge or gave testimony in a Board-conducted hearing.

Refusing to bargain with the representative of the employees

An employee or a labor organization has 6 months from the date of the employer's alleged unfair labor practice to file a charge with the Board. (In Section 10, the Act empowers the Board to prevent unfair labor practices and to require remedial action, including reinstatement of illegally discharged workers, with or without back pay, if the unfair labor practice charge is upheld.)

Section 7 is applicable to union-organizing campaigns and also to situations in the absence of a union in which employees band together for purposes of mutual aid and protection. For example, an employer was found guilty of an unfair labor practice for discharging two employees on a construction site who refused to work while it was raining. The employees argued that the work would be dangerous while it was raining and stated that they would resume working when the rain stopped. The supervisor fired the employees, and they, in turn, filed an unfair labor practice charge with the Board. The Board upheld the charge because the employees were engaged in protected, concerted activities for their mutual aid and protection as guaranteed in Section 7; it ordered the employees reinstated with back pay.[2] A union did not represent the employees on the job site. Thus, contrary to popular belief, employees of institutions subject to the National Labor Relations Act enjoy the protection of the Act regardless of the question of unionization.

Taft–Hartley amended Section 7 to grant employees the right to refrain from unionization. Section 8 was also amended to include union unfair labor practices. Among these were the following:

Restraining or coercing employees in the exercise of their rights guaranteed in Section 7

Refusing to bargain collectively with an employer.

Charging excessive or discriminatory union initiation fees and dues

Causing or attempting to cause an employer to pay for services not performed

Engaging in various kinds of secondary boycott activity which involves striking or placing other economic pressure on an employer to force it to cease doing business with another employer

The Taft–Hartley amendments also provide a definition of professional employees in Section 2(12) and, in Section 9(b), give professional employees the right to be represented separately for purposes of unionization, rather than to be included in a bargaining unit with other employees. In Section 2(2), the federal government, states and their political subdivisions, and voluntary nonprofit health-care institutions are excluded from the coverage of the Act, although the latter's exclusion was removed with passage of the 1974 Health Care Amendments. Section 14(a) provides that employers are not obliged to recognize nor to bargain with a unit of supervisory employees. Section 14(b) allows individual states to enact laws prohibiting compulsory union membership. These laws are known as *right-to-work* laws and will be discussed more fully later in this chapter.

The Labor–Management Reporting and Disclosure Act

Enacted in 1959, The Labor–Management Reporting and Disclosure Act was primarily concerned with the internal affairs of unions, although it did contain some amendments to the National Labor Relations Act. Primarily, the amendments modified Section 8. Unions could not picket for more than 30 days for the purpose of obtaining recognition from an employer, and contract clauses that allow union members to refuse to work with nonunion goods were prohibited.

The 1974 Health Care Amendments

Prior to the enactment of Public Law 93-360 in 1974, the nation's nonprofit health-care institutions were excluded from the coverage of the National Labor Relations Act. In Section 2(2) of the National Labor Relations Act, these institutions were excluded from the definition of employers subject to the Act along with the federal government and states and their political subdivisions. In essence, one of the primary features of the 1974 Health Care Amendments was to amend Section 2(2) so that nonprofit health-care institutions were not contained in the grouping of employers excluded from the coverage of the Act.

There are several other features of the 1974 Health Care Amendments that are unique to a health-care setting:

1. In initial contract bargaining, a 30-day written notice of the existence of a labor dispute must be given to the other party involved in the negotiation, to the Federal Mediation and Conciliation Service (an agency of the federal government) and to any appropriate state agency (such as a state labor relations board) before the party serving the notice may engage in a legal strike, in the case of the union, or a lock out of the employees, in the case of the health care institution.[11]
2. A written notice of the union's intent to strike or picket the health care institution must be served to a responsible official of the institution

and to the Federal Mediation and Conciliation Service at least 10 days prior to the commencement of such activity of the strike for picketing to be legal.[12]

The general counsel of the NLRB, in an advisory memorandum, determined that these two sections should be read in tandem, based upon the legislative history of the Act.[13] Thus, in initial bargaining, a total of 40 days must elapse after the notice of the existence of a labor dispute has been communicated to the appropriate parties before a union may legally strike or picket. An employee who violates these provisions loses the protections against employer discipline afforded employees by the National Labor Relations Act.

3. In private health care settings in which a union-management contract is presently in effect, a party seeking to terminate or modify the existing contract must serve a written notice of the existence of a labor dispute to the other party at least 90 days before a legal work stoppage can take place and must notify the Federal Mediation and Conciliation Service and any appropriate state agency at least 60 days prior to the commencement of a work stoppage.[11]
4. Union and management are *required* to participate in negotiation meetings requested by the Federal Mediation and Conciliation Service.[14]
5. The Director of the Federal Mediation and Conciliation Service is empowered to appoint a Board of Inquiry in the event that a strike or lockout or a threatened strike or lockout will interrupt the delivery of health care services for an entire locality or geographic area. The Board of Inquiry is to be appointed within 15 days of the receipt of the notice of a labor dispute by the Federal Mediation and Conciliation Service and the Board of Inquiry is to issue a nonbinding report of the facts of the dispute and the positions of the respective parties to the Director of the FMCS within 15 days.[14]

Effective August 1, 1979, the FMCS issued new regulations, which afford labor and management jointly an opportunity to nominate persons for a board of inquiry, if the nominations are received by the FMCS before the notice of the existence of a dispute is served.[5] The FMCS will also defer to a privately agreed upon fact-finding procedure established by labor and management and will decline to appoint a board of inquiry if

a. The fact-finding procedure is automatically invoked at a specified time;
b. The fact-finding procedure provides a

permanent method of selecting the impartial fact-finding person or board;

c. The fact-finding procedure provides that strikes or lockouts will not occur except by mutual agreement prior to, during and for a period of seven days after the completion of the fact-finding procedure; and

d. The person or board conducting the fact-finding procedure makes a written report to labor and management containing the findings of fact and recommendations for settling the dispute and submits a copy to the FMCS.

The FMCS will also decline to appoint a board of inquiry if labor and management have agreed to an interest-arbitration procedure and the procedure meets the following conditions:

e. Except by mutual agreement, the procedure must provide that a work stoppage will not ensue and conditions of employment will not change during the contract negotiations and the time period during which the interest arbitration is conducted;

f. The award of the interest arbitrator or arbitration panel is final and binding on both parties;

g. The procedure contains a fixed method for selecting the interest arbitrator or arbitration panel;

h. The procedure provides that the award of the interest arbitrator or arbitration panel must be in writing.

The overriding concern of the Congress in passing these amendments was to ensure the continuity of patient care. Thus the "ally doctrine" does not apply if a hospital accepts patients transferred from a hospital that is being struck. Under any other circumstances, the acceptance of work normally performed by the striking employees of a struck employer by a neutral employer makes the neutral employer an "ally" of the struck employer. The neutral or "ally" employer may then be legally picketed by the striking employees of another employer.

UNIONS

Why Do Workers Join?

Unless belonging to a union is part of a family tradition, most workers probably know very little about a union and the process of unionization. What, then, is the catalyst that propels employees to seek union-

ization? Unfortunately, there is not a single explanation of the dynamics of unionization. This section outlines some of the factors that may cause employees to seek unionization.[20]

Personal Factors

A sense of dissatisfaction with elements of the job and the employing institution often acts as a stimulus for unionization, especially if the employee perceives that attempts to eliminate dissatisfactions through existing organizational channels would be fruitless. Pay, quality of supervision, the level of fringe benefits, general working conditions in the laboratory, the organization's rules and policies and the perceived fairness of their administration and enforcement, and the pattern of interpersonal interactions in the laboratory are variables that may lead to dissatisfaction. Employees make a number of comparisons based upon these variables. First, they compare them in light of their own perceived competence and self-image, and they compare the levels of each of the variables that they perceive they need or deserve and the levels of each that they actually receive. They also compare the levels of these variables that they receive with the levels received by other medical technologists in the laboratory and with other occupational groups in the workplace. They also compare the levels of these benefits with medical technologists employed in other health-care institutions and with other occupational groups in the community.

The perceptions of the individuals, while important, do not lead directly to unionization. Unless the individual perceives or knows that other medical technologists share some of the same concerns, the individual acting alone will probably not attempt to seek union representation and in fact may leave the organization. However, as employees interact with each other on and off the job, the sharing of perceived similar dissatisfactions begins to build a critical mass of similarly held beliefs and opinions.[1] Once the critical mass is developed, a group that develops its own norms, values, and sanctions is established. If the group perceives that its dissatisfactions cannot be remedied through existing organizational channels, it may seek outside assistance. It is quite easy for this group to become the union's internal organizing committee, since it is this group that establishes the norms of behavior for its members and the sanctions against nonmembers.

The Image of the Union

Even though all the necessary ingredients of individual and group attitudes may seem to be present for a successful union-organizing campaign, this does not ensure that the organizing campaign will result in unionization. An important ingredient is the image of the union that seeks to represent the employees, both its general image as a union and its specific image as an effective representative of medical technologists as professionals.

It would be very difficult for a traditional blue-collar union to be perceived as an effective representative of what are essentially white-collar professionals. Medical technologists might very well question whether such a union would understand the professional issues that confront the occupational group. On the other hand, a union that has traditionally represented white-collar professionals might be perceived as acceptable, especially if it demonstrates an understanding and knowledge of the professional concerns of medical technologists and if it demonstrates that such concerns can be successfully negotiated with the employer through collective bargaining.

A union perceived as being corrupt and engaging in questionable practices might also be perceived as unacceptable to medical technologists, whereas a union that does not have such a history of adverse publicity might be considered more acceptable.

Although this short discussion by no means includes all the factors that lead to unionization and is not supported by empirical evidence, it does attempt to make the supervisor aware of some of the factors that enter into the decision of employees to seek unionization. The view that medical technologists have of their supervisor is important. The supervisor is one of them, although at the same time a management representative of the employing institution. If the supervisor is perceived by his employees as effectively representing their personal and professional interests, there will probably not be an effort to unionize. If the supervisor is perceived as representing the employing institution to the detriment of the personal and professional interests of the medical technologists, the supervisor may be perceived as ineffective, and a more effective representative, a union, may be sought.

The Bargaining Unit

If employees seek to be represented by a union for purposes of collective bargaining, usually they will not be voluntarily recognized by the employer. The union must therefore resort to the procedures promulgated by the NLRB to obtain an election for union representation [6] Suppose the employees of a nonunion employer wish to be represented by a union. The union will ask them to sign *authoriza-*

tion cards, cards that state that the employee wishes to be represented for purposes of collective bargaining by the union named on the cards. From the occupational groups the union seeks to represent, the union must have 30% of the employees sign authorization cards before the board will honor a petition for a union-representation election. In its petition, the union must specify the occupational groups it seeks to represent. This is the start of defining an appropriate *bargaining unit,* the occupational groups of employees the union seeks to represent. The bargaining unit is important because it determines the persons who will be eligible to vote in a union-representation election and the persons who will be covered by the labor–management contract should the union be successful in winning the election and in negotiating an agreement with the employer.

Regardless of the union's proposed bargaining unit, the final responsibility for determining an appropriate bargaining unit lies with the NLRB.[16] An employer may also challenge the appropriateness of a bargaining unit in a hearing conducted by the board. The employer may want the bargaining unit expanded to include occupational groups perceived not to be in favor of unionization. The main factors considered by the board, other than the pleadings of labor and management, are (1) the history of collective bargaining in the industry and the occupational groups represented; (2) the community of interest among employees, such as common pay plans, interdependent work, and common supervision; and (3) the desires of the employees.[8] After the determination of an appropriate bargaining unit, the board conducts a secret-ballot election among the employees in the bargaining unit. The union must obtain a majority of the votes cast to carry the election and to be certified as the exclusive representative of the employees for purposes of collective bargaining.

It is important in health-care settings to understand that there may be multiple appropriate bargaining units in an employing institution. Congress, in the deliberations that led to the passage of the Act, recognized that a large number of different occupational groups are employed in health-care institutions and that many of these groups have their own professional membership organizations. The Congress, therefore, stated that the board should avoid a proliferation of bargaining units in health-care settings. In general, the board will allow up to six different bargaining units in a health-care institution:[7]

1. Physicians
2. Registered nurses

3. Other professional employees
4. Technical employees
5. Service and maintenance employees
6. Business office clerical employees

However, that the board allows up to six bargaining units in health-care institutions does not mean that the board is required to acknowledge six individual bargaining units. In one instance, the board merged registered nurses and other professional employees into a single bargaining unit.

Once the bargaining unit is determined, the NLRB schedules an election. The election is held at a place and time to afford maximum participation by the affected employees in voting for or against union representation. Only those employees who are in the bargaining unit are eligible to vote. Notices will be posted at the employer's place of business, usually on bulletin boards, informing employees of the occupational groups in the bargaining unit and the date, time, and place of the election. The election is by secret ballot, and the union must have a majority of the votes cast in order to win and to be certified by the NLRB as the bargaining representative. If the employer carries the election, another election cannot be held in that bargaining unit for a period of 12 months.

If the union carries the election, then the issue of whether or not compulsory union membership will be required of members of the bargaining unit must be decided, according to a number of factors. First, the National Labor Relations Act, as amended by Taft–Hartley in Section 8(a)(3), states that nothing in the law prohibits an employer and a labor organization from negotiating a contract clause that requires union membership, provided that a minimum period of 30 days has elapsed since the employee was hired or the contract clause has been put into effect. Thus, in the first instance, a contract clause that requires union membership is a subject of negotiations, as is the length of the probationary period before an individual is required to join the union. This arrangement is known as a *union-shop clause*. Whether the union is able to obtain such a clause in the contract depends on the strength of the union (the percentage of the employees in the bargaining unit who have voluntarily joined the union) and the union's willingness to strike over the issue.

Although federal labor law does not prohibit such contract clauses, Section 14(b) of the Taft–Hartley amendments allows an individual state or United States territory to enact legislation that prohibits the enforcement of a compulsory union membership contract clause. These right-to-work laws have been enacted in 20 states. Thus, in these states, union membership is strictly voluntary. As a result, the bargaining unit is composed of union members and persons who refrain from union membership. However, the contract negotiated by the union, in all other respects, applies to the bargaining unit, and both union and nonunion members are subject to its terms and provisions. A union is prohibited from negotiating contract clauses that discriminate against nonunion members of the bargaining unit and must provide representation for nonunion members of the bargaining unit in grievance and arbitration hearings. The reason is that the union, by virtue of winning an election to represent employees for collective bargaining, is certified as the representative of the bargaining unit under Section 9(a) of the National Labor Relations Act.

Because of the prohibitions against compulsory union membership and the realization that nonunion members of a bargaining unit benefit from union representation, some states, especially as part of their state labor relations laws for public employees, enable a union to collect some specified portion of the monthly union dues from nonunion members of the bargaining unit. These are alternately called *agency-shop* or *fair-share laws;* the amount of the monthly financial contribution required from nonunion members of the bargaining unit varies among the states.

As part of the 1974 Health Care Amendments to the National Labor Relations Act, the Congress, in Section 19, stated that persons included in bargaining units in voluntary nonprofit health-care institutions who had religious objections to joining or financially contributing to a union would not be required to do so, even if a compulsory membership clause was contained in the collective-bargaining agreement. Rather, these persons may contribute the equivalent of the monthly union dues to a nonreligious, nonprofit charitable organization. More recently, the Congress enacted legislation that extended this right to employees of institutions other than voluntary nonprofit health-care institutions. However, in this case, the union is allowed to seek reimbursement for expenses incurred in representing such employees in collective bargaining or contract administration. On December 29, 1980, President Jimmy Carter signed a bill that extended the coverage of Section 19 to all workers.[18]

The Collective-Bargaining Process

Collective bargaining is characterized by negotiations between the union and the employer in an attempt to establish the wages, hours of work, and other terms and conditions of employment in a contract for a specified time period. It is through negotiations that labor and management make known their respective interests. The National Labor Relations Act, as amended, requires the parties to meet at reasonable times and bargain in good faith concerning wages, hours, and other conditions of employment.[17] However, the law does not require that the parties reach an agreement.

Some items of interest to either of the parties are considered to be mandatory subjects of bargaining, meaning that labor or management cannot seek to establish them unilaterally, and neither of the parties can refuse to discuss them. Examples of such items are wages, pensions, fringe benefits, vacations, holidays, work rules, the definition of bargaining-unit work, seniority, promotions, transfers, safety and health provisions, a procedure for the discussion of grievances, the arbitration of unresolved disputes, performance appraisals, and others. If either one of the parties expresses an interest in these issues, the other party is obligated to discuss them, although the two may not be able to reach an agreement.

Although collective bargaining negotiations have historically been characterized by an adversarial relationship between labor and management, some issues are of concern to both parties. For example, there is interest by labor, management, and the government in increasing productivity. Much interest is being expressed in newer labor–management techniques, such as quality circles, which are used in Japan. As a result, some United States companies and unions have begun to experiment with similar concepts. If they are successful, they will eventually permeate all industrial sectors of the economy, including health-care institutions.

The following areas of interest, by no means an inclusive listing of the items contained in all collective-bargaining agreements, provide an overview of the basic elements of a collective-bargaining agreement. Questions are also raised that must be considered by the laboratory supervisor. Finally, there are given examples of how some of these issues are being addressed in some existing labor–management agreements.

Wages

Wages are a critical component of the labor–management negotiation. They are of concern to the laboratory supervisor and to the institution, for they represent a cost that to some degree must be controlled. They are also of concern to the union,

for they are a benefit to its members. The credibility of the union is enhanced if it can negotiate an increase that is perceived by members to be more than management would grant voluntarily.

Wages include direct pay and a variety of fringe benefits, which are all costs to the employer. Fringe benefits include such items as pensions, health insurance, disability insurance, and premium pay for overtime and shift differentials. The laboratory supervisor must be concerned with these costs because they become part of the laboratory budget. However, the laboratory must do more than simply attempt to control these costs. The supervisor must assess the impact that wages and fringe benefits will have on the retention of present employees and the recruitment of future employees. To accomplish this, the supervisor must be aware of the wage structure of other laboratories and health-care institutions in the geographical area. Today it is not uncommon for the laboratory supervisor to be required to know the pay structure of alternative occupations open to medical technologists with comparable skills or with minimal additional knowledge or training.

Primarily to retain present staff and to recruit qualified medical technologists competitively, the laboratory supervisor must have direct communication with the management personnel responsible for negotiating with the union. The cost of retaining employees must be evaluated against its alternative —employee turnover and the costs of seeking replacements. There are costs associated with advertising open positions, with using supervisory time to interview applicants, and with the administrative overhead of adding new employees to the payroll. If employee turnover requires that other medical technologists work overtime, then premium pay for the hours of overtime should be taken into account. If this resulting overtime occurs too frequently or the duration of each occurrence is long, there will be a cost associated with declining employee morale. Thus, the laboratory supervisor's role is not simply one of controlling costs. By necessity, it must include a realistic assessment of the impact of the institution's ability to retain and attract qualified employees.

Hours of Work

Hours of work, which are normally discussed in negotiations between labor and management, are also important to the laboratory supervisor because of the impact they have on staffing patterns. The supervisor, after all, is responsible for planning, organizing, and directing the accomplishment of work. Most employees will want to work a 40-hour week. The supervisor must consider how long each shift will be, on what day the workweek will begin, whether the workweek will begin on the same day for everyone, whether there will be overlapping shifts to cover peak loads in hospital admissions, whether weekends will be covered by part-time employees or by staggered workweeks of full-time employees, and a number of other issues. These schedules must, in turn, be coordinated with other departments in health-care institutions.

At present, the laboratory supervisor must to some extent consider the desires of employees. The supervisor may have to introduce some variation of flextime, such as 4-days-on/4-days-off or 7-days-on/7-days-off. In this event, the length of the daily shift must be extended, which may entail some amount of premium pay and should concern the supervisor from the standpoint of employee fatigue.

Working Conditions

Working conditions also encompass a wide variety of issues. For example, if the laboratory is large enough and has sufficient volume, will it be departmentalized, and if so, will employees be allowed to rotate among departments to reduce boredom? Will present employees be given preference over outside applicants for openings? Will employees be given the opportunity to transfer to openings on another shift? How will a determination be made if two qualified employees request a shift transfer to a single open position? How much latitude will employees be given to trade with one another? How will promotional opportunities be determined? These questions may be raised during contract negotiations.

Another aspect of working conditions is paid vacations and holidays. To some degree, this will be determined by the policy-makers in higher management. However, the laboratory manager should discuss these issues and their impact on the management of the laboratory with higher management. The supervisor should also have some knowledge of the practices of other laboratories and health-care institutions in the area.

The laboratory supervisor may by now realize that many of the same issues must be confronted whether or not there is a union representing the employees. The difference is that if a union is involved, these issues will be subject to negotiations between labor and management, rather than unilaterally determined by the supervisor. Once they are incorporated in the labor–management agreement, these issues cannot be unilaterally changed by management.

Although it is not common, some contracts enable either of the parties to reopen negotiations on any portion or section of the contract by giving the other party a notice of such intent. If this is to be allowed, there is usually a specific clause in the contract that states this right as well as the amount of advance notice that must be given. Another means of accomplishing the change of a contract clause during the life of a contract is to amend the contract with a letter of agreement concerning a specific issue. Again, however, both labor and management must agree to such a procedure in addition to the content of the change. This second method has appeared in the current economic climate when companies ask employees to forego a scheduled wage increase or to take actual reductions in pay to help the company remain solvent and competitive. In the final analysis, whether such procedures for change are to be included in the contract or are to be accomplished through a letter of agreement depends upon whether labor and management prefer to institute procedures for change or would rather invoke them only when confronted with a crisis.

Contract Administration

The most conscientious labor and management negotiators cannot write a perfect contract. The contract must be worded so that it can be applied in a variety of situations. The negotiations cannot possibly envision all the problems that may arise during the life of the contract. Different people will interpret the contract differently. For instance, it is not uncommon for a contract to contain a clause on promotion that gives the promotion to the senior employee (in terms of length of employment) who bids on the job, provided the senior employee is reasonably qualified. The first issue, seniority, may be resolved by consulting employment records. The second issue, being reasonably qualified, is not so easily resolved. A union might interpret it to mean having skill and ability. Management may interpret it to mean having efficiency and dependability in addition to skill and ability. Thus, management may want to deny a promotion to someone because of a record of tardiness and absenteeism. The union may argue that management should handle absenteeism and tardiness through its rules and disciplinary procedures and not through the denial of a promotion. Issues such as this are normally resolved through a formal procedure in which an individual employee may allege that management has violated the labor–management agreement. This process is referred to as *contract administration* and is composed of a grievance procedure that includes arbitration as the terminal step. The purpose of such a procedure is to provide a mechanism for resolving day-to-day differences between labor and management without the union's having to resort to a work stoppage. In most labor–management contracts, the union surrenders its right to strike during the life of the contract in return for a grievance procedure and arbitration.

The grievance procedure is a series of steps or meetings through which an employee's complaint may move in an attempt to resolve it. The initial step of a grievance procedure is normally a verbal discussion of the complaint between the employee and the supervisor with or without a representative of the union being present. The union representative at this step is normally called the *union steward* and is the union's counterpart to the first-line supervisor. Whether or not the union representative is present depends upon the wishes of the employee. Under the National Labor Relations Act, the employee has a right to representation by the union, and the union has the obligation to represent all employees in the defined bargaining unit if requested to do so.

Contracts usually specify a given time period, from the date of the action by management that is alleged to violate the contract, within which the allegation must be brought to the attention of management. The length of this period is subject to negotiations and is sometimes as long as 45 days. Regardless of the merits of the employee's complaint, this first step is important in having the employee verbalize the dissatisfaction. Equally important is the manner in which the employee's immediate supervisor conducts this meeting. Even through the allegation may involve the immediate supervisor, the supervisor must listen to the complaint as a member of management and must not be personally offended by the employee's complaint. The supervisor may be uncertain whether the complaint has merit or may need time to further investigate the complaint, but the contract usually allows a given number of days before which the management representative must answer the complaint. This time should be used by the supervisor to discuss the complaint with higher-level supervision or with the personnel department. Since management has the responsibility of ensuring that policies and rules are applied consistently and fairly throughout the organization, the supervisor should not hesitate to consult with other levels of management. If the grievance is denied, the union will satisfy itself that the employee's complaint has no merit before it will decide not to appeal the grievance. The contract normally specifies a period of time within which the union may appeal a grievance.

Managers are sometimes perplexed that a union will defend an employee when it seems obvious to management that an employee should be disciplined or discharged. This is a result of the manager's failure to understand the moral and legal role of the union as a representative of the employee. In many instances, the union may be aware of the employee's violation of a rule or policy. The union may also have cautioned the employee that continued infractions of the rules and policies of the institution might result in discipline or discharge. The union, by filing a grievance, may simply want to review management's decision process to ensure that management has applied its rules, policies, and discipline fairly and consistently; that management has followed its own policies in carrying out the discipline; and that the discipline is not more harsh than the offense. The union may object to the strength of the discipline or the manner in which management applied its rules and policies, rather than whether or not the employee should have been disciplined. If it did not challenge management in this manner, the union would be perceived by its own members as not properly representing them. It would also violate its legal duty to fairly represent the employees in the bargaining unit. Supervisors should understand that this is one of the legitimate roles of the union and expect that the union will challenge many of management's decisions.

To continue with the grievance procedure, labor and management negotiate several steps or meetings during which their respective representatives will attempt to resolve the grievance. Each step is characterized by time limits for the union's appeal of the grievance and for management's response after the grievance has been discussed. Each step is also characterized by the addition of higher levels of decision-makers by both labor and management. For example, the final step of the grievance procedure prior to arbitration might involve the hospital administrator in addition to the personnel manager, the laboratory supervisor, and the first-line supervisor for management. The union might be represented by a representative of the national union, the local union president, the grievance committee chairman, the union steward, and the employee.

What if a resolution is not reached during these meetings? The majority of union–management contracts provide that the union may appeal to arbitration. *Arbitration* is the process whereby an impartial third party is selected to hear the facts pertaining to the dispute and each party's position and then render a final and binding decision. The arbitrator is jointly selected by labor and management and is knowledgeable about labor–management contracts and labor–management relations. There are some full-time arbitrators, but most are fully employed elsewhere. Many arbitrators are practicing attorneys, professors of law or industrial relations, or former employees of agencies of government involved in the labor-relations process.

Two important aspects of the arbitration process should be mentioned. First, if the contract provides for the arbitration of all disputes that arise during the life of the contract, the federal courts will enforce arbitration; that is, if the contract contains an arbitration clause for all disputes and the union appeals a grievance to arbitration, management cannot refuse arbitration simply because it views the employee's complaint as frivolous. In order to avoid arbitration, management would have to show that the issue is not covered by the language of the contract. The decision of whether or not the dispute is subject to arbitration is the province of the arbitrator. The arbitrator will decide the merits of the grievance, and the award will be final and binding.[19]

One final word on contract administration can be offered. The supervisor must work within the framework of institutional policy for the handling of grievances. The institution may elect to allow supervisors to evaluate and settle employee complaints, or it may choose to centralize this function in the personnel division to ensure uniformity. The supervisor should be aware of the institution's policy.

Management's Rights

Almost all labor–management contracts have a *management's rights clause*. It may range from a brief paragraph to several pages in length. Essentially, a management's rights clause states that management has the sole right and prerogative to unilaterally make decisions concerning the operation of the institution except as it may be limited by the labor–management agreement. These rights usually include, among others, the right to hire, fire, suspend, and discharge for just cause; the right to temporarily assign, promote, or discharge employees according to the needs of the business; and the right to determine the methods of work. The right to suspend and discharge employees for just cause is vitally important, for a union will many times challenge a suspension or discharge for lack of just cause. An employee who has been improperly terminated may be reinstated to the former position by an arbitrator. The arbitrator may also direct remedial action, such as full pay for all time lost and restoration of all benefits that resulted from an improper discharge.

Because of the length of time required to process a grievance to arbitration, which exposes the institution to greater remedial legal liability, some contracts now provide for an expedited grievance procedure for cases that involve discharge and lengthy suspensions. The accused employee is suspended for a short period of time subject to discharge at the end of that time. The union is notified of the institution's action. If the employee believes that management's action is improper, the employee may file a grievance, and a meeting with all the parties involved is scheduled during the period of suspension and prior to the employee's termination. At this meeting, management will consider the employee's and the union's arguments that the suspension or discharge is unwarranted. This meeting provides an immediate, high-level management review of the discharge and speeds the invocation of arbitration by the union, thereby reducing the institution's potential liability should the arbitrator judge management's action to have been improper.

REFERENCES

1. Antony J: Management and Machiavelli. New York, Bantam Books, 1968
2. Brown & Root, Inc., 246 NLRB 132 (1979)
3. Butte Medical Properties, 168 NLRB 266 (1967) and University Nursing Homes, Inc., 168 NLRB 53 (1967)
4. Civil Service Reform Act, 95 Stat. 454
5. FMCS Services in Health Care Industry Labor Disputes. Code of Federal Regulations, Vol 29, Part 1420
6. McGuiness KC: How to Take a Case before the National Labor Relations Board. Washington, DC, Bureau of National Affairs, 1976
7. Morales G: Unit appropriateness in health care institutions. Labor Law J March, pp 174–179, 1979
8. Morris CJ (ed): The Developing Labor Law: The Board, The Courts and the National Labor Relations Act. Washington, DC, Bureau of National Affairs, 1971
9. National Labor Relations Act, 49 Stat. 449, as amended by Public Law No. 101, 80th Cong., 1st sess., 1947; Public Law No. 257, 86th Cong., 1st sess., 1959; and Public Law No. 360, 93rd Cong., 2d sess., 1974. Hereinafter referred to the NLRA
10. NLRA, Sec. 2(2)
11. NLRA, Sec. 8(d)(A), 8(d)(B), 8(d)(C)
12. NLRA, Sec. 8(g)
13. NLRA: Guidelines issued by the General Counsel of the National Labor Relations Board for use of board regional offices in unfair labor practice cases arising under the 1974 nonprofit hospital amendments to the Taft–Hartley Act. In Labor Relations Yearbook, pp 343–365. Washington, DC, Bureau of National Affairs, 1974
14. NLRA, Sec. 213
15. NLRA, Sec. 3
16. NLRA, Sec. 9(b) and 9(c)
17. NLRA, Sec. 8(d)
18. Public Law No. 96-593
19. Textile Workers v. Lincoln Mills, 353 U.S. 448 (1957); United

Steelworkers of America v. Warrior and Gulf Navigation Co., 363 U.S. 574 (1960); United Steelworkers of America v. Enterprise Wheel and Car Corp., 363 U.S. 593 (1960); United Steelworkers of America v. American Mfg. Co., 363 U.S. 564 (1960)

20. van de Vall M: Labor Organizations: A Macro- and Micro-Sociological Analysis on a Comparative Basis. London, Cambridge University Press, 1970

ANNOTATED BIBLIOGRAPHY

Elkowi F, Elkowi E: How Arbitration Works. Washington, The Bureau of National Affairs Inc., n.d.

    Written by practicing arbitrators, this volume is an invaluable aid to supervisors in understanding the rulings of arbitrators on various issues covered by labor–management agreements. It should assist supervisors in evaluating grievances brought forward by employees.

Fein M: Motivation for work. In Dubin R (ed): Handbook of Work, Organization and Society, pp 465–530. Chicago, Rand McNally & Company, 1976.

    Primarily concerned with the effect of payment systems upon motivation, this reference nevertheless contains a description of the function of a union in representing employees. It offers a different view of the nature of motivation and a description of the experiences of companions using different payment systems.

Grievance Guide. Washington, The Bureau of National Affairs Inc., n.d.

    A synthesis of rulings of arbitrators on various elements of labor-management contracts. A valuable aid to supervisors because of the policy statements that introduce each topic.

Updated periodically, it should be of assistance to supervisors in evaluating employee grievances.

Miller RU: Hospitals. In Somers GG (ed): Collective Bargaining: Contemporary American Experience, pp 375–434. Madison, Industrial Relations Research Association, 1980

    This resource includes a good description of the development of unions in the health-care industry. It also includes a description of the unions active in organizing health-care personnel and the history of their involvement.

Morris CR (ed): The Developing Labor Law: The Board, The Courts and the National Labor Relations Act. Washington, The Bureau of National Affairs, Inc., 1971.

    This is possibly the most comprehensive work available on the legal aspects of labor–management relations. Updated by annual supplements, the volumes synthesize the major legal developments in labor management relations. The reader, therefore, should be prepared to research case reports to fully comprehend the rulings of the National Labor Relations Board and the courts.

Sovereign KL, Bognanno M: Positive contract administration. In Yoder D, Heneman HG (eds): Employee and Labor Relations, Vol III, ASPA Handbook of Personnel and Industrial Relations, pp 7.145–7.182. Washington, The Bureau of National Affairs Inc., 1976

    This resource provides a comprehensive discussion of grievances and the role of the union and managerial personnel. It includes a "how-to" section for first-line supervisors. Many of the prescriptions offered apply to employer–employee relations with or without a union.

Tannenbaum AS: Unions. In March JG (ed): Handbook of Organizations, pp 710–763. Chicago, Rand McNally & Company, 1965

    An overview of the structure and functioning of unions, this reference provides a description of internal union processes, which filter into the relationship between management and the union.

part four

Essentials of
Effective
Laboratory
Operation

sixteen

Quality Control and Method Evaluation

John A. Lott

QUALITY CONTROL OF CLINICAL LABORATORY PERFORMANCE

Quality control encompasses each step of the chain of events from the preparation of the patient and collection of the sample to the delivery of the result to the clinician. Every action in the chain of events must be scrutinized to ensure that optimal *patient care* is achieved. It is clearly not enough to monitor only within-laboratory analytic performance.

The following interlinked items detail the points where quality control is important:

- Training and experience of technical and clerical laboratory personnel.
- Level of supervision of the clinical laboratory.
- Training and experience of phlebotomist.
- Patient preparation before acquiring specimens.
- Collection, transportation, and handling of specimens.
- Storage of specimens if analysis is delayed.
- Time between collection and analysis.
- Instrument maintenance and checks on instrument functions.
- Quality of reagents, kits, and analytic materials; quality of standards and controls.
- Thorough evaluation of any new methods and procedures.

- Quality of the laboratory environment.
- Cleanliness of collection vessels, laboratory glassware, and equipment.
- Adequacy of procedure manuals, within-laboratory policy manuals, and instructions.
- Adequacy of controls and reference specimens in verifying levels of analytic performance.
- Assessment of analytic variability by an adequate reference specimen method.
- Participation in external quality control surveys.
- Policy on extreme values for patients, *i.e.,* "panic values."
- Optimum result reporting and delivery.
- Correctness of reference ("normal") ranges.
- Interpretive reporting for certain tests.
- Patient record-keeping.
- Long-term patient and control record storage.
- Laboratory computerization and integration with hospital's computer.
- Continuing education of entire professional staff.

Training and Experience of Laboratory Personnel

The article "Laboratory Personnel: The Most Important Aspect of Quality Control" speaks to this point.[31] It is impossible to have consistently good laboratory performance with inadequately trained personnel. Laboratory personnel must have the necessary technical skills; but probably more important, they must have good judgment. Judgment is acquired and cannot be taught. Good judgment includes

- Recognizing that the specimens are from *patients* and erroneous laboratory data can have unpleasant and serious consequences for the patient, such as unnecessary diagnostic procedures, extra days in the hospital, mistaken or missed diagnoses, and so forth.
- Being able to communicate to the other providers of health care in a professional and helpful way to the furtherance of patient care.
- Identifying and correcting lapses in laboratory performance such as mistaken values.
- Alerting physicians at once when extremely abnormal results are observed in the laboratory and identifying a possible life-threatening situation.
- Having a willingness to provide extra effort and time when the situation demands it with ill patients, unusual cases.
- Recognizing the need to keep professionally alert and informed on new developments in the field.

Within-Laboratory Quality Control

The increasing sophistication of medicine has placed greater demands on clinical laboratories for reliable analyses. More sensitive and specific laboratory tests have simplified diagnostic medicine and provided signals of diseases earlier in their course.

Quality-control programs provide a mechanism by which the analytic performance of clinical laboratories may be *evaluated, documented,* and *improved.* A quality-control program should contain the following elements:

- The precision of the method over the entire analytic range of both normal and abnormal results is known.
- Simple statistical calculations are made on the control results to give means, standard deviations (SD), and coefficients of variation (CV) of all analytic procedures.
- Control charts, *e.g.,* Levey–Jennings (L–J) charts, are prepared, kept up-to-date, and are displayed prominently in the laboratory. The control charts contain "warning limits" and "action limits" to assist the technical staff in decision-making.

- A set of rules, *e.g.,* the Shewhart multirule method, is in place to guide the technical staff in deciding whether or not patient results are acceptable.
- Continuous monitoring of analytic performance is carried out by introducing fictitious patient specimens into the laboratory in addition to the control specimens known to the analysts.
- The entire laboratory staff is responsible for the entry of quality-control data onto suitable record forms or into a computerized quality-control system.
- Certain individuals are responsible for collation of data, for long-term record-keeping, and for record storage and retrieval.
- The corrective actions in cases of "out-of-control" situations are defined, and the role of the various levels of laboratory personnel in correcting such problems is clearly delineated.
- Individuals who have problems performing a given procedure are identified, not for punitive purposes, but rather for initiating retraining.

The Reference Sample Method of Quality Control

The reference sample method is the most efficient and widely used system of quality control in clinical laboratories. Controls that mimic patient specimens are analyzed repeatedly within day and between days. The reference sample method can be used for evaluation of laboratory performance based on the repeatability of the results and the proximity of the results to the true values. In addition, it can monitor interlaboratory variability when identical specimens or sets of specimens are sent to a group of laboratories.

Commercially Available Controls

Purchased controls have the advantage of convenience. They cannot be used uncritically; criteria for selection must include qualitative characteristics, concentration, stability, and cost.

QUALITATIVE CHARACTERISTICS. Quality control materials must mimic patient specimens as closely as possible, whether they are whole blood, plasma, serum, urine, body fluids, or other patient-derived materials. A basic assumption of all quality-control specimens is that the repeatability and accuracy obtained with control materials is the same as that obtained with patient specimens. If this assumption is correct, the laboratory has an estimate of how well it is performing analyses of patient specimens. Often, nonhuman quality-control materials must be used. For example, because of the difficulty in obtaining human tissue enzymes, animal enzymes are commonly used to fortify control sera. Porcine heart creatine kinase (CK) resembles human skeletal muscle CK[29]; however, calf intestinal alkaline phosphatase (ALP), a common source of ALP, is very different from ALP derived from human liver.[32]

Lyophilization tends to denature proteins; for example, albumin exhibits changed dye-binding characteristics after lyophilization. Liquid controls containing ethylene glycol are unsuitable for analytic systems employing dialysis[33]; however, they are very convenient and may be less costly than lyophilized controls, because there is less waste. Another advantage is better reproducibility of their target values; the variable associated with reconstitution is absent.

CONCENTRATIONS OF ANALYTES IN CONTROLS. Control sera should have concentrations or activities based on the following considerations. Methods should be monitored at decision points. For example, hemoglobin, leukocyte count, serum glucose, iron, protein, PCO_2, calcium, digoxin, cortisol, alkaline phosphatase, potassium, magnesium, and most drugs have more than one value where therapeutic, diagnostic, or management decisions are made. Controls should be available with concentrations close to decision values. Other tests such as creatinine, aspartate aminotransferase (AST), and lactate dehydrogenase (LDH) have only one decision region. Here, fewer controls are needed. Bilirubin has decision points for newborns different from that for adults, and the quality control needs are more complex.

Most methods in clinical chemistry are designed to cover a wide dynamic range of concentrations. If possible, controls should be used to monitor the stability of the dynamic range or when a loss in precision has occurred at medically important or decision values.

INTERRELATED CONCENTRATIONS IN CONTROLS. Commercially prepared quality-control materials that are prepared in sets of two or three should have the concentrations of analytes present in known interrelationships. If the concentrations of the common analytes are present in known ratios, then additional information is obtained in their analysis. For example, a set of controls could have glucose concentrations of 50, 100, 200, and 400 mg/dl. The instru-

ment's response would be graphed versus the expected concentration to prepare the "operational line" for glucose (see below). Much more quality-control information is available from an operational line than from repetitive analyses of unrelated controls.[8]

ACCURACY OF CONTROLS. The true concentration of an analyte in a control can only be estimated. A few analytes such as calcium[5] and glucose[30] have "reference methods" by which reliable values can be determined. Reference methods have undergone extensive scrutiny; their bias, variability, source of interferences, and so forth, are known. Nearly all the other common analytes have well-established methods of tested reliability.[23] Control materials should have only *one* concentration for most analytes. The pressure of the marketplace has created a preposterous situation for some manufacturers of control sera. Ortho Diagnostic Systems, of Raritan, New Jersey, for example, lists 47 results for glucose for its "QCS Normal" control. For the same control, the listed glucose values range from 83 to 130 mg/dl, a spread of 47 mg, or 57% of the lower value. Laboratories want to be "in control" for their method; yet they miss the much more serious problem of a substantial bias from the true value.

Frequency of Analysis of Control Sera

How often should patient specimens be interspersed with control materials? The frequency of analysis of controls is dictated by the variability of the test and what is acceptable "drift." The definition of *drift* in turn describes a "batch" of specimens. With this gestalt, drift is acceptable; during the analysis of a batch of specimens, controls are analyzed along with the specimens in the batch.

The definition of acceptable drift is subjective, but it should include what is medically acceptable. Acceptable drift has been defined as the percent biologic variation times the upper reference limit in the units of the test.[23] The calculated acceptable drift will be greater with tests that show large intrapersonal variability like leukocyte count, cholesterol, and CK; the acceptable drift will be smaller for tests like hemoglobin, pH and calcium where the intrapersonal variability is small.

On a practical basis, a batch is 5 to 10 specimens for methods using an ion-specific electrode, flame photometry, or atomic absorption measurements; it is 15 to 20 specimens for spectrophotometry, blood cell counters, or many multichannel chemistry instruments. Some instruments, like the Kodak Ektachem 700, are very stable, and the analyses of as few as one or two controls in an 8-hour day suffice.

Determination of Laboratory Variation

Levey-Jennings Charts

The most widely used system of quality control employs the reference sample system.[18] Here, quality-control specimens are analyzed singly or in replicate on each day specimens are run, and the mean and SD are calculated. Two equations can be used to calculate the SD:

1. $SD = [\text{Sum of all (Value } i - \text{Mean})^2/(n-1)]^{1/2}$

Where (Value i − Mean) is the deviation of the ith value from the mean, and n is the number of values. The square root of the entire term equals the SD.

2. $SD = [n(\text{Sum Value } i^2) -$
   $(\text{Sum Value } i)^2/n(n-1)]^{1/2}$

Where (Sum Value i^2) is the sum of the squares of the values. (Sum Value i)^2 is the sum of the values squared, and n has the same meaning as before.

The second equation is more convenient to use with computers and is used with all hand calculators that have the SD function. With equation 2, the individual points need not be stored by the computer.

When new quality-control materials are introduced, it is necessary to establish what the acceptable SD will be. This can *only* be done when

- The method has good stability and the values are not drifting up or down, as determined with an established control material.
- The laboratory experiences a period of "good performance" where there are few outliers, and the procedure is well controlled.
- An adequate amount of data has been collected. In general, for small sets of data, as n increases, the SD increases. Ideally, n should be very large, perhaps 400. For practical purposes, the SD can be calculated if 30 to 50 values are available. With a small sample, the SD may have to be revised as additional data are collected.
- The data must have a reasonably Gaussian distribution. L–J charts assume the baseline data is Gaussian; if not, new data become uninterpretable.

Use of L–J Charts

Stable Performance

A typical L–J chart is shown in Figure 16-1. Here, two control results are graphed each day on separate charts, and the data for 1 month are displayed. Re-

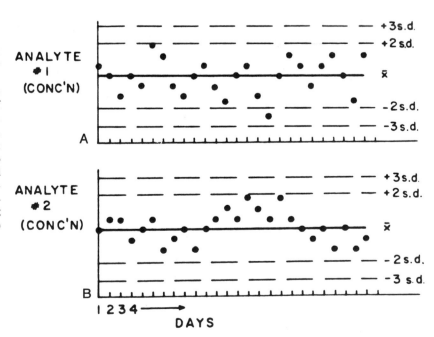

FIGURE 16-1. A Levey–Jennings chart showing the distributions of quality control data using limits that include day-to-day variability. (*A*) The data are randomly distributed between the limits. (*B*) Over a short period of time, the data are clustered well within the designated limits. However, small shifts occur from time to time, causing the data to range between the designated limits. (From Grannis GF, Caragher TE: Quality-control program in clinical chemistry. CRC Crit Rev Clin Lab Sci 7:327, 1977)

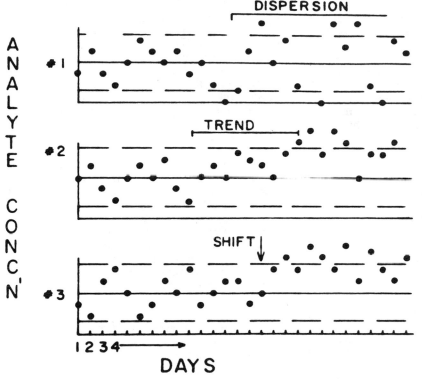

FIGURE 16-2. Examples of three types of changes in quality control data. Chart #1 illustrates dispersion of data characterized by an increased frequency of both high and low outliers. A frequent cause of such dispersion is loss of precision of an automatic dispenser. Chart #2 illustrates a trend in the data. Over a period of days, the determined values drift progressively from the prior mean value. Trends are commonly caused by deterioration of instrumental components and by changes in analytic standards. Chart #3 illustrates an abrupt shift in the data to a new mean value. Shifts are commonly caused by changes in analytic systems, such as replacement of components or use of a different lot of standards or reagents. (From Grannis GF, Caragher TE: Quality-control program in clinical chemistry. CRC Crit Rev Clin Lab Sci 7:327, 1977)

sults outside of ±2 SD are termed "warning limits," and those outside of ±3 SD are designated as "action limits." If the mean and SD of the control were established during a period of stability, and if the procedure remained stable, new quality control data could be used for judging current performance. If the results follow a Gaussian pattern, 68.3% of the values will fall within ±1 SD, 95.5% will fall within ±2 SD, and 99.7% will fall within ±3 SD. One in 20 results should be expected to fall outside of ±2 SD, and only 3 per 1000 should fall outside of ±3 SD. Values outside of ±3 SD should always be questioned, because they are so rare and usually point out unacceptable analytic variability. If a small sample were used to establish the SD, more outliers would be expected. A small shift in values will result in more outliers if the variance is small.

Allen and co-workers[1] found that if the control was known to the analyst, the SDs were generally smaller than when the controls were "blind," that is, disguised as a patient specimen. If generally true, the implication of this finding is that the actual performance on patient specimens is worse than what is determined with quality-control schemes.

Dispersion or Contraction

A change in precision causes increased dispersion or contraction of the spread of the data. Increased dispersion is shown in Figure 16-2, *Chart 1*; there are a host of reasons for worsening precision, which is usually apparent from an L–J chart. Some causes are more or new individuals performing tests, inattention to critical steps of procedure, unstable line voltage, greater variability in pipetting specimens and/or reagents, and so forth.

Trends

Trends in quality-control data are shown in Figure 16-2, *Chart 2*. Trends are commonly caused by a gradual change in standards, reagents, instrument condition, and so forth. L–J charts are excellent for detecting trends. A trend is always a signal for remedial action and is apparent when at least ten consecutive values are above or below the mean.

Shifts

Shifts as shown in Figure 16-2, *Chart 3,* are commonly caused by the introduction of new standards, reagents, and methods. Shifts caused by a remedy of an unsatisfactory situation are unavoidable and at times desirable. Small trends or shifts within acceptable limits are not a problem.

With many contemporary instruments, for example, the Coulter Stacker, Beckman ICS, Kodak Ektachem 700, and others, the L–J chart often shows tight clusters of data and significant shifts when new lots of reagent or calibrations are introduced. The analytic range, including the shifts, may be narrow; so that shifts of this nature are unimportant.

LONG-TERM DATA RECORDS. L–J charts show long-term trends very well. In Figure 16-3A, monthly CVs are shown for glucose data from the clinical chemistry laboratory of The Ohio State University Hospitals covering a period of 18 years. Each of the data points is the mean of 100 or more values at concentrations of 80 to 100 mg/dl. With improving technology, the CVs have become narrower. From 1967 to late 1974, the Technicon AutoAnalyzer (Techicon Corporation, Tarrytown, NY) ferricyanide method was used; monthly CVs were in the 5% to 6% range with occasional months where the CV was close to 9%. Between late 1974 and late 1979, glucose was analyzed on the Technicon SMA-6 with a glucose oxidase method[28]; the precision improved, and the CVs were typically near 4%.

In June of 1981, we started using the Beckman Astra-8 and a glucose oxidase-oxygen electrode method and observed a further improvement in precision. CVs are now in the 2% region, that is, a fourfold improvement in precision over the time period shown in Figure 16-3A.

Similar long-term data for serum cholesterol are shown in Figure 16-3B. Here, each point represents the mean of 25 to 30 values at concentrations of 250 to 300 mg/dl. A ferric chloride-H_2SO_4 method was used from 1967 to late 1977. CVs averaged 4% to 5%; however, there were months with considerably greater variability. Since late 1977 to the present, a cholesterol oxidase method has been employed on the Abbott ABA-100 Analyzer (Abbott Laboratories, North Chicago, Illinois). The precision of the automated enzymatic method is clearly better than that of the manual procedure.

Serum sodium data is shown in Figure 16-3C. A flame photometer was used until 1969, and an automated flame thereafter. An ion-specific electrode was introduced in 1981.

Application of Shewhart Control Rules

Westgard described a series of control rules for use in the clinical laboratory to judge if data are acceptable.[38] Certain managerial decisions must be made before the Westgard system can be implemented: a

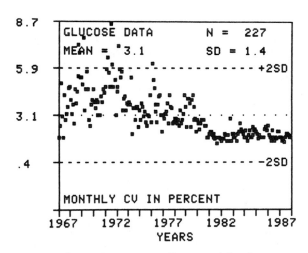

FIGURE 16-3A. Long-term quality control data for serum glucose obtained in the clinical laboratories of Ohio State University. The monthly mean CVs are shown for controls with glucose concentration between 80 mg/dL and 100 mg/dL. There is a clear trend toward better performance between 1967 and 1987.

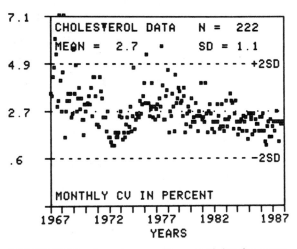

FIGURE 16-3B. Long-term quality control data for serum cholesterol. The monthly mean CVs are shown for controls with cholesterol concentrations between 250 mg/dL and 300 mg/dL. There is distinct improvement in precision over the 20-year period.

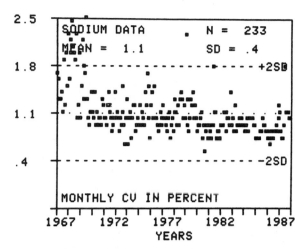

2.5

SODIUM DATA   N = 233

MEAN = 1.1   SD = .4

1.8 ---------------------------------- +2SD

1.1 ----

.4 ---------------------------------- -2SD

MONTHLY CV IN PERCENT

1967   1972   1977   1982   1987

YEARS

FIGURE 16-3C. Long-term quality control data for serum sodium concentrations between 150 mmol/L and 150 mmol/L. There is some narrowing for the CVs over the 20-year period, but this is less dramatic than for glucose or cholesterol.

decision is needed on how many controls are to be analyzed with each batch of specimens, what is the desirable error detection rate, and what is the acceptable false rejection rate of otherwise acceptable data.

Development of the Model

The number of control specimens analyzed per batch and the *laboratory-determined* acceptable SD determine the probability of detecting error (P_{ed}) and the probability of false rejection (P_{fr}) of acceptable data. Two extremes are easily imagined: Several controls are analyzed with every batch, and the acceptable SD limits are extremely narrow. The (P_{ed}) will be close to one; however, P_{fr} will be unacceptably large. Conversely, with very few controls and wide acceptable SD limits, P_{ed} and P_{fr} will be low; many errors will be missed. Clearly, a middle ground is needed. P_{ed} and P_{fr} are defined as

$$P_{ed} = (\text{Proper rejection})/(\text{Proper rejection} + \text{False acceptance})$$

$$P_{fr} = (\text{False rejection})/(\text{False rejection} + \text{Proper acceptance})$$

Westgard has defined the predictive value of a quality control scheme to accept data or to reject it as being erroneous. Also described are the theoretic bases of the Shewhart multirule system.[37,40–43]

Application of the Shewhart Model

Two controls are analyzed with each batch of specimens, and the results are recorded on an L–J chart. It is assumed the SD limits are appropriate as described above. A decision for acceptance or rejection of a batch of results is based on the following set of rules:

1_{2s} Rule: The run is accepted when both control results are within 2 SD limits from the mean value.

1_{3s} Rule: The run is considered out of control when one of the control results exceeds the ±3 SD limits.

2_{2s} Rule: The run is rejected when both controls exceed their mean value +2 SD or the mean −2 SD limits.

R_{4s} Rule: The run is rejected when one control result exceeds a mean value +2 SD limit and the other exceeds the mean −2 SD limit or when the range of a group of controls exceeds 4 SD.

4_{1s} Rule: The run is rejected when four *consecutive* control results exceed the mean +1 SD or the mean −1 SD.

10_{x} Rule: The run is rejected when the last ten consecutive control results fall on the same side of the mean.

A violation of the 1_{3s} or R_{4s} control rules generally indicates random error. Violations of the 2_{2s}, 4_{1s} or 10_{x} rules are indicative of systematic error; however, violation of the 1_{3s} rule also points to a large systematic error. The multirule Shewhart procedure could be used with manual calculations; a computer makes the implementation more efficient.

Flow Diagram of Multirule Shewhart Procedure

A flow diagram applying the above model is shown in Figure 16-4.[38] Analysis of control data with a computer is straightforward, using a proper algorithm based on the flow diagram. The mean and SD of the control must be well established before this procedure can be applied.

Criticism of the L–J Method

The ability of L–J charts and/or the Shewhart multirule method to detect increasing dispersion, shifts, trends, and so forth, depends on the SD of the method. If the procedure has a broad "acceptable" range, then small increases in imprecision, shifts, or trends will probably be lost in the overall scatter of

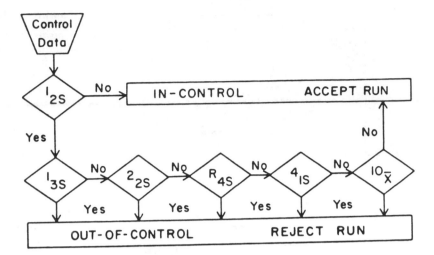

FIGURE 16-4. Logic diagram for applying a series of control rules in the multirule Shewhart procedure. (From Westgard JO, Barry PL, Hunt MR: A multirule Shewhart chart for quality control in clinical chemistry: Clin Chem 27:493, 1981)

the data. Amador showed that sudden new biases had to be 1.5 times the SD before they became obvious.[2] Imprecise methods tend to lull the analyst into a false sense of confidence; shifts, trends, and the like, occur, but the method remains "in control."

L–J chart limits cannot be based solely on statistical criteria developed during periods of "good performance." Grannis and Caragher recommended that the allowable limits (of error) *a priori* be based on ±2.2 SD developed during an "extended period of good performance."[13] They also recommended that the limits undergo periodic review and be "revised downwards whenever possible." When the laboratory was showing better performance, they recommended that the allowable limits (*e.g.,* ±2.2 SD) should be narrowed.

These recommendations must be revised in terms of current technology and *medical needs*. If only statistical criteria are used such as ±2.2 SD, a preposterous situation can develop: Highly precise methods will, by definition, have small limits; outliers, deemed medically unimportant, will create unnecessary concern, reanalysis, and so forth. Less precise methods will have broader quality control limits; here an outlier of the same magnitude as above will be inside the acceptable limits. In general, with narrower ±2 SD limits, there will be more frequent outliers.[11]

The relationship between outlier and quality control limits is given in Figure 16-5. Assume that a small sample is taken from a large population of values, for example, ±2 SD is calculated from ten replicate determinations of a control and found to be 0.5 units. The true SD for the entire population is

1 unit; that is, the sample has grossly underestimated the *true* SD of the population. This procedure is now put into routine use, and the acceptable quality control limits are set at ±1 unit. During the early application of the method, the laboratorians quickly find that many of the analyses of the same control yield values outside of the acceptable limits, in fact, nearly 32% of the results, are "out of control."

The causes of the above are that an inadequate sampling of the population—that is, too few

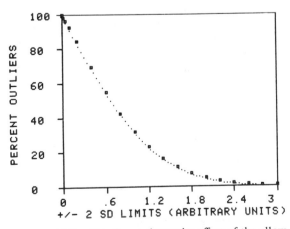

FIGURE 16-5. This figure shows the effect of the allowable control range and the percent of outliers. As the allowed range is narrowed, there is a sharp increase in the number of outliers. In some instances, the allowable limits are too narrow, resulting in unnecessary reanalyses of specimens.

replicates—was used to establish the quality control limits—and that the limits are much too narrow. In the above example, the true ±2 SD limits were from −2 to +2 units; smaller limits will yield many more outliers, as is shown in Figure 16-5. Sometimes even with a large sample, the limits are set to an unrealistically small value, particularly with the newer and more precise technology.

ALLOWABLE ERROR IN THE MEDICAL NEEDS CONTEXT

Defining Allowable Error

Allowable error means a deviation of the determined value from the true value. Bias can be estimated by repetitive analysis of specimens with a *known* content of analyte. Unfortunately, most of the time the true value or a good estimate of the true value is not known. Total error includes both bias, which we assume is known, and random analytic variation. The above is better stated as "What is allowable analytic variation?" Barnett used expert clinicians and users of clinical laboratory data to define acceptable error[4]; his approach has been updated and extended.[34] Barnett's method is reasonable, and the analytic requirements were linked to the clinical setting. In general, the medically useful precision limits were broader than current state-of-the-art analytic precisions.

Other criteria that have been suggested are "Tonk's rule" or one-fourth of the reference range or ±10%, whichever is smaller.[35] Cotlove and coworkers suggested that the "tolerable" analytic variability was 50% of the total biologic variation;[9] the latter is defined as combination of interpersonal and intrapersonal variability.[16]

Glick[10] recommended that the random error be no greater than 20% of the population-based reference or therapeutic range *or* no greater than 60% of the "medical decision range." For glucose, typical population limits are 65 to 115 mg/dl; 20% of this range is 10 mg/dl. At 120 mg/dl glucose, the medical decision range could be ±20 mg/dl; 60% of the decision range would be 12 mg/dl. Lindberg and Watson used a "loss to society" approach of a false diagnosis owing to laboratory error[20]; improvements in laboratory precision result in less loss to society. They concluded that there is no simple answer as to what is medically acceptable imprecision; the circumstances under which the test is used dictate what is acceptable. Their approach is described in more detail below.

Effect of Changing Precision on Predictive Value

Allowable error can be calculated for a specific test and purpose with the use of one of three models described by Harris.[15] The first model deals with population screening to detect a biochemical abnormality. The effect of a change in precision on the predictive value of an abnormal test result is calculated; a subjective decision remains as to what loss is acceptable in the predictive value of a result. In population screening studies, the precision needs are less stringent; the within-laboratory variability is small, compared with interindividual variability for most tests. Table 16-1 shows acceptable imprecision for a variety of tests, according to several authors. Notice that the issue of *accuracy* has not been addressed. The values in Table 16-1 are reasonable target values for CVs in population studies.

In the second case, Harris examines the effect of improved precision (the reverse is also possible) on the ability to detect abnormal values in a single person. Sharp decision boundaries are defined where the results are abnormal, and estimates are made whether a new value is truly outside these limits.

In the last case, Harris examines the effects of changes in precision on the ability to detect short-term or long-term trends of an analyte in one person. Within-person short-term monitoring is the most demanding situation for the laboratory; there the greatest precision is required. For example, in a patient being treated for possible acute rejection following renal transplantation, small changes in the serum creatinine, as little as 0.2 mg/dl, become important.[24] A serum creatinine increase of 0.2 mg/dl in a renal transplant recipient can result in changes in clinical management. Another example is a patient with a possible problem with internal bleeding. Here changes of 0.3 to 0.5 g/dl in hemoglobin become important, and the laboratory must be as precise as possible.

As described by Campbell and Owen,[6] Glick,[10] and Harris,[15] the allowable limit of error should be determined by the diagnostic application and certain other factors, as described below. There is no *single* acceptable analytic error for any test.

Cost to Society of Missed Diagnoses

"Allowable error" will always have a subjective component. What costs to society are acceptable? With overlapping populations, false-positive and false negative are inevitable; the key issues are

Table 16-1
Medically Acceptable Imprecision Stated as %CV

Test	Concentration or Activity	Tonks[35]	Harris[15]	Skendzel[34]	Barnett[4]
Acid phosphate		10			
Albumin	3.5 g/dl		3.9		7.1
Amylase	100 U/l	10			
AST (SGOT)	30 U/l			26	
Bicarbonate	25 mmol/l		4.2		
Bilirubin	1 mg/dl			23	20
total	20 mg/dl			5	7.5
Calcium	11 mg/dl	3.0	1.7	5	2.3
Chloride	90 mmol/l				2.2
	110 mmol/l	2.0	1.4		1.8
Cholesterol	250 mg/dl	5.0	6.4	12	8.0
Creatinine	1.0 mg/dl	5.0		17	
Glucose	100 mg/dl	5.0	5.6	11	5.0
	120 mg/dl				4.2
Globulin	3.5 g/dl				7.1
Hemoglobin	11 g/dl				4.8
Iron	150 mg/dl			17	26.6
LD (LDH)	200 u/l		9.0		
Lipase	100 u/l	10			
Mg	2 mmol/l		1.6		
pH(arterial)	7.4	2.0			
Phosphorus	4.5 mg/dl	5.0	7.5	14	5.6
PO_2	80 mm	10			
PO_2	40 mm	10			
Potassium	3.0 mmol/l			5	8.3
	6.0 mmol/l	4.4	5.0		4.2
Protein	7.0 g/dl	3.5	2.8		4.3
Sodium	130 mmol/l	2.0		2.7	1.5
	150 mmol/l				1.3
Triglycerides	130 mg/dl			16	
Thyroxine	6 mg/dl			17.2	
Urea nitrogen	27 mg/dl	6.0	11.9	19	7.4
Uric acid	6 mg/dl		10.1	7.3	8.3

where the decision point or cutoff value is defined and the allowance for analytic variability at this decision point.

Lindberg and Watson described the diagnosis of acute appendicitis as a test case.[20] It is desirable to have very few false-negative results; a false-negative result carries greater weight than a false-positive result. Operating on a few patients with a normal appendix is acceptable because the cost to society of a missed diagnosis leading to a ruptured appendix, peritonitis, and so forth, is much greater. The relative weights of false-positive and false-negative errors are subjective. Where is the line to be drawn?

An example in which the laboratory plays a large role is in the diagnosis of neonatal hypothyroidism. A false-negative diagnosis carries a much greater cost than a false-positive one; a large number of false-positive results are an acceptable cost. If we assume that the test for thyroxine (T_4) is the primary screening test, then the decision point to identify "abnormal" newborns is set to allow for considerable analytic variation. The test must be as sensitive as possible at the cost of specificity. The hypothyroid and euthyroid neonates will have overlapping T_4 values; the cutoff point should be set to include all the hypothyroid cases *plus* 4 SD of the analytic variation. If a T_4 value of 4 µg/dl includes all hypothyroid cases and the SD of the method is 0.5 µg/dl, then the decision point is 6 µg/dl; infants with a T_4 value below 6 µg/dl receive further testing.

The last example is a hospitalized patient who is known to have diabetes mellitus. If the laboratory variability is so great that the high glucose result is incorrectly reported as normal, then the test result is falsely negative. The cost to society of the false-negative result is probably minimal because of the likelihood of further testing. The cost of a false-positive and that of a false-negative result appear to be the same.

Variables Affecting Allowable Error

Degree of Overlap

In instances of greatly overlapping population of well and sick, less laboratory imprecision is acceptable than in nonoverlapping cases. A change in precision in a test for patients in the overlap region has much more effect on the predictive value of a positive test (PV[+]) as compared with the same test with a value at a decision point for nonoverlapping populations.

Disease Prevalence

In overlapping populations, disease prevalence is a major factor in determining PV(|) (see Table 16-2); the PV(+) may be such that the test is not worth doing regardless of the analytic variability. Watson and Tang showed that serum acid phosphatase had no value as a screening test for prostatic cancer[36]; the PV(+) was low because of considerable overlap and low prevalence. Obviously, a PV(+) of 50% or less is no better than a guess, though "educated."

Biologic Variability

The data in Table 16-2 assume an overlap of 2.3% of the well and sick.[23] A decrease in precision has its greatest effect on PV(+) for tests that have a small interpersonal biologic variability (C_B). Calcium has a C_B of about 1%; it shows the most rapid decline in PV(+) with a decreasing prevalence. For glucose and urea nitrogen, which have much larger C_B values, the PV(+) at 10% prevalence is nearly twice that of calcium.

Summary

Medically acceptable error is a subjective value. However, certain circumstances require highly pre-

---

Table 16-2
Effect of Prevalence and Change in Precision on PV(+)

Test	C_B*	C'_A/C_A†	PV(+)‡	PV(+)	PV(+)
(Prevalence)			(50%)	(10%)	(1%)
Any	29%	1.0	97.7	82.5	30.0
Calcium	0.6%	1.9	87.1	42.9	6.4
Glucose	9.6%	1.5	97.6	81.9	29.1
Urea nitrogen	16.8%	2.3	97.1	78.8	25.3

*Percent interpersonal biological variability.
†Ratio of "poor" to "good" precision.
‡Predictive value of a positive test at indicated prevalence.
(Adapted from Lott JA, Abbott LB, Koch DD: An evaluation of the DuPont aca IV: Does it meet medical needs? Clin Chem 31:281, 1985.)

cise laboratory values, and/or a large number of false-positive results are acceptable:

- The overlap between the well and sick populations is small. An example is a borderline increase of serum gastrin in a patient with Zollinger–Ellison syndrome. A decision must be made regarding further testing. False-positive results are acceptable because of the serious consequences of missing a treatable case.
- The prevalence of disease is low. An example is neonatal hypothyroidism. Screening tests must be both sensitive and precise, and one must accept a significant number of false-positive results.
- The within-person biologic variability is small. Renal transplant patients, if they are stable, show only small changes in serum creatinine. A precise test is needed to detect an upward trend in the serum creatinine.[24]

INTERLABORATORY SURVEYS

Interlaboratory proficiency surveys, or laboratory improvement programs (a better term), provide quality-control and management information for participants. Because many laboratories analyze the same material, group mean values can be determined that are generally excellent estimates of the true value if the cohort is large. From survey data, a participating laboratory can determine whether its values are biased relative to those of peer laboratories using the same method of whether the laboratory's variability is generally larger than that of the peer group.

Most surveys report the methods being used, precision data, and how many participants are using a particular method. This provides management information; laboratories tend to abandon obsolete methods or those that give results that are consistently different from the consensus mean. Finally, surveys provide information on the state-of-the-art of common analyses and can provide the basis for goal-setting or improvements in methodology. Based on survey data, improved performance in the determination of serum calcium, creatinine, and thyroxin were recommended in a symposium on analytic goals.[3] Target values for improvement are shown in Figure 16-6; calcium and creatinine are analytes that require further attention to improve precision.

Professional Organizations Providing Surveys

Three professional groups provide external proficiency surveys in clinical chemistry. The largest survey by far is that of the College of American Pathologists (CAP). Theirs is the most comprehensive evaluation of the common and unusual tests performed in clinical laboratories. The American Association for Clinical Chemistry Survey is limited to therapeutic drugs; it has a continuing education component dealing with the use of drugs, toxicity,

FIGURE 16-6. Some analytical goals for clinical analytes. For some tests, *e.g.,* urea, analytical goals have been met. For others, *e.g.,* thyroxine and creatinine, more work is needed to improve analytical precision. (From College of American Pathologists: Aspen Conference on Analytical Goals, p 5. College of American Pathologists, Skokie, IL, 1976).

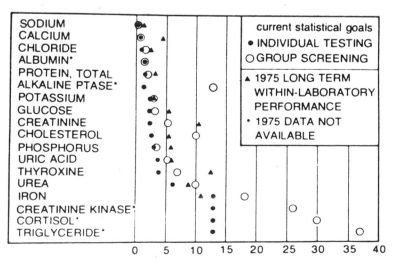

ANALYTICAL COEFFICIENT OF VARIATION

Interlaboratory Surveys Provided by Professional and Governmental Agencies

PROFESSIONAL GROUP SURVEYS

1. *American Association of Bioanalysts*
   Comprehensive surveys in chemistry, hematology, immunohematology, microbiology, urinalysis, etc.

   Report includes:
   Laboratory's value and SD
   Participant mean
   Method code

   Proficiency Testing Service
   205 West Levee
   Brownsville, TX 78520
   (512) 546-5315

2. *American Association for Clinical Chemistry*
   Therapeutic drug monitoring survey

   Report includes:
   Laboratory's value and SD
   All methods—mean
   Most widely used methods
   Continuing education modules

   AACC Proficiency Surveys
   1725 K Street NW
   Washington, DC 20006
   (202) 857-0717

3. *College of American Pathologists* (National and Regional Programs)
   Broad program for all clinical laboratory disciplines:
   Basic and comprehensive chemistry
   Blood gases and critical care
   Cerebrospinal fluid
   Electrophoresis: enzymes, hemoglobin, lipids, proteins, amniotic fluid
   Enzymes
   Instruments: spectrophotometers, balances, pH meters
   Ligands
   Therapeutic drugs
   Urine chemistry and toxicology

   Report typically includes:
   Laboratory's value and SD
   All methods mean
   Most widely used methods

   College of American Pathologists Survey Programs
   5202 Old Orchard Road
   Skokie, IL 60077
   (312) 966-5700

GOVERNMENT: FEDERAL

4. *Centers for Disease Control*
   Neonatal screening:
   Phenylalanine, T_4, TSH
   Blood lead

   Report includes:
   Laboratory's value and SD
   All methods mean

   Performance Evaluation Branch
   CDC
   Atlanta, GA 30333
   (404) 329-3877

GOVERNMENT: STATE

5. *Contact your state department of health or related agency.*

methods, pharmacokinetics, and so forth. The American Association of Bioanalysts provides surveys with a broad menu of tests (see listing above).

Government Agencies Providing Surveys

The largest government survey is prepared by the Centers for Disease Control (CDC). Their menu is fairly comprehensive, although smaller than that of the CAP. Many state health departments and regulatory agencies provide surveys. Prominent among these are the programs in New York, Georgia, and Wisconsin (see listing above).

Commercial Surveys

Manufacturers of control materials have provided proficiency surveys. Because the availability of these programs changes frequently, laboratories should discuss their needs with manufacturers' representatives.

CAP Fixed Criteria for Proficiency Testing

The usual protocol for evaluating interlaboratory quality control data in proficiency surveys was to calculate the means and SDs (usually after exclusion of extreme outliers) and then to grade the participants by statistical tests. Values outside of ±2 SD were graded as marginal or unacceptable. Certain instruments were developed recently that are highly precise; for participants with these devices, an odd situation developed: Peer groups using these instruments generally had small SDs, and the "acceptable" limits of ±2 SD became very narrow indeed, in fact, much narrower than for most older analyzers. Thus, the virtuous were being punished, and a remedy was needed. The answer was fixed limits of acceptable values; these are given in Table 16-3. The limits are quite broad and approximate what would be acceptable for population screening.

RESOLVING ANALYTICAL ERRORS

When an out-of-control situation arises in the laboratory, it is often difficult to identify the problem as having to do with instrumentation, reagents, or inappropriate standardization. The use of interrelated

specimens in a *constant,* pooled human serum matrix can often resolve the problem. The advantages of these materials are several:

- Only the analytes of interest vary from specimen to specimen; the concentrations of protein, other analytes, and possible interferents are constant.
- They are prepared from pooled serum; therefore they mimic patient specimens closely.
- Reference-grade materials can be used as the supplement for some analytes; with careful weighing, the concentration added to the pool can be calculated.
- More than one analyte can be checked at a time. If an enzyme is being investigated, the supplement can contain a simple analyte such as NaCl in addition to the enzyme. If on analysis for Na^+ or Cl^- the expected linear relationships are obtained, then the specimens were prepared correctly. If the enzyme results are unsatisfactory, the problem

Table 16-3
CAP Fixed Criteria for Survey Analytes

Test	Example Concentration or Activity	Acceptable ± in Units	Performance* ± in Percent
Albumin	4.0 g/dl	0.2 g/dl	6.7%
Calcium	10 mg/dl	1.0 mg/dl	—
Chloride	100 mmol/l	5.0 mmol/l	—
Cholesterol	250 mg/dl	—	15%
Creatinine	1.2 mg/dl	0.2 mg/dl	9.9%
Glucose	100 mg/dl	6.6 mg/dl	13.3%
Phosphorus	4 mg/dl	0.3 mg/dl	10.7%
Potassium	3.5 mmol/l	0.5 mmol/l	—
Protein, total	7 g/dl	—	5.8%
Sodium	140 mmol/l	4.0 mmol/l	—
Urea nitrogen	20 mg/dl	2.0 mg/dl	8.8%
Uric acid	6 mg/dl	—	16.7%
ALT	<0.5 × ULN†		100%
AST	>0.5 but <1 × ULN		
CK			50%
LD	>1 × ULN		25%

*Whichever is greater of two criteria.
†Multiple of upper limit of normal.

lies not with the specimens, but with the method, instrument, or some other factor.

The procedure that follows could be observed in any laboratory for resolving an analytic problem. The supplementing material need not be highly purified; crude organ extracts can be used successfully for enzyme tests. For simple analytes like Na^+, Cl^-, glucose, uric acid, pure materials should be used because they will permit a calculation of the expected "delta" values as described below.

Example Case

In the example here, uric acid is used as the test analyte being investigated. Creatinine has been added to the supplement to permit checking if the specimens have been prepared properly.

Preparation of Interrelated Specimens with Uric Acid Supplement

Pool about 60 ml of fresh patient serum. Use only clean, nonturbid, nonhemolyzed, nonicteric sera. Strain through gauze for removal of small fibrin clots. This is the *base pool.*

Prepare the uric acid supplementing solution. Prepare on the day of use; do *not* add formaldehyde if a uricase method is being used.

Uric acid (reagent grade or equivalent)	100 mg (weigh to nearest 0.1 mg)
Creatinine	100 mg (weigh to nearest 0.1 mg)
Lithium carbonate	100 mg
Dist. H_2O, enough to make	100 ml of solution

Dissolve the Li_2CO_3 in 80 ml H_2O, add the uric acid and creatinine, dissolve, and bring to 100 ml in a volumetric flask with distilled water. Prepare two pools as follows:

Pool A: 25 ml base pool + 2 ml supplement (1 mg uric acid + 1 mg creatine/ml)

Pool B: 25 ml base pool + 2 ml 154 mmol/l NaCl (saline)

Note: The *concentration* of the uric acid in the supplement is about 10 to 20 times normal, and the *volume* of the supplement used is about 5% to 10% of the total volume of *Pool A*. The volume of the supplement is kept low to prevent excessive dilution of the base pool matrix.

Prepare *interrelated specimens* as follows:

Specimen number	1	2	3	4	5	6
Pool A, ml (or parts)	5	4	3	2	1	0
Pool B, ml (or parts)	0	1	2	3	4	5
Total volume (or parts)	5	5	5	5	5	5

- Note that the *matrix* of the interrelated specimens is constant.
- The *difference* in uric acid and creatinine concentration, that is, delta concentration between adjacent specimens, is constant if the specimens have been prepared properly.

Analysis

Analyze the specimens for uric acid and creatinine. If an independent method is available for uric acid, use it also for the six interrelated specimens.

Calculations

The values determined by analysis for samples 1 to 6 are used in the calculations. Incorrect values for uric acid as determined by analysis do not render the method useless; the data are still usable, although of lesser value.

Calculate the expected values as follows:

$$\text{Pool A concentration} = \frac{25(\text{concentration base pool}) + 2\,(\text{concentration supplement})}{27}$$

$$\text{Pool B concentration} = \frac{25(\text{concentration base pool}) + 0}{27}$$

Sample 1 = Pool A

$$\text{Sample 2} = \frac{80\,(\text{Pool A concentration} + 20\,(\text{Pool B concentration})}{100}$$

$$\text{Sample 3} = \frac{60\,(\text{Pool A concentration} + 40\,(\text{Pool B concentration})}{100}$$

and so forth.

The delta values are simply the difference in concentration of uric acid or creatine of adjacent specimens, that is,

$$\text{Delta 1, uric acid} = \text{uric acid}_1 - \text{uric acid}_2$$

$$\text{Delta 2, uric acid} = \text{uric acid}_2 - \text{uric acid}_3,$$
and so forth.

Data Analysis

If the deltas for the control analyte, creatinine, are very similar, and the found values are very close to the expected values, then the specimens were properly prepared. If the deltas for the test analyte, uric acid, are

- highly variable, the method has poor precision.
- increasing with increasing concentration of uric acid, the method has a positive proportional bias.
- decreasing with increasing concentration of uric acid, the method has a negative proportional bias.

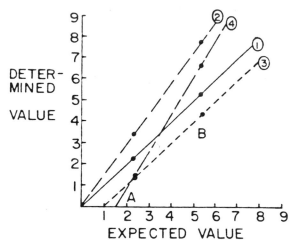

FIGURE 16-7. Illustration of some possible operational lines. When determined values are compared to expected values, the results should ideally correspond and fall along Line 1. Actual results may fall along Lines 2, 3, 4, depending on the standard curve used for the determination. The data illustrate typical "operational lines" for analytical procedures. The operational lines can indicate specific kinds of method misstandardization. See Table 16-5 for analyses of the operational lines. (From Grannis GF, Gruemer H-D, Lott JA et al: Proficiency evaluation of clinical chemistry laboratories. Clin Chem 18:222,1972)

If a plot of found concentration of uric acid versus percent pool A in the specimens is not straight, then the response is nonlinear, or there is a loss of linearity at higher concentrations.

Operational Lines

The analytic results for tests fall on an "operational line," which is a plot of found (Y) versus expected (X) analytic values.[14] Typical operational lines are shown in Figure 16-7; they can be of great help in diagnosing analytic problems. Ideally, the operational line should have a slope of 1.00 and an intercept of zero.

Preparation of Operational Lines

How are operational lines determined? A simple procedure is to analyze CAP survey serum or other serum-based material of *known* content and the calibrating materials being used by the laboratory. CAP survey serum has been analyzed by thousands of laboratories; the values can be assumed to be correct or are an excellent estimate of the true values. Some examples of CAP data from the 1986 C-D Comprehensive Chemistry Survey are given in Table 16-4. Results for the well-accepted methods are shown and the mean of all results; the means are extremely close, which supports the premise that extreme outliers become unimportant when the cohort is large.

A plot of the results from the known material (Y) versus the calibrators (X) used in the laboratory produces the operational line. Grannis showed that laboratories produced the expected relationships of interrelated survey specimens, suggesting that the mean values of all laboratories are excellent estimates of the true values.[12] For serum calcium, the mean survey results by atomic absorption agreed with the values determined by the National Bureau of Standards using an exacting method.[12] Assuming the survey specimens have not deteriorated, they are the most widely available materials that mimic patient specimens and for which an excellent estimate of the true value of the concentrations of the common analytes is available.

Analysis of Operational Lines

The types of operational lines in Figure 16-7 are summarized in Table 16-5. For line 2, the mirror image about line 1 could be imagined; that is, all values are too low by a proportional amount because of standards that are more concentrated than

Table 16-4
Data from CAP 1986 C–D Comprehensive Chemistry Survey

Analyte	No. Laboratories	Method	C-16		C-17	
			Mean	%CV	Mean	%CV
Albumin	3818	All	4.4	4.8	2.8	7.3
	2389	Automated BCG*	4.4	4.5	2.8	7.9
Bilirubin, total	5732	All	6.1	7 0	1.1	15
	2008	Automated J–G	6.1	5.8	1.0	12
Calcium	5440	All	13.9	3.9	8.8	4.1
	4628	Automated cresolphthalein	13.9	4.0	8.8	4.0
Creatinine	6018	All	5.3	5.7	1.0	11
	4290	Automated alkaline picrate	5.2	5.2	1.0	10
Glucose	6506	All	311	4.3	104	5.1
	2838	Automated hexokinase UV	313	3.9	105	4.7
Potassium	6290	All	6.6	3.0	3.6	3.1
	2665	ISE, diluted	6.5	2.0	3.5	2.6
Urea N	6179	All	50	6.7	14	10
	3380	Urease/GLDH	50	5.7	14	8.0
Cholesterol	4702	All	297	5.9	306	6.0
	4459	Automated, enzymatic	296	5.9	309	5.9

*Abbreviations: BCG, bromcresol green; J–G, Jendrassik–Grof; UV, ultraviolet. ISE, ion-specific electrode; GLDH, glutamate dehydrogenase.

believed. Line 4 occurs in an interesting way with instruments using single point calibration if the baseline is misset.[22] Only results at the calibration point, or close to it, will be correct; if the baseline is set at 95%, rather than 100% T, then all results below the standard will be too high, and all results above the standard will be too low. The error is not proportional to concentration but is related to it in a complex way by the following equations:

$$\% \, Error = [(A_{observed} - A_{correct})/A_{correct}] \times 100$$

$$\% \, Error = Ab[(1 - Cu/Cs)/As(Cu/Cs)] \times 100$$

Ab is the absorbance setting of the baseline, As is the absorbance of the standard, Cs is the concentration of the standard, and Cu is the concentration of the unknown.

The absorbance of the standard plays a role; the worst errors occur with specimens less concentrated than the standard and with a standard having a low absorbance.[22]

LABORATORY MISTAKES

Defining Blunders

A mistake, or blunder, as distinct from analytic error, can result in grossly incorrect results leaving the laboratory. Much attention has been given to improving precision; the worst culprit—mistakes—deserves more attention in the laboratory. Typically, physicians are more aware of laboratory mistakes than the laboratory staff.

Blunder Detection

Grannis and co-workers estimated the mistake rate in a clinical chemistry laboratory based on suspect values coming to the quality-control section.[14] Mistakes were confirmed before they were counted, and the rate was 3.5% for the laboratory and 0.2% for the quality-control section. Northam estimated

Table 16-5
Analysis of Operational Lines in Figure 16-7

Line No.	Possible Problem(s)	Constant Bias	Proportional Bias
1	None	No	No
2	Standards less concentrated than believed: incorrect preparation, dilution, decomposition, etc.	No	Yes
3	Inappropriate blank, all values too low by a fixed amount	Yes	No
4	Use of single point calibration and inappropriate baseline; could also be combination of 2 and 3 above	Yes	Yes
5	Nonlinear response; loss of analytic sensitivity (line not shown)	No	?

errors from a proficiency survey[31]: 13% of the outliers were more than 10 SD from the mean, 22% were between 5 and 10 SDs, and 65% were between 3.2 and 5 SDs from the mean. A 5-SD error for sodium was 11 mmol/l. Some of the "worst" laboratories had a blunder rate of 10%.

In the CAP Enzyme Survey, specimen mix-ups are readily detected, because the results from a set of specimens within a mailing must be in a known sequence of increasing or decreasing values. Lott and co-workers estimated the blunder rate in the CAP Enzyme Survey at 4.1%; the mistakes probably occurred because of specimen mix-ups.[25]

Types of Mistakes

Grannis and co-workers provided a rather complete list of typical blunders.[14] The most serious blunders were mislabeling and misplacing specimens in an analyzer tray. The latter error can affect *all* of the specimens in the tray. Other types of mistakes were chart-reading errors, calculation errors, errors due to inappropriate reagents or standards, errors due to neglect, unrecognized instrument problems, and mentally calculated results.

Reducing Laboratory Mistakes

Is a 3% to 4% mistake rate the irreducible minimum? For a clinical laboratory of our size, performing 6 million tests a year, this means 240,000 mistakes a year, or 657 a day! On the basis of our observations and those of Northam, we suggest that the following procedures be implemented to reduce blunders:

- Specimen labeling is done at the bedside with a machine-readable label.
- The labeled specimen is sampled; transfer tubes—"take-off" tubes and the like—are never used in the laboratory.
- The laboratory has a computerized information system for test requisitioning, accessioning, interfacing of equipment, reporting, log generation, inquiry, test requisitioning, and so forth.
- As much automation is present as is consistent with the size of the laboratory.
- Manual pipetting is not done, and dilutions are never made. When the instrument encounters an out-of-range specimen, the instrument automatically makes a dilution and reanalyzes the specimen.
- Reagents are labeled with machine-readable tags; the instrument checks the validity of the reagent vessel and its expected contents.
- Real-time feedback of out-of-control results for proficiency specimens are available through the computer system.
- The number of steps or procedures between receipt of the specimen (or its collection) and the delivery of the report are kept to an absolute minimum.[14]
- Manual calculations are never performed, and hand-held calculators are forbidden. Only laboratory computer-controlled calculations are performed with suitable safeguards in the computer program.
- Real-time checks of today's patient results against previous results are made to identify impossible or erroneous values.[17]
- Multivariate computer checks are made of

single results and sets of results for flagging impossible values or unlikely data, for example, high calcium *and* high phosphorus levels, low sodium *and* high chloride levels.[19]
- The laboratory staff is well trained and highly motivated to provide the best laboratory services possible. They can quickly identify unlikely results or unusual situations.[21]
- Preemployment testing is done to identify individuals who are likely to make transcription errors and similar mistakes.
- The automated equipment has an elaborate system of self-diagnostic steps and internal checks to detect malfunctions.

METHOD EVALUATION

Selection of a new method for any test in a clinical laboratory is a vital aspect of quality control. Discussed here are primarily procedures that give a numeric result; however, some of the concepts are applicable to qualitative methods. The reasons for establishing a new test fall into two categories: (1) the test is new to the laboratory, or (2) the new test replaces an existing method.

Old methods are replaced for a host of reasons: the old procedure may be obsolete, *e.g.,* glucose by neocuproine; it may have poor clinical sensitivity or specificity, *e.g.,* the thymol turbidity test; it requires too large a specimen, *e.g.,* the Technicon SMA-12; it has poor accuracy, *e.g.,* the titan yellow method for magnesium; it has poor precision, *e.g.,* the olive oil emulsion method for lipase; the reagents are poisonous or carcinogenic, *e.g.,* the NaCN–urea method for uric acid or the use of *o*-toluidine or benzidine. Many other reasons can be given for abandoning older procedures.

Before a new method is chosen, considerations of convenience, cost, and so forth, should be made. Listed at the top of the right-hand column are the most important factors that should be pondered before a new procedure is implemented in the laboratory.

Method Comparison Studies

Clinical laboratorians are typically conservative; they want some assurance that the results of tests they are reporting are "correct." A new or replacement test can be judged for correctness only with considerable difficulty. A utopian and largely impossible procedure is to compare the new and old methods with many specimens from patients with a great variety of disorders, the same receiving a long

---

Checklist for New Methods

PATIENT-RELATED FACTORS

Clinical sensitivity and specificity
Volume of specimen required
Difficulty in obtaining specimen
Accuracy and precision
Freedom from interferences

LABORATORY-PERSONNEL FACTORS

Complexity of test or instrument
Dynamic range of test
Safety: carcinogens, poisons, radionuclides
Throughput/automation
Convenience for one or many tests
Performed by all personnel on any shift

FISCAL FACTORS

Costs of materials, instrument, service, utilities, personnel, maintenance contracts, etc.
Increase or decrease costs in implementing new test

---

list of drugs, and patients of all ages and of both sexes, including newborns and children. Furthermore, the new test is compared with the contemporary "gold standard"; the latter may be extremely cumbersome and costly to carry out, *e.g.,* isotope dilution—mass spectrometry.

In the real world some compromises must be made; nevertheless, a logical and cost-effective evaluation is possible.

Selection of a Reference Method

The most difficult aspect of method evaluation is judging accuracy. Absolute accuracy is unknowable; however, in some instances, good estimates of "truth" are possible. A few tests have been investigated in great detail, and reference methods exist that give excellent estimates of the true value if the details of the methods are adhered to with great care. They are bilirubin, calcium chloride, cholesterol, glucose, hemoglobin, potassium, protein (total), sodium, and urea nitrogen. At the other extreme are tests for immunoglobulins, many hormones, trace elements such as Al and Cr, coagulation factors, and other minor metabolites, where there is extreme disagreement among various methods and no reference methods exist.

Comparison Studies

Assume that a reference method or a well-accepted procedure exists that will serve as the anchor for the new method. The reference method need not be a "routine" method; that is, it could be one that is used only for comparison purposes. Required are patient specimens that cover the dynamic range of the test. Preferably, the specimens should come from the well and sick and should include most or all of the clinical cases for which the test is designed. The specimens are analyzed by the new and reference procedures, preferably in duplicate, and graphed.

Typical X–Y charts are shown in Figure 16-8.[26] Here the reference titration method for serum lipase is compared to three candidate methods. Graphing the data is *always* necessary; statistical evaluation, as discussed below, is necessary but insufficient. Graphs will reveal the degree of dispersion, disagreement, nonlinearity, gross errors, and slope and/or intercept errors. Some of these factors will not be apparent from the usual statistical calculations.

Statistical Tests of Comparison Data

Westgard and Hunt[44] evaluated the commonly performed statistical tests; the tests with the greatest information content are the slope and intercept of the least-squares regression line and the SD of the scatter (in the Y direction), that is, $Sy \cdot x$.

The student-paired t test and the correlation coefficient contain little information or are impossible to evaluate (see Table 16–6).

SLOPE OF THE LINE. A sample regression plot is here as Figure 16-9. The slope of the line is a measure of proportional bias. Assuming that there are no gross outliers, a slope greater than 1 means the Y values are generally higher. A slope of 1.11 means the Y values are on average 11% higher than the X values.

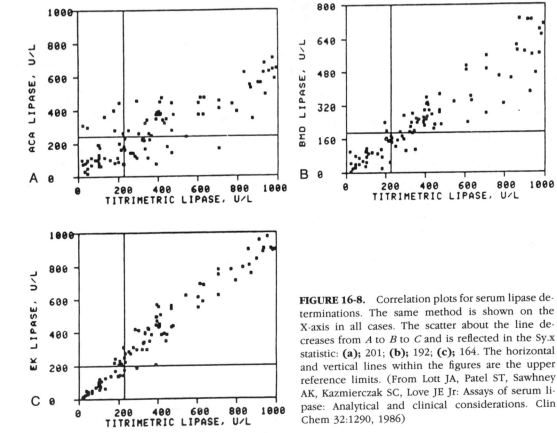

FIGURE 16-8. Correlation plots for serum lipase determinations. The same method is shown on the X-axis in all cases. The scatter about the line decreases from A to B to C and is reflected in the Sy.x statistic: **(a)**; 201; **(b)**; 192; **(c)**; 164. The horizontal and vertical lines within the figures are the upper reference limits. (From Lott JA, Patel ST, Sawhney AK, Kazmierczak SC, Love JE Jr: Assays of serum lipase: Analytical and clinical considerations. Clin Chem 32:1290, 1986)

Table 16-6
Value of Statistical Tests in Method Comparison Studies

Statistical Test	Type of Error Detected		
	Random	Constant	Proportional
Slope of line	No	No	Yes
Y intercept of line	No	Yes	No
Sy·x	Yes	No	No
Correlation coefficient (r)	Yes	No	No

(Adapted from Westgard JO, Hunt MR: Use and interpretation of common statistical tests in method-comparison studies. Clin Chem 19:49, 1973)

INTERCEPT OF THE LINE. The equation for the line in Figure 16-9 is

$$Y = 1.11X + 12$$

The method has a constant bias, and all Y values are at least 12 units higher than the X values.

STANDARD ERROR, Sy·x. The best-fit line to the paired data is shown in Figure 16-9. Vertical bars could be drawn to indicate the deviation of each point from the line in the Y direction. The mean bar length is proportional to the $Sy·x$ statistic, and it is a measure of the scatter about the line. If all the points fit exactly in the line, $Sy·x$ would be zero.

CORRELATION COEFFICIENT (r). This statistic is frequently quoted but poorly understood. An r value close to 1 does *not* mean agreement, only that the values go up and down in tandem. It is possible to have a huge proportional or constant bias and still have a near-perfect r. In Figure 16-9, r is 0.9967.

Caragher and Grannis showed graphically that the r value is highly dependent on the distribution of the data: If a few outliers on the 45-degree line are added to a random cluster of data about the line, the r value increases dramatically.[7] In short, the r statistic is largely inappropriate and uninterpretable for method comparison data.

Estimates of Accuracy

Determinations of accuracy are difficult; at best, an estimate can be made. To judge accuracy, a "gold standard" method must be available. A material that mimics patient specimens closely and that contains a *known* quantity of the analyte under study is also helpful. In Table 16-7 are shown some methods that have been used to estimate accuracy, how good these methods are, and how difficult it is to carry out the indicated study.

Estimates of Precision

Measuring the precision of a new method is straightforward. Control materials at two or more

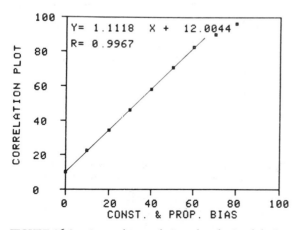

FIGURE 16-9. A sample correlation plot obtained during a method-comparison study. The regression equation, $Y = mX + b$, is shown at the top. There is a proportional bias (m) of about 11% and a constant bias (b) of 12 units. Note the r value, which is very close to 1 despite the proportional and constant bias and a loss of linearity above about 60 units.

Table 16-7
Judging the Accuracy of a New Method

Approach	Value	Difficulty in Performing
Comparison with "definitive method"	Best	Extremely difficult
Comparison with "reference method"	Excellent	Difficult
Analysis of specimens with known values	Good	Easy
Comparison to routine method	Fair or poor	Easy
Recovery studies	Fair	Easy

concentrations are analyzed at least ten times on 10 successive days. The within-day and between-day SDs are calculated, and L–J charts can be prepared and analyzed as described earlier.

Interference and Recovery Studies

The study of potential interferents, if properly done, is generally quite elaborate.[27,28] The number of drugs in common use is huge, and seriously ill individuals typically receive 8 to 12 different medications. An interference study should include the effects of lipemia, icterus, and hemolysis. Lipemia should be due to endogenous hypertriglyceridemia and not added milk or cream! Also, bilirubin should be added from patients' specimens; adding bilirubin from an alkaline solution does not represent the endogenous form.

A study of drugs should include the 20 or so most frequently prescribed agents[27]; obviously, all drugs cannot be examined.

A recovery study should be performed with the technique of interrelated specimens, as described earlier. Ideally, adding the analyte to the blood or serum specimen should not change the endogenous matrix.

Judging the Acceptability of a Method

The procedure described below as a case study follows the approach of Westgard and co-workers.[39] Before this can be used, one must know the medically acceptable error or maxium error from the true value; an estimate of the true value must also be available.

A Case Study of Method Acceptability

Work through the problem below; the answers follow.

A new uric acid Test method is to be evaluated. The Test method uses uricase coupled to an insoluble matrix plus an electrode that determines oxygen consumption as in the following reaction:

$$\text{Uric acid} + 2\ H_2O + O_2 \xrightarrow{\text{uricase}} \text{allantoin} + CO_2O + H_2O_2$$

The reference method also uses the above reaction, but a colorimetric end-point. The reference method is considered to be reliable and is believed to give accurate results.

DATA.

1. The medically acceptable error over the analytic range of 3 to 12 mg/dl is ±10% (CV). Thus, at 5 mg/dl, the allowable error is ±0.5 mg/dl.
2. A control serum analyzed 34 times over a period of 1 month with the Test method gives

   Mean 5.2 ± 0.14 (SD) mg/dl

3. Linear regression analysis of the Test method with the reference method on 50 patient specimens gives

   $Y\,(\text{Ref}) = mX\,(\text{Test}) + b$ (m = slope, $b = Y$ intercept)

   $Y = 1.02\ X + 0.10$

At 5 mg/dl for Test, the reference method gives:

$$y = 1.02\ (5.0) + 0.10 = \underline{5.2}\ \text{mg/dl}$$

Thus, the Test method has a proportional error of 2% (slope of 1.02) and a constant error of 0.10 mg/dl (intercept of 0.10).

Is the Test method acceptable? (See answers below.)

(a) Randon Error (*RE*)

   $RE = 2(\text{SD}) = \underline{\quad}$ mg/dl (Use SD determined from control)

Random error is *acceptable/not acceptable*, because it is *less than/greater than* allowable error of 0.5 mg/dl.

(b) Systematic Error (*SE*)

   $SE = Found - Correct$

   $5.20 - 5.00 = \underline{\quad}$ mg/dl

Systematic error is *acceptable/not acceptable*, because it is *less than/greater than* allowable error 0.5 mg/dl.

(c) Total Error (TE) = *RE* + *SE*

   $TE = \underline{\quad}$ mg/dl + $\underline{\quad}$ mg/dl

   $TE = \underline{\quad}$ mg/dl

Total error is *acceptable/not acceptable*, because it is *less than/greater than* allowable error of 0.5 mg/dl

ANSWERS.

(a) $RE = 0.28$, acceptable, less than.

(b) $SE = 0.20$, acceptable, less than.

(c) $TE = 0.48$, acceptable, less than.

CONCLUSION. The Test method is acceptable; the total error is less than the medically acceptable error.

REFERENCES

1. Allen IR, Earp R, Farrell EC Jr, et al: Analytical bias in a quality control scheme. Clin Chem 15:1039, 1969
2. Amador E: Quality control by the reference sample method. Am J Clin Pathol 50:360, 1968
3. Aspen Conference on Analytical Goals. College of American Pathologists, Skokie, IL p 5, 1976
4. Barnett RN: Medical significance of laboratory results. Am J Clin Pathol 50:671, 1968
5. Cali JP, Mandel J, Moore L et al: A referee method for the determination of calcium in serum. NBS Spec. Publ. 260–36, US Dept. of Commerce, National Bureau of Standards. Cat. No. C13.10:260. Washington, DC, US Government Printing Office, 1972
6. Campbell DG, Owen JA: Clinical laboratory error in perspective. Clin Biochem 1:3, 1968
7. Caragher TE, Grannis GF: Design of quality-control specimens for use with a small multi-channel analyzer. Clin Chem 23:2011, 1977
8. Caragher TE, Grannis GF: Performance evaluation of multi-channel analyzers by use of linearly-related survey specimens. Clin Chem 24:403, 1978
9. Catlove E, Harris EK, Williams GZ: Biological and analytic components of variation in long-term studies of serum constituents in normal subjects: III. Physiological and medical implications. Clin Chem 16:1028, 1970
10. Glick JH: Expression of random analytical error as a percentage of the range of clinical interest. Clin Chem 22:475, 1976
11. Gooszen JAH: The use of control charts in the clinical laboratory. Clin Chim Acta 5:431, 1960
12. Grannis GF: Studies of the reliability of constituent target values established in a large inter-laboratory survey. Clin Chem 22:1027, 1976
13. Grannis GF, Caragher TE: Quality-control programs in clinical chemistry. CRC Crit Rev Clin Lab Sci 7:327, 1977
14. Grannis GF, Gruemer H-D, Lott JA, et al: Proficiency evaluation of clinical chemistry laboratories. Clin Chem 18:222, 1972
15. Harris EK: Statistical principles underlying analytic goal-setting in clinical chemistry. Am J Clin Pathol 72:374, 1979
16. Harris EK, Kanofsky P, Shakarji G, et al: Biological and analytical components of variation in long-term studies of serum constituents in normal subjects: II. Estimating biological components of variation. Clin Chem 16:1022, 1970
17. Ladenson JH: Patients as their own controls: Use of the computer to identify "laboratory error." Clin Chem 21:1648, 1975
18. Levey S, Jennings EF: The use of control charts in the clinical laboratory. Am J Clin Pathol 20:1059, 1950
19. Lindberg DAB, Vanpeenen HS, Couch RD: Patterns in clinical chemistry. Am J Clin Pathol 44:315, 1965
20. Lindberg DAB, Watson FR: Imprecision of laboratory determinations and diagnostic accuracy: Theoretical considerations. Meth Inform Med 13:151, 1974
21. Lott JA: Laboratory personnel: The most important aspect of quality control. Med Instrument 8:22, 1974
22. Lott JA: Hazards of incorrect use of the calibration wheel and single-point calibration. Lab Med 8:25, 1977
23. Lott JA, Abbott LB, Koch DD: An evaluation of the DuPont aca IV: Does it meet medical needs? Clin Chem 31:281, 1985
24. Lott JA, Hebert LA, Baer SG: Use of computer graphics to assess trends in glomerular filtration rate (GFR) from sequential serum creatinine values. J Med Tech 1:361, 1984
25. Lott JA, O'Donnell NJ, Grannis GF: Interlaboratory survey of enzyme analyses: III. Does College of American Pathologists' Survey Serum mimic clinical specimens? Am J Clin Pathol 76:554, 1981
26. Lott JA, Patel ST, Sawhney AK, Kazmierczak SC, Love JE Jr: Assays of serum lipase: Analytical and clinical considerations. Clin Chem 32:1290, 1986
27. Lott JA, Stephan VA, Pritchard KA Jr: Evaluation of the Coomassie Brilliant Blue G-250 method for urinary protein. Clin Chem 29:1046, 1983
28. Lott JA, Turner K: Evaluation of Trinder's glucose oxidase method for measuring glucose in serum and urine. Clin Chem 21:1754, 1975
29. Lott JA, Wenger WC, Massion CG, et al: Interlaboratory survey of enzyme analyses: IV. Human versus porcine tissue as source of creatine kinase for survey serum. Am J Clin Pathol 78:626, 1982
30. Neese JW, Duncan P, Bayse D, et al: Development and evaluation of a hexokinase/glucose-6 phosphate dehydrogenase procedure for use as a national glucose reference method. HEW Publication No. (CDC) 778830, Centers for Disease Control, Atlanta, 1976
31. Northam BE: Whither automation? Ann Clin Biochem 18:189, 1981
32. O'Donnell NJ, Lott JA: Intralaboratory survey of alkaline phosphatase methods. Am J Clin Pathol 76:567, 1981
33. Pope WT, Caragher TE, Grannis GF: An evaluation of ethylene glycol-based liquid specimens for use in quality control. Clin Chem 25:413, 1979
34. Skendzel LP, Barnett RN, Platt R: Medically useful criteria for analytic performance of laboratory tests. Am J Clin Pathol 83:200, 1985
35. Tonks DB: A study of the accuracy and precision of clinical chemistry determinations in 170 Canadian laboratories. Clin Chem 9:217, 1963
36. Watson RA, Tang DB: The predictive value of prostatic acid phosphatase as a screening test for prostatic cancer. N Engl J Med 303:497, 1980
37. Westgard JO: An internal quality control system for the assessment of quality and the assurance of test rules. Scand J Clin Lab Invest 44:315, 1984
38. Westgard JO, Barry PL, Hunt MR: A multi-rule Shewhart chart for quality control in clinical chemistry. Clin Chem 27:493, 1981
39. Westgard JO, Carey RN, Wold S: Criteria for judging precision and accuracy in method development and evaluation. Clin Chem 20:825, 1974

40. Westgard JO, Falk H, Groth T: Influence of a between-run component of variation, choice of control limits, and shape of error distribution on the performance characteristics of rules for internal quality control. Clin Chem 25:394, 1979

41. Westgard JO, Groth T: Power functions for statistical control rules. Clin Chem 25:863, 1979

42. Westgard JO, Groth T, Aronsson T, et al: Performance characteristics of rules for internal quality control: Probabilities for false rejection and error detection. Clin Chem 23:1857, 1977

43. Westgard JO, Groth T, DeVerdier CH: Principles of developing improved quality control procedures. Scand J Clin Invest (Suppl 172) 44:19, 1984

44. Westgard JO, Hunt MR: Use and interpretation of common statistical tests in method-comparison studies: Clin Chem 19:49, 1973

seventeen

Laboratory Requisitions and Reporting of Results

Doris A. Johnson

THE REQUEST

An efficient requisitioning system is a well-defined communication system by which a physician's request for specific laboratory tests for a specific patient is received by laboratory personnel within a short period of time in a manner that allows few translation errors. A written request on a properly designed form is preferable to a verbal or telephoned request. The request form must be designed to meet the specific needs of the institution or practice and can vary from a very simple written request to printed forms that serve not only as requests but provide for test-result reporting and patient billing. Factors that have an impact on decisions regarding the requisitioning system include type of institution or practice; number of types of tests ordered; where the request is initiated; where the request is received; related systems, such as reporting and billing; existing institutional policies; requirements of external agencies for accreditation; and regulation by state and/or federal government.

Accrediting agencies have addressed requisitioning and reporting. The Joint Commission on Accreditation of Healthcare Organizations (JCAHO), 1986, Pathology and Medical Laboratory Services, Standard PA 3) states,[2] "Channels of communications within the pathology and medical laboratory services, with other departments/services of the hospital and the medical staff and with outside ser

vices and agencies, are appropriate for the size and complexity of the hospital." Required characteristics of this standard are as follows:

All requests for laboratory tests are made in writing or by electronic means. Orders or requisitions for inpatient and ambulatory care patient services must clearly identify the patient, the requesting individual, the tests required, any special handling required, the date and, when relevant, the time the specimen was collected, and the date and time the request and/or specimen reached the laboratory. Requests for examinations of surgical specimens contain a concise statement of the reason for the examination. The laboratory performs tests and examines specimens on the written request of individuals authorized by the medical staff to order such evaluations and receive the results; those physicians or dentists who are not members of the medical staff but who have authorization from the medical staff and administration to request such support services from the hospital; and to the extent permitted by law, other persons authorized by the hospital and licensed to engage in direct treatment of patients.

There are some general criteria for the requisition. The requisition should be easily recognizable by shape or color and easy to use; it should be printed in readable type, with a listing of all frequently requested tests, and provide adequate space for indicating the choice of test, so that check marks

(*Text continues on p 291*)

LINCOLN CLINIC, P.C. ● 3145 "O" STREET ● LINCOLN, NE 68501 ● P.O. BOX 81009

| TICKET NUMBER | PATIENT'S NAME | SERVICE | DR. NO. | DOCTOR'S NAME | NEW |
| | LAST | F | | | RET. |

HISTORY NUMBER

BILLING NAME A

CHECK DIGIT

BILLING NUMBER

✔	PANEL OR PROFILE		FEE	✔
	Chemistry Profile	80013		Amy
	Lipoprotein Profile	83716		Bili
	Coagulation Panel	85342		Bili
	Protein Profile	84166		Ca
	Liver Profile	80006		Ch
	Hematology Profile	85011		C
	URINALYSIS			
	Routine, Complete	81000		
	Chemical, Qual	81005		
	Microscopic, Only	81015		
	FUNCTION TESTS			
	E.C.G.	93000		
	E.C.G., Exercise	93020		
	Gastric Analysis c̄ Hist.	82935		
	Vital Capacity, Total TMBC	94010		
	Vital Capacity, Total	94150		
	Vital Capacity, Fev	94160		
	Max. Breath. Cap.	94200		
	Max. Ex. Fl. Rt.	94210		
	IMMUNOHEMATOLOGY			
	Bl. Gp. & ABO	86060		
	Rh	86100		
	Antibody Titer Screen	86020		
	Coombs, Dir.	86250		
	Coombs, Ind.	86260		
	HEMATOLOGY			
	CBC	85010		
	WBC	85030		
	Differential	85040		
	RBC	85020		
	Hemoglobin	85050		
	Hematocrit	85055		
	Platelets	85590		
	Sed Rate	85651		
	Reticulocyte Ct.	85640		
	L. E. Cell Prep.	86380		
	Pro. Time	85610		
	P.T.T.	85730		
	Coag Time (Lee - White)	85345		
	RBC Fragility	85620		
	HGB. Electrophoresis	83020		
	Eosin. Ct.	85350		
	MISCELLANEOUS			
	Semen Eval	89320		
	Cytology, Pap	88100		
	Allergy Smear	86383		
	Sweat Test	89960		
	Synovial Fluid Ex	89330		
	Blood Drawing	89230		
	House Call	89398		

LC-160

SPECIAL REQUEST — Please Check Tests Desired

MICROBIOLOGY REQUEST

Source □ Throat □ Sputum □ Urine □ Stool □ CSF □ Abcess □ Wound □ G.U.

□ Skin Scraping □ Other

Request □ Smear (Grams) □ Smear (Acid-Fast) □ Wet Mount □ Mycology Mount

□ Culture □ Sensitivity □ Colony Count □ Fluorescent Antibody

Tenative Dx:

Duration of Infection:

Other Pertinent Information: Treatment:

ELECTROPHORESIS REQUEST

Specimen: □ Serum □ Urine □ C.S.F. □ Other

Request: □ Protein Profile (E.P.-I.E.P.-IQ) □ Electro. Only □ Immunoelectrophoresis Only

□ Immunoglobulin Quant. Only □ Other

Clinical Information:

Patient			History #		Dr.

LINCOLN CLINIC, P.C. — CLINICAL LABORATORIES   Technologist

Mid. Exp. F.R. (MMEF)

		Normal Value			Normal Value	Glucose Tol. B	U	B	U
Bilirubin, Direct	Mg %		Lipids, Total	Mg %		Fasting		2 Hr.	
Bilirubin, Indirect	Mg %		Triglycerides	Mg %		½ Hr.		3 Hr.	
Bilirubin, Total	Mg %		Amylase			1 Hr.		4 Hr.	
Calcium	Mg %		Lipase						
Cholesterol	Mg %		C.P.K.						
Creatinine	Mg %		LDH						
Glucose	Mg %		SGOT						
Iron	Mcg %		SGPT						
IBC	Mcg %		HBDH						
Protein	Gm %		Alk. Phos.						
Phosphorus	Mg %		Acid Phos.						
Urea Nitrogen	Mg %		T7						
Uric Acid	Mg %		T4						
Sodium	MEq/L		T3						
Potassium	MEq/L		17ketogenic						
Chloride	MEq/L		17keto						

LC-B 1-71   **BIOCHEMISTRY**   Date

FIGURE 17-1. Multipurpose request forms with check-off sections for easy use may be provided to the physician with every patient chart. The laboratory makes the appropriate reporting form, such as the biochemistry example. Note that the most commonly specified tests are printed on the face of the form with space provided for the specification of any unlisted test. (Forms courtesy of Lincoln Clinic, P.C., Lincoln, Nebraska, and Woehrmyer Printing Co., Denver, Colorado)

THIRD PART IS A FILE COPY FOR THE REQUESTING LABORATORY   65825

BLOOD CHEMISTRY
URINE CHEMISTRY

REGIONAL LABORATORY SECTION
Department of Pathology — UNMC

Call Results When
Available to: _____
Name _____
No. _____

| Name | | Age | Sex | Date Received | | Date Reported |

| Date Collected | For Urine Date Completed | Time: | AM PM | Laboratory |

| Physician: | Vol. (Urine) _____ ml / _____ hr. |

UNIVERSITY HEALTH CENTER
LABORATORY
15TH AND U ST.
LINCOLN, NE   68500

✓	BLOOD CHEMISTRY			NORMAL VALUES
	Australian Antigen (HBAg) NR	POS		Non-Reactive
	Carcinoembryonic Antigen Indirect Direct	ng/ml		With Report
	Carotene	mcg/dl		70–250 mcg/dl
	Cortisol 8 AM	mcg/dl		4–18 mcg/dl
	4 PM	mcg/dl		2–10 mcg/dl
	Digitoxin	ng/ml		2 6 mg/dl
	Dilantin	mcg/ml		Therapeutic: 15–40 mcg/ml
	Estriol	ng/ml		With Report
	Folic Acid			With Report
	Follicle Stimulating Hormone (FSH)	ng/ml/hr		Male: 300–1200 ng/ml Female: 0–80 ng/dl
	Growth Hormone	ng/dl		Therapeutic: 10–20 mcg/ml Toxic >20 mcg/ml
	Human Chorionic	mcg/ml		2–10 mcIu/ml
	Insulin	mcIu/ml		
	Thyroid Stimulating Hormone	ng/dl		40–170 ng/dl
	Triiodothyronine (T3 by RIA)	pg/ml		200–900 pg/ml
	Vitamin B12			
	OTHER			

URINE CHEMISTRY			
	mcg/24 hrs	<125 mcg/24 hrs
Catacholamines, Free	mcg/24 hrs	<100 mcg/24 hrs
Cortisol	mg/24 hrs	>40% decrease from established values suggests fetal distress
Estriol	mg/24 hrs	Adults: <1.3 mg/24 hrs, Equivocal 1.3-2.5 mg/24 hrs
Metanephrines, Total		Negative
Neurometabolic Screen	mg/24 hrs	Adults: 0.2-3.5 mg/24 hrs
Pregnanetriol	mg/24 hrs	Adults: 2-9 mg/24 hrs
Vanilmandelic acid	gm/5 hrs	Adults: > 4 gm/5 hrs
D-Xylose		
OTHER		

BC-2

ORIGINAL

REGIONAL LABORATORY COPY

REQUESTING LABORATORY COPY

ACCOUNTING COPY

BILLING COPY

FIGURE 17-2. Multitest request form folded to show the number of carbon copies provided. (Form courtesy of Regional Laboratory Section, University of Nebraska Medical Center, Omaha)

ROCHE

ROCHE BIOMEDICAL LABORATORIES, INC.

Wichita, KS (316) 686-7161
(800) 362-2660 Kansas
(800) 835-2361 Outside Kansas
Lincoln, NE (402) 464-8268
Kansas City, MO (816) 361-7777
Topeka, KS (913) 357-6284

W2

Client
UNIVERSITY HEALTH CENTER
BUSINESS SERVICES, RM 209
15TH AND U STREETS

LINCOLN, NE 68508

Other tests not listed	Clinical history, special instructions	Client number	Chart Number	Order Number
1.		/	/	
2.		Date collected / /	Time collected AM PM	Physicians name
3.		PATIENT NAME (Last, first)		
4.		Age	Sex	Hours fasting	24 - Hour Urine volume ml

Remove Center Labels First

E053924-4 EC53924-4 E053924-4

E053924-4 EC53924-4 E053924-4

Specimen Codes - Check Directory of Services for specimen requirements
S = Serum or centrifuged serum separator tube
L = EDTA whole blood (lavender)
t = Aliquot of 24 hour urine
B = Sodium Citrate (light blue)
G = Sodium Flouride (gray)
Gr = Heparinized (green)
* = Frozen in plastic tubes
Sl = Slides
U = 12 ml random
RT = Maintain at room temperature
P = Plasma
Y = ACD whole blood (yellow)

PATIENT OR THIRD PARTY BILLING INFORMATION

BILL TO:
☐ ACCOUNT ☐ MEDICARE ☐ MEDICAID
☐ PATIENT ☐ BLUE SHIELD ☐ OTHER

Certificate Number

Name of Responsible Party	Street Address	City	State	Zip	Phone ( )

Medicare Number	Medicaid Number	Blue Shield Subscriber Number	Patient/Subscriber Relationship ☐ Self ☐ Spouse ☐ Dependent

Diagnosis	Physician's Name	Patient's Date of Birth

PROFILES				INDIVIDUAL TESTS				
91025-7	Diagnostic Profile	S	82150-4	Amylase	S	83540-5	Iron	S
91000-0	Health Survey	S	86350-6	ANA	S	83550-4	Iron, IBC, % Saturation	S
- - - -	Profile Options		86260-7	Antibody Screen	S, L	83620-5	LDH	S
75900-1	Amylase	S	84520-6	BUN	S	75477-0	LDL	S
75901-9	CBC	L, Sl	75519-9	CA-125	S	83655-1	Lead	L
75240-2	CBC without Diff	L	82310-4	Calcium	S	83690-8	Lipase	S
75902-7	CPK	S	75145-3	Carbamazepine (Tegretol)	S	80919-4	Lipoprotein Phenotype	S
75903-5	Direct Bilirubin	S	82950-7	CBC	L, Sl	83725-2	Lithium	S
72306-4	Fructosamine	S	82959-8	CBC without Diff (Hemogram)	L	75052-1	Luteinizing Hormone	S
75904-3	HDL	S	75011-7	CEA, Roche	P-2L	83735-1	Magnesium	S
75905-0	IBC and % Saturation	S	82385-6	Cholesterol	S	75186-7	Marijuana Screen	U
75906-8	RA Factor	S	92012-4	Cholesterol and Triglycerides	S	86300-1	Mononucleosis Screen	S
75907-6	RPR	S	86155-9	Cold Agglutinins	S - RT	82205-6	Phenobarbital	S
75908-4	T₄	S	82015-9	Cortisol _____ A.M.	S	85580-9	Platelet Count	L
75909-2	T₇ (includes T₄ + T₃U)	S	75320-2	Cortisol _____ P.M.	S	75086-9	Potassium	S
76832-5	Urinalysis	U	82550-5	CPK	S	75252-7	Pregnancy Test, Serum	S
			82565-3	Creatinine	S	83160-2	Pregnancy Test, Urine	
82206-4	Drug Abuse Screen	U	82903-6	Creatinine Clearance	t, S	75030-7	Progesterone	S
82922-6	Electrolytes	S	86140-1	CRP	S	75082-8	Prolactin	S
92004-1	Inflammatory Study	S	82657-8	Digitoxin	S	84065-2	Prostatic Acid Phos., RIA	S*
			82656-0	Digoxin	S	82914-3	Protein Electrophoresis	S
INDICATE PROFILE LETTER OR NUMERAL			82655-2	Dilantin	S	- - - -	☐ if abnormal, IEP	
(See back for some options)			77116-2	Flecainide	G	85610-4	Prothrombin Time	P-B
			72305-6	Fructosamine	S	75053-9	Quinidine	S
Customized Profile _____			73311-3	FSH	S	86360-5	RA Factor	S
Drug Analysis _____				Glucose	G or S	85640-1	Reticulocyte Count	L
Executive Profile _____				Glucose _____ hr. p.p.	S	86410-8	RPR	S
Hepatitis Profile _____		S	9433X-X	Glucose Tolerance	S	86399-3	Rubella Immune Status	S
Lipid Profile _____		S	- - - -	_____ hr. _____ # specimens		85650-0	Sedimentation Rate	L
Liver Profile _____		S	75205-5	HCG-Beta, Quant	S	84455-5	SGOT (AST)	S
Prenatal Profile _____		S, L	75229-5	HDL	S	84465-4	SGPT (ALT)	S
Rheumatoid Profile _____		S	75279-0	Hemoglobin A1c	L	75047-1	T₃ RIA	S
Thyroid Panel _____		S	77005-7	HTLV-III Antibody	S	83440-8	T₃ Uptake	S
			85353-1	IgE	S	83455-6	T₄ (Thyroxine)	S
			86330-8	Immunoglobulins (G,A,M)	S			

92009-0	T₇ (Free Thyroxine Index)	S
73406-1	Testosterone	S
75083-6	Theophylline	S
84475-3	Triglycerides	S
75085-1	TSH	S
86057-7	Type and Rh	S, L
84550-3	Uric Acid	S
82991-1	Urinalysis	U
74587-7	Vitamin B12	S
92057-9	Vitamin B12 and Folate	S*
72000-3	Venipuncture	

MICROBIOLOGY		
87100-4	Acid Fast Culture and Smear	
87101-2	Blood Culture	
76400-1	Chlamydia/EIA	
- - - -	Source _____	
87060-0	Fungus Culture	
87009-7	Fungus KOH Prep	
87052-7	General Culture	
- - - -	Source _____	
87008-9	Genital Culture Screen (GC)	
87003-0	Gram Stain	
- - - -	Source _____	
87038-6	Herpes EIA/Culture	
87013-9	Ova and Parasites	
87053-5	Salmonella/Shigella Screen	
87054-3	Sputum Culture	
87001-4	Strep Screen (Throat)	
87007-1	Stool Culture, Comprehensive	
87010-5	Upper Respiratory Tract Cult.	
87055-0	Urine Culture, Comprehensive	
87011-3	Urine Culture, Screen	
87056-8	Urogenital Culture	
75497-8	Urogenital GC/EIA	

Front

288

PROFILES
REFER TO DIRECTORY OF SERVICES FOR FURTHER INFORMATION

DIAGNOSTIC PROFILE (Multi-Chem) 91025-7

A/G Ratio
Albumin
Alkaline Phosphatase
ALT (SGPT)
AST (SGOT)
BUN
BUN/Creatinine Ratio
Calcium
Chloride
Cholesterol
Creatinine
GGT
Globulin
Glucose
Iron
LDH
Phosphorus
Potassium
Sodium
Total Bilirubin
Total Protein
Triglycerides
Uric Acid

HEALTH SURVEY 91000-0

Albumin
Alkaline Phosphatase
AST (SGOT)
BUN
Calcium
Cholesterol
Glucose
LDH
Phosphorus
Total Bilirubin
Total Protein
Uric Acid

DRUG ABUSE SCREEN, URINE 82206-4

*Amphetamines
*Barbiturates
*Benzodiazepines
Cannabinoids
Cocaine/Metabolite
Methaqualone (Quaalude®)
*Opiates
Phencyclidine (PCP)
*Reported as a class

EXECUTIVE PROFILE A 91004-2

Health Survey
T₄
CBC

EXECUTIVE PROFILE B 93004-0

Diagnostic Profile
T₄
CBC

EXECUTIVE PROFILE C 92103-1

Diagnostic Profile
CBC
HDL
RPR
T₄
Urinalysis

HEPATITIS PROFILE I (DIAGNOSTIC) 87043-6

HBsAg
Anti-HBc, IgM
Anti-HAV, IgM

**HEPATITIS PROFILE II
(DIAGNOSTIC FOLLOW-UP) 87044-4**

HBeAg
Anti-HBe
Anti-HBs

**HEPATITIS PROFILE III
(PATIENT MANAGEMENT) 87045-1**

HBsAg
Anti-HBe
HBeAg

**HEPATITIS PROFILE IV
(IMMUNE STATUS) 87046-9**

Anti-HAV, Total
Anti-HBs
Anti-HBc, Total

HEPATITIS PROFILE V (A PANEL) 87047-7

Antibody to HAV, IgG/IgM
Differentiation

HEPATITIS PROFILE VI (B PANEL) 87048-5

HBsAg
Anti-HBs, Total
Anti-HBc, Total
Anti-HBc, IgM
HBeAg
Anti-HBe

HEPATITIS PROFILE VII 87049-3

A + B Panels

INFLAMMATORY STUDY 92004-1

A/G Ratio
Albumin
ANA
CRP
Globulin
RA Factor
Streptococcal Exoantigens
Total Protein
Uric Acid

LIPID PROFILE A 80919-4

Cholesterol
Triglycerides
Lipoprotein Phenotype

LIPID PROFILE B 92085-0

Cholesterol
Triglycerides
HDL
LDL
VLDL
Risk Index

LIPID PROFILE C 92106-4

Cholesterol
Triglycerides
HDL
LDL
Risk Index
Lipoprotein Phenotype

LIVER PROFILE A (Liver Study) 92010-8

Albumin	Cholesterol
Alkaline Phosphatase	GGT
ALT (SGPT)	LDH
AST (SGOT)	Protein, Total
Bilirubin	

LIVER PROFILE B 92104-9

Profile A
Protein Electrophoresis

PRENATAL PROFILE A (Prenatal #5) 91101-6

ABO Grouping and Rh Typing
Antibody Screen (includes ID and titer
on clinically significant antibodies)
CBC without differential
Syphilis Serology

PRENATAL PROFILE B (Prenatal #6) 91102-4

Profile A
Rubella Antibodies, HAI, Quant.

PRENATAL PROFILE C 92087-6

ABO Grouping and Rh Typing
Antibody Screen (includes ID and titer
on clinically significant antibodies)
Syphilis Serology

PRENATAL PROFILE D (Prenatal #4) 91100-8

Profile C
Rubella Antibodies, HAI, Quant.

THYROID PANEL A (EUTHYROID) (T7) 92009-0

T3 Uptake
T4
T7 (Free Thyroxine Index)

THYROID PANEL B (HYPOTHYROID) 92072-8

T7 (Free Thyroxine Index)
TSH (Thyroid Stimulating Hormone)

THYROID PANEL C (HYPERTHYROID) 92105-6

T7 (Free Thyroxine Index)
T3, RIA

Back

FIGURE 17-3. Multitest request form (front and back) with peel-away numbers for specimen identification. (Form courtesy Roche Biomedical Laboratories, Inc., Wichita, Kansas)

TISSUE EXAMINATION REQUISITION
(Please Type or Print Plainly)

TO: PATHOLOGY CONSULTANTS, INC.
3333 East Central, Suite 721
Wichita, Kansas 67208
316-681-2741
CLIA 15-1025   Medicare: 17-8048
Shelby Rose, M.D., F.C.A.P.
Director

Patient Information

Name _____

Address _____

City - State _____

Phone _____ Age _____ Sex _____

Physician _____ Hospital/Clinic _____

Address _____

Diagnosis _____

Specimen _____

Date Obtained _____

Duration _____

Bill: Doctor ☐   Clinic ☐   Patient ☐

REQUISITION NUMBER	PATIENT NAME	PHYSICIAN	NO.
55006			55006
PATHOLOGY CONSULTANTS, INC.	PATIENT NAME	PHYSICIAN	NO. 55006
WICHITA, KANSAS	PATIENT NAME	PHYSICIAN	NO. 55006
316-681-2741			

Part 1

PRINT FIRMLY   2784

78621

pci

PATHOLOGY CONSULTANTS, INC.
3333 East Central, Suite 721
Wichita, Kansas 67208
316-681-2741
CLIA 15-1025   Medicare 17-8048
Shelby Rose, M.D., F.C.A.P., Director

NAME _____ PHONE _____

ADDRESS _____

CITY
STATE _____ ZIP _____ PHYSICIAN _____

HOSPITAL/CLINIC _____

SOURCE _____

DATE OBTAINED _____ LMP _____

MEDICATIONS _____

RADIATION _____

LAST PAP: Date _____

RESULT _____

OTHER HISTORY _____

DATE OF BIRTH _____

RESULTS	
☐ Negative	Cytology # _____
☐ See Below	

MEDICARE-MEDICAID REQUIREMENTS

Date of Birth _____
(MONTH)   (DAY)   (YEAR)

Medicare #'s _____

Medicaid #'s _____

SEND BILL TO: Doctor ☐   Hospital ☐   Clinic ☐   Patient ☐

☐ Cytogram

PARABASALS __/__ INTERMEDIATES __/__ SUPERFICIALS

☐ Cells of Endocervical Origin Not Seen

Shelby Rose, M.D., Pathologist

CYTOLOGY REPORT FORM

Part 2

FIGURE 17-4. Specific information must be provided with requests for cytology and tissue examinations. (Forms courtesy Pathology Counsultants, Inc., Wichita, Kansas)

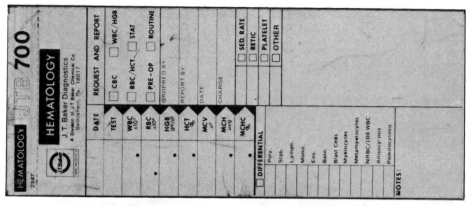

FIGURE 17-5. Multitest request forms of noncarbon paper provide the report copy, file copy, and a copy for the requesting physician. Note the test identification numbers. (Forms courtesy J. T. Baker Diagnostics, Bethlehem, Pennsylvania, and the State of Nebraska Department of Health Laboratories, Lincoln, Nebraska)

do not overlap. There should be space for patient identification, date, time received in the laboratory, and name of the person requesting the test. The name and address of the laboratory may be printed on the requisition and a space provided for listing a reference laboratory. Additional space may be provided for pertinent clinical information such as that required by laboratories that perform viral and rickettsial tests. A space should be provided for the addition of tests that are not printed on the form.

Institutional policies and computer capabilities may dictate other criteria for requisitioning. Multipart forms have been popular, especially for laboratories that have combined requisitioning with reporting and/or billing. Nursing or clerical personnel who transcribe the physician's orders and initiate requests may desire to keep a copy of the request in the initiating area. Physicians' offices or clinic laboratories that do limited testing may find

that one request form will meet their needs; whereas larger private, hospital, or independent laboratories need request forms for each department within the laboratory or for each group of related tests. There have been reports of success with a check-off test-order sheet/computer-card request system.[4] In that system, the physician checks the tests desired on the order sheet, and a nurse transcribes the orders on a computer card, which will print labels and work lists in the laboratory. It is estimated that this system works for 95% to 98% of all tests ordered in an institution. Before making a final decision regarding the format of the requisition, a multidisciplinary committee should review the proposed form. All of the user groups should be represented.

Request forms may be purchased from a commercial company or printed to order by a private printing company. Factors that need to be taken into

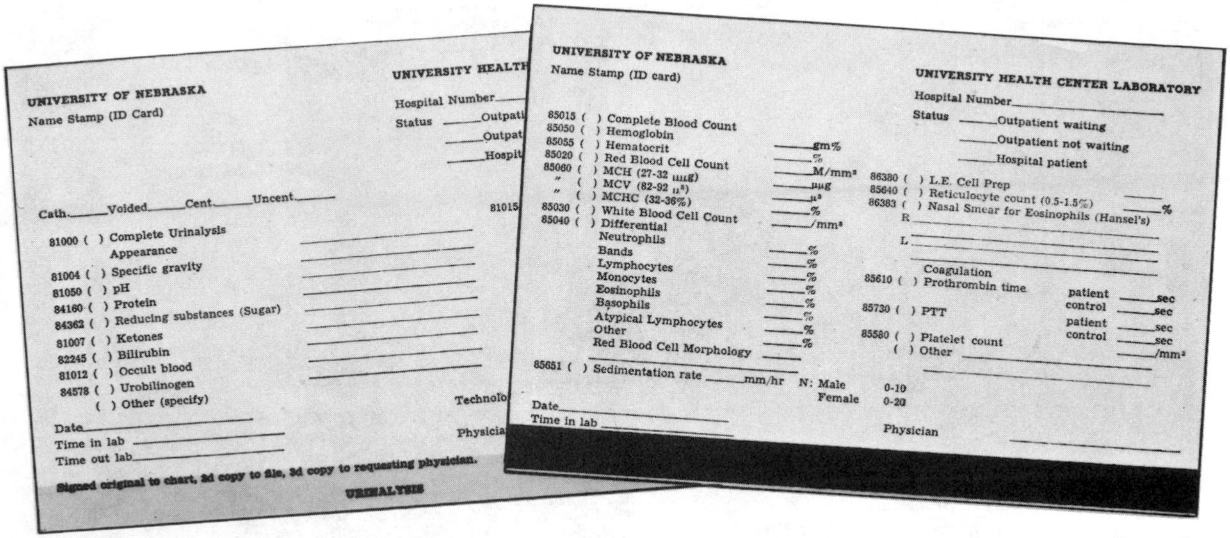

UNIVERSITY OF NEBRASKA
Name Stamp (ID Card)
UNIVERSITY HEALTH
Hospital Number
Status ___Outpati ___Outpat ___Hospit
Cath.___ Voided___ Cent.___ Uncent.___
81000 ( ) Complete Urinalysis
Appearance
81004 ( ) Specific gravity
81050 ( ) pH
84160 ( ) Protein
84362 ( ) Reducing substances (Sugar)
81007 ( ) Ketones
82245 ( ) Bilirubin
81012 ( ) Occult blood
84578 ( ) Urobilinogen
( ) Other (specify)
Date
Time in lab
Time out lab
Technolo
Physicia
Signed original to chart, 2d copy to file, 3d copy to requesting physician.
URINALYSIS

UNIVERSITY OF NEBRASKA
Name Stamp (ID card)
UNIVERSITY HEALTH CENTER LABORATORY
Hospital Number
Status ___Outpatient waiting ___Outpatient not waiting ___Hospital patient
85015 ( ) Complete Blood Count
85050 ( ) Hemoglobin ___gm%
85055 ( ) Hematocrit ___%
85020 ( ) Red Blood Cell Count ___M/mm³
85060 ( ) MCH (27-32 μμg) ___μμg
" ( ) MCV (82-92 μ³) ___μ³
" ( ) MCHC (32-36%) ___%
85030 ( ) White Blood Cell Count ___/mm³
85040 ( ) Differential
Neutrophils ___%
Bands ___%
Lymphocytes ___%
Monocytes ___%
Eosinophils ___%
Basophils ___%
Atypical Lymphocytes ___%
Other ___%
Red Blood Cell Morphology
85651 ( ) Sedimentation rate ___mm/hr N: Male 0-10 Female 0-20
Date
Time in lab
86380 ( ) L.E. Cell Prep
85640 ( ) Reticulocyte count (0.5-1.5%) ___%
86383 ( ) Nasal Smear for Eosinophils (Hansel's)
R
L
Coagulation
85610 ( ) Prothrombin time patient ___sec control ___sec
85730 ( ) PTT patient ___sec control ___sec
85580 ( ) Platelet count ___/mm³
( ) Other
Physician

FIGURE 17-6. Hecon printer card report forms and computer-card-size forms for manual reporting are among the most commonly used report forms. (Forms courtesy The University Health Center. University of Nebraska, Lincoln, Nebraska)

consideration are cost, institutional policies, the possibility of modifying a commercial form to fit a particular need, and whether or not the commercial forms can be purchased with the name and the address of the laboratory printed on them.

A plan for implementation should be developed. It should include orientation for all of the individuals who will be initiating requests and allow for revision after a specified period of usage.

Figures 17-1–17-5 provide numerous examples of multipurpose, multitest, and computer requisitions that may be used in effectively communicating laboratory requests.

THE REPORT

General considerations for report forms include adequate space for test results and reference values; the time test was reported; the date; the technologist's initials; and if appropriate, the name of the reference laboratory. Abnormal results should stand out clearly.

The Joint Commission on Accreditation of Hospitals (JCAH, 1986, Pathology and Medical Laboratory Services, Standard PA 3 Required Characteristics) states[2]

> Communication systems within pathology and medical laboratory services and between it and other departments/services efficiently accomplishes both the urgent and the regular transfer of information. The laboratory report includes the date and time of reporting and the condition of any unsatisfactory specimen. A system assures the ability to identify the individual responsible for performing or completing the procedure used. Criteria are established for the immediate notification of the practitioner responsible for the care of the patient when critical limits of specified test results are exceeded.

Standard PA 4 also refers to required characteristics for records and reports:[2]

> Authenticated, dated reports of all examinations performed by the pathology and medical laboratory services are made part of the patient's medical record. The director of the pathology and medical laboratory services is responsible for all hospital laboratory reports. When tests are performed in a reference laboratory, the name of the laboratory performing the test is included in the report placed in the patient's medical record. Reports of all anatomic and clinical laboratory tests and examinations performed are readily available to the individual ordering the tests. The hospital assures that the reports are filed promptly in the patient's medical record. Report forms are designed to facilitate comparison of each determination with pertinent reference values and sequential and related analysis. The requirement for providing reference values may be met by including in the medical record a current listing of such values approved by the direc-

(Text continues on p 297)

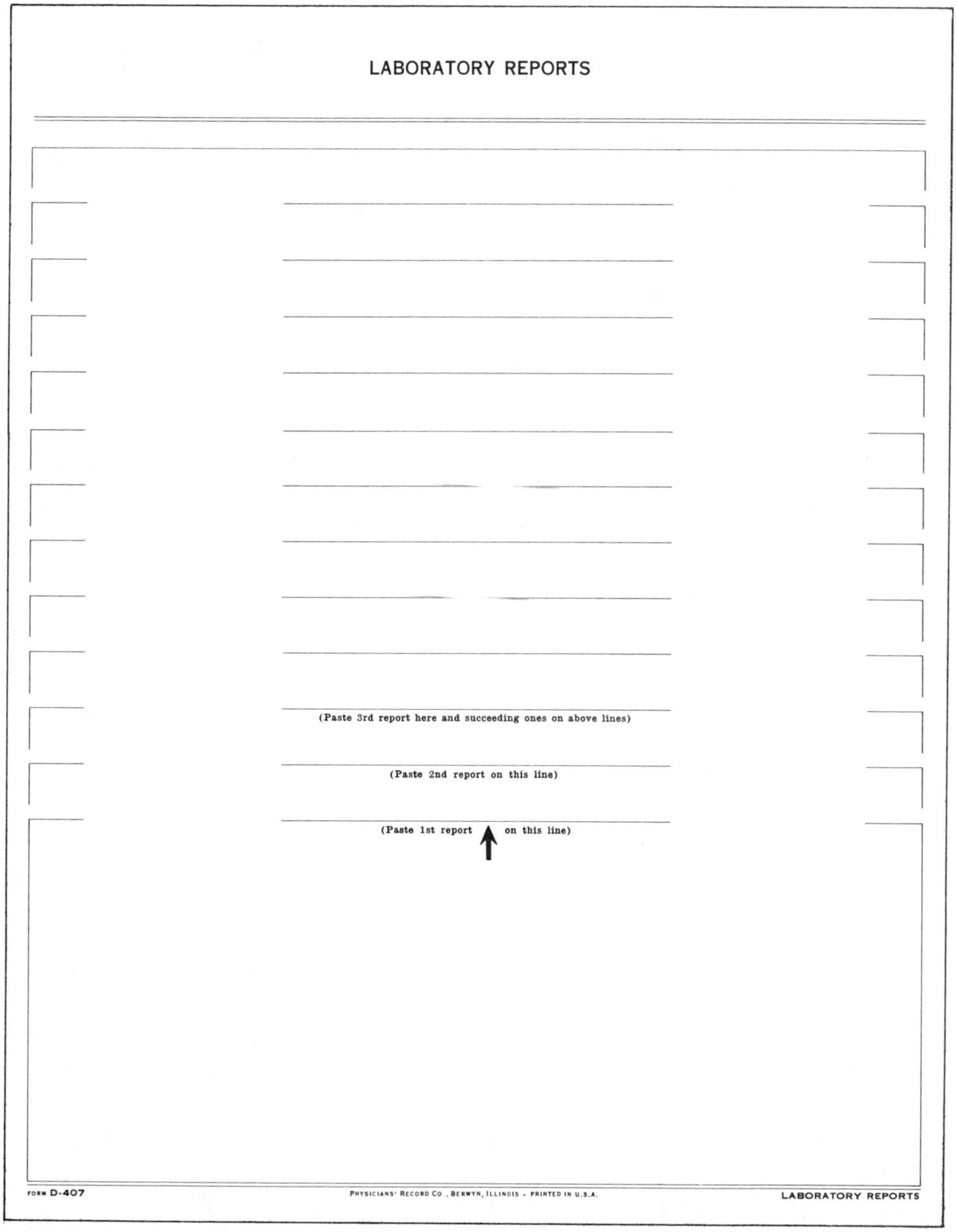

LABORATORY REPORTS

(Paste 3rd report here and succeeding ones on above lines)

(Paste 2nd report on this line)

(Paste 1st report ⬆ on this line)

FORM D-407   PHYSICIANS' RECORD CO., BERWYN, ILLINOIS · PRINTED IN U.S.A.   LABORATORY REPORTS

FIGURE 17-7.   Record sheets that have pressure-sensitive strips for the attachment of reports provide for sequential layering. (Form courtesy Physicians' Record Co., Berwyn, Illinois)

505862 4722102

** FINAL REPORT **

CHART#
@@YR @ 2/27/87   @@HF
6053833   0:00HRS

ROCHE
ROCHE BIOMEDICAL LABORATORIES, INC.
SUBSIDIARY OF HOFFMANN-LA ROCHE, INC.

WICHITA	316-686-7161	IN KANSAS	800-362-2660
KANSAS CITY	816-361-7777	NATIONALLY	800-835-2361
LINCOLN	402-464-8268		

TEST	RESULT	USUAL RANGE - UNITS	TEST	LO	NORMAL	HI
GLUCOSE	90	60-125 MG/DL	GLUCOSE		*	
BUN	13	7-26 MG/DL	BUN		*-	
CREATININE	0.7	0.5-1.5 MG/DL	CREAT		*--	
SODIUM	141	135-148 MEQ/L	SODIUM		*	
POTASSIUM	4.2	3.5-5.5 MEQ/L	POTASSIUM		*-	
CHLORIDE	103	94-109 MEQ/L	CHLORIDE		-*	
TRIGLYCERIDE	92	10-190 MG/DL	TRIGLYCER		*	
URIC ACID	3.5	2.2-9.0 MG/DL	URIC ACID		*---	
CALCIUM	8.9	8.5-10.6 MG/DL	CALCIUM		*--	
PHOSPHORUS	3.9	2.5-4.5 MG/DL	PHOS		--*	
TOTAL PROTEIN	6.0	6.0-8.5 G/DL	T PROTEIN		*-----	
ALBUMIN	4.0	3.5-5.5 G/DL	ALBUMIN		*--	
CHOLESTEROL	162	115-295 MG/DL	CHOLESTER		*--	
BILIRUBIN, TOTAL	0.5	0.1-1.2 MG/DL	T BILI		*-	
ALKALINE PHOSPHATASE	67	20-125 U/L	ALK PHOS		*	
SGOT (AST)	28	0-50 U/L	SGOT		*	
SGPT (ALT)	17	0-50 U/L	SGPT		*-	
GGTP	16	0-65 U/L	GGTP		*--	
LDH	230	100-250 U/L	LDH		---*	
IRON	136	40-180 MCG/DL	IRON		-*	
GLOBULIN	2.0	1.5-4.5 G/DL	GLOBULIN		*----	
A/G RATIO	2.0	1.1-2.5	A/G RATIO		-*	
BUN/CREATININE RATIO	18.6	5.0-50.0	BUN/CREAT		*--	
	*********					
IRON CONTENT	136	40-180 UG/DL	IRON		-*	
IRON BINDING CAP	330	250-450 UG/DL	TIBC		*-	
	*********					
HDL - SERUM	47	MALE: 30-65 MG/DL	HDL		*	
		FEMALE: 35-85 MG/DL				

LOW VALUES INDICATE INCREASED RISK
HIGH VALUES INDICATE REDUCED RISK

ROCHE BIOMEDICAL LABS
P. O. BOX 2858
WICHITA, KANSAS 67201

PHILLIP M. ALLEN. MD., DIRECTOR

UNIVERSITY HEALTH CENTER
BUSINESS SERVICES, RM 209
15TH AND U STREETS

LINCOLN, NE   68508

A

MEDICARE 17-8041
CDC 15-1014

FIGURE 17-8.   Computer printouts (**A, B, C**) provide test results, specimen-collection times, normal values, and a column to indicate whether the test values are within normal limits, high, or low. (Form courtesy Roche Biomedical Laboratories, Inc., Wichita, Kansas)

SPECIMEN #	TYPE	PRIMARY LAB	REPORT STATUS					Roche Biomedical Laboratories, Inc.

SPECIMEN # 057-135-0064-1   **TYPE** R   **PRIMARY LAB** BN   **REPORT STATUS** PRELIM PG 1

ADDITIONAL INFORMATION

PATIENT NAME ... I   **SEX** F   **AGE (YR./MOS.)**

PT. ADD.

DATE OF SPECIMEN	DATE RECEIVED	DATE REPORTED	
02/26/87	03/04/87	03/05/87	0758

ROCHE Roche Biomedical Laboratories, Inc.

CLINICAL INFORMATION

PHYSICIAN ID. 922 74   PATIENT ID. 910354

ACCOUNT
ROCHE BIOMEDICAL LABS   15400030
911 NORTH HILLSIDE   90
911 NORTH HILLSIDE   90
WICHITA   , KS   67214-
316-686-7161

TEST	RESULT		LIMITS	LAB
CBC & DIFFERENTIAL				
MONOCYTES	8	%	0 - 10	BN
MONOCYTES (ABSOLUTE VALUE)	0.4	X1000/CMM	0.0 - 0.8	BN
PLEASE NOTE NORMAL CHANGE: PLATELET COUNT CHANGE TO 140-440 X1000/CMM				
URINALYSIS, ROUTINE				
SPECIFIC GRAVITY	1.007		1.010 - 1.030	BN
PH	7		5 - 7	BN
URINE COLOR	YELLOW		YELLOW	BN
APPEARANCE	CLEAR		CLEAR	BN
WBC ESTERASE	TRACE		NEGATIVE	BN
PROTEIN	NEGATIVE		NEGATIVE	BN
GLUCOSE	NEGATIVE		NEGATIVE	BN
ACETONE	NEGATIVE		NEGATIVE	BN
OCCULT BLOOD	TRACE		NEGATIVE	BN
MICROSCOPIC EXAMINATION	.			BN
WBC/HPF	0-1			BN
RBC/HPF	0-1			BN
EPITHELIAL CELLS	FEW			BN
BACTERIA	FEW			BN
MUCOUS	SLIGHT			BN
CALCIUM OXALATE CRYSTALS	FEW			BN
THYROID PROFILE A				
MULTI-24				
OSMOLALITY, CALCULATED	313 H	MOSM/KG	275 - 305	
BUN/CREATININE RATIO	12			
LDL CHOLESTEROL, CALCULATED	250 H	MG/DL	60 - 210	
AN AVERAGE HDL VALUE OF 45 MG/DL IS ASSUMED				

PATIENT NAME   PATIENT ID.   (BOX) SPEC. NO.   SPEC. DATE

BONE		ELECTROLYTES			HEART		LIVER				LIPIDS	
Calcium mg/dl (8.5-10.6)	Phosphorus mg/dl (2.5-4.5)	Sodium mEq/L (135-148)	Potassium mEq/L (3.5-5.5)	Chloride mEq/L (94-109)	LDH IU/L (100-250)	SGOT IU/L (0-50)	T. Bili mg/dl (0.1-1.2)	GGT (IU/L) (M 0-65) (F 0-45)	SGPT IU/L (0-50)	Alk. Phos. IU/L (20-125)	Cholesterol mg/dl (115-295)	Triglycerides mg/dl (10-190)

PROTEIN				KIDNEY		THYROID				MISCELLANEOUS		
T. Protein g/dl (6.0-8.5)	Globulin g/dl (1.5-4.5)	Albumin g/dl (3.5-5.5)	A/G Ratio g/dl (1.1-2.5)	BUN mg/dl (7-26)	Creatinine mg/dl (0.5-1.5)	T4 μg/dl (4.5-12.5)	T3 Uptake % (35-45)	Free T4 Index (1.6-5.6)	TSH μIU/ml (<5.0)	Uric Acid mg/dl (M 3.9-9.0) (F 2.2-7.7)	Glucose mg/dl <50 yrs. (60-115)	Iron μg/dl (40-180)

HEMATOLOGY														
RBC x10⁶/mm³ (M 4.3-5.9) (F 3.5-5.5)	HGB g/dl (M13.9-18.0) (F 12.0-16.0)	HCT % (M 39-55) (F 36-48)	MCV μ³ (80-100)	MCH μμg (26-34)	MCHC % (31-37)	Platelets x 10³/mm³ (140-440)	WBC x 10³/mm³ (4.0-10.5)	Polys (45-75%) (1.5-8.0)	Bands (0-5%)	Metas (0%)	Lymphs (20-45%) (0.8-3.2)	Mono (20-45%) (0.8-3.2)	EOS (0-6%) (0-0.5)	BASO (0-2%) (0-0.1)

%

ABSOLUTE VALUES

RESULTS ARE FLAGGED IN ACCORDANCE WITH AGE DEPENDENT REFERENCE RANGES WHICH ARE SUMMARIZED ON THE BACK OF THIS REPORT.
*A comment applied to this test has been printed in the body of the Report.   REPORT

B

(continued)

TEST	RESULT	LIMITS	LAB

FOR THE LDL CALCULATION WHEN TESTING FOR HDL IS NOT REQUESTED.

DIRECTOR: JAMES B POWELL MD

FINAL REPORT WILL FOLLOW

IF YOU HAVE ANY QUESTIONS CONTACT - BRANCH: 919-584-5171 LAB: 919-584-5171

PATIENT NAME DUMMY , 1	PATIENT ID. 910354	SPEC. NO. 0571850066-1	SPEC. DATE 02/26/87

BONE / ELECTROLYTES / HEART / LIVER / LIPIDS

Calcium mg/dl (8.5-10.6)	Phosphorus mg/dl (2.5-4.5)	Sodium mEq/L (135-148)	Potassium mEq/L (3.5-5.5)	Chloride mEq/L (94-109)	LDH IU/L (100-250)	SGOT IU/L (0-50)	T. Bili mg/dl (0.1-1.2)	GGT (IU/L) (M 0-65) (F 0-45)	SGPT IU/L (0-50)	Alk. Phos. IU/L (20-125)	Cholesterol mg/dl (115-295)	Triglycerides mg/dl (10-190)
10.0		152	4.0	110	151	30	1.5	39	21	111	334	192
		HIGH		HIGH			HIGH				HIGH	HIGH

PROTEIN / KIDNEY / THYROID / MISCELLANEOUS

T. Protein g/dl (6.0-8.5)	Globulin g/dl (1.5-4.5)	Albumin g/dl (3.5-5.5)	A/G Ratio g/dl (1.1-2.5)	BUN mg/dl (7-26)	Creatinine mg/dl (0.5-1.5)	T4 µg/dl (4.5-12.5)	T3 Uptake % (35-45)	Free T4 Index (1.6-5.6)	TSH µIU/ml (<5.0)	Uric Acid mg/dl (M 3.9-9.0) (F 2.2-7.7)	Glucose mg/dl <50 yrs. (60-115)	Iron µg/dl (40-180)
7.7	3.2	4.5	1.4	15	1.2	8.3	40	3.3		7.7	95	

HEMATOLOGY

RBC x10⁶/mm³ (M 4.3-5.9) (F 3.5-5.5)	HGB g/dl (M13.9-18.0) (F 12.0-16.0)	HCT % (M 39-55) (F 36-48)	MCV µ³ (80-100)	MCH µµg (26-34)	MCHC % (31-37)	Platelets x10³/mm³ (140-440)	WBC x10³/mm³ (4.0-10.5)	Polys (45-75%) (1.5-8.0)	Bands (0-5%)	Metas (0%)	Lympha (20-45%) (0.8-3.2)	Mono (20-45%) (0.8-3.2)	EOS (0-5%) (0-0.5)	BASO (0-2%) (0-0.1)	
5.14	15.2	45.9	89	29.5	33.1	174	5.4	61			26		4	1	%
								3.3			1.4		0.2	0.0	ABSOLUTE VALUES

C

RESULTS ARE FLAGGED IN ACCORDANCE WITH AGE DEPENDENT REFERENCE RANGES WHICH ARE SUMMARIZED ON THE BACK OF THIS REPORT.
*A comment applied to this test has been printed in the body of the Report.

REPORT

tor of the clinical laboratory. Reports of quantitative analysis include the units of concentration or activity. The basis upon which the reference values in use was established is available to medical staff members upon request.

The pathology and medical laboratory services maintain a record of the daily accession of specimens and an appropriate system for identification of each. The record includes at least the laboratory and patient identification; the identification of the practitioner ordering the test or evaluation; the date and, when relevant, time of specimen collection and receipt; the reason for any unsatisfactory specimen; the test or evaluation performed; the result; and the date and time of reporting to the requesting practitioner or patient care unit.

Duplicate copies of all anatomic and clinical laboratory tests and examinations performed are retained in the laboratory in a readily retrievable manner. Requirements for record retention are determined by applicable law and regulation, and by local needs, but are in effect for at least two years.

Federal regulations have an impact upon those institutions or persons who receive payment from Medicare and Medicaid. It is stated in the regulations for the management of independent laboratories[3] that normal ranges of values must be available upon request. This is interpreted to mean that normal values must be on the report.

Patient information, including name, room number or address, hospital number, age, and sex, must appear on each laboratory report. It is helpful if all of the patient information is in the same place on all of the report forms. If identification cards are made for the patients, the requisition or report form may have a space provided for imprinting the name and other information from the identification card.

Reports must be legible, and all recorded results must be reviewed for error. Diamond[1] defined the report as the object of all quality control and added that reports are not reliable or valuable unless they are comprehensible and timely. It is of little value to have a rapid testing system if there is an appreciable time lag between the recording of the result and the actual charting of the result on the medical record.

Reporting may be on a single form or on any number of forms. Most laboratories have found it convenient to develop report forms for each department within the laboratory. Report forms may be designed for special groups of tests, such as chemistry profiles. Report forms can be any size desired; however, most forms are computer-card size, 8.3 cm by 18.7 cm, letter size, 21.5 cm by 28 cm, or half-letter size, 14 cm by 21.5 cm.

Multicopy forms can provide as many as five legible copies. The original becomes the chart copy, and the copies may be used for the laboratory file copy, physician's copy, accounting copy, and billing copy. Use of the multicopy form as the request form and report form reduces paperwork and transcription errors.

Time received and time reported can be stamped on the side of the form if desired; however, it is more convenient if there is a special place for this on every form. In addition, there may be a space provided for indicating telephoned reports.

Clinical laboratories that serve as reference laboratories or provide laboratory service for outpatients need requisitions and report forms that have adequate space for the name and address of the referring physician. The forms may be designed so that the name and address of the referring physician will show when the report is put into a window envelope, thus avoiding additional clerical work.

Reference laboratories frequently report test results by telephone, especially results that are out of the normal range. It is very important to know who receives the call and that he has the correct information. It is appropriate to ask the receiver to read the report back to the caller. Telephone report pads are helpful if a large number of test results are frequently telephoned. The tests, including normal ranges, may be printed on the pad so that limited conversation and recording are required.

The laboratory report becomes part of the medical record. There are a number of ways that it can be charted in the medical record. Filing envelopes or jackets may be placed in the record. The report forms can then be filed in these jackets. Such a system does not provide for an orderly review of laboratory tests from several days as does sequential layering of laboratory reports or cumulative computer printouts. Sheets that have pressure-sensitive adhesive areas for layering report forms may be purchased. The report forms may also have adhesive material on the back so that they can be attached easily to a special form in the medical record. (See Figures 17-6, 17-7, and 17-8 for examples of multipurpose, multitest, and computer report forms for communicating laboratory results.)

Highly efficient data systems have been developed to help the clinical laboratorian meet the ever-increasing demand for test results. Such systems reduce the time lag between requests and reports, reduce paperwork, and contribute significantly to better laboratory management. A computer system may be used to provide a daily printout of test results and, in addition, may be programmed to print out cumulative test results and flag abnormal results.

Information regarding data-processing systems is provided in Chapter 18. There is also an in-depth coverage of that subject in Henry's *Todd-Sanford-Davidsohn Clinical Diagnosis and Management by Laboratory Methods*, which is listed in the bibliography.

Requisitioning and reporting systems, however carefully devised, are not permanent. A good system will provide for feedback and a periodic review so that the system can be modified to function in the ever-changing environment of the clinical laboratory.

REFERENCES

1. Diamond I: Quality Control Revisited. Pathologist 34:333–336, July 1980
2. Joint Commission on Accreditation of Hospitals: Accreditation Manual for Hospitals. Chicago, Joint Commission on Accreditation of Hospitals, 1986
3. Medicare Regulations, 42CFR Part 405. Subpart Condition 6, Management of Independent Laboratories (405.1613), 1966
4. Ostrin S, Ring A: Streamline ordering with an all-in-one request form. Med Lab Observer 9:56–58, 1977

ANNOTATED BIBLIOGRAPHY

Halper H, Foster H, Gayer G: Laboratory Regulation Manual. Washington, DC, O'Connor & Hannon, 1976

This is a composite of regulations that impact upon the clinical laboratory.

McLendon W: Communications and data processing. In Henry J (ed): Todd-Sanford-Davidsohn Clinical Diagnosis and Management by Laboratory Methods. Philadelphia, WB Saunders, 1979

This book lists essential components of requisitioning and reporting, with an emphasis on data processing and telecommunications.

eighteen

Computers and Laboratory Information Systems

John R. Svirbely
Jack W. Smith, Jr.
Carl E. Speicher

Clinical laboratories perform the laboratory tests requested by physicians. They must generate the right data, on the right person, and deliver it to a locatable place, within a medically useful period of time. Many kinds of tests are performed, several of which must be available 24 hours a day. This results in a considerable flow of information into, through, and out of the laboratory.

The collection and communication of information by the clinical laboratories may be viewed as two separate processing cycles (Fig. 18-1), one being an extralaboratory communication cycle and the other an intralaboratory analysis cycle. The extralaboratory cycle consists of afferent and efferent limbs. The afferent limb involves specimen/request collection and delivery, and the efferent limb consists of report collection and delivery to the physician. The intralaboratory cycle involves accessioning test requests and patient specimens, dividing the specimens into aliquots, delivering them to the appropriate work station, performing the test, and preparing the report of the results. The organization of a laboratory profoundly affects the information flow within the laboratory.

Computers were introduced into clinical laboratories during the 1960s to aid in the information-processing task. Today, computers are extensively distributed and integrated in the clinical laboratory. They serve an essential role in information processing and are expected to have an increasingly larger role in the future. This chapter is an overview of how the modern laboratory information system (LIS) utilizes computerization for efficient information management. We will first discuss the problems encountered in information processing before the advent of computers. We will then cover the "classic" roles for computers in the laboratory, as well as the newer roles computers have today. Finally, we will discuss how to select a laboratory information system.

PROBLEMS IN INFORMATION HANDLING PRIOR TO COMPUTERIZATION

Manual information systems can function adequately when the work load is limited in volume and the timeliness of the results is unimportant. However, for the last three decades there has been a relatively constant rate of increase in the number of tests performed annually, and there has been a greater need for urgency in reporting these results.

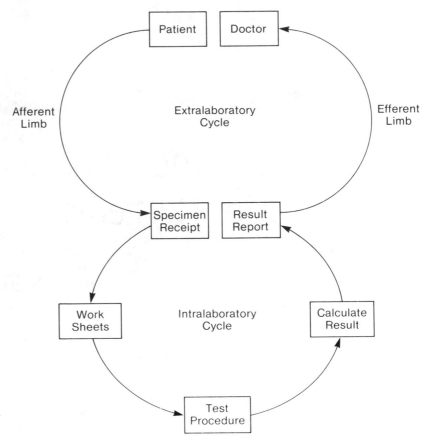

FIGURE 18-1. The laboratory information cycles.

By the late 1950s laboratories were already finding themselves unable to handle the constantly rising work load. Most test procedures in the clinical laboratories at that time were done individually, by hand. In addition, much of the clerical work associated with the tests was done by the same technologist who was performing the test. For each test, several stages were involved in information handling, each of which could delay processing or result in an error. Particularly troublesome were specimen misidentification, transcription errors, illegible handwriting, and misplaced reports.

There was hope that the introduction of automated analytic instruments would solve some of these problems. However, because data could be generated in large amounts very rapidly, the capacity of the data-interpretive processes within the laboratory was easily overwhelmed. Rather than simplifying the situation, test automation contributed to further decompensation. The emergence of automated information processing was necessitated.

OVERVIEW OF COMPUTER SYSTEMS

A computer alone does not constitute an LIS. An LIS consists of computer hardware, software, data, and personnel.

Computer hardware consists of the actual computer machinery. The central processing unit (CPU) is where the principal computer operations are actually performed. Data being sent to or received from the CPU is stored in memory, which is very fast but typically of a finite size. Larger amounts of data require slower storage devices, such as magnetic disks, magnetic tapes, and, more recently, laser disks. Users can directly access computers by means of terminals, such as the cathode ray tube (CRT), which may be directly connected to the computer if nearby, or may make use of modulating–demodulating devices (modems) if remote from the computer. Information stored in the computer is output on printers, which range in their capabilities in speed and readability. Instruments can directly deliver data into the computer by means of instrument "interfaces." Computers can be connected to each other over communication networks, which use sophisticated protocols for exchange of information.

Software consists of the commands by which the hardware is controlled and directed. Computers operate by means of a binary code (0, or *off;* 1, or *on*); however, the actual language used by the machine (machine code) is both difficult and time-consuming for people. This has necessitated development of "high-level" languages, such as FORTRAN or PASCAL, which are easier for programmers to use, but whose commands must be translated by the computer into a machine code that it can understand. The operating system is the software that allocates system resources among the different processes running at the same time. Software packages, such as an LIS, consist of a number (often very large) of programs written in high- or low-level language to implement certain desired functions. The functional implemented in an LIS will be discussed in the next section.

Data are the actual information the computer uses or generates in its computations. Data may be acquired by direct manual entry, but are more often input over instrument interfaces. This information can be stored on various kinds of hardware devices, the choice of which depends on how much data must be stored, how fast it must be retrieved, how often it will be accessed, and how long it needs to be available. Because patient information is confidential and may be of a sensitive nature, special provisions for data security are required, as will be discussed in the next section.

Specially trained personnel are required for optimal computer system operation. The system manager is the director for the computer system; he interfaces with hospital administrators, allocates resources, and directs projects. Programmers develop and maintain software programs. System analysts interface between system users and programmers, in order to design the applications that will be implemented by the programmers. Operators are the persons who perform the actual maintenance functions for the system.

THE FUNDAMENTAL FUNCTIONS OF THE LIS

An LIS must be capable of performing many different functions. We will describe these in relation to their location in the laboratory information cycles, as shown in Figure 18-1.

The LIS and the Extralaboratory Cycle — Afferent Limb

The afferent limb of the extralaboratory information cycle involves test ordering and the delivery of the necessary specimens to the laboratory. Test ordering minimally requires completion of a test requisition form (paper or computer-based) with sufficient information to identify the patient uniquely (full name and a unique identification number), indicate the type of determinations required, and indicate the person to whom the results should be reported. After a test is ordered, specimens should be correctly collected, labeled, and then transported to the laboratory.

The most important problem in this cycle involves specimen and patient identification. No completely reliable, generally accepted, and cost-effective system for specimen and patient identification is available. Identification of blood products with bar-coded labels has been widely used in blood banks; but despite their great potential, the use of bar-coded patient identification systems has not become widespread. In most laboratories patient identification still requires that the specimen collection personnel either read the patient's identification bracelet or ask the patient his name and birth date.

In other ways, however, the LIS can simplify the afferent limb for the laboratory. By referring to centralized patient demographic (admission–discharge–transfer, or ADT) information, the LIS can update patient status and location on an ongoing basis. This permits accurate collection of specimens, as well as reports of results, with a minimum of delays and errors. Much of the information required to complete a test requisition can be automatically retrieved from this source.

Direct communication links between patient care units and the laboratory computer greatly improve the test-ordering process, in comparison with older, manual methods. The ability of patient care units to order tests and to obtain results by such links improves handling of information transfer, particularly in emergency situations.

For nonemergency situations, the LIS can use requisition data to prepare collection lists for specimen collection personnel; such lists permit more efficient specimen collection and result in fewer collection errors. By synchronizing specimen collection times throughout an institution, maximum advantage can be taken of economics of scale in high throughput laboratory instrumentation with laboratory personnel resources adjusted for peak periods. This can provide a cost effective and acceptable turnaround time for the majority of test requests.

The Intralaboratory Cycle — Clerical Functions

Within the laboratory, there are many clerical duties associated with performing tests. First, test requests must be tabulated and arrangements made for specimen collection. When a specimen is received in the laboratory, it is assigned a unique identifier (accessioned) and entered in the laboratory record system. The specimen is then divided into appropriate aliquots, which are distributed with work sheets to the different analytic work stations. After tests are performed and the results are verified, reports are generated in a useful format and delivered to the appropriate physician offices and patient locations. Finally, any inquiries concerning pending or incomplete procedures must be answered, whereas completed reports must be placed in archival storage.

Reduction in clerical errors and improvement in efficiency were some of the first improvements noted with the introduction of computers into the laboratory. The LIS can integrate the accessioning process, generation of work sheets, and result collection. An essential feature is the ability to maintain a tracking log for each test request, which contains the data entered on that request at each stage of processing. This record maintains the connection of the specimen to the patient, permits interim status inquiries, and is needed for data interpretation. Later we shall further discuss the role of the LIS in reporting results.

The Intralaboratory Cycle — Data Acquisition and Manipulation for Quantitative Tests

Laboratories can be roughly divided into two kinds, based on the general nature of the results that they generate. One kind, for example, the chemistry or hematology laboratory, generates data that are primarily numeric in nature and are the result of quantitative analyses. The second kind, for example, the microbiology or surgical pathology laboratory, generates primarily descriptive results, which are expressed in varying amounts of text. The success of computers in data handling has varied because of this essential difference in the type of data generated.

Some of the earliest uses of computers in the laboratory involved their use for data acquisition from laboratory instruments. The advent of semiautomated and then automated instruments, which were capable of performing multiple analyses on single specimen, made the ability to collect and store the increased amount of data in a similarly automated way desirable, thereby eliminating human error and time delays associated with data collection and entry. The first attempts at data acquisition used off-line input with marksense or punched cards and some human coding of instrument outputs. Subsequent instruments produced output on a machine-readable medium that could later be fed into a computer. Later, direct instrument–computer interfaces, for which the computer uses the analog output from instruments to obtain digitalized results, were used for data input. The earliest success with this direct interface was achieved with the AutoAnalyzer (Technicon Corporation), the IL flame photometer, and the Coulter blood cell analyzer. Once data was stored in the computer, it was a simple matter to perform data manipulation, with curve interpolation, statistical calculation, or other mathematic functions being used to generate analyte results directly from raw data. The combination of automated analyses and automated data handling allowed development of powerful instruments that permit a very high volume of testing to be performed.

Let us examine more closely how the typical on-line instrument interface transmits data in real time via a direct hardware connection without human intervention. In the AutoAnalyzer (Fig. 18-2), the transmittance of light through a solution is measured by an electronic detector, which generates a voltage. The peak value of this voltage is directly proportional to the amount of the analyte being measured, with the proportionality factor determined by testing a series of standard solutions and generating a working curve. To determine the analyte value, a computer must digitalize the voltage over time (analog-to-digital conversion). The peak value may then be found by making use of various peak detection algorithms that make use of curvature parameters such as slope changes or derivatives of the input. This value is then interpolated to a working curve for obtaining a result, which may be subjected to further calculations for a final determination of the actual analyte value. The data acquisition computer must have a list of how to associate each peak with a specimen type and the analyte being measured. This is traditionally accomplished by inputting loading lists that specify the identity of each sample as "patient specimen," "test standard," or "quality assurance sample." In this way the on-line interface can convert data in a "raw" form (varying voltage) to a digital analyte value, which can be stored.

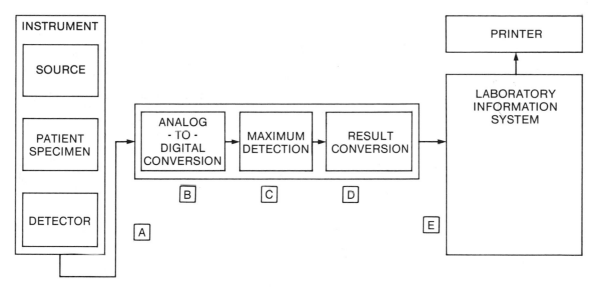

FIGURE 18-2.   Data requisition from an analytical instrument. Data from an on-line instrument is processed in the following steps:
- A. Instrument output
- B. Analog-to-digital conversion
- C. Maximum (peak) detection
- D. Result calculation (converting test data to an analyte value). The amount of a substance can be determined by interpolating the slope of its reactivity curve to a working curve made by testing standard solutions of known activity.
- E. Storage in the central LIS

The intermediate processing steps (B–D) involved in converting instrument output initially were located in the central LIS computer, but they now are often located in the instruments themselves.

The data acquisition interface was originally achieved in the central laboratory computer. However, developments in computer interfacing have taken it out of the central computer and placed it directly in the instrument. Many automated instruments come now equipped with preprocessors that convert the raw data generated by the instrument into data results, which are output in a uniform digital format. Indeed, other aspects of data handling can now be achieved locally in the instruments themselves.

A computer may be used as a process controller for the mechanical operation of the instruments as well as for data handling. In 1970 the first computer-controlled laboratory instrument, the Automated Clinical Analyzer (ACA, DuPont) was made available. It incorporated a hard-wired computer to control instrument function as well as to calculate results from raw data and output results for direct reporting. Size and price reductions have hastened the incorporation of computers into laboratory instruments to control instrumentation components,

to acquire and process data, and to format instrumental output. Since then, the trend is toward highly automated, intelligent, stand-alone instrument systems with dedicated processing and control computers.

The Intralaboratory Cycle — Data Acquisition and Manipulation in Descriptive Domains

Computerization has been slower and more difficult in laboratory divisions like microbiology and the anatomic pathology services, where data are nonnumeric in nature. This has not been due to a lack of effort, for the advantages of computerized information processing in these domains were appreciated early, but rather to certain features of the domains that have limited development of computerized systems. Specimens analyzed in these laboratories may undergo many nonautomated processing and interpretive steps; these may take varying periods of time — days, weeks, even months — to complete. In addition, their reports make use of a nonstandard terminology and use variable amounts of natural language text ("free text") in nonstandard formats. These make data storage and retrieval more difficult than for the quantitative domains.

Word processing, combined with coded text retrieval, has been used in such laboratory areas. The development of standardized coding schemes such as SNOMED (*S*ystematized *No*menclature of *Med*icine) have partially resolved some of the problems with nonstandard terminology. These coding schemes provide a way to index and retrieve specimens numerically on the basis of descriptors, such as anatomic location, diagnosis, or cause. Although widely employed, this approach suffers from the general problems of any controlled vocabulary indexing scheme, where the text being indexed may be subject to multiple interpretations or for which the indexers may not be exact. This is especially true when a laboratory modifies index terms to meet its own particular operation. Another approach to the terminology problem entails free text entry, with indexing based upon the use of all uncommon words (key words in context, or KWIC). However, these systems have not gained wide popularity.

Status-of-specimen processing, whereby specimens are tracked through the laboratory, and which assures that appropriate information is associated with the specimen at each stage of processing, is often a problem for computerized systems handling descriptive domains. Because no standard terminology has emerged to describe all of the steps involved, the LIS vendors may adopt an idiosyncratic terminology or format for describing specimen-processing status. This may force a laboratory to make compromises, such as a compromise between making extensive changes in the LIS system to match its operation and making changes in a laboratory's internal procedures to match the system.

The Intralaboratory Cycle — Data Storage and Retrieval

Today, the wide choice of ways to store information has greatly reduced storage and retrieval problems. The best decision for a laboratory requires consideration of the constraints in cost, ease of use, and space. Peripheral storage devices such as magnetic discs offer more rapid retrieval at a higher cost; many laboratories use these modalities for short-term or frequently queried domains. Many laboratories still rely on paper records or magnetic tapes for long-term retrieval; however, this practice often is plagued by storage problems and inefficient retrieval. The availability of other media, such as microfiche, provides for useful and economic alternatives.

Descriptive domains are problematic for both memory-storage and result retrieval because (1) the amount of text required to report a case is unpredictable at the time of specimen receipt; (2) a relatively long and variable period is required for specimen processing (24 hours or more in anatomic pathology, 24 hours to 3 or more weeks in microbiology); and (3) the steps in specimen processing can vary considerably and unpredictably, depending on interpretations made at various stages of specimen processing — for example, a sputum Gram stain and smear showing no organisms and salivary contamination may not be processed further, whereas one showing white cells and a uniform collection of gram-negative organisms will be cultured on a variety of media, with any isolated organisms tested for antibiotic sensitivities. The LIS must be capable of handling these complex storage requirements.

Although the length of time that records must be stored varies for each laboratory, there has been a tendency toward longer periods of storage. Records must be retained for specified periods as stipulated by government regulatory agencies. Stored data can be used for purposes such as replacing lost reports or noting patient trends over long periods of time. Many laboratories, particularly at larger teaching institutions, use records for educational and research purposes. Most laboratories store their reports for at least 1 year; exceptions include blood banks, which must keep blood product records for 5 years, and anatomic pathology services, which often keep their records indefinitely.

It is important to guarantee the confidentiality and security of patient data because of the economic, social, and legal consequences of access by unauthorized persons. The conflict to be resolved is between the need for ease of access dictated by the demands of medical practice and the need to limit access by security measures. Most LISs offer several different levels of protection through the use of passwords and access-limited accounts. In addition, users may be distinguished by what functions they can use in their interaction with the LIS. Typically, physicians have "read-only" access, laboratory technologists have "read and write" access, and supervisory personnel have full privileges.

The Intralaboratory Cycle — Quality Assurance Functions

Quality assurance (quality control) is an essential concern of any laboratory. Its purpose is to monitor the quality of work produced by the laboratory, and thus to ensure that high standards in practice are adhered to. Quality assurance involves several different functions whose common goal is that they permit better laboratory service. Examination of quality-assurance records is an important part of laboratory licensure, while statistics based on quality-control data permits comparison of different laboratories. The LIS can help in quality assurance by storing the various records required and by statistical analysis of control samples.

Repetitive analysis of standard samples with known composition is a standard quality assurance activity and is done for two reasons. Results obtained on control samples included within a particular analytic procedure permit the technologist to verify that the data generated during that particular examination are valid. Statistical analysis of control sample data over longer periods of time can be used for evaluation of the laboratory's accuracy and precision and can detect trends in data due to problems in instruments or reagents (Fig. 18-3).

The "delta" check is a consistency check that involves the review of those test results that exhibit a statistically significant difference from previous analyses performed on the same patient. If a reasonable explanation for this difference cannot be found in the patient's medical condition, then review of other samples analyzed at the same time is performed. This may result in detection of sample mixups, contamination, or reagent errors that otherwise might not be evident. A similar procedure is the absolute limit check, in which test results beyond certain limits are reviewed.

Quality assurance involves maintaining a series of different records. All the equipment and most of the utilities in the laboratory need to be monitored, with the records required for inspections. Each piece of equipment in the laboratory must be maintained; time and personnel must be scheduled for this task. Reagents must be assayed to verify that they are properly prepared and labeled. These and other records are handled much better and with more accuracy in a computerized LIS than by manual systems.

The Extralaboratory Cycle — Reporting Along the Efferent Loop

Once analysis is complete, the results need to be delivered to the ordering physician. Reports need to be a concise, readable, chronologic representation of information if they are to be interpretable. The LIS can not only generate standard report forms but can present the same information in alternative representations that may be more useful in a given situation (Fig. 18-4). Interim reports permit delivery of information about test results as they become available, rather than delaying the report for completion of all the requested testing. Cumulative reports summarize all the information on a patient over a given period of time, with information arranged by related data items. Physician reports summarize the data on all of the patients of a particular physician. Ward reports similarly can be useful, especially if they list the work still waiting to be performed.

Delivery of laboratory reports is often among the greatest problems faced by laboratory directors. Verbal reports are subject to misinterpretation or incomplete data transferral, and manual report de-

(*Text continues on p 308*)

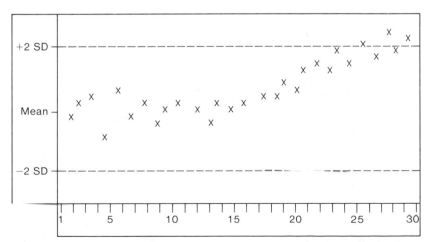

FIGURE 18-3. Analysis of quality assurance data. Several different statistical analyses may be performed on the results found for control samples of known composition. One of the simplest is the Levey-Jennings Statistical Plot. In this plot, the distribution of values about the mean is observed for patterns (dispersion, shifts, trends) that may be due to methodological problems. In the example shown, the results are "in control" during the first half of the month. However, there is an upward trend in the second half of the month, which may indicate an underlying technical problem.

```
OHIO STATE U HOSP              CUMULATIVE REPORT          1417 07/15/86   PG  1
CARL SPEICHER MD LAB DIR NS: U10E   ROOM: 1001 1   H#:
                            DOB: 02/20/1940  SEX: M   R#:
DR: D0349                                             NAME:


        ***********************  H E M A T O L O G Y  ***********************
        TEST:    WBC      RBC    HEMOGLOBN HEMATOCRT    MCV      MCH      MCHC
        LO-HI:   5-10    4.6-6.2   14-18     40-54     82-99    27-31    32-36
        UNITS: THOU/CMM MIL/CMM   GM/DL       %          FL       PG     GM/DL


   R07/13/86    10.9  *   4.59 *   13.7  *   39.6  *    86       29.8     34.6
     1205HR
  \R07/15/86    10.6  *   4.80     14.1      41.0       85       29.4     34.4
  \  1230HR


        TEST:   RDW
        LO-HI: 11.5-14.5
        UNITS:    %

   R07/13/86    13.5
     1205HR
  \R07/15/86    13.4
  \  1230HR

        *********************  D I F F E R E N T I A L  *********************
        TEST:MYEL META BAND  SEG  LYM  MON  EO  BASO COLR SIZE MORP  PLT
        LO:                   50   25   1    0    0
        HI:                   70   40   8    4    2
        UNITS:  %    %    %   %    %    %    %    %
   R07/13/86 0    0    0   81 * 14 * 4    1    0   NMRK NMRK NMRK INCR
     1205HR
  \R07/15/86PEND PEND PEND PEND PEND PEND PEND PEND PEND PEND PEND PEND
  \  1230HR

        ******************  R O U T I N E   C H E M I S T R Y  ****************
        TEST:  GLUCOSE
        LO-HI:  65-115
        UNITS:  MG/DL


   R07/12/86     86
     0915HR
   R07/13/86     86
     0844HR


        ************************  C O M P L E M E N T  ***********************
        TEST:    C3       C4     CH 50
        LO-HI:  97-155   13-44   70-206
        UNITS:  MG/DL    MG/DL  CH50 UNITS

  \R07/14/86    151       30     PENDING
  \  1805HR




        INCR   =  INCREASED
        NMRK   =  NOT REMARKABLE


A                                END OF REPORT                       PG   1
```

FIGURE 18-4. Laboratory result reporting. Many different types of laboratory result formats are visible. (**A**): The cumulative report allows reporting of results in a concise format, with related tests clustered and accompanied by the normal ranges. (**B**): The interpretive report presents the results of one or more related tests and an interpretation based upon those results.

General Consultation Request

The Ohio State University Hospitals

To ___IMMUNOLOGY___ **Date** _____   DOE, JANE
(Physician and/or service)   900-01-9109

☐ **Outpatient**   ☐ **Inpatient**

Provisional Diagnosis:

Reason for Referral:

HEPATITIS PROFILE TESTING

(Use reverse side if necessary) _____ **M.D.**

Report and Opinion of Consultant

Date ___9/10/88___

HEPATITIS PROFILE 1. (DIAGNOSTIC)

PATIENT I.D.

NAME DOE, JANE   DATE
HOSPITAL #   900-01-9109   SPECIMEN # U 2 W

TEST: TEST RESULTS:

HBAG (HB-S-AG)   POSITIVE *
HBCB (HB-C-AB)   POSITIVE *
HAMB (HA-IGM-AB)   NEGATIVE

INTERPRETATION:

SEROLOGICAL EVIDENCE FOR RECENT HEPATITIS-B INFECTION, SUGGEST
RETEST SPECIMEN IN 10-12 WEEKS FOR ANTIBODY TO HEPATITIS-B
SURFACE ANTIGEN (HBAB).

(Use reverse side if necessary) _____ **M.D.**

The Ohio State University
Form 3352 Rev 6/78
(4610011)

1-4 \   **Consults**

B

livery can result in a significant percentage of lost or misplaced reports. As an alternative to these report delivery methods, various transmission devices for communication with the laboratory have been utilized, particularly to key areas such as the emergency room and intensive care units. While pneumatic tube delivery to selected stations has advantages over manual transmission, it is also restricted and expensive. The use of teleprocessing between the laboratory and the wards has greatly improved the ability of laboratories to deliver results rapidly and accurately.

Due to the increases in both the type and the amount of data being generated, it is becoming less acceptable to simply report test result data. One of the most important developments in laboratory medicine has been the interpretive reporting of test results, which is an attempt to transform data into relevant information pertinent to health care. Several workers have presented schemes for interpreting laboratory data with computers. One method has been the implementation of computer-assisted strategies to aid clinical decision-making and highlight important information on recurring patterns and associations of laboratory measurements. Simple attempts in this direction have been made in the past, by (1) marking abnormal results, providing reference values adjacent to test results, grouping data by system or organs; (2) displaying data in more informative ways; (3) computer-generating diagnostic possibilities; (4) making interpretive comments; (5) suggesting additional studies or performing additional studies automatically; and (6) providing reminders when certain clinical situations occur.

Others have attempted to discover relationships in data that are useful for clinical problem-solving, employing various forms of analysis such as multivariate analysis, numeric taxonomy, and discriminant functions. However, recent surveys of interpretive reporting in clinical pathology indicate that although there is a wide variety of interpretive reports currently in use, few are integrated directly into the LIS. To work effectively, the LIS will need to incorporate data retrieval with computer decision aids for interpretive reporting.

CURRENT AND FUTURE REQUIREMENTS FOR LABORATORY INFORMATION SYSTEMS

Modern clinical laboratories must be cost-effective, and being cost-effective requires greater efficiency in all stages of management. Moreover, providing clinicians with laboratory results in formats that aid decision-making can improve patient care. Because many departments in the health-care system not only need to share information but also are computerized, there is an increasing need for "networking" the hospital computers, resulting in highly distributed computer systems.

Cost-Effectiveness

In the past, most hospital laboratories were revenue-generating operations. Today, because of changes in reimbursement legislation, laboratories are facing a conflict between the need to reduce total operating costs and the need to meet the continuing rise in demand for services. It will be an economic necessity that automation, miniaturization, systemization, and computerized information handling in laboratories continue to evolve. There are at least three major ways that the LIS can help contain costs.

First, because personnel costs for wages and benefits represent a significant proportion of any laboratory budget, LIS functions that result in savings in labor will be beneficial. The LIS has proven cost-effective in the performance of numerous clerical functions, such as data collection and report preparation. It may be expected that there will be continued improvements of basic functions, while there is an expansion in analytic and administrative functions.

Second, an LIS can contribute to the decentralization of the clinical laboratories, a process that will result in a significant reduction in transportation time and costs. In the past it was desirable to maintain centralized laboratories, because large automated analyzers were expensive and needed to be operated by highly trained individuals. Newer instruments can perform an increasing number of measurements on smaller samples, and their cost and complexity in operation are decreasing. These instruments employ built-in microcomputers, which control operation and provide digital outputs of fully processed data for direct display or transmission to other computers. With the increasing availability of such instruments, physical dispersion of laboratory testing to other areas is likely, especially where there is high laboratory usage and demand for fast turnaround times. Another development that will contribute to further distribution of chemical analysis is the implantable biosensor. These instruments will provide real-time biochemical information on the patient, without the need for directly collecting specimens or waiting for test results. As the laboratory services become more physically distributed, there will be greater need for flexible distribution of laboratory data, of the information derived from those data, and of analytic information about the different laboratory procedures.

Finally, the LIS can reduce laboratory testing costs by reducing the number of tests performed. More extensive networking of LISs, with creation of regional data banks and long-term storage, would reduce the amount of duplicate testing performed on patients, particularly those transferred between care facilities. By automatic ordering of additional laboratory tests based on symptoms, diagnoses, or screening test results, it is possible to reduce replicate testing and to shorten patient hospital stays.

Management Support Functions

Careful management of clinical laboratories is required for efficient operation. Many of the tasks required are amenable to information-processing techniques.

Personnel management is a very important function, particularly in large laboratories that provide continuous operation throughout the day. In order to perform this task intelligently, one must perform work-load and work-flow analyses. These studies permit each procedure to be reviewed as to the number of times that it was performed, who performed it, and to what extent usage patterns may be changing. This information allows for optimalizing productivity in the laboratory. The College of American Pathologists (CAP) standardized a work-load measurement system in 1978 that has been widely accepted. Under this system, each determination or test procedure is assigned a unit value, which has been determined from time-motion studies done in several laboratories. Each unit represents a minute of clerical or technical time, and reflects the amount of time required to perform the

test; this value may be weighted by considerations such as the method used and the degree of automation involved. The number of tests performed ("raw count") multiplied by the procedure's unit value gives the total work load due to that test. From this information the productivity of each part of a laboratory can be quantitated. Changes in personnel allocation can be made based on analysis of these values. In addition to these calculations, computers can monitor parameters such as laboratory turnaround time or usage volume (Fig. 18-5), in order to maintain efficient service.

Fiscal control is another management activity. Budgets for personnel and purchase of capital equipment or reagents need to be calculated. The billing for the testing performed must be recorded and collected. The LIS significantly reduces errors and decreases the time involved in billing, when compared with manual systems. At the same time, it increases the recovery of charges and permits a greater flexibility in test ordering by allowing tests to be ordered in different combinations.

Inventory control poses a significant problem in certain laboratories.

The blood bank needs to maintain careful inventory of all available blood products, not only within the blood bank itself but also in peripheral storage sites such as in the operating suite. The blood bank is required by regulations to maintain exact records for all specimens received, tests performed, blood products transfused, and adverse reactions reported. Microbiology and other laboratories may similarly maintain large inventories of frozen organisms or cells. Database capabilities in the LIS can greatly simplify the paperwork entailed in such data storage situations.

Managers must ensure that the laboratories meet licensure requirements and regulations, which have been increasing since the passage of the Clinical Laboratories Improvement Act of 1967. Currently several general agencies inspect and cer-

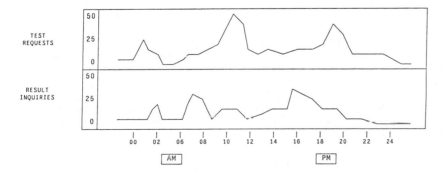

TEST REQUESTS

RESULT INQUIRIES

FIGURE 18-5. Assistance for making management decisions. The LIS computer can be used to monitor test ordering and test result inquiry patterns. This information can be used to determine staffing for periods of more critical need. In this example, maximum staffing for logging test results should be planned to cover the hours of 1 A.M., AND 7 P.M.

tify clinical laboratories, notably the Joint Committee for Accreditation of Hospitals and CAP. In addition, some laboratory divisions are inspected by specialty organizations such as the American Association of Blood Banks and the Nuclear Regulatory Commission. These groups all set certain standards for test performance and for the laboratory work environment. By maintaining records and manuals, the LIS can greatly simplify the clerical labor involved in preparing for laboratory inspections.

Decision Support Aids

In the future computers will be increasingly used to assist physicians in the ordering and the interpretation of laboratory test data. Not only is the sheer volume of laboratory testing already beyond the capacity of humans to assimilate it, but the knowledge required to effectively use it is vast and constantly increasing. The combination of these factors has caused clinicians either to underutilize or to misinterpret a large proportion of the laboratory data from their patients. It has been shown that

1. A high percentage of significantly abnormal laboratory results have no measurable effect on physician decisions.
2. A significant disparity exists between the criteria that physicians use to determine whether a laboratory measurement has changed and the analytic limitations for detecting such a change, based on the underlying methodology.
3. Laboratory utilization differs significantly between physicians managing patients with similar diagnoses.

A number of recent studies have supported the thesis that current laboratory utilization is less than ideal and suggest that it is often both inappropriate and excessive.

Improvements in the capabilities of the LIS for data retrieval and manipulation can be employed to make patient data more interpretable. The benefits of being able to interpret a patient's results in reference to precisely defined populations matched to the patient's personal characteristics or to the patient's prior data have long been appreciated. By being able to store and collate large amounts of information, the LIS can provide a greater ability to define the normal and abnormal values for the body's chemical constituents. Correction of patient results for the influence of drugs and physiologic abnormalities will become possible through alter-

ing or rejecting affected test data. The development of information systems banks in such areas as the causes of specific laboratory abnormalities will allow retrieval of otherwise relatively inaccessible information. Information services from the laboratory such as on-line assistance for test interpretation should become commonplace.

The decision models used in the past have paralleled the mathematic models most popular in computer-assisted diagnostic systems: Baye's theorem, decision analysis, algorithms, or sequential branching strategies. Knowledge-based LIS decision support modules incorporating the techniques of artificial intelligence are just beginning to emerge. We expect that knowledge-based expert systems will increasingly be incorporated into the LIS. Expert systems technology has been applied in a limited way to some laboratory interpretation tasks already and reached sufficient maturity to be incorporated in commercial products. For example, the EXPERT language has been used for construction of a series of decision-making models for endocrinology, serum protein analysis, and interpretation of a select number of enzyme tests. Several of these modules are now available as add-ons for a commercially available serum protein electrophoresis instrument.

Distributed Computing Systems

In the past many LISs were designed to run on a single, stand-alone minicomputer, which handled all of the information system functions. This choice was dictated by the available computer technology. However, for efficient laboratory operation, more flexible computational abilities and communication links between the individual laboratory divisions are required. Laboratory divisions require communication links with other hospital services outside the laboratory (Fig. 18-6). The needs for communication to acquire and disseminate data are compatible with the use of distributed computing through networked computers. Much of the data required for efficient operation could be obtained by communication with sophisticated data-processing modules embedded in laboratory instruments and with on-line data sources located outside of the actual laboratory (the hospital information system, or HIS).

One view of an organizational hierarchy of computers is that of three tiers of computing (Fig. 18-7). One level consists of the central hospital computer (or a distributed network of computers utilized by other departments), which handles pa-

Hospital Division	Laboratory	Information
ER, ICU, OR, wards	Blood Bank Chemistry Hematology Microbiology Surgical Pathology	Blood product usage Chemical analyses Blood indices Culture results Tissue diagnoses
Monitoring services (Epidemiology, Tumor Registry, etc.)	Microbiology Surgical Pathology	Bacterial isolates Tumor diagnoses
Support Services (Pharmacy, Sterile Supply, etc.)	Chemistry Microbiology	Drug levels Drug adverse effect Sterility checks Drug susceptibility

FIGURE 18-6. Some examples of the communication exchanges between laboratory divisions and different hospital departments.

FIGURE 18-7. Organization of an information system into tiers.

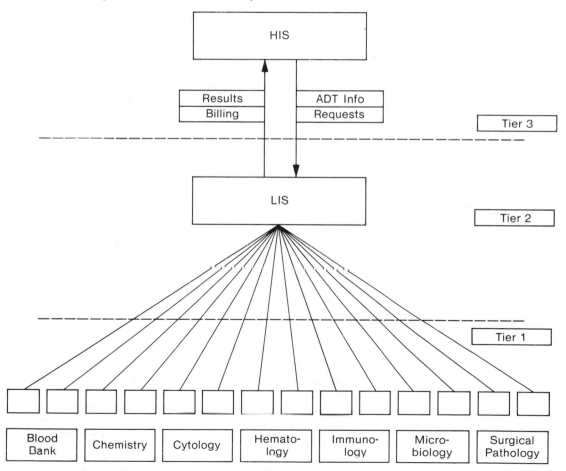

tient demographics, result reporting, and billing. The next level is a centralized laboratory computer, which collates data and maintains centralized patient records and permits interlaboratory communication. At the lower level, microcomputers and minicomputers are dispersed in the divisional laboratories; these locally process data and transmit it to the central computer for further processing and merging with patient data.

In the future, the HIS will probably be a high distributed computing environment with networking of specialized computers in the different patient care areas. The LIS will likewise be a distributed computer network, with the microcomputers in instruments communicating with more powerful processors that collate data, generate reports, perform data correlations, and execute medical-interpretive functions. The LIS will interface to other hospital data sources, not only for the transmission of laboratory data, but also for collection of the necessary data required for more detailed interpretive functions.

CHOOSING AN LIS

Choosing an LIS involves addressing the following major issues:

1. Is it really necessary?
2. What needs to be computerized and to what extent?
3. What resources, particularly how much money, are available?
4. Should system development be done in-house or by an outside vendor?
5. Will the system interface with other computer systems, either internal or external to the laboratory?
6. What guidelines are to be used assessing the different options?

Necessity of Computerization

Before computerization is decided upon as a solution to a problem, it is first necessary to decide exactly what problems are to be addressed and what benefits are to be achieved by computerization. Simply putting something on a computer may not make a problem any more solvable or easy to deal with, because many problems are not optimally handled by computer. A systems analysis should therefore be performed to define the problems to be considered for computerization and to help in deciding what options are available for their solution.

Some Benefits of a Computerized Laboratory Information System

Decrease in turnaround time

Decrease in clerical errors and loss of results

Decrease in boring and tedious jobs

Flexibility in report formats and interpretations

Increased accuracy in patient and research data retrieval

Increased accuracy in billing information

Increased accuracy in quality control data and inventory records

Increased efficiency and productivity of technologists

Optimalization of work flow and organization

A comparison off the expected cost for an LIS to its potential benefits is a fundamental question in determining the need for computerization. The potential benefits of a LIS can be great, as shown above. However, the cost of most systems is also great, because it includes not only the expense of the system but also personnel and supply costs. Many laboratory directors and health-care officials have expressed dissatisfaction at the economic impact of computers in laboratory medicine, citing the failure to see any drop in laboratory expenses since the introduction of their use. However, evaluation of the direct and indirect economic impacts of a laboratory information system does not support this view. The direct economic impact of such systems includes decreased data handling expenses, greater personnel productivity, and greater control over finances, particularly with regard to recoverable charges. The indirect economic impact includes improved patient care and improved laboratory morale. When evaluating the economic impact of an information system, one must examine factors that affect laboratory expenses (inflation, billing practices of the institution) and reevaluate managerial decisions that may be resulting in a failure to use the system optimally.

Extent of Computerization

Key factors in determining the choice of an LIS are the size of the laboratory, the size of the hospital in which the laboratory is located, and whether the entire laboratory or only some of its divisions are to be computerized. In general, options for a small laboratory in a small hospital are more extensive than for a large laboratory in a large teaching hospital.

For most laboratories, a single integrated computer system is preferable to several different systems, because an integrated system is usually easier to manage. A single system requires less redundancy in training of personnel, fewer supply-storage problems, simpler exchange of data, and better data integration. However, because of economic or other practical considerations, compromises may be required.

Available Resources

Based on what goals are decided on, sufficient resources must be available. Requirements for a computer system include the following:

A proper environment
Proper support personnel
Proper training of laboratory personnel
An adequate budget
Support from the administration

If any of these requirements is inadequate, it is better to reevaluate goals than to proceed with computerization.

In-House Versus Vendor System Development

An LIS may be developed either through in-house ("do-it-yourself") development or by purchase from a commercial software vendor of a "turnkey" system. In-house LIS development typically utilizes personnel and hardware of an already existing hospital computer system. Although this approach would seem to be effective use of available computer resources, many of these systems have failed. This is because of the difficulty of the task as well as the need to maintain software for long periods by persons familiar with the unique features of the system. Moreover, much of the work required is duplication of efforts done by other ("reinventing the wheel").

The majority of laboratories use vendor-developed commercial systems, specifically designed for use in the clinical laboratory. These "turnkey" systems derive their name from the theory that one can purchase an entire computer system, have it installed, and begin operation by simply "turning the key." There are several advantages to this approach of LIS development. The extremely high cost involved in the development of a computer system is

distributed among the many users, as is the cost of software maintenance and updating. Groups of system users can solve common problems, advise the vendor about the needs for improvements in programs, and develop new computer programs. However, several potential problems can occur if a turnkey system is purchased (as listed below). Most of these problems are well-known, so that the hazards can be minimized. For example, most vendors offer more flexibility in system function, through the use of modular programs and of table-driven system definitions. Still, every system has problems, and therefore a careful comparison between potential choices is necessary.

Evaluation of each prospective vendor provided system should include the following:

Interviewing other users of the LIS, especially those with laboratories and hospitals similar in size to one's own hospital
Visiting one or more sites where the LIS is installed
Having an on-site demonstration of the system
Clarifying what is provided by the vendor for each level of support, with a review of the contract by a lawyer
Checking on the viability of the vendor and the stability of the programming support staff.

In general, it is advisable to avoid using a system that integrates the hardware of several manufacturers and to avoid being the first laboratory to use a new computer system (or to implement a major software change).

Integration with Other Computer Systems

Interfacing the LIS with other computers over a network is desirable for both medical and fiscal management, because it allows both transfer of ADT and billing information and rapid exchange of information. If interfacing is a possibility, it is important to know which machines will be communicating and what information is to be exchanged. It is essential

---

Some Hazards of Vendor Systems

Restriction in computer choices to those dictated by the vendor
A loss of flexibility in laboratory operations
The expense to modify and to maintain changes
Dependence on the vendor's commercial viability

to know whether the LIS hardware allows interfacing and how accessible the data is for exchange.

Comparison of Options

The choice of an LIS from among the alternative systems requires a careful evaluation of the systems, with comparison of the laboratory's information-processing needs with the functions provided by the different systems available.

This process has been greatly simplified by independent evaluations, which exhaustively compare the features of the commercial systems. The MedSy and Johnson reports are two early comparisons; CAP and the American Society of Clinical Pathologists maintain information on computer systems.

BIBLIOGRAPHY

Aller RD, Elevitch FR: Symposium in the Clinical Laboratory, Clinics in Laboratory Medicine, Vol 3, Philadelphia, WB Saunders, 1983

Chou D, McLendon WW: Information management. In Henry JB (ed): Todd-Sanford-Davidsohn Clinical Diagnosis and Management by Laboratory Methods, 17th ed, pp 1401–1415.

Grams RR (ed): The MedSy Report on Clinical Laboratory Computer Systems. Medical Systems Research, Inc, Gainesville Florida, 1981

Grams RR, Peck GC: National Survey of Hospital Data Processing — 1985. J Med Syst 10:423–568, 1986

Griesser G, Jardel JP et al (eds): Data Protection in Health Information Systems. North Holland, New York, 1983

Heusghem C, Albert A, Benson ES: Advanced Interpretation of Clinical Laboratory Data. New York, Marcel Dekker, 1982

Johnson JL: Achieving the Optimum Information System for the Laboratory. J. Lloyd Johnson Associates, Northbrook, Illinois, 1975

Speicher CE, Smith JW: Choosing Effective Laboratory Tests. Philadelphia, WB Saunders, 1983

Statland BE, Burke WP, Galen RS: Quantitative Approaches Used in Evaluating Laboratory Measurements and Other Clinical Data. Philadelphia, WB Saunders, 1979

nineteen

Concepts of Preventive Maintenance for Laboratory Instrumentation

Judith Thompson
Peggy Prinz Luebbert

The establishment and documentation of preventive maintenance programs has become a responsibility of pathologists, clinical chemists, and medical technologists as a result of requirements by accrediting agencies. Preventive maintenance should also be considered from a practical point of view. A patient's treatment is often dependent upon quick turnaround time for critical laboratory tests; so any type of equipment malfunction could potentially affect patient care. When an instrument malfunctions, it is very expensive for a laboratory to maintain backup equipment or send tests to another laboratory.

The purpose of a preventive maintenance program is to ensure that equipment operates properly and safely. Yapit described a comprehensive system of preventive maintenance, including instrument manuals, troubleshooting specialists, and breakdown/repair documentation that resulted in a 54% reduction in downtime.[11] This can be accomplished by checking critical operating characteristics of an instrument and performing the recommended maintenance on a scheduled basis. Preventive maintenance can be divided into two categories: function

verification, which includes checks and tests to ensure that an instrument is working properly and is correctly calibrated; and maintenance, which includes replacement, adjustment, or repair to prolong the life of an instrument and prevent mechanical malfunctions.[6] When developing and organizing a preventive maintenance program, the following should be considered:

Government and accrediting agency requirements
Instrument selection and implementation
Documentation
Performance responsibility of personnel

GOVERNMENT AND ACCREDITING AGENCY REQUIREMENTS

At this time there is no government legislation specifically requiring all laboratories to have a preventive maintenance program. The Clinical Laboratory Improvement Act of 1967 (CLIA '67) requires that laboratories licensed for interstate commerce maintain records, equipment, and facilities necessary for effective operation of the laboratory. The Health Care Financing Administration (HCFA) regulates, inspects, and licenses laboratories that are covered by CLIA '67. The Centers for Disease Control (CDC) evaluates the HCFA program by unannounced laboratory inspections. The HCFA recognizes both Joint Commission on Accreditation of Healthcare Organizations (JCAHO) and College of American Pathologists (CAP) accreditation as assurance of compliance with regulations. These accrediting agencies have specific requirements for preventive maintenance programs. The JCAHO outlines general guidelines requiring a system of periodic maintenance, inspection, and performance testing for all equipment and instruments with appropriate documentation.[1] The CAP requires a detailed program of preventive maintenance with documentation and provides the laboratory with a checklist of requirements that must be met upon inspection.[4] This checklist covers instrument operating characteristics, interval of inspection and maintenance, tolerance limits, and documentation. Meeting requirements for accreditation is not a major task if a laboratory establishes a preventive maintenance program following these guidelines and maintains documentation on a routine basis.[4]

INSTRUMENT SELECTION AND IMPLEMENTATION

Preventive maintenance programs begin by selecting instruments that will operative effectively for a reasonable period of time. The routine operation of the instrument should be considered. Is it an instrument that will be used by many people and operated 24 hours a day, or is it a highly specialized instrument that will be used infrequently? Before purchasing an instrument, inquiries should be made at laboratories using similar equipment regarding the performance record of their particular instrument and the quality of service provided by the manufacturer.

When the decision has been made to purchase an instrument, specific items should be outlined in the purchase contract. These should include installation of the instrument, training of personnel, and an evaluation period (generally 30 to 60 days) during which the instrument can be returned at no cost if it does not meet expected performance.

As soon as an instrument is delivered and installed, it should be evaluated. Before the evaluation it is important to define specific operating characteristics with tolerable limits or performance for acceptance. The manufacturer's operation manual is a good reference source, as are publications on laboratory instrumentation. These publications list function checks needed and frequency of performance.[2, 10] After the instrument has been evaluated and has met the criteria for acceptance, it can be implemented for routine use. At this time a preventive maintenance program for the instrument should be initiated. The operating parameters and tolerance limits that have been defined in the initial evaluation can be incorporated into the program.

For some instruments commercial service is required as part of the routine preventive maintenance program. For example, cleaning the objectives, oiling, and aligning a microscope require skill and should not be attempted by an untrained person. Also, analytic balances should be cleaned and calibrated annually by a qualified service agent. Service contracts can be purchased for more sophisticated instruments that may include routine calibration and maintenance. When considering a service contract, one should note whether parts, labor, travel, emergency service, and calibration are covered. Also, the availability of competent in-house service personnel should be considered.

An important aspect of implementing a new instrument into routine use is training of personnel.[8] This can be accomplished in several ways. The company representative who installs an instrument generally will give basic instructions on use and care. Often the manufacturer holds an instrument training program at its applications laboratory for technologists. The training session and expenses can be included as part of the initial purchase agreement. In-house continuing education sessions are an effective way of informing groups of technologists about the underlying principles and operation of the instrument and preventive maintenance procedures. An obvious source of instruction, but one that is frequently overlooked, is the operation manual provided with the instrument. It contains basic operating instructions, maintenance, and a troubleshooting guide. The operation manual and warranty should always be kept in a convenient location near the instrument.

When an instrument has been carefully chosen, its operating characteristics evaluated, its operators well-trained, and preventive maintenance regularly performed, it should perform well for its expected lifetime.

DOCUMENTATION

The key to a good preventive maintenance program is organization. This includes developing protocols for function checks and routine maintenance for each instrument, performing these checks at scheduled intervals, and carefully documenting this information and any repair work or service done to the instrument.[3] It is important for these records to be complete and kept up to date.

Organization of a program begins with a careful inventory of all equipment and instrumentation. This inventory can be in the form of a card file, notebook, or computer listing. It should include the following information for each item of equipment: name of instrument, manufacturer, model number, serial number, inventory number, purchase date and price, service representative, and service phone numbers. It also may be helpful to include a list of spare parts with part description number, price, and vendor (Fig. 19-1). A copy of the list of spare parts should also be filed with the inventory control department of the laboratory.

After all equipment has been itemized, an outline of function checks and routine maintenance must be developed for each instrument (Table 19-1). The instrument operation manual contains a list of necessary function checks, a maintenance protocol, and a troubleshooting guide. If the operation manual has been misplaced, it can be replaced by contacting the manufacturer's headquarters. Other sources of information are also available.[2,10]

After the function checks and routine maintenance requirements have been outlined, a written protocol should be developed. This should include performance criteria as well as concise, step-by-step instructions covering each item in the outline. Performance criteria for each function check can be obtained from the operation manual or other reference sources.[6, 10] Also, information from an in-house evaluation of the instrument can be used. This written protocol should also include a brief troubleshooting guide or referral to the troubleshooting guide in the operation manual. A typical written maintenance protocol for wavelength calibration check, using the holmium oxide filter from the Chemetrics Spectro-Standard set, is listed below:

1. Turn operation switch ON, tungsten lamp ON, filter to appropriate setting for wavelength being checked, lamp selector to VISIBLE, sensitivity to HIGH.
2. Read instructions included with Chemetrics Standard set on handling of filters.
3. Place holmium oxide filter in cell holder of spectrophotometer.
4. Set wavelength on spectrophotometer at 536 nm.

5. Turn operation switch to METER. Adjust transmittance to approximately 50% T.
6. Slowly change the wavelength on either side of the selected value until a minimum % T value is obtained. (Do final rotating of knob in clockwise direction to eliminate backlash error.)
7. Wavelength of minimum % T should correspond to specific holmium oxide value within the tolerances specified by the spectrophotometer manufacturer (± 0.5 nm). If adjustment is required, see operation manual.

A system of charts and records should also be developed. Each laboratory can devise charts that best suit its needs. A good chart should include a title, date, results of a function check, comments, and a place for the technologist's and reviewer's initials. It is also helpful to include the established performance limits so the technologist can immediately see whether the day's reading is acceptable. The chart should be simple, well-organized, and permit easy and rapid review of equipment function (Fig. 19-2).

A maintenance schedule should be established and incorporated into the routine work load. Many different types of reminder techniques have been developed.[9,7] Specific tasks may be assigned to a work unit or person; and a reminder system of calendars, charts, and file cards can be developed (Fig.19-3). Provision should also be made for doing critical function checks and maintenance on weekends and during the evening and night shift. The checklists as well as charts and written protocols should be kept on the bench next to the instrument so that the technologist has easy access to them.

(*Text continues on p 321*)

Table 19-1
Spectrophotometer Maintenance Outline

Function Verification

1. Check linearity with NBS standard weekly.
2. Check wavelength calibration monthly.
3. Check for stray light monthly.

Routine Maintenance

1. Check cuvette well weekly.
2. Dust optical surfaces weekly.
3. Check excitor lamp monthly.
4. Check silica gel monthly

(front side)

INVENTORY RECORD CARD

Name of Instrument:_____
Laboratory Location:_____
Model Number:_____
Serial Number:_____
Inventory Number:_____
Manufacturer:_____
Purchase Date:_____
Purchase Price:_____
Service Representative:_____
Service Phone Number:_____

(back side)

SPARE PARTS

Description	Order Number	Price	Vendor

FIGURE 19-1. Inventory record card (5 in x 7 in).

Daily refrigerator/freezer temperatures _____ 19 _____

Room # _____ Refrigerator or freezer # _____

Limits: ± 5°C of assigned temperature _____

Reviewed by _____

Date	Initial	Temperature	Comments	Date	Initial	Temperature	Comments
1				16			
2				17			
3				18			
4				19			
5				20			
6				21			
7				22			
8				23			
9				24			
10				25			
11				26			
12				27			
13				28			
14				29			
15				30			

FIGURE 19-2. Daily maintenance chart.

A troubleshooting log for each instrument must be maintained. The following should be included: problem, action taken, comments, date, and technologist's initials (Fig. 19-4). When the service representative repairs the instrument, this information can be obtained from the customer's copy of the service report.

It may be beneficial to incorporate a survey program into the preventive maintenance program.[5] The CAP conducts an instrument survey program, which can be used for comparison of instrument performance with established standards and other laboratories. Check samples are provided for spectrophotometers, analytic balances, and pH meters. Each participating laboratory receives a summary of all data obtained for the check sample, as well as educational material outlining procedures for calibration and performance validation.

PERFORMANCE RESPONSIBILITY

Responsibility and accountability for a preventive maintenance program begin with the technologist at the bench. Before attempting to use an instrument, the technologist must learn the operation of the instrument, its performance capabilities, preventive maintenance protocol, documentation, and simple troubleshooting. This is accomplished by on-the job training, continuing education seminars,

WEEK I			DATE	INITIALS
Clean Mechanical Pipettes				
Clean Heat Sealers				
Check and Clean Balances				
Platelet Quality Control (4 units/month)				
Temp of Incoming Shipment	Source	Temp		
WEEK II				
Clean All Microscopes				
JHH Platelet Culture—Unit #				
Donor Arm Culture—Unit #				
Check and Clean Refrigerated Centrifuges				
Temp of Incoming Shipment	Source	Temp		
WEEK III				
Check Refrigerator & Freezer Alarms				
Temp of Incoming Shipment	Source	Temp		
WEEK IV				
Check FFP and Cryo				
Check Thermometers Against Standard				
Check Heat Blocks and Water Baths				
Check Agglutination Viewing Mirrors				
Check Platelet Rotator				
Temp of Incoming Shipment	Source	Temp		

FIGURE 19-3. Monthly maintenance and quality control chart. (Baldwin M, Barrasso C: The development and operation of an efficient laboratory preventive maintenance program. Am J Med Technol 45:216–218, 1979)

manufacturer's training programs, and reading the operation manual provided with the instrument. The technologist performs the daily function verification and routine maintenance for the instrument. Each time an instrument reading is taken, it should be compared with established performance criteria. If the reading exceeds these limits, the technologist should perform simple troubleshooting to restore

instrument function or notify the supervisor so that appropriate action can be taken. This should be carefully documented in the troubleshooting log by recording the problems, corrective action, date, and technologist's initials.

The department supervisor is responsible for coordination and review of the preventive maintenance program. The supervisor should designate

Date:_____

Technologist:_____

Service Representative:_____

Costs:_____

Problem:_____

_____

_____

_____

_____

Action Taken:_____

_____

_____

_____

Comments:_____

_____

_____

_____

_____

_____

FIGURE 19-4. Trouble-shooting log and repair record.

specific maintenance assignments and provide a schedule with effective reminders for bench technologists. Preventive maintenance should be scheduled during a time when the instrument is not heavily used. These assignments should be given to a specific person or work unit, which provides a system of accountability. The supervisor should review all records on a monthly basis to ensure that the procedures are being carried out, identify potential problems, and review corrective action. The supervisor usually initiates all repair work and sees that it is documented.

A full-time or part-time instrumentation technologist can be very beneficial. This position can be effective for a small laboratory that does not have access to biomedical engineers or for a large laboratory that has a wide variety of equipment requiring one person to effectively coordinate and maintain the preventive maintenance program. General qualifications for this position include a medical technology background with a special interest in instrumentation and electronics. This person should be responsible for all preventive maintenance and troubleshooting for equipment. He should be able to provide emergency repairs, communicate with the service representative, maintain an inventory of spare parts, supervise the maintenance program, and instruct technologists and students on the care

and troubleshooting of laboratory instrumentation. Having an instrumentation technologist coordinate the preventive maintenance program can result in repair-cost savings and reduction of instrument downtime.

Most large hospitals and institutions have biomedical engineers responsible for general repair and maintenance of all hospital instrumentation. They provide a useful service to the laboratory by repairing common instruments, such as centrifuges and water baths; installing replacement parts; and doing emergency repair. Plant maintenance engineers can be called upon to provide service for refrigerators and freezers.

Generally, all instrument manufacturers have field service representatives who have been trained to repair their instruments. They provide service on a request basis as well as initial set-up and testing of a new instrument. Their services can also be covered by a service contract. When a service representative is called for instrument repair, the laboratory should explain the problem, how it was identified, and what initial repair work has been done. When field service is necessary, the service representative should be prompt, answering the call within 24 hours if the problem is acute and affecting patient care. When the service representative arrives, the laboratory should have someone available to explain the problem and provide necessary assistance. After the repair work has been done, the representative should fill out a field service report, listing the problem, work done, and cost (parts, labor, travel). These services may be covered by a warranty or service contract or paid by individual call. Good communication between the representative and customer is important for good service.

BENEFITS OF PREVENTIVE MAINTENANCE

The preventive maintenance program should be periodically reviewed for the frequency and cost of repairs for each instrument. The program should be analyzed for determining whether (1) a change should be made in preventive maintenance frequency or inspection points; (2) certain preventive maintenance checks should be discontinued for equipment needing infrequent repair; (3) modification, overhaul, or replacement of equipment is needed owing to the increasing costs of the maintenance and repairs; and (4) a service contract is cost-effective. A preventive maintenance program is cost-effective when repairs and adjustments are made at a convenient time instead of when a breakdown occurs. This decreases the number of outside service calls, lowers repair costs, and decreases equipment downtime. A well-organized preventive maintenance program can provide additional benefits to the laboratory. A good program improves the morale and self-confidence of the technologists by giving them a working knowledge of how to use and take care of instruments. It also reduces the frustration caused by an inefficiently operating instrument. The technologist will have the confidence needed for accurate laboratory results when he know his instrument is performing at the desired levels of precision and accuracy.

REFERENCES

1. Accreditation Manual for Hospitals. Chicago, Joint Commission of Hospitals, 1980
2. A Guide on Laboratory Administration. Publication VIII, Maintenance. Laboratory Consultation Office, Bureau of Laboratories, Centers for Disease Control, Atlanta, 1976
3. Baldwin M, Barrasso C: The development and operation of an efficient laboratory preventive maintenance program. Am J Med Technol 45:216–218, 1979
4. College of American Pathologists Inspection Checklist. Chicago, Commission on Inspection and Accreditation, College of American Pathologists, 1980
5. Hamill RD: Quality control in the laboratory. Clin Toxicol 12, No. (2):213–217, 1978
6. Hamlin WB, Duckworth JK, Gilmer PR, et al: Laboratory Instrumentation Maintenance Manual. Chicago, College of American Pathologists, 1977
7. Jaglinski K: A flexible reminder system for preventative maintenance. MLO 8(5):79–86, 1976
8. Lee LW (ed): Elementary Principles of Laboratory Instruments, 4th ed, pp 287–289. St Louis, CV Mosby, 1978
9. McDonald CW: Keeping track of preventive maintenance. MLO 12(3):77–84, 1980
10. Ottaviano PJ, DiSalvo AF: Quality Control in the Clinical Laboratory: A Procedural Text, pp 9–16. Baltimore, University Park Press, 1977
11. Yapit MK: Keeping your instruments happy. MLO 15(11):33–39, 1983

ANNOTATED BIBLIOGRAPHY

Accreditation Manual for Hospitals. Chicago, Joint Commission of Hospitals, 1980

In this manual, the Joint Commission of Hospitals lists general requirements for an accredited preventive maintenance program. It outlines a basic system of periodic maintenance, inspection, and performance testing for most equipment and instruments used in the clinical laboratory. It also describes the appropriate documentation needed for an acceptable program.

A Guide on Laboratory Administration. Publication VIII, Maintenance. Atlanta, Laboratory Management Consultation Office, Bureau of Laboratories, Centers for Disease Control, 1976

The benefits of preventive maintenance on laboratory instruments are outlined in this section of the guide published by Health and Human Services, the Centers for Disease Control. A detailed description on how to set up and evaluate a successful preventive maintenance program is also discussed. The appendices in this section include an example of a preventive maintenance card, recommended preventive maintenance check points, and frequencies of inspection for 11 laboratory instruments.

Hamlin WB, Duckworth JK, Gilmer PR et al: Laboratory Instrument Maintenance Manual, Chicago, College of American Pathologists, 1977

This manual provides basic information on two important aspects of instrument quality control: function verification and preventive maintenance. A specific format for each instrument or general category of instrument is used to describe principles of operation, installation requirements, suggested function verification, and preventive maintenance activities.

twenty

Basics of Clinical Laboratory Safety

M. Robert Hicks

The goal of a laboratory safety program is to provide the facility, equipment, training, and atmosphere necessary for employees to have a healthful place in which to complete their tasks in an efficient manner. This responsibility must be assured by the employer and has been assigned to him by law under the Occupational Safety and Health Act (OSHA) of 1970.[35] This law, however, does not in itself produce a safe work place. It only stipulates what an employee has a right to expect of the employer as far as workplace safety is concerned and who is responsible if accidents occur. Workplace safety is the result of the education and cooperation of all parties involved and demands action to sustain it.

In any situation where hazardous materials are involved, special precautions must be taken to safeguard those who are directly involved with the handling and processing of the compounds.[31] Where these materials are in the form of waste products, the well-being of safety of the general public must also be considered. The proper disposal of waste material is of utmost concern when it contains infectious, flammable, toxic, and radioactive substances. These materials can be hazardous to all who become contaminated with them. For this reason, these substances must be treated to be rendered harmless or diluted to safe levels before disposal. Some radioactive wastes may need to be isolated from the environment. Organic compounds and solvents should be burned, thus converted to

carbon dioxide and water. Compounds that are extremely toxic or that may become concentrated in nature should be reclaimed. In this way the workplace, the population, and the environment is protected.

The first step in dealing with a hazardous situation is to identify the dangerous steps and materials that are present in it. In the laboratory, this requires thorough knowledge of the procedure, instrumentation, sample to be analyzed, and miscellaneous equipment that may be used. The knowledge must cover instrument operation and all reagents employed, as well as the procedures for disposal of any chemical or waste product. Only when knowledge is coupled with a fair amount of common sense is it possible to make intelligent safety policies. Arbitrary rules by the uninformed all too often breed contempt for any policy.

HAZARDS OF THE WORKPLACE

A hazard of the workplace can be identified as anything that can cause injury or illness to the employee or the general public. Because of the many procedures, instruments, reagents, and types of samples analyzed, the hazards in the laboratory are many and varied.

Another cause of accidents is the thoughtlessness of people. The personal habits of some can be hazardous to them and to others around them. This complicates a safety program, and one must plan for the unknown as well as the known.[14] When employees are not able to correct their dangerous work habits, they may have to be removed from their area; and when employees are unwilling to make corrections, their attitude must be considered as grounds for disciplinary action, transfer, or dismissal.

Mechanical Hazards

Although the clinical laboratory does not have the heavy machinery normally associated with mechanical hazards, dangerous conditions are always present with some instruments and can develop with the misuse of others. For this reason, one should be ever mindful of the fact that carelessness breeds accidents.

Blenders and centrifuges are used routinely without problems, but these instruments can be extremely dangerous when normal care is not exercised in their use. When one is preparing emulsions of biologic specimens, blender speeds are very high; and rotor knife blades, when uncovered, can mutilate fingers as well as blend solutions. Aerosols can also be released when sealed blender chambers are not used or when the blender chamber ruptures. For this reason, blenders and homogenizers should be used in a hood or safety cabinet so that the user is protected and spills can be controlled.

The centrifuge is probably the most frequently used instrument in the clinical laboratory; and if it is not guarded by very strong side walls and heavy, locking covers, accidents that should be nothing more than nerve-wracking episodes can be very serious, if not fatal. Most of the problems with the centrifuge stem from the construction of the horizontal heads where the carriers fit into place and with the balancing of the load. When the carriers of a horizontal-head centrifuge are hung in position at 0 rpm, the cups are in the vertical position. As the motor starts up and the speed increases, however, the carriers will rotate to a horizontal position. When the carriers are not in the correct position, or when they are binding because of damage to the head, they can turn out of the holding slots and crash against the side of the centrifuge. The same thing can happen when the wrong head or wrong cups are used and the carriers swing out against the side of the centrifuge. These problems generally develop after the head has been sprung out of shape and the trunnion rings and cups have come off the heads before high speed is attained. A far more serious accident can happen when the heads have

been weakened or the safe speed or load has been exceeded. When this happens, the trunnion rings, cups, and load will fly loose after revolutions per minute have been reached. These missiles can then penetrate the sides of the centrifuge and destroy anything in a wide arc. Any of these accidents can spill or propel hazardous aerosols into the surrounding area to complicate the first accident.

The centrifugation of volatile organic solvents presents special problems of fire and explosion when sufficient organic vapors are released. Centrifugation of volatile organic solvents requires a centrifuge designed for use in hazardous atmospheres. General ventilation should be sufficient to dilute and remove any escaping vapors from the flammable liquids. Refrigeration could also be of some help in reducing volatility of the liquid.

One aspect of compressed gas in cylinders that must be considered as a mechanical hazard in transportation and careless handling. The tanks must have the screw caps on at all times when they are not in use, because the caps protect the valves at the top of the tanks. Also, the tanks should be fastened in place in an upright position by a strap or chain. When transported, they should be moved by cart and held in place by a strap.[37] These precautions are necessary because the internal pressures of the tanks can be as high as 2200 psi, which is sufficient to propel the tanks like a rocket.[14] Runaway tanks have been known to generate enough energy to damage a cement-block wall. If the tank is filled with a flammable gas, this destruction can be compounded by fire or explosion.

Electrical Hazards

One of the hazards of any area is the possibility of electrical current passing through a person. When the amount of current is enough to cause a physiologic change or a physical sensation, it is referred to as *shock*. The safe limits for this kind of current flow in specific circumstances has been determined and reported by the Association for the Advancement of Medical Instrumentation.[1] This value has been set at 500 μamp for laboratory instruments not used in patient contact. Any instrument not meeting this requirement should be taken out of service until this hazard has been corrected.

The loss or absence of a third-wire ground on any instrument must not be overlooked either by accident or by intention, because this can result in personal injury as well as property damage. For this reason, certain electrical checks should be made whenever electrical circuits have been changed or altered and at regular intervals thereafter. These checks are as follows:

Third-wire ground must be intact

Polarity must not be reversed

Minimum tension must be applied to all electrical outlet contacts

Correct voltage must be applied to outlet

Current leakage must be under 500 μamp

Power cord insulation must not be broken or frayed

Infectious Hazards

Pathogenic microorganisms whose presence may or may not be suspected can cause infectious hazards. If one is working in microbiology, mycology, or virology, one is almost always alert to the possibility of pathogenic organisms being present, and the routine technique is set up to handle these situations. However, the careless person, the thoughtless slip in technique, the poor safety procedure, or the unexpected pathogen has caused unnecessary infections of laboratory personnel.[15,24,47] For this reason, certain precautions must be taken to eliminate or at least decrease the potential of microbiologic infections of the work place.

The handling of known infectious materials is generally automatic and done without incident when thoughtful precautions are taken. These precautions must be specifically instituted to ensure the safe handling of the materials without employee infection. This is especially true in the handling of cultures of pathologic organisms and viruses. Spills of these materials must be cleaned up, and the area sterilized with chemical disinfectant. In the past, samples taken from any patient in isolation would be collected with isolation techniques—the samples labeled with a special alert marker, such as isolation, hepatitis, or blood—and "body fluid precautions."[46] If the samples were divided or placed in different containers, the special markers would be placed on these tubes as well, so that all health-care workers would be warned that special precautions should be taken to protect the hands and body from infectious hazard. This type of labeling was recommended in place of labels using specific disease names. This type of labeling alerts the health-care worker *and* protects the confidentiality of the patient and the report.[30] Recent information on the exposure of health-care workers to hepatitis and AIDS[17,28] has indicated that the health-care worker cannot depend on this type of warning system before using protective measures. For this reason, the Centers for Disease Control (CDC) issued recommendations for prevention of human immunodeficiency virus (HIV) and hepatitis B virus (HBV) transmission in health-care settings.[29] These were followed by a joint advisory notice from the Department of Labor and the Department of Health and Human Services on protection against occupational exposure to HBV and HIV.[34] OSHA has also warned that health-care institutions not heeding these precautions will be subject to prosecution and fines.[48]

The new CDC Blood and Body Fluid Precautions for Laboratories stipulate that the blood and body fluids of all patients are to be considered infectious. Thus, hand, face, and body barrier precautions must be used by all health-care workers when contact with nonintact skin, mucous membranes, or blood and body fluids is anticipated. These barriers are gowns, masks, eye shields, gloves, coats, and aprons. Biologic hoods may also be needed when droplets may be produced in certain procedures. Gloves must be removed and hands washed after the handling of samples. Coats, aprons, and other protective devices should not be worn out of the area of use. (See Blood and Body Fluid Precautions for Laboratories).

Work areas where infectious materials are handled must be cleaned daily with a disinfectant that is effective against HBV and HIV and bacteria.[2,4,7,36] These viruses, with their many and varied routes of infection, have become most troublesome infectious agents for the hospital laboratory.[4,39,41,46] For this reason, it has become necessary to clean all laboratory work bench areas with a disinfectant solution that is capable of destroying bacteria, viruses, rickettsiae, and fungi. A very good disinfectant can be prepared by diluting household bleach (5.25%) 1:10 in 0.07% non-ionic detergent.[7,25,41,46] This solution is unstable and corrosive to metals; therefore, it must be made up often, and care must be exercised in its application. This material also combines with protein, so that an excess of the halide must be used. We have found that this bleach solution in detergent works well, and because of economy and ease of use, this solution is used to wash all laboratory work benches and to mop all laboratory floors every day. This solution will spot clothes and will irritate skin. For this reason, care must be taken so that it does not get into the eyes; and the hands should be washed after using.

Sampling of this material must be done by pipetting devices that preclude pipetting by mouth. Special precautions must be taken so that the work space is not contaminated by the material. The sampling tips from the pipetting systems must be collected in specially marked containers for proper disposal. After the procedure has been completed, all disposable material should be placed in a specially marked disposal system. Items that are not disposable should be cleaned in bleach solution or sterilized before washing.

Exposure in the laboratory to pathogenic microorganisms can happen by a number of means. It is possible to be infected by other routes, and the disease produced may be difficult to diagnose, because of the fact that symptoms are atypical. The occurrence of the infection, however, depends on the virulence of the infecting agent and the susceptibility of the host being infected. The possible routes of infection are described below:

Airborne routes are created through occurrences such as spills or breaking of containers, which propel infectious agents into the air. Removing caps from tubes, heating liquids on inoculating needles too rapidly, and breakages in centrifuges can also cause aerosols to be formed.

Ingestion may occur through the practice of mouth pipetting and failure to wash the hands after handling specimens or cultures.

Direct inoculation is a result of broken glassware, needles, and syringes.

Skin contact may be a route, even though infectious agents will not normally penetrate the skin. Small cuts or scratches of the skin and conjunctiva of the eye may admit organisms.

The transportation of possible infectious material presents special problems in preserving the condition of the specimen as well as in ensuring the safety of all handling it. Special packaging and marking must be used[5,43] to protect the specimen from breakage and to alert others of the hazards associated with the contents. These specimens, as defined by the Public Health Service Interstate Quarantine Regulations and by the Department of Transportation, are subject to minimum packaging requirements of the Public Health Service. A National Committee for Clinical Laboratory Standards (NCCLS) has also proposed a standard for the collection, processing, preservation, packaging, and shipping of these materials.[43]

BLOOD AND BODY FLUIDS PRECAUTIONS FOR LABORATORIES

These policies have been adapted from those recommended by the CDC in *Morbidity and Mortality Weekly Report*[29]:

1. All health-care workers should routinely use appropriate barrier precautions to prevent skin and mucous-membrane exposure when contact with blood or other body fluids of any patient is anticipated. Gloves should be worn for touching blood and body fluids, mucous membranes, or nonintact skin of all patients, for handling items or surfaces soiled with blood fluids, and for performing venipuncture and other vascular access procedures. Gloves should be changed after contact with each patient. Masks and protective eyewear or face shields should be worn during procedures that are likely to generate droplets of blood or other body fluids to prevent exposure of mucous membranes of the mouth, nose, and eyes. Gowns or aprons should be worn during procedures that are likely to generate splashes of blood or other body fluids.

2. Hands and other skin surfaces should be washed immediately and thoroughly if contaminated with blood or other body fluids. Hands should be washed immediately after gloves are removed.

3. All health-care workers should take precautions to prevent injuries caused by needles, scalpels, and other sharp instruments or devices during procedures; when cleaning used instruments; during disposal of used needles; and when handling sharp instruments after procedures. Needles should not be recapped or bent after use. All sharps should be disposed of in puncture resistant containers for disposal. These items should be disposed of in a manner so that they may not be reused.

4. All specimens of blood and body fluids should be collected in a sealable primary container that will not leak. Care should be taken that the outside surface of the container is not contaminated. Contaminated containers should be placed in a sealable secondary container for prevention of more contamination. These tubes should be decontaminated when they reach the laboratory processing area.

5. All persons handling blood and body fluids should wear gloves. Masks and protective eyewear should be worn if mucous-membrane contact with blood or body fluids is anticipated. Gloves should be removed, discarded, and the hands should be washed after completion of specimen processing.

6. Biologic safety cabinets may be needed with

procedures that have a high potential for generating droplets.

7. Use mechanical pipetting devices, not mouth pipetting.
8. Use of needles and syringes must be limited to situations in which there is no alternative.
9. General precautions should be taken with laboratory work surfaces.
10. General precautions should be taken with contaminated materials.
11. Scientific equipment that has been contaminated must be cleaned and decontaminated before being repaired or shipped out for repair.
12. Each and every person should wash his hands after completing laboratory activities and should remove protective clothing before leaving the laboratory.
13. Pregnant women are not known to be at greater risk of contracting HIV infection than others; however, when HIV infection develops during pregnancy, the infant is at risk of infection resulting from perinatal transmission. Because of this risk, pregnant health-care workers should be especially familiar with and strictly follow precautions to minimize the risk of infection.

Chemical Hazards

Even though many chemicals are considered to be completely safe, the term *safe* must be qualified to some extent by how the chemicals are to be used. We may say that sodium chloride is a safe chemical, but no one would want salt tossed into his eyes. However, if a small amount of salt is dissolved in water, the resulting solution becomes an excellent eyewash. In the first instance the salt crystals are sharp, and the strong salt will burn the eyes. In the second instance, the weak salt solution, if isotonic, would be soothing to the eyes. This illustration, although very simple, helps to demonstrate the fact that usage and conditions of usage will affect the safety of the chemical. For this reason, it is imperative that one become familiar with the physical properties, chemical properties, and physical effects of the compounds with which he is dealing. The OSHA has published a list of compounds and chemicals with which restricted exposure is necessary.[8,9,33] These compounds are listed with exposure limits as well as routes of exposure. A more complete listing of these chemicals, including the waste disposal procedures, threshold limit values, National Fire Prevention Association (NFPA) coding

system, and pertinent physical properties, are provided by the Manufacturing Chemists Association.[26] Exposure limits are to be used as a guide for the safe use of these chemicals. Personal exposure levels should be determined when usage is started and checked routinely thereafter to ensure that safe levels are not exceeded. The routine monitoring of xylene and formaldehyde (formalin) vapors in the laboratory and morgue is needed to guard against over exposure to these commonly used chemicals.[10,27,42] If exposure levels are excessive, ventilation must be increased, or special carbon filtration hoods should be used to remove organic vapors.

Carcinogenic Chemicals

The *chemical carcinogen* is one which has been demonstrated to cause tumors in mammalian species by induction of a tumor type normally seen or by the appearance of such tumors at an earlier time than would be otherwise expected. By definition, these compounds may produce tumors in man. For this reason, it is important that special precautions be taken. The National Institutes of Health issued working guidelines and general safety principles for these compounds when fourteen such chemicals were listed in 1973.[6] Of these chemicals, benzidine, 3,3-dichlorobenzidine, β-naphthylamine, and 4-dimethylaminoazobenzene have been used to some extent in the clinical laboratory. Benzidine and benzidine dihydrochloride, both extensively used in the laboratory, were listed as carcinogens in 1972.[21] Benzene is now listed, and maximum limits of exposure have been set.[33] Some questions also have been raised as to the carcinogenic properties of carbon tetrachloride[22] and chloroform.[23]

Because of the possible carcinogenic properties of these chemicals to man, as well as the toxic properties of the compounds, it is reasonable to discontinue using those for which substitutes can be found and to follow strict guidelines for usage and disposal and not exceed the permissible exposure limits for those that must be used.[26,33] In that the effect of these agents is long term, control practices included in the National Cancer Institute Safety Standards involve special work procedures, environmental control techniques, and a health surveillance program. These are meant to supplement conventional safety programs and are designed to

Prevent exposure of personnel

Limit access of chemical agents to authorized personnel only

Prohibit access of these chemical agents to unauthorized personnel by strict traffic control

Prevent environmental contamination with strict waste disposal techniques

Protect the laboratory worker from exposure to chemical agents.

Corrosive Chemicals

The corrosive chemicals, acid and alkalies, are capable of destroying material by altering the chemical nature of the material. An example of this type of reaction is treating zinc metal with hydrochloric acid to produce zinc chloride, which is soluble in water. The metal has been destroyed with no visible trace unless the water is evaporated; then the zinc chloride remains as a white crystalline material. Another example would be the destruction of human tissue by sulfuric acid. When sulfuric acid contacts the skin, a slight warming sensation is felt after about two to three seconds, and this warming sensation increases with time. If the acid is washed off within that first two-to-three-second period, no significant burn is likely, but as the acid is washed off with water, more burning will be felt because more heat will be released as the acid reacts with the water. This reaction must be expected, and no matter how much the burning increases, continue to wash the area with copius amounts of water. A slight burn will probably show only a red coloration, but as the reaction continues, blistering will take place. If the reaction continues, the skin and underlying tissue will char. With other chemicals, such as picric acid, nitric acid, phenol, silver nitrate, and sodium hydroxide, slightly differing colors and sensations may be exhibited, but the end-product, tissue destruction, is the same. The speed of the reaction from chemical to chemical may vary, but the extent of the burn will be directly proportional to the time the agent is in contact with the skin: the longer the reaction, the greater the damage. Thus it is imperative that physical exposure to corrosive materials be prevented; but if it should occur, the area of exposure must be washed immediately. Another important precaution to take when using acids is to wear protective clothing.

Some simple rules for controlling corrosive chemical accidents are as follows:

1. Always use the special rubber or plastic acid carriers to transport corrosive chemicals.
2. Never pipette these chemicals by mouth.
3. Always use protective clothing, aprons, and face masks when handling concentrated acids and alkalies.
4. Make sure the safety showers, hand sprays, and eyewash systems are in working condition.
5. Never wear sandals or open-toed shoes while working with corrosive chemicals.
6. Never wear contact lenses without a face mask while handling corrosive chemicals.
7. In case of corrosive spills to the body, get under the safety shower and disrobe immediately while the water is running. Remember that any clothing held firmly against the body will tend to hold the corrosive chemicals against the skin.

Flammable Chemicals

Although we tend to think of flammable chemicals as liquids, these reagents can be gases, liquids, or solids. In order to use these chemicals safely, one must be familiar with their physical states, with how readily those states can change with the environment, and with how easily the substances can be ignited and how explosively they will burn. This information is published by the NFPA[12] and is readily available from other laboratory safety books.[26,27,45]

In considering the flammability of a substance, we are considering the probability that the material will be ignited. In order for something to be ignited, three conditions must be met: (1) there must be a spark or heat source; (2) the material must be in a form that is readily ignitable (vaporized); and (3) enough air must be available to support combustion.

In considering ways to decrease the fire hazard, again consider these three conditions. The oxygen or air supply cannot be altered permanently, although it may be altered in localized areas when fighting fires. The source of the ignition can be controlled. In areas where flammable vapors and gases are present, or likely to be present, all spark-causing relays, switches, motors, or hot plates must be eliminated or sealed off from these elements. This is not easy to do, and static electricity is even harder to control. If heating is necessary, only water or steam heat should be used. The third part of this triangle is probably the most easily controlled: flammable gas should not be allowed to escape into the laboratory area. If there is any chance that flammable vapor or gas might escape during a procedure, work must be done in the fume hood. An added precaution in controlling the flammable vapors in the work area is to make sure flammable liquids are always kept in safe storage areas. If extremely volatile liquids (*e.g.,* ether) are used, storage in safety or explosion-proof refrigerators may be necessary.

Safe storage of flammable liquids and gases means storage in approved storage cabinets or closets.[13,19] These safety storage cabinets are of double-walled steel construction and provide good storage for limited amounts of flammable liquids. With this type of storage unit, our laboratory has been able to eliminate all supplies of flammable liquids from the laboratory work bench. No amount of flammable liquid is left out when not in immediate use.

There are a number of flammable reagents that are in the solid state. Even though these reagents are not as likely to produce flammable vapors and are, therefore, less likely to contribute to the vapor hazards, they are flammable and should be stored in safe storage areas. Some of these reagents are explosive and can be set off by impact or friction. Picric acid, dinitrobenzenes, 2,4-dinitrophenol, and 2,4-dinitrotoluene are explosive solids that require extreme caution in handling. These reagents should be stored in a safe area removed from other flammable compounds, because they may explode and detonate other chemicals. Picric acid has 1% water added and is usually quite safe. Only when this reagent is dehydrated does it become explosive. For this reason, it should be stored away from other flammable reagents and kept tightly capped at all times. Some of the peroxides of ether are also explosive and can be set off by impact, shaking, or friction. Therefore, special care must be taken to set up and enforce strict dating procedures for these reagents. Ethyl ether, isopropyl ether, dioxane, tetrahydrofuran, and other alkyl ethers tend to form unstable peroxides, which may detonate with extreme violence.[44] We note in red the day we open this type of reagent and discard it within 1 month if it is not completely used.

Another potentially explosive agent, sodium azide, is a chemical preservative that is used in many kits containing protein agents. It is a good preservative that does not generally interfere with the planned reaction. In the past, this reagent was used extensively in saline-diluting fluids. It does not have explosive capability in itself, but it reacts with copper and lead in the sewer systems to form a very unstable compound that will explode by friction or concussion when the sewer drains are repaired.[49] The National Institute for Occupational Safety and Health (NIOSH) sent out an alert in August 1976[3] on the explosive hazard of copper and lead azide forming in sewer drains. This same alert recommended that these lines be flushed with water several times a day and that the copper, brass, and lead sections of the sewer be eliminated. We have found glass and plastic replacement lines and continuous flush to work very well. Lines that have already been contaminated should be flushed with 10% sodium hydroxide.[13,38] Because of these problems, azide-free cell-counting fluid is now available and widely used. The replacement of the azide with other reagents and pharmaceuticals was studied by the College of American Pathologists and others, and the consensus of opinion was that sodium azide is a useful and technically sound preservative that need not be replaced if handled with appropriate precautions.[20] When the proper precautions are followed, no problems should be encountered.

Toxic Chemicals

Toxicity is the potential of a substance to cause injury by direct chemical action on the body tissues and organs. This toxic or harmful effect on body tissues is caused by interference with the function of the cells of the body tissues. The localized effects will be seen at the place of contact. The most common of these sites would be the skin, eyes, nose, throat, and lungs when the chemicals are air droplets. When the chemicals are swallowed, the effect will be in the mouth, throat, stomach, and intestines. Systemic injuries can be produced in any body organs after the toxic element has been absorbed into the blood-stream.

It is generally accepted that when we speak of a toxic chemical, we are speaking of a substance that is toxic in small quantities. This assumption is not always correct, because concentration must be considered with toxicity. Any substance can be toxic to the human body if the dose is large enough. This is true even for the chemicals that are essential for life to exist. It is also true that some compounds are toxic in very low doses. Many medicines have great therapeutic value at one concentration and toxic effects at only slightly higher levels. These toxic levels must be known and referred to when chemicals are used or disposed of, because these data must control usage and the means of disposal. Some of the extremely hazardous compounds that may be found in the laboratory are beryllium and its salts, bromine, chloracetec acid, *m*-dinitrobenzene fluorine, hydrofluoric acid, and mixtures of sulfuric and nitric acid. These chemicals should be used with extreme caution, and access to them and the area of their use should be restricted. Special disposal procedures must be followed.[26,45] These chemicals can cause death despite medical treatment. There are also more than 30 chemicals that are commonly found in the clinical laboratories that can cause serious injury despite medical treatment.

Burns

For our purposes here, we shall consider a *burn* to be the damage or destruction of tissue by chemical or thermal means. Thermal means shall include both hot and cold, because some very cold substances can produce burns. Chemical burns have been mentioned previously and will not be discussed here.

In discussing thermal burns and how to prevent them, we must consider ways and means of preventing the rapid transfer of thermal energy. This thermal energy may be in the form of light when one is working with ultraviolet lamps, deuterium lamps, or lasers. These instruments are capable of producing large amounts of radiant energy in the form of light. If this energy is emitted in the ultraviolet range, it cannot be seen; so one does not have a visible means of determining that a hazard exists. For this reason, special goggles should be used for eye protection when one is working with any of these light sources. Standard glass lenses will also absorb these rays; so people wearing regular glass lenses are protected from harmful ultraviolet radiation. If a technologist is working with lasers emitting energy in the visual or near ultraviolet range, he should wear neutral density filter lenses or special lenses that will filter out or decrease the light emitted.

Wounds

Severe wounds generally do not occur in the hospital laboratory. The main problem in the laboratory or in the hospital is the infection potential created by sores, cuts, or puncturing of the skin. Two sources of severe cuts are from broken glassware and microtome blades. Because of the continuous problems with infected cuts from broken glassware, it has become necessary to provide special disposal for broken glass and to make it mandatory that all broken glassware be discarded in the special container immediately. The glass in this container should be transported to the landfill in that same container and buried. If your institution has an approved incinerator, this glass can be melted down, and the glass slag can be discarded with the rest of the ashes. Microtome blades are extremely sharp and must be kept cased when not in use. About the only protection one has when using these instruments is the presence of mind to keep hands off the knife edge. Any distraction while one is working with the microtome, such as loud noises, visiting, or listening to the radio, should not be tolerated.

Puncture wounds seem to be endemic to the clinical laboratory, especially in the area of phlebotomy. After blood is drawn from a patient, the phlebotomist must remove the tourniquet, cover the needle, and discard the needle while holding onto the tubes of blood. If a tube of blood slips or if the phlebotomist is distracted at this time, an accident involving the sharp end of a contaminated needle can occur. If needles are to be recapped, a special hand-shielding clamp[32] should be used to protect the hand, or the needle and syringe should be discarded without recapping the needle.[36] The combative patient can be a problem, because he might "explode" at a moment when the needle is uncovered; the phlebotomist might lose his composure and stick himself. In this way the phlebotomist can be inoculated with bacteria from his own skin or from the patient. New students are prone to stick themselves when they uncover the needle just before venipuncture. In these cases, an accident seems to happen because of nervous stress. For this reason, it is essential that the teaching supervisors instill self-confidence as well as knowledge when working with new students. The experienced phlebotomist should not allow himself to be distracted while working with the patient, because this can result in sample mix-up as well as accidents involving both patient and phlebotomist.

SAFETY PRECAUTIONS

There are certain specific practices for personal hygiene and safety that require special attention by hospital laboratory personnel. The following safety precautions are listed in numeric order so that they may be employed as a checklist:

1. No food or drink shall be kept in the laboratory or in the laboratory refrigerator.
2. No food or drink shall be consumed in the laboratory.
3. Lipstick and other cosmetics shall not be kept or used in the laboratory.
4. No smoking shall be allowed in the laboratory.
5. Nervous habits, such as biting fingernails, chewing toothpicks, or chewing pencils, must be discouraged. Placing anything in or near the mouth may serve to transfer an infectious organism into the mouth.
6. Hands should be washed after handling a contaminated specimen, before eating, or before applying cosmetics.
7. Special protective coats, gowns, aprons, gloves, or masks should not be worn out of the laboratory.
8. Sharp objects should be disposed of properly.
9. Needles should be placed in special containers and sterilized before disposal.

Incineration will sterilize as well as destroy these items so that others cannot use or puncture themselves on them.

10. Centrifuges must not be opened while still in motion.
11. Special goggles should be available and used when one is working with ultraviolet light sources.
12. Hazardous fumes or gas is not to be tolerated in the work area.
13. All chipped and cracked glassware should be taken out of service.
14. Mercury should be properly stored, and all spills cleaned up immediately.
15. All biohazard spills should be disinfected and cleaned up promptly.
16. All flammables should be kept in proper storage areas and properly disposed of.
17. Ether should be dated and disposed of promptly after outdating.
18. Refrigerators should be marked either explosion hazard or explosion-proof and used properly. Remember that the safety refrigerator is adequate when the source of fumes is inside and not outside the box.
19. Hazardous chemicals should be properly stored.
20. Acids and corrosive chemicals should be carried in safety buckets.
21. Spill buckets should be available in all areas.
22. Eyewash units and safety showers should be available and in working order.
23. Fume hoods should be available and in working order.
24. Safety pipette bulbs should be available and used.
25. Air-breathing units, if needed, should be available and in working order.
26. Work benches should be swabbed daily with bleach solution or other suitable disinfectants.
27. The laboratory environment should be kept clean and damp-mopped with a disinfectant.
28. Toxic solvents, such as toluene, xylene, chlorinated hydrocarbons, diethylamine, and other solvents having a health hazard rating of 3 or above, should be used only in the chemical hood.
29. Proper fire extinguishers should be available and maintained.
30. Fire blankets should be available.
31. Fire evacuation routes should be posted.
32. If radioactive isotopes are used, the area should be properly posted, radiation exposures monitored, records kept, and mouth-pipetting prohibited.

Hazard Labeling System

The storage of chemicals, specimens, and cultures in the clinical laboratory poses some special problems for those who must work with them. It is well understood that these items must be labeled as to the contents, but the listing of contents alone is not sufficient information for those who are not familiar with the reagent or specimen. All specimens must be clearly labeled as to contents and then dated. The labeling of reagents is even more critical, and any reagent that has lost its label must be discarded. Reagent labels, at the very least, must indicate the contents, date of preparation, and expiration. There is more information needed if one is to safely handle these chemicals. Certain chemical and physical properties have been compiled and tabulated in a simple numeric form to give firemen some general information as to the hazards that may be present during emergency situations in the laboratory. This information is listed by five numerals (zero through four) indicating the severity of hazards with respect to health, fire, and reactivity of the chemical (Fig. 20-1). This information has been combined into a special hazard label (Fig. 20-2) to be applied to all reagents and chemicals.[40] If a labeling system such as this is not used, a reagent list for each laboratory should be prepared. This list should contain the previously noted information as well as data on the permissible limits for human exposure and for disposal. An excellent source for this data is prepared by the Manufacturing Chemists Association.[26] The information should be posted on the entrance to each laboratory using the special NFPA hazard warning emblem (Fig. 20-1). this emblem is a square label with three colored square patches—blue, red, and yellow—placed in three of the corners. It should be posted so that the red patch is at the top. The numeric hazard information is printed in the respective colored squares: the numeral for health hazard information is printed on the blue patch, fire hazard on the red patch, and reactivity hazard on the yellow patch. When many chemicals are present in a laboratory room, a work list should be prepared of all the chemicals showing the numeral for each of the three hazards. The highest numeral for each hazard should be printed on the respective colored patches. In this way, anyone entering the room can tell at a glance what chemical hazards may be encountered.

A special symbol has been prepared as a warning concerning a biologic hazard (Fig. 20-3); it is fluorescent orange or red in color.[5,7] This symbol should be used to signify the actual or potential presence of a biohazard and to identify equipment,

FIGURE 20-1. Hazard label with NFPA health, fire, and reactivity code numbers. The color blocks are blue, red, and yellow respectively.

FIGURE 20-2. Chemical reagent label with health, fire, and reactivity hazard code. (From Scheffler GL: Laboratory safety. In Bond RG, DeRoos RL: Environmental Health and Safety in Health-Care Facilities. New York, Macmillan, 1973)

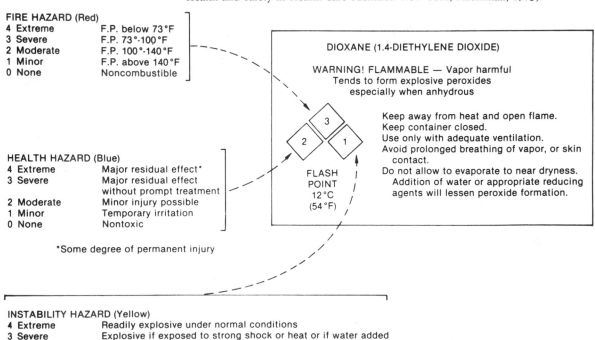

FIRE HAZARD (Red)
4	Extreme	F.P. below 73°F
3	Severe	F.P. 73°-100°F
2	Moderate	F.P. 100°-140°F
1	Minor	F.P. above 140°F
0	None	Noncombustible

HEALTH HAZARD (Blue)
4	Extreme	Major residual effect*
3	Severe	Major residual effect without prompt treatment
2	Moderate	Minor injury possible
1	Minor	Temporary irritation
0	None	Nontoxic

*Some degree of permanent injury

DIOXANE (1.4-DIETHYLENE DIOXIDE)

WARNING! FLAMMABLE — Vapor harmful
Tends to form explosive peroxides
especially when anhydrous

Keep away from heat and open flame.
Keep container closed.
Use only with adequate ventilation.
Avoid prolonged breathing of vapor, or skin contact.
Do not allow to evaporate to near dryness.
Addition of water or appropriate reducing agents will lessen peroxide formation.

FLASH POINT
12°C
(54°F)

INSTABILITY HAZARD (Yellow)
4	Extreme	Readily explosive under normal conditions
3	Severe	Explosive if exposed to strong shock or heat or if water added
2	Moderate	Normally unstable, or violently reactive with water
1	Minor	Unstable at elevated temperatures, or reacts with water
0	None	Normally stable

FIGURE 20-3. Biohazard warning symbol. The color should be a fluorescent orange or red.

containers, rooms, materials, experimental animals, or combinations thereof that contain or are contaminated with viable hazardous agents.[7,8] Where possible, this symbol should be posted with the single, open-ended circle pointed upward and the other two forming the base. Pertinent information concerning identity of the hazard, name of responsible party, and precautionary information may be associated with, but not imposed upon, the symbol. This symbol, with directory information, can serve to warn the uninformed against unauthorized admittance.

Hazard Identification Signals

The hazard signals just discussed were established by the NFPA, which identifies hazards as follows[11]:

IDENTIFICATION OF HEALTH HAZARD (BLUE)

4. Materials that on very short exposure could cause death or major injury even though prompt medical treatment were given
3. Materials that on short exposure could cause serious temporary or residual injury even though prompt medical treatment were given
2. Materials that on intense or continued exposure could cause temporary incapacitation or possible residual injury unless prompt medical treatment were given
1. Materials that on exposure would cause irritation but only minor residual injury if no treatment were given
0. Materials that on exposure under fire conditions would offer no hazard beyond that of ordinary combustible materials

IDENTIFICATION OF FLAMMABILITY (RED)

4. Materials that will rapidly or completely vaporize at atmospheric pressure and normal ambient temperature or that are readily dispersed in air and will burn readily
3. Liquids and solids that can be ignited under almost all ambient temperature conditions
2. Materials that must be moderately heated or exposed to relatively high ambient temperature before ignition can occur
1. Materials that must be preheated before ignition can occur
0. Materials that will not burn

IDENTIFICATION OF REACTIVITY (YELLOW)

4. Materials that are readily capable of detonating or of explosive decomposition or reaction at normal temperatures and pressures
3. Materials that are capable of detonation or explosive reaction but require a strong initiation source or that must be heated under confinement before initiation or that react explosively with water
2. Materials that are normally unstable and readily undergo violent chemical change but do not detonate; also, materials that may react violently with water or that may form potentially explosive mixtures with water
1. Materials that are normally stable but that can become unstable at elevated temperatures and pressures; also, materials that may react with water with some release of energy, but not violently
0. Materials that are normally stable, even under fire exposure conditions, and that are not reactive with water

SPECIAL SYMBOLS

P: Polymerizes
W: Reacts violently with water

Although these special symbols are listed under flammability, they would appear in a separate place on a special label.

Safety Cabinets

Biologic safety cabinets are the principle equipment used to provide physical containment of specimen and protection to personnel.[25] There are three major types of biologic safety cabinets used in the microbiologic laboratory: the Class I cabinet, the Class II cabinet, and the Class III cabinet. These cabinets provide differing kinds of protection as far as user, environment, and experiment are concerned. Therefore, the kind of protection needed will dictate to a great extent the type of cabinet needed.

The Class I biologic safety cabinet is set up to draw room air away from the user, over the specimen, and out through the HEPA filter. This filtered air is then vented into building air supply or outside. This system will provide protection for the user and the environment; however, the user's hands and arms are not protected, and quick movement may also let microorganisms and moist droplets escape to the user's body. For this reason, the user must be protected by special clothing and gloves when using this type of device.

The Class II biologic safety cabinet, commonly known as a laminar-flow cabinet, is set up so that HEPA-filtered air is circulated down inside the front surface of the cabinet, over the work area, filtered again, and exhausted from the unit. Different models of these cabinets will exhaust the air into the room or outside. These units will provide protection to the user, the environment, and the experiment. The front panel has an open access window, the same as the Class I cabinets, so these units are therefore partial containment devices.

The Class III biologic safety cabinet is a totally enclosed, ventilated cabinet of gas-tight construction. Operational access is through attached rubber gloves. When in operation, this cabinet is maintained under negative pressure of at least 0.5 inch of water. Air is drawn through HEPA filters and exhausted out through HEPA filters. This unit provides the possibility of pretreatment of specimen entering the cabinet and of waste before disposal. Thus, there should be no possibility of specimen contamination by outside air or environmental contamination by the specimen waste. The Class III cabinet provides the highest level of personnel and environmental protection, with sample protection at a high level. However, this protection can be compromised by puncture of the gloves or by accidents that create positive pressure in the cabinet.

The protection capabilities of the biologic safety cabinets are dependent upon their proper use and adequate functioning. The choice of the proper safety cabinet to do the required task, the correct operating procedure, and the adequate functioning of the unit must be considered in any hazardous situation. For this reason, it is imperative that functional checks be made on the units at regular intervals.[25]

Fume Hoods

The laboratory fume hoods come in three basic designs: conventional, bypass, and add-air. Fume hoods may be constructed of wood, fiberglass, sheet steel, stainless steel, epoxy, or cement. The front entrance is controlled by a sliding door that is raised and lowered. Air enters at the front under the sliding door (sash). The baffle at the back directs air along a specific flow pattern. This flow pattern is generally back and up, so that the air is always moving away from the user. The air velocity is controlled by a blower system mounted outside or on top of the fume hood. If negative air pressure is desired throughout the system, the blower system must be placed outside on the roof of the building. The type of construction material will be determined by the expected use of the hood: if flammable agents are to be used, the construction must be of fire-resistant material. The same is true of chemical resistance for such chemicals as organic solvents, acids, and alkalies. When flammable agents are to be used, the lighting and blower system must be vapor-proof. All utility controls—gas, air, vacuum, power, and water—should be located externally. Perchloric acid use dictates that the hood be constructed of 316 stainless steel and be equipped with a special blower air-ejector system.

The conventional fume hood may be constructed of any of various materials. Room air enters at the front and moves back and up inside the hood. The velocity of this air will be changed as the front sash is moved up and down. The air to be exhausted is derived totally from within the room.

The bypass fume hood operates as does the conventional system; but there is an air bypass constructed into the top front portion of the hood, so that the air velocity will not change when the sash is lowered. This type of construction is desirable when a fragile apparatus is used in the hood. This type of airflow has some definite advantages when varying airflow patterns may interfere with instruments placed within the hood. These hoods are constructed of the same materials as the conventional systems and airflow patterns are somewhat similar. Again, the airflow is coming totally from within the room.

The add-air fume hood adds another definite advantage. This system has the means of bringing outside air into the hood, rather than taking all of its air from the room. This unit can bring in up to 50% of the air it uses from the outside, but this requires an extra blower and vent. Because of this extra blower and venting, the initial cost will be greater;

but total operating costs could be lower because less heated or cooled air is lost.

As with the safety cabinets, the operation of these units must be checked regularly. For general laboratory use, the face velocities should be at least 100 ft/min. This is for corrosive and moderately toxic materials that have a threshold limit value (TLV) of 10 to 10,000 ppm. When materials having higher toxicity levels (TLV less than 10 ppm) are to be used, face velocity should be increased to 150 ft/min. From the above data, it can be seen that the safety factor provided by these hoods is subject to the face velocities and that these should be checked at regularly scheduled intervals.

Disposal of Hazardous Materials

A hazardous waste management system has been set up by the federal government.[8,10] Although it deals primarily with the wastes generated by industry, it is expected that a similar system will be applied to the hazardous wastes, solid and liquid, generated by the hospital laboratory.[16,18] The federal system stipulates that a generator of hazardous waste material must have a waste disposal number and that the waste material must be packaged and contained in a specified manner. The processors or the disposers of this material are required to obtain a permit, and the method of final disposition is specified.

If there is any question of infectious hazards in laboratory waste, the material should be incinerated or sterilized before disposal and then need not be considered a hazardous waste. Organic waste materials that can be burned should be incinerated, because this will produce complete oxidation of the material, converting it to carbon dioxide and water. Thus, the material would be put back into nature's cycle.

In the disposal of flammable material, one must consider the quantity of the material and whether it is soluble in water, liquids, or solids. In dealing with small spills, one should absorb the material on paper or some other porous material and burn all of the material. This should be done in an incinerator. If the flammable material is also toxic or will produce or emit toxic substances when heated or burned, it should be burned in an incinerator with afterburners and scrubbers. When large quantities of materials are involved, they should be burned. Small quantities of very volatile material, such as ether, can be evaporated and vented out the fume hood. Larger volumes should be burned. Small amounts of water-soluble materials may be flushed down the sewer with excess water. Small amounts of flammable solids may be burned with excess porous material or dissolved in an excess of organic solvents and injected into an incinerator.

Some chemical companies have included pertinent information in their catalogues on disposal of specific hazardous materials. This information is also sent to chemical users in the form of material safety date sheets. More information is available from the Manufacturing Chemists Association.[26] The organic chemicals that are not flammable should be recovered or returned to the manufacturer for reprocessing.

For the disposal of toxic materials that are flammable, burning in an incinerator equipped with afterburners and scrubbers is the method of choice. Those materials that are not flammable should be chemically converted to nontoxic substances, reprocessed and recovered, or disposed of as hazardous substances, with the laws governing this type of disposal taken into consideration.[8,9,10] It may be advantageous to consider the services of a commercial disposal company. There are some substances that must be cleaned up and recovered. One such element (mercury) is used commonly in the clinical laboratory and is very toxic in all forms. Mercury, or its salt, has been used as a disinfectant, colorimetric reagent, and in pressure- and temperature-measuring devices. Whenever spilled, mercury should be picked up immediately by suction through a small capillary and placed in a covered container. This recovered mercury should be saved for cleaning and reuse. The use of mercury thermometers in ovens should be discontinued. It is very unlikely that the spilled mercury in an oven will, or can be, cleaned up. This mercury under high temperature will vaporize and contaminate the laboratory at an even faster rate than when left on the bench top or on the floor. Special mercury vacuum cleaners are available for picking up mercury from the floors, tables, bench tops, and even sewer and sink traps.

Infectious materials should not be deposited directly into a solid waste disposal system (landfill). This means of disposal can place high concentrations of pathogenic microorganisms into small areas that can be stirred up by mechanical equipment, humans, and animals at the time of disposal or at a later date.[47] For this reason, the material should first be treated by a suitable disinfectant, autoclaved, or incinerated. Then it can be disposed of in the same way as any solid waste. Urine and fecal material remaining after chemical analysis should be deposited in the sewer. All of the materials used during blood collection and processing must be considered an infectious hazard. Therefore, the syringes (plastic), needles, blood tubes, blood clots, and serum should be disinfected by chemical treatment, autoclaved, or incinerated before disposal. Needles should be placed in special protective containers after use so that the unwary are protected. Incineration is a good means of disposal for these items.

Broken glass is one of the worst offenders in accidental cuts. For this reason, broken glassware should be placed in specially marked and covered containers. The glass can then be taken directly to the landfill in the special receptacle, which limits the possibility of accidental wounds. Cracked and broken glassware should be removed from service immediately and discarded or repaired.

Emergency Procedures

Emergency planning for a hospital must consider both internal and external disasters as well as the smaller accidents within the institution; the laboratory must consider these plans when forming its own policies. Here we shall consider only planning for the laboratory in handling emergencies within that area.

The most obvious planning should cover fire and explosion. This planning must also concern everyone in the institution; but when the emergency arises in the laboratory, one must respond wisely and quickly. One's response at this time can affect the safety of all concerned. When this type of disaster occurs, everyone in the laboratory must accept the responsibility for turning in the alarm, helping others escape, and fighting the fire if needed. This type of response requires that one know the following:

Where the fire alarm pull station is located and how to use it

Where the fire extinguishers are located, which kind to use, and how to use them

Where the proper exit routes are located; these should be posted so that all can see them

Which members of the staff are working in your area and where they should be

Where the fire blankets are and how to use them

In the case of electrical shock and chemical spills, one needs to know the following:

The location of the main power switches for his area

The location of the chemical spill buckets and how to use them

The location of the air filters or the air breathing devices and how to use them

How to dispose of the waste after the spill is cleaned up

How to isolate the area if toxic fumes are involved

Accident Reports

Accident reports should be filled out and signed by the respective supervisors. Suitable forms are available from the insurance company, the state Department of Labor, or the institution. The purpose of these reports is not only to provide information in case of workmen's compensation, but also to provide information to the safety committee on how the accident happened. This part of the report must be studied by the safety committee in its efforts to improve safety. One should remember that accidents are happenings that are out of the ordinary, and they may or may not produce injury. Accident reports should be made on all accidents. In this way, it is possible for situations to be corrected before injury takes place. The reports should include the following information:

Persons involved

Injury and to whom

Treatment given

Time of accident

Location of accident

Cause of accident

Instrument or machine involved

Comments of those involved

Safety Committee

The safety committee personnel should be responsible people with good judgment who have the respect of the administration as well as their peers. Their function should be to recommend policy, promote safety standards, advise, and instruct the staff and students. Their responsibility should be to the chairman of the department or the director, and their recommendations should be made to him. They should encourage suggestions from their fellow laboratory workers and should be willing to listen, no matter how trivial a problem may seem at the time. If fellow workers are scorned or made light of, they will be less likely to report an accident or seek advice again.

REFERENCES

1. American National Standard: Safe Current Limits for Electromedical Apparatus. Arlington, Association for the Advancement of Medical Instrumentation, 1978
2. Blumberg JM. Laboratory safety. Pathologist 28:39, 1974
3. Current Intelligence Bulletin 13. Explosive Azide Hazard. (NIOSH Communication) August, 1976
4. Duckworth JK: Clinical laboratory precautions against viral hepatitis. Pathologist 30:412, 1976
5. Federal Register 37:127, June 30, 1972
6. Federal Register 38:10929, 1973
7. Federal Register Part II, 41:27926, 1976
8. Federal Register 45:33122, 1980
9. Federal Register 45:12722, 1980
10. Federal Register 51:142, 1986
11. Fire Hazards of Materials. Identification System for NFPA #704M. Boston, National Fire Protection Association, 1969
12. Fire Hazard Properties of Flammable Liquids. Gases, Volatile Solids. Boston, NFPA, 1969
13. Fisher Safety Manual. St Louis, Fisher Scientific Co, 1979
14. Flury PA: Look out for hidden laboratory hazards. MLO 9:73, 1977
15. Follow-up on laboratory-associated typhoid fever. MMWR 28:50, 1979
16. Guarnieri M, Guarnieri SR: Laboratory regulations: Protection or problems? MLO 11:93, 1979
17. Handsfield HH, Cummings MJ, Swenson PD: Prevalence of antibody to human immunodeficiency virus and hepatitis B surface antigen in plasma samples submitted to a hospital laboratory: Implications for handling specimens. JAMA 258:3395, 1987
18. Hazardous waste disposal: A new regulatory headache, Washington Report. MLO 11:23, 1979
19. How to Handle Flammable Liquids Safely. Des Plaines, IL, Justrite Manufacturing Co, 1977
20. I & A Newsletter, Vol 8, p 3. Skokie, IL, College of American Pathologists, 1980
21. Evaluation of Carcinogenic Risk of Chemicals to Man. IARC Monogr 1:80, 1971
22. Evaluation of Carcinogenic Risk of Chemicals to Man. IARC Monogr 20:371, 1979
23. Evaluation of Carcinogenic Risk of Chemicals to Man. IARC Monogr 20:401, 1979
24. Laboratory associated typhoid fever. MMWR 28:44, 1979
25. Laboratory Safety Monograph. Supplement to the Guidelines for Recombinant DNA Research. Bethesda, National Institutes of Health, July 1978
26. Manufacturing Chemists Association: Guide for Safety in the Chemical Laboratory, 2nd ed. New York, Van Nostrand Reinhold, 1972
27. Misiak PM, Miceli JN: Toxic effects of formaldehyde. Laboratory Management 25:63, 1986
28. MMWR 36:285, 1987
29. MMWR Supplement 36:2S, 1987
30. National Intelligence Report: Lawsuits Likely Against Labs Which Carelessly Handle AIDS Screening Test Results. Washington, G-2 Reports, February 26, 1986
31. NCCLS: Clinical Laboratory Hazardous Waste. NCCLS Document GP5-P, Vol 6, No. 15, 1986
32. Nixon AD, Officer JA, Law R, Cleland JF, Goldwater PN: Simple device to prevent accidental needle-prick injuries. Lancet 1(8486):888, 1986
33. OSHA Safety and Health Standards (29 CFR 1910). U.S. Department of Labor, Occupational Safety and Health Administration OSHA 2206, Revised. Washington, U.S. Government Printing Office, 1978
34. Protection against Occupational Exposure to Hepatitis B Virus (HBV) and Human Immunodeficiency Virus (HIV). Joint Advisory Notice Department Labor/Department of Health and Human Services, October 19, 1987
35. Public Law 91-596, Occupational Safety and Health Act. Washington, U.S. Government Printing Office, 1970
36. Recommendations for preventing transmission of infection with human T-lymphotropic virus type III/lymphadenopathy-associated virus in the workplace. MMWR 34:681, 1985
37. Safe Handling of Compressed Gases in Laboratory and Plant. East Rutherford, Matheson Gas Products, 1974
38. Safety Management (CDC 22). Atlanta, Centers for Disease Control, 1976
39. Saslow AR, Immarino R: Viral hepatitis in clinical chemistry laboratory workers. Clin Chem 20:514, 1974
40. Scheffler GL: Laboratory safety. In Bond RG, Michaelsen GS, DeRoos RL (eds): Environmental Health and Safety in Health-Care Facilities. New York, Macmillan, 1973
41. Skinhoj P: Occupational risks in Danish clinical laboratories. Scand J Clin Lab Invest 33:27, 1974
42. Spaul WA, Branscomb F: Formaldehyde exposures at work and home. U.S. Navy Medicine 77:11, 1986
43. Standard Procedures for the Handling and Transport of Domestic Diagnostic Specimens and Etiologic Agents. NCCLS Approved Standards: ASH-5. Villanova, National Committee for Clinical Laboratory Standards, 1980
44. Steer NV: Control of hazards from peroxides in ethers. J Chem Educ 41:68, 1964
45. Steer NV: Handbook of Laboratory Safety, 2nd ed. Cleveland, Chemical Rubber Co, 1971
46. Tierno PM: Preventing acquisition of human immunodeficiency virus in the safe handling of AIDS specimens. Lab Med 17:696, 1986
47. Vesley D, Greene VW: Sterilization and cleaning techniques. In Bond RG, Michaelsen GS, DeRoos RL (eds): Environmental Health and Safety in Health-Care Facilities. New York, Macmillan, 1973
48. Washington Report, OSHA Puts Teeth into AIDS Prevention Guidelines. MLO 19, No. 11, 1987
49. Wear JO: Azide hazards with automatic blood cell counters. J Chem Educ 52:A23, 1975

ANNOTATED BIBLIOGRAPHY

Block SS (ed): Disinfection, Sterilization and Preservation, 2nd ed. Philadelphia, Lea & Febiger, 1977

This reference contains methods and procedures for controlling bacteria, fungi, viruses, protozoa, and helminths by chemical and physical methods.

Flury PA: Environmental Health and Safety in the Hospital Laboratory. Springfield, IL, Charles C Thomas, 1978

Complete with discussions about pertinent OSHA standards, this safety reference is especially useful for ideas regarding preparation of safety guidelines, tables, and manuals.

Fuscaldo AA (ed): Laboratory Safety, Theory and Practice. New York, Academic Press, 1980

This reference contains an excellent discussion of the many aspects of laboratory safety.

twenty-one

Laboratory Accreditation, Licensure, and Regulation

Donald A. Senhauser

The earlier edition of this chapter began by noting that there had been a marked increase in credentialing and licensure activity affecting clinical laboratories and their personnel. This development was attributed to the marked increase in the volume of laboratory testing as well as the critical importance such testing had assumed in the scientific and highly technologic practice of medicine.

The time since that edition was published has seen accelerating regulatory activity, not only affecting clinical laboratories, but the entire health-care delivery system. Although some of this regulatory thrust is the result of advancing technology and increased utilization, much of it stems from efforts to contain the ever-spiraling costs of health care by a debt-ridden government and from the new wave of consumerism that has swept the country. There is widespread public concern over the real or perceived danger that the quality of medical care is eroding in the face of severe cost-containment measures, the liability crisis, and resource limitations placed on the health-care delivery system. As noted in a recent editorial by Dennis S. O'Leary, these concerns have resulted in a public demand for greater accountability by hospitals, physicians, and others (including clinical laboratories) involved in providing health-care services.[5] This public pressure has magnified the ever more complex interactions among federal and state lawmakers, regulators, credentialing agencies, and professional societies. These interactions have created a plethora of laws and regulations that are constantly changing with time and locale, to the confusion of most laboratorians. Because the details change from year to year and locale to locale, this chapter will attempt to deal with the general principles of accreditation and regulation. Each reader should understand the importance of carefully familiarizing oneself with the local, state, and federal regulations as well as the voluntary credentialing activities that apply to a specific laboratory and locale, especially when one assumes an administrative position in the organization.

DEFINITIONS

A major source of difficulty in understanding the process of laboratory regulation and accreditation is the imprecise definition of the terms used in discussing these complex issues. Therefore, we will begin this discussion by defining several key terms, using those developed by Schenken[8] in an earlier edition of this book, with slight modifications.

ACCREDITATION. The process by which an agency or organization evaluates and recognizes a program of study or an activity in an institution as meeting certain predetermined standards is called *accreditation*. Standards are usually defined in terms of physical plant, governing body, administration, medical and other staff, and scope and organization of services. Accreditation is usually granted by a private or professional organization created for the purpose of assuring the public of the quality of the accredited. Accreditation is a procedure of voluntary self-regulation by professional peer groups in contrast to review and regulation by governmental agencies. Accreditation standards and individual performance with respect to such standards are not always available to the public. However, in some situations, government agencies recognize accreditation in lieu of, accept it as the basis of, or require it as a condition of licensure or participation in public health and welfare programs. Public or private payment programs often require accreditation as a condition of reimbursement for covered services. Accreditation may either be permanent once obtained or limited to a specific period of time. Unlike licensure, accreditation is not a condition of *lawful* practice, but is intended as an assurance of high-quality practice, although where payment is effectively predicated on accreditation, it may have the same effect as licensure.

CERTIFICATION. The process by which a nongovernmental body or association grants recognition to an individual or an entity such as a laboratory that has met certain predetermined qualifications specified by that agency or organization is called *certification.* It is voluntary and carries no legal sanction.

CREDENTIALING. The broad generic term *credentialing* may be defined as the formal recognition of professional or technical competence. When applied to health manpower, it takes three forms: licensure of individuals or organizations by government, certification of individuals by voluntary agencies, and accreditation of organizations or programs by voluntary associations or agencies. A task force of the American Council of Education has proposed the following principles for credentialing:

1. Credentialing should seek to minimize risks to the public health, safety, and welfare by identifying the qualified.
2. Credentialing, which recognizes and encourages pride and accomplishment and the mastery of knowledge and skills, is in the public interest because it contributes to the advancement of society and improvement of the human condition.
3. Mandatory credentialing should be exercised only when there is a relationship demonstrable to public health and safety.

4. Credentialing is involved substantially with the system of economic and social rewards in the society. Therefore, it is incumbent upon all credentialing systems to recognize pertinent requisites regardless of how and where they are achieved.
5. Credentialing activities of agencies and institutions, whether they are governmentally or publicly controlled or sponsored by occupational and professional organizations, substantially intersect the public interest. Their policy-making and governing boards, therefore, should be representative of broad social interests.
6. Credentialing ultimately related to the health and safety of the public should periodically require proof that the credentialed still possess the necessary requisites and have kept pace with advances in the field.

Because these six principles were drawn up by a group to fit the broadest spectrum of public interest, they do not specifically represent the thinking of any particular health-care profession or organization. This is especially true of the principles dealing with the measurement of recertification and continuing competence in the practice of the various health-care professions. However, they do encompass the major general components of the credentialing process.

LICENSE. A *license* is permission granted to an individual or organization by competent authority, usually governmental, to engage in a practice, occupation, or activity defined legally to be otherwise unlawful. Licensure is the process by which the license is granted. Because a license is needed to begin lawful practice, it is usually granted on the basis of examination or proof of education, rather than on measures of performance. The license, when given, is usually permanent but may be conditioned on annual payment of fee, proof of continuing education, or proof of competence. Commonly accepted grounds for revocation of a license include incompetence, commission of a crime (whether or not related to the licensed practice), or moral turpitude. Possession of a medical license from one state may (by reciprocity) or may not suffice to obtain a license from another. There is no national licensure system for health professionals, although requirements from one state to another are often so nearly standardized as to constitute such a licensing system.

Licensing acts are designed to protect the public from incompetent practitioners, and consequently such acts must contain a realistic definition of the practice they seek to regulate. Licensing boards are, by their very nature, consumer-advocacy boards. They have basically two functions: (1) to establish entry-level standards that will assure safe practice and (2) to monitor the continued competency and ethicality of the licensee's practice.

REGULATION. The intervention of government in the health-care or other service market to control entry into or change the behavior of participants in that marketplace through specification of rules for the participants is called *regulation*. This does not usually include programs that seek to change behavior through financing mechanisms or incentives. It does not include private accreditation programs, although they may be relied upon by government regulatory programs. Regulatory programs can be described in terms of what is regulated (*e.g.,* charges or costs), who is regulated (*e.g.,* hospitals), who regulates (*e.g.,* state government), and how the regulation is carried out (*e.g.,* prospective rate review). Regulatory programs may include certification, registration, licensure, certificate of need, or other measurements. Regulation is also a synonym for a rule published by the executive branch, and its agencies, of the federal, state, or local government, which implements a law passed by that government's legislative body(s).

INSPECTION AND ACCREDITATION OF CLINICAL LABORATORIES

Inspection and accreditation programs for clinical laboratories have been well established for a number of years. A number of voluntary professional associations have developed laboratory accreditation programs that have been a major factor in the attainment of the high standards of quality that characterize laboratory medicine in the United States today. Several of the larger programs will be described in the following sections in some detail, because almost any clinical laboratory will be participating in one or another of these programs.

Laboratory Accreditation Program of the College of American Pathologists

The Laboratory Accreditation Program (LAP) of the College of American Pathologists (CAP) came into being in November 1961 when an *ad hoc* committee on laboratory accreditation and the Board of Governors of the College implemented a program for the voluntary inspection and accreditation of clinical laboratories, which primarily focused on the

hospital laboratories. This program had its genesis in the growing hospital accreditation program of the Joint Commission on Accreditation of Hospitals (JCAH), which from its very inception in 1924 had included clinical laboratory services in its standards.[7] Over the years, as clinical laboratories grew in size, sophistication, and complexity, it became increasingly clear that the general JCAH inspection was inadequate to ensure the highest laboratory standards, and that a specialized accreditation program was needed. CAP responded to this need with its laboratory accreditation program; and from its beginnings in 1961, it has developed into the largest voluntary laboratory improvement program in the world.

Under the CAP program, standards of performance were developed and an inspection process initiated that was modified and updated through constant education and performance review over the years. In 1984, the CAP board of governors requested that the Commission on Laboratory Accreditation review the standards in light of the increasing emphasis on quality assurance and outcome measurement as well as the greater diversity of laboratories participating in the accreditation program. After 3 years of study, review, and revision, CAP published a new manual of standards, in which the standards of performance have been reduced from eight to five. The effective date for implementation of the new standards was July 1, 1987.[10] The key provisions of these standards deal with (1) amplification of the laboratory director's responsibilities; (2) quality assurance (in response to the JCAH thrust in this arena); (3) uniform standards for all laboratories; (4) ancillary testing programs; and (5) adoption of a standard format for all technical procedure manuals.

The CAP accreditation program continues to be a voluntary program with heavy emphasis on improvement through peer review and education. The heart of the program is the corps of trained volunteer inspectors who are practicing pathologists and medical technologists. The program is organized into ten geographic regions, each in charge of a commissioner appointed by the College. The regional commissioner is responsible for selection and training of the inspectors and coordination of the on-site inspection process of the laboratories within his region. The success of the program was recognized by Congress when it passed the Clinical Laboratories Improvement Act of 1967 (CLIA '67), which reflected in its legislative history that the College's accreditation program was "equivalent or more stringent than" the requirements set forth in the federal regulation governing laboratories under the Medicare program. However, it must be emphasized that the College's program is *voluntary* and that improvement comes through education and the desire for professional self-improvement, not legislative coercion. However, the withdrawal of College accreditation may have serious consequences, especially for hospital laboratories inspected by the JCAH for Medicare certification and for those independent laboratories using the CAP program in lieu of CLIA '67 inspection.

The new standards are supplemented by an extensive, published, and verified checklist that is used by each outside inspector and the subject laboratory to review laboratory performance on site in great detail. These checklists are developed and approved by the various CAP Scientific Resource Committees, which cover each laboratory discipline, and represent the state of the art in each subspecialty of laboratory medicine. The checklists are being constantly revised in response to the burgeoning scope of laboratory testing, as well as to ongoing feedback from the inspectors in the field.

Joint Commission on Accreditation of Hospitals

The JCAH is an outgrowth of a hospital standardization program of the American College of Surgeons (ACS) that was launched in 1917, funded by a gift from the Carnegie Foundation. The early emphasis was on the adoption of a uniform medical record format that would facilitate accurate recording of the patient's clinical course in order to measure surgical outcomes or clinical course. The ACS recognized that such a program also involved setting standards for hospital services and in 1924 published five minimum standards for hospitals in the College Bulletin. The early history of this accreditation program is well presented by Roberts and associates.[7] Even then, one of the five standards was concerned with the availability and function of clinical laboratory and pathology services in the hospital. In 1950, the size and scope of the inspection program had grown beyond the resources of one organization to sustain it, and after extensive negotiations, an organization was created whose sole purpose was to encourage the voluntary attainment of uniformly high standards of hospital care. The organization was named the Joint Commission on Accreditation of Hospitals, and the founding sponsors were the American College of Surgeons, the American College of Physicians, the American Medical Association, the Canadian Medical Association, and the American Hospital Association. The JCAH began to offer accreditation to hospitals in January 1953. Later the Canadian Medical Association withdrew,

and the American Dental Association was added to the organization in 1980.

The JCAH surveys over 3500 hospitals a year and has its own full-time field staff to carry out this mission. The inspection process is based on an accreditation manual that the JCAH reviews, updates, and revises and that includes standards for all hospital departments, including pathology and medical laboratory services. In 1979, recognizing the complexity and growth of laboratory medicine, the JCAH entered into discussions with CAP concerning the need to update and refine the standards the JCAH had adopted for hospital laboratories. The result of these discussions was an agreement whereby the College would assist the JCAH in training inspectors for hospital laboratories, and the JCAH would waive its inspection of the hospital laboratory during the course of the general survey of the hospital departments if the laboratory had been previously accredited by the CAP. Major exceptions to this waiver are in the area of safety and quality assurance, where the JCAH team continues its jurisdiction as part of the overall survey of the hospital. In addition, the JCAH has developed mechanisms for surveying hospitals with laboratories who do not participate in the College inspection and accreditation program. These joint arrangements between the JCAH and the College have resulted in the Joint Commission developing standards and a checklist of questions that closely follow the format of the College inspection checklists.

In 1965, the Medicare law, PL 89-97 was enacted. Written into the Medicare law were standards of patient care that had to be maintained or achieved if a hospital wished to participate in this major federal health-care reimbursement program. The law recognized that the voluntary program of the JCAH was widely accepted as the norm in the delivery of quality hospital services to the patient. Hence, hospitals accredited by the Joint Commission were automatically deemed to be in compliance with federal Medicare conditions of participation and thus eligible for reimbursement under Medicare without further inspection by a government agency. This legislative language is the source of the term *deemed status* used to describe certain voluntary programs of inspection and accreditation, such as the JCAH program, that meet or exceed federal standards. In turn, by agreement between the JCAH and the Health Care Financing Administration (HCFA), the agency responsible for the administration of the Medicare program, the College Laboratory Accreditation Program has received "sub-deemed" status to accommodate its role in the JCAH program. Those hospitals and other health-care facilities not in the JCAH program are directly inspected by an agency of the federal government or its designee.

The American Association of Blood Banks

The final voluntary inspection and accreditation program that will be briefly discussed is that of the American Association of Blood Banks (AABB), which has been actively evaluating and accrediting blood banks and hospital transfusion services since 1957.

The inspection process is based on the *Standards for Blood Banks and Transfusion Services* manual developed by the Committee on Standards of the AABB. The 12th edition of the standards was published in early 1987.[9] During the 30 years of its existence, the standards manual has come to be recognized as the single most authoritative source for evaluating the practice of blood banking and transfusion medicine. The 12th edition contains major changes in the standards for donor testing, labeling, and record-keeping. An updated section addresses the prevention of transfusion-associated infectious diseases such as the acquired immunodeficiency syndrome (AIDS) and non-A, non-B hepatitis. This enhancement reflects the growing recognition and concern with this major public health problem.

The standards manual begins with a general policies section, in which the requirement is made that the AABB *Technical Manual* be followed as the operational policy of the blood bank. There follow detailed sections on donor and donor blood procedures, plasmapheresis operations, including therapeutic plasmapheresis and exchange and cytopheresis. Compatibility testing and recipient evaluation are covered, as well as standards for evaluation of transfusion complications. Finally, histocompatibility testing and organ transplantation are thoroughly covered in the 12th edition, accommodating to this new and important technology.

Voluntary inspectors are screened and appointed by the AABB and almost always are recognized as persons with considerable knowledge in the field. These inspectors conduct an on-site review of the facilities and services of a blood bank or transfusion service using a published checklist designed to elicit the degree to which the facilities are operating in compliance with the standards. Outside quality assurance (proficiency testing) is required. Following the on-site inspection, the AABB communicates to the facility whether or not it has been approved. Approval is withheld until deficiencies (if any) noted by the inspector have been corrected or commented upon by the transfusion service within a limited time period.

Many hospital transfusion services are inspected by both the AABB and the CAP during its accreditation inspection of the clinical laboratory. In addition, the Food and Drug Administration (FDA) has the legal authority to inspect hospital blood banks by its own standards, but has generally limited its activities to freestanding facilities that only obtain and process blood and blood products from donors. Much of the potential for confusion and misunderstanding among these parties is dealt with through the appointment of liaison members from the College, the FDA, and the American Red Cross, and the Department of Defense to the committee on standards of the AABB.

FEDERAL AND STATE REGULATION OF CLINICAL LABORATORIES

Medicare Regulations

Unlike the *voluntary* inspection and accreditation programs described above, which evolved from the desire of the laboratory professionals themselves to improve medical care through *peer* review systems initiated and maintained by their professional societies, the federal and state governments can mandate inspection and standards programs through their powers to license and/or reimburse health-care facilities, including clinical laboratories. Such power is derived from the enactment of laws by the various legislative bodies under their duty to protect the public health, safety and welfare.

Several state legislatures, notably New York and California, had done so prior to the entry of the federal government into the health-care arena in a major way after the enactment of Medicare and Medicaid (Title XVIII and XIX of the Social Security Act). The Medicare regulatory program was based on the statutory authority (the Social Security Act of 1965) given to the Secretary to set standards to assure the health and safety of Medicare (and Medicaid) beneficiaries. As a result of these laws, the Secretary of the Department of Health and Human Services (DHHS, formerly Department of Health, Education, and Welfare [DHEW]), through the regulatory agencies within the Department, developed standards of health care for all clinical laboratories operating in inpatient and outpatient settings, including independent (freestanding) laboratories. The major exemptions within this law were for clinical laboratories operated by a licensed physician, osteopath, dentist, podiatrist, or group thereof, that performed laboratory tests or procedures solely as an adjunct to the treatment of their own patients. The power to regulate clinical laboratories derives not only from statutory authority but also through the mechanism known as "conditions of participation in the Medicare/Medicaid program" under which a health-care facility (including clinical laboratories) can be barred from receiving reimbursement for services rendered to the beneficiaries of these entitlement programs—certainly a powerful sanction.

The Medicare regulations for clinical laboratories, as they have evolved since 1965, basically cover standards for personnel, record-keeping, management, safety, and internal and external quality-control systems, including proficiency testing. The standards for each type of laboratory are reasonably uniform, with the exception of those for independent laboratories that have more detailed personnel standards, including those for the director, technical supervisor, general supervisor, technologist, and technician. In addition, independent laboratories, unlike hospital laboratories that are approved as part of the overall facility, are approved by specialty and subspecialty activity, *i.e.,* chemistry, radioimmunoassay, and so forth.

The regulatory structure begun in 1965 was based on a combination of several model state regulatory programs and the accreditation programs of the private sector, such as those of the CAP and JCAH. Thus, there is considerable overlap and commonality among the quality-assurance aspects of these programs. Medicare regulations have been promulgated and expanded each year since 1965, increasing in complexity and detail. Such changes and updates are published in the Code of Federal Regulations (CFR).[1]

Clinical Laboratory Improvement Act of 1967

After the Medicare/Medicaid laboratory standards programs were put in place in 1965, the perception developed in Congress that problems existed in the quality of services provided to Medicare recipients by clinical laboratories, especially those engaged in interstate commerce. The Congress attempted to solve these perceived problems, unfortunately not through the Medicare regulatory mechanisms already in place, but by passing CLIA '67. This broad act defined a clinical laboratory as follows:

> . . . A facility for the biological, microbiological, serological, chemical, immunohematological, hematological, biophysical, cytological, pathological, or other examination of material derived from the human body, or for the purpose of providing information for the diagnosis, prevention or treatment of any disease or impairment of, or the assessment of the health of man.

The provisions contained in CLIA '67 were limited to those laboratories that were engaged in interstate commerce. Such laboratories are defined in this act as those accepting more than 100 specimens during each year in each category of testing listed in the definition. Laboratories receiving less than 100 specimens can obtain a letter of exemption on application to the Centers for Disease Control (CDC) in Atlanta. As in the case of the Medicare regulations, medical office laboratories were exempted from this law.

Laboratories that were deemed to be in interstate commerce were prohibited from operating in that sphere unless they obtained an appropriate *license* issued by the Secretary of the DHEW (now DHHS) or his designee. CLIA '67, which was passed to ensure the quality of the clinical laboratories engaged in interstate commerce, was significantly different from the Medicare regulations in that sanctions were not based on reimbursement denial, but rather on the power of *licensure*. The act also differed from Medicare in that it provided for regulation by individual test, rather than an entire facility. While many of the standards promulgated under CLIA '67 were essentially the same as those for independent laboratories under Medicare, there were significant differences. One notable difference was the requirement that laboratories licensed under CLIA '67 were required to participate successfully in a proficiency testing program operated by the CDC. The power to license interstate laboratories was also delegated to the CDC, which administered the program.

The upshot of the passage of CLIA '67 was that the government found itself administering two separate regulatory programs for clinical laboratories. Although the regulations governing these programs overlapped considerably, there were significant differences, which over the years have been complicated by shifting authority among various and often rival agencies within the government delegated to administer the laws (especially Medicare). The magnitude of these differences is exemplified by the fact that the regulations for each are promulgated in different parts of the CFR. Thus, the regulations implementing CLIA '67 are published in an entirely different section of Part 74, Title 42, of the CFR.[2] For an excellent account of the evolution of federal regulation of clinical laboratories, the reader is referred to a recent review by Edinger.[3]

State Regulation of Clinical Laboratories

Adding to the complexities caused by the dual nature of the federal regulation of clinical laboratories is the fact that both Medicare and CLIA '67 mandate that all participating laboratory facilities must be in compliance with the state and local laws of the locality in which they operate. These laws may include personnel licensure, facility licensure, fire safety requirements, and other related health and safety requirements. For example, 26 states have licensure or other types of requirements for clinical laboratories or their personnel.[3] Over half the states have regulations governing independent laboratories. Many states have proficiency testing programs. Federal clinical laboratory regulation review for Medicare/Medicaid programs is delegated to the state health departments in at least 40 states, under contract with the federal government. Because local regulation varies widely from state to state and even major cities within a state, this federal deference to local law has added to the already confusing laboratory regulatory climate. Yearly modification of old regulations and promulgation of new rules at the local, state, and federal level contribute further to the difficulty.

The Regulatory Climate Today

Laboratory medicine has become one of the most heavily regulated sectors of the health-care system under the intervention by the federal government. The welter of rules and regulations has been confounded by jurisdictional disputes not only among federal agencies, but state and local governments as well. This Babel of divided and conflicting authority has been further confused by a series of major reorganizations that the Public Health Service, the DHHS, and the Social Security Administration (SSA) have undergone since 1972, during which time a number of different agencies were involved in the responsibility for laboratory regulation under Medicare and CLIA '67. Agencies were shifted from one department of the government to another, transformed into new entities with different names, and at times given entirely new authority for regulatory and reimbursement functions. Some indication of the magnitude of such changes is the fact that the entire DHEW became DHHS, losing jurisdiction over education and gaining certain agencies concerned with Medicare from the SSA. This divided and confused authority led to serious contention not only among the various regulatory agencies but also spread to the various laboratory constituencies in the private sector that were the subject of the regulations. Such contention remains today, especially in the areas of proficiency testing and personnel standards affecting clinical laboratory operation.

In 1978, a reorganizational change took place within the DHHS that would have a profound impact on the effectiveness and efficiency of the Medicare regulatory programs, including those effecting clinical laboratory medicine. This change created an agency, the Health Care Financing Administration (HCFA), in which the regulatory, financing (reimbursement) and enforcement activities for the Medicare/Medicaid programs were removed from several agencies and departments (such as the SSA), which previously had divided such authority, and were combined into the new agency. This powerful agency came under the purview of the Secretary for Health and Human Services (HHS). Since its formation, the HCFA has had a tremendous influence on shaping the whole health care delivery system, including laboratory medicine.

Today, the HCFA is charged with the administration of both the Medicare and CLIA '67 regulatory programs for clinical laboratories. It has inherited a confused, contentious, and sometimes adversarial climate due to the years of conflicting and overlapping jurisdiction of the laboratory regulatory programs described above.

Under HCFA, the regulatory thrust of the 1980s is clearly to provide increased uniformity between the Medicare and CLIA '67 regulatory programs, in cooperation with the private sector. However, such efforts have been hampered by the overriding necessity to implement cost-containment measures affecting clinical laboratories that have been mandated by the budget reduction measures instituted by Congress every year since 1982. This cascade of draconian cost-containment measures passed by Congress since that time has magnified the difficulties between the agency and its various constituencies in the private sector. Reimbursement issues frequently seem to override the concern for the quality of laboratory services, which is the stated goal of both the public and the private sector. Such emphasis on cost containment is understandable when one realizes that there are now 12,000 federally regulated clinical laboratories that are participating in an "industry" that is producing an estimated $15 to $20 billion worth of services each year,[6] with much of this cost borne by Medicare/Medicaid and other health and welfare programs of the federal and state governments. Nonetheless, the implementation of cost-containment measures frequently works at cross-purposes to the goal of uniformity and deregulation.

A recent example of this situation is the effort by the HCFA to simplify some of the detailed technical standards found in the present regulations in support of the Administration's deregulatory policy.[4] Due to pressure from the Office of Management and Budget (OMB), driven by budgetary considerations, and applied through the Office of the Secretary of HHS, this effort to deregulate and simplify some technical regulations became entangled in regulatory language that included major changes in laboratory personnel standards as well. The regulatory changes would make Medicare hospital standards universal in all clinical laboratories. This proposal for such a major change in personnel standards, made without seeking prior consultation with the private sector, has created great perturbation among the several professional organizations with an interest in specific personnel standards, thus making the promulgation of any deregulatory changes problematic and unpredictable, even though badly needed.

Thus, deregulation and elimination of costly duplication of regulatory programs are being carried out in an atmosphere that is charged with rapid technologic change, cost-containment issues, and the conflicting needs of the private sector being regulated. The regulatory areas currently under review include personnel, proficiency testing, quality control, management, program administration, and hearing procedures. As attempts are made to achieve uniformity between Medicare and CLIA '67 regulations, additional efforts must also be made to reconcile the primary goal of the private sector, which is to achieve excellence by education through voluntary peer-review and accreditation programs, and the regulatory requirements of the federal standards programs that seek quality assurance and cost-containment through a system of rules and regulations enforced by sanctions. It remains to be seen whether this task can be successfully carried out.

It should be clear to the reader from the above passages that understanding the impact of regulatory activity on the operation of a clinical laboratory is a necessity for successful administration. It should also be apparent that this subject is exceedingly complex and undergoing constant change and revision. Perhaps the only "given" for a laboratory administrator is that the issues of accreditation, regulation, and licensure will play an increasingly important role in decision-making in the future, whatever the setting of the clinical laboratory. Regulation has and will have a profound fiscal impact on the laboratory as well.

It behooves the successful laboratory director to be knowledgeable concerning, and keep abreast of, the specific licensure and regulatory requirements that pertain to the laboratory. Fortunately, there is enough overlap between the federal and state regulations concerning quality assurance and the various voluntary laboratory accreditation programs, such as those of the CAP and the AABB, that strict adherence to such voluntary programs in the operation of a laboratory will provide the basis for successful participation in most federal and state regulatory programs, in addition to ensuring high-quality output from the laboratory, which contributes to excellent patient care.

However, especially in the areas of licensure and reimbursement, the director/administrator must keep abreast of the specific requirements of state and federal agencies. The complexity and constant changes in these regulations make this a difficult and onerous task. It can be made less so by maintaining a constant and ongoing contact with one's state public health agency and especially with the headquarters staff of the professional laboratory organizations such as the CAP, the American Society of Clinical Pathologists, the Clinical Laboratory Management Association, and the American Society for Medical Technology. These organizations maintain expert staffs, knowledgeable in government affairs, regulation, and reimbursement issues, in order to assist their members. Another important source of information is the local and regional Medicare intermediary and/or carrier, especially for information regarding rules for reimbursement. The laboratory administrator/director should keep orderly, up-to-date files of the publications, newsletters, and so forth, of these private and governmental agencies close at hand.

Obviously, if the laboratory is planning a new venture such as promoting outside reference testing, spinning off an independent laboratory division, or engaging in interstate commerce, the impact of the applicable state and federal regulations on such activities must be an important part of the planning process.

REFERENCES

1. Code of Federal Regulations: Public Health: Title 42, Parts 74, 405.1310 et seq, 405.1128 and 482.27. Washington, D.C., U.S. Government Printing Office, 1987
2. Code of Federal Regulations: Public Health: Title 42, Part 74, 62–75. Washington, DC, U.S. Government Printing Office, 1985

3. Edinger SE: Evolution and future directions of the federal regulation of clinical laboratories. J Med Technol 1:776–786, 1984

4. HCFA to Open Up Laboratory Personnel Standards. Washington Report V(3):2–3. Washington, DC, American Society of Clinical Pathologists, 1987

5. O'Leary DS: The Joint Commission looks to the future. JAMA 258:951–952, 1987

6. Report of the Laboratory Task Force (on Clinical Laboratory Reimbursement). Baltimore, Department of Health and Human Services, Health Care Financing Administration, 1984

7. Roberts JS, Cook JG, Redman RR: A history of the Joint Commission on Accreditation of Hospitals. Jama 258:936–940, 1987

8. Schenken JR: Laboratory accreditation, licensure and regulation. In Snyder JR (ed): Administration and Supervision in Laboratory Medicine, pp 360–362. Philadelphia, JB Lippincott, 1983

9. Standards for Blood Banks and Transfusion Services. Arlington, Committee on Standards, American Association of Blood Banks, 1987

10. Standards for Laboratory Accreditation: Chicago, Commission on Laboratory Accreditation, College of American Pathologists, 1987

twenty-two

Laboratory Inspection as a Management Tool

John C. Neff

This chapter addresses laboratory inspection, a part of the accreditation process, as a management tool. Participation in an accreditation program is a real opportunity to improve laboratory services and should be viewed in this manner, rather than as a mere means of fulfilling an onerous requirement. Laboratory inspection requires a close look at detailed procedures and policies established to enable both the laboratory and the institution as a whole to provide quality patient care. Laboratory directors and supervisors often assume that once a procedure or policy is in place, operations are routinely carried out in accord with these plans. As a result of preparing for and experiencing an accreditation inspection, many a laboratory director and manager learned a great deal about their own laboratory— much of which they did not realize they did not know.[2]

The discussion in this chapter rests on the following thesis: involvement in laboratory inspection and accreditation is one of the most valuable management tools the director or administrator possesses. Consider with what the full-time manager or administrator is confronted and what usually takes up most working hours: organization, motivation, the delegation of authority, managing conflict, personnel administration, medicolegal concerns, fiscal management. A thorough involvement in the laboratory accreditation process may be the single most comprehensive method available to help the man-ager stay current with what is actually happening, technically, at the bench level. A lack of knowledge of the technical mission and problems confronting the laboratory is a criticism frequently leveled at upper management and in many instances is justified. Participation in the laboratory accreditation process not only fulfills requirements that must be met from a service perspective but also forms the centerpiece of effective and successful laboratory management in the delivery of quality patient care. Laboratory accreditation inspection is a program for laboratory improvement.

ACCREDITING AGENCIES THAT INSPECT CLINICAL LABORATORIES

Accreditation programs are basically methods of voluntary self-regulation whereby a private agency, through the judicious application of standards, grants accreditation to an organization, thus assuring the public of quality and safety. Although such accreditation does not have the force of law (such as licensure), accreditation, certification, licensure, and credentialing are often so intertwined that it is difficult to be sure that they are in fact separate processes. Consider, for example, that a Medicare license is compulsory if health-care institutions or laboratories are to be reimbursed by the federal government (these monies may account for as much as 30% of the revenue of some health-care organizations and laboratories); yet the federal Medicare program (compulsory) will under some circumstances accept Joint Commission on Accreditation of Healthcare Organizations (JCAHO) and College of American Pathologists (CAP) Laboratory Accreditation Program (LAP) accreditation (voluntary). The interconnection should be obvious.

Table 22-1 lists organizations and agencies that are involved in hospital and laboratory accreditation and regulations. Some inspections are mandatory and thus involve legal license, and others involve voluntary types of accreditation. The individuals, inspectors, accreditors, licensors, regulators, and so forth, that represent these agencies or organizations (whose jurisdictions frequently overlap) have nothing directly to do with what occurs technically or from a real-time management standpoint, in the day-to-day operation of a laboratory. However, in a very real way it can be said that they allow the work to be done, ensure that the work performed in the laboratory does not endanger the public, permit the laboratory to state that its mission is carried out adequately or in an excellent fashion, and in many instances allow the laboratory or the health-care institution to be paid for the work that it does.

Chapter 21 described CAP/LAP, accreditation by the JCAH, now known as the Joint Commission on Accreditation of Health Care Organizations (JCAHO),[5] and accreditation by the American Association of Blood Banks (AABB). For both scope and detail in comprehensive clinical laboratory inspection, the CAP/LAP and JCAHO standards are comparable. (See Appendix 22-A and Appendix 22-B at the end of this chapter.) This chapter focuses on the CAP/LAP because it is one of the largest in the world and has been in existence in the United States for the longest period of time.

CAP LABORATORY ACCREDITATION PROGRAM

It is appropriate to emphasize that the CAP/LAP is a part of the total activity of the CAP. It is a part of an organizational structure that receives input from several sources within the College (Fig. 22-1). The CAP is divided into a number of councils. The LAP is in the Council on Quality Assurance, whose structure can be outlined as follows:

Council on Quality Assurance
    Laboratory Accreditation Commission
    CAP Working Committees with the Centers for Disease Control (CDC), Health Care Financing Administration (HCFA), JCAH, and industry

Table 22-1
Types of Accreditation of Approval for Hospitals and Laboratories

Organization/ Agency	Status	Hospital	Laboratory	Comments
JCAHO	Voluntary	+	+	Usually 3 years' duration. Will accept CAP accreditation
CAP/LAP	Voluntary		+	2 years' duration; may be used for purposes of CLIA '67 accreditation
Medicare	Compulsory when applicable		+	Accepts JCAHO, JCAHO/CAP or CAP accreditation for laboratory only
State licensing	Compulsory	+	+	Various state organizations
AABB	Voluntary		+	Blood banks only; acceptance by some in lieu of state organizations
CDC	Compulsory		+	Laboratories involved in interstate commerce; inspection by HCFA; may accept CAP program
FDA	Compulsory		+	Blood banks; animal facilities
NRC	Compulsory		+	Usually under state regulatory agency

Abbreviations: JCAHO, Joint Commission on the Accreditation of Healthcare Organizations; CAP/LAP, College of American Pathologists/ Laboratory Accreditation Program; CDC, Centers for Disease Control; AABB, American Association of Blood Banks; FDA, Federal Drug Administration; NRC, Nuclear Regulatory Commission; CLIA, Clinical Laboratory Improvement Act; HCFA, Health Care Financing Administration.

CAP COUNCIL AS IT RELATES TO THE
CLINICAL LABORATORY ACCREDITATION PROGRAM

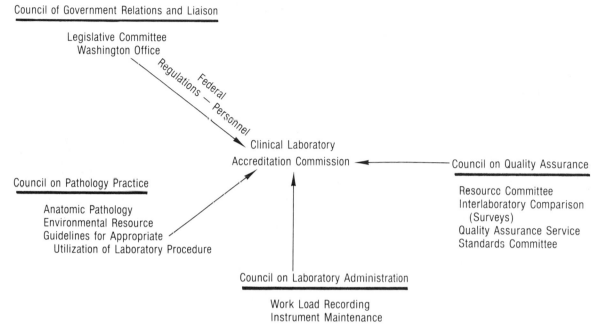

FIGURE 22-1. CAP Council structure as it relates to the clinical laboratory accreditation program.

Policy Committee
Standards Committee
Publications Committee
    Water
    Fire
    Newsletter
    Seminar Manual
Seminar Committee
Safety
Standards Committee
Surveys—proficiency testing; interlaboratory comparison program
Quality Assurance Service (QAS)—internal, day-to-day quality control
Resource Committees
    Blood Banking
    Hematology
    Chemistry
    Toxicology
    Therapeutic Drug Monitoring

    Microbiology
    Nuclear Medicine
    Diagnostic Immunology

In addition, there are other councils and committees in the College that coordinate the efforts of the total program in laboratory improvement.

Goals of the Program

Consistent with the original purpose of the Laboratory Accreditation Program, most goals and objectives of the Commission on Clinical Laboratory Accreditation are oriented toward laboratory improvements. Some of the objectives are as follows[4]:

- To be an educational program that provides a mechanism for introducing new ideas and new technology and provides appropriate credit for continuing education.
- To develop recommendations that will assist the laboratory in providing a safe working

environment and satisfactory working conditions for laboratory employees.

- To conduct a program that encompasses and encourages modern quality-assurance techniques, that is relevant and practical, that does not include unnecessary testing, that is unencumbered with unnecessary regulatory or bureaucratic requirements, and that is based upon scientific need, not supposition.
- To operate a program that will encompass the state of the art with respect to professional consensus standards.
- To serve as consultants to laboratory directors on problems of laboratory standards and practice.

Management Responsibilities Under the CAP Program

Management has specific responsibilities with relation to the CAP Accreditation Program.[6] These can be divided into the following categories, not necessarily in the order of their importance:

Communication
Personnel
Instrument function checks and preventive maintenance
Internal and external quality control and quality assurance
Documentation and supervision of the various quality-control activities
Safety

Accreditation Standards Applied in Inspection

Each of the aforementioned management responsibilities are evaluated during the inspection process by comparison with the published standards. The inspection process maximizes two-way consultation. The inspector's major responsibilities are those of evaluation and education. The laboratory agrees to hold itself to five generic standards having to do with personnel, facilities, quality assurance, quality control, and process. These standards have been changed a number of times since the inception of the LAP/CAP in 1961; the revised 1988 standards are reproduced here (see Appendix 22-A for interpretation):

STANDARD I: DIRECTOR AND PERSONNEL REQUIREMENTS

The pathology or medical laboratory service shall be directed by a physician or doctoral scientist qualified to assume professional, scientific, consultative, organizational, administrative, and educational responsibility for the service. Generally, it is medically preferable that the director be a board-certified pathologist. The director shall have sufficient authority to implement and maintain the standards.

When a nonpathologist physician or doctoral scientist serves as director, such individual must be qualified by virtue of documented training, expertise, and experience in the areas of analytical testing offered by the laboratory. Where the functions of the laboratory so require, the services of a qualified consulting pathologist shall be retained. In all facilities where anatomic pathology services are provided, a pathologist shall perform such services.

Special function laboratories shall be directed by either a physician who is qualified to assume professional responsibility for the special function laboratory or a qualified doctoral scientist with documented training, expertise, and experience in the appropriate specific clinical discipline and area of testing.

The location, organization, or ownership of the laboratory shall not alter the requirements of this standard, its interpretation, or its application.

STANDARD II: RESOURCES AND FACILITIES

The pathology service shall have sufficient and appropriate space, equipment, facilities, and supplies for the performance of the required volume of work with accuracy, precision, efficiency, and safety. In addition, the pathology service shall have effective methods for communication to ensure prompt and reliable reporting. There shall be appropriate record storage and retrieval.

STANDARD III: QUALITY ASSURANCE

There shall be an ongoing quality assurance program to monitor and evaluate objectively the quality and appropriateness of the care and treatment provided to patients by the pathology service, to pursue opportunities to improve patient care, and to identify and resolve problems.

STANDARD IV: QUALITY CONTROL

Each pathology service shall have a quality control system that demonstrates the reliability and medical usefulness of laboratory data.

STANDARD V: INSPECTION REQUIREMENTS

A pathology service which desires accreditation shall undergo periodic inspections and evaluations as determined by the Commission on Laboratory Accreditation of the College of American Pathologists.

Adherence to these standards is monitored by the inspector by referring to over 1600 questions, occurring in 15 booklets (checklists). Each booklet of questions is designed to evaluate a particular part of the laboratory, *i.e.,* the general laboratory, the laboratory information system, hematology, anatomic pathology and cytology, blood bank, diagnostic immunology, syphilis serology, and so forth. The construction of the checklists is overseen by a number of resource committees working under the Commission on Laboratory Accreditation (see Fig. 22-1). The membership of these resource committees (chemistry, toxicology, hematology, nuclear medicine) is drawn from the very best practitioners of laboratory medicine in the United States and Canada.

Steps in the Accreditation Process

The steps in the accreditation process are as follows[4]:

1. Prior to the initial application, it is assumed that the laboratory has obtained the CAP *Standards for Accreditation of Medical Laboratories* and the checklists. These are available from the CAP headquarters office. Most laboratories review the standards, then inspect their own facility, using the checklist. This can be accomplished in whatever way is convenient. The pathology staff, pathology residents, section supervisors, and technologists should be involved so that they can become familiar with the checklist. Then any obvious corrections can be made.
2. If the laboratory chooses to apply for accreditation by the CAP, it contacts the CAP headquarters office, Laboratory Accreditation Department, to request an application; completes the necessary paperwork; and submits the appropriate fees.
3. Upon receipt of the application questionnaire and director's statements, the CAP Central Office notifies the appropriate regional or state commissioner that the applying laboratory is ready for inspection. The commissioner then appoints an inspector to visit the laboratory and notifies the CAP Central Office. The inspector/inspection team reviews the data and contacts the laboratory director to arrange for the inspection data and discusses the particulars of the visit.

4. All inspection visits are announced. The on-site inspection is customarily scheduled about 6 weeks from the time the application forms are received from the applying laboratory. The information included in the *Inspector's Manual,*[3,7] supplied as part of the inspection packet, should be followed by the inspector/team. During the on-site visit, the inspector (or inspection team) meets with the laboratory director and department or section heads for a preliminary orientation. A brief visit and discussion with the hospital administrator and chief of staff is also customary. The inspector (or inspection team) then conducts a complete inspection of the laboratory, answering all questions in the appropriate checklists.
5. When the inspection has been completed, the inspector (or inspection team) meets with the laboratory director and staff for a summation conference and complete review of the inspection findings. All deficiencies noted should be discussed in detail, and any misinterpretations or similar errors should be resolved, if possible.
6. Following completion of the on-site visit, the inspector (or leader of the inspection team) forwards the completed checklists as well as a completed "Inspector's Supplemental Report" form to the CAP Computer Center, where a computer-generated list of deficiencies (along with explanatory commentaries, which include recommended corrective actions and pertinent references) is printed. This list is sent to the regional commissioner, along with the "Inspector's Supplemental Report."
7. The commissioner reviews these materials and sends a copy of the list of deficiencies (with commentaries) noted in the inspection report to the inspected laboratory, requesting that any deficiencies noted be corrected and that each corrective action be documented within 30 days.
8. The laboratory returns its response, along with documentation of corrected deficiencies, to the regional commissioner for final review.
9. The regional commissioner recommends accreditation or denial of accreditation, but official accreditation or denial of accreditation are actions taken by the total commission at its regularly scheduled meetings.

The fact that the director must reply, in the initial application, to all standards, coupled with the fact that all inspections are announced, and finally that the director and institution are given 30 days to announce corrective actions taken on all deficiencies, ensures that the laboratory and institution fully understand the deliberately set high standards and are given every opportunity to comply with them.

Programs/Services Integral to the Operation of a Laboratory Accreditation Program (CAP)

Standards and a checklist for use by inspectors are supplemented by other publications and programs for integral for a successful laboratory accreditation program. Publications include *Guidelines for Laboratory Safety, Reagent Water Specifications, Laboratory Instrument Verification and Maintenance Manual,* and the adoption of standard guidelines for the design, preparation, and production of laboratory manuals.

Two other programs, the Quality Assurance Service (QAS) and the Proficiency Survey Program, are also important to laboratory accreditation. The QAS is a comprehensive data-processing service for the management of daily quality control, through intralaboratory and interlaboratory comparisons. *Unassayed* materials are processed daily in the user's laboratory, along with patient control and standard specimens. Results are sent to the CAP Computer Center, after which the participant receives not only precision day-to-day comparison data but comparisons of performance by procedure, instrument, similar laboratories, and so forth. (This service is thus more appropriately termed a *quality-control,* rather than a *quality-assurance* service.) The QAS has as its goal the provision of internal precise results.

Assayed materials, the referent values of which have been determined by reference laboratories, are provided on a timely basis to participants in the Proficiency Survey Program. The size of a laboratory's proficiency survey depends upon the magnitude of its operation and its level of sophistication. Basic surveys, large hospital surveys, and a variety of special surveys are available. Results are compared with those of the reference laboratories, and extensive survey comments are provided with computer-generated printout. In 1981 the CAP published a compilation of 10 years of data from the CAP Clinical Laboratory Improvement programs. This publication, *DATA ReCAP: 1970–1980,* is a compilation of measurements in the areas of clinical chemistry, hematology, immunohematology, microbiology, and immunology and documents laboratory performance spanning the decade.[1] Additionally, it is indicative of the state of the art of laboratory medicine in these disciplines in 1980. This publication is

an indispensable document for those who wish to learn about the development and current state of the art and practice of laboratory medicine; and it further serves as a benchmark for those developing new assays and instrumentation in laboratory medicine.

QUALITY ASSURANCE — A COMMENT

It is appropriate to comment on the new Standard III of the CAP/LAP because it is likely to have profound influence on the practice of laboratory medicine, as well as the activity of many laboratory administrators and directors. This standard mandates the establishment of an ongoing quality assurance program designed to monitor and evaluate objectively and systematically the quality and appropriateness of the care and treatment provided to patients by the pathology service, and to pursue opportunities to improve patient care.

The concepts of quality control and quality assurance are frequently confused. *Quality control* is most appropriately termed process control and is the goal of programs such as the proficiency surveys. Basically, it refers to everything that is done inside the laboratory to ensure accurate, precise results in a safe environment. It is a surveillance process designed to detect, reduce, and correct deficiencies in the analytic process. As such, it is the most fundamental obligation of the laboratory; however, its procedures and processes do not necessarily indicate how this surveillance affects patient care.

Quality assurance might be briefly defined as what one does outside of the laboratory with data that has been generated in an accurate, precise, and safe manner, to ensure excellence in patient care. Quality assurance is basically an outcome-oriented process, the goal of which is to ensure that all pathology services have been accomplished in a manner appropriate to maintaining excellence in medical care. This standard is in keeping with the most recent developments in the JCAHO accreditation process, in which quality assurance (outcome evaluation) is given major emphasis.

Many would say that all of the temperature checks, delta checks, surveys, control specimens, procedure manuals, and in-service education sessions (all aspects of quality or process control) naturally lead to an effective quality-assurance system. It is, however, one thing to be assured that a laboratory is producing accurate and precise potassium or carcinoembryonic antigen (CEA) measurements; it quite another to assess their appropriateness and relevance in patient care and patient outcome. A word of warning: because the laboratory produces readily quantifiable data, it may be all too easy to assume that the laboratory alone should be the "policeman" in how those data are used. Although quality control is the sole prerogative of the laboratory, quality assurance is a process that the laboratory can carry out only in cooperation with other services within the hospital (see Chap. 23). Thus, the laboratory manager will be extensively involved in these cooperative efforts. For example, a quality-assurance study of serum potassium measurements will involve not only the laboratory (specimen pickup times, turnaround time, and so forth) but possibly the hospital computer system, the nursing service, the medical, surgical, and pediatric services, and a number of morbidity and mortality committees within the institution.

PREPARING FOR AN ACCREDITATION INSPECTION

Preparing the clinical laboratory for an accreditation inspection can be stressful. This stress can be reduced and the inspection experience turned into a valuable management exercise if the preparation is a communal effort.[2] All section heads and supervisors should receive copies of the appropriate checklists and deficiencies noted from previous inspections. This allows an opportunity for correction of obvious deficiencies.

Diamond and Hamlin offer the following suggestions, not in any specific order, to be attended to in the inspection preparation[2]:

Clean and organize the laboratory. Have the laboratory cleaned—shelves, cupboards, refrigerators, floors, toilets—everything. If necessary, arrange a schedule with housekeeping for walls, shelves, and windows. Then clean the drawers and cabinets. Make sure they contain only what they should. A tape embosser and a role of tape will do wonders for designating contents. Remove all unused equipment and cartons. If you are forced into floor storage, raise it on wooden platforms to avoid wet-mopping damage. Get rid of clutter. If necessary, rent some storage space; but whatever is retained on site should be straightened and smartened.

Check materials for outdates. Check chemicals and reagents for container and label integrity and appropriate dating. If you are saving outdated material, sequester it, and write a brief note explaining its presence.

Review procedures for purchasing and storing of supplies. The inspector should see evidence of inventory control.

Review quality-control records documentation. A significant part of the accreditation inspection is concerned with records and documentation, and a major part of inspection difficulties arises from the absence or incompleteness of records. First and foremost should be the statements of quality-control policies and procedures for each laboratory section. Although these may be centralized, they should be available to the inspector as he begins his sectional inspection. These statements should include a definition of the limits of acceptable performance and what one does when those limits are exceeded. In laboratories of pathologic anatomy, microbiology, and other areas producing judgmental data, a quality-control statement requires considerable thought. In any event, these statements provide the inspector with the internal yardstick against which performance is measured.

Review proficiency results. Of equal importance are the results of proficiency testing. Again, centralized or not, they must be available to the inspector as the sectional inspection begins. These records must show evidence of dated review and documented corrective actions when indicated. In preparing for the inspection, the manager does well to review the material personally.

Make instrument maintenance records available. Instrument maintenance records must be available and conveniently accessible. If Engineering is responsible for this activity and maintaining the records, have the records in the laboratory at the time of the inspection, rather than sending the inspector to their location. Go over these records carefully. Do they record actual data or just check marks? Are there written standards for acceptable performance? If outside firms are servicing equipment, do you have a protocol of what they do and the defined limits of acceptable performance? Are temperature records in a uniform format, and are the limits of tolerance stated? Is there some indication of actions taken when specified limits are exceeded? In any event, have the records assembled, legible, and backed by protocol. The same applies to records for grounding checks for equipment and circuits.

Review procedure manuals. Procedure manuals should be reviewed for undated or unattributable annotations and calibration curves. Has every procedure been approved and recently reviewed? Wisdom dictates that obsolete procedures be removed. Take a very close look at package inserts. If they are in the manual, ask why they are there and whether they are in fact the procedure. If they are not the exact procedure as performed, this is a deficiency that the inspector will not overlook. Have your water check data available along with the testing protocol. Beware of check marks without the supporting procedure!

Have personnel records available and up-to-date. Many laboratories have a problem with personnel records, because in some hospitals the personnel department keeps all data. The inspector will wish to spot-check for job descriptions, performance evaluations, continuing education records, and credential validation. Either have the records available in the laboratory, or ensure that the inspector's visit to the Personnel Department does not waste time.

Review safety documents and practices. The inspector will want to see the Safety Manual, waste disposal procedures, and fire policies. Make sure personnel know what is in them, and that there is evidence that every new employee reads them. Go through your laboratories for incompatibilities: wires and water (get wires off the floor), food and infectious agents (coffee makers, cups, saucers, silverware), volatiles and strong acids, flammables and flames, and ether and closed spaces. Check fire equipment (any blankets in those boxes?), posted fire routes, and posted fire instructions. Challenge your personnel at random to tell what they would do in case of fire.

SUMMARY

Preparing for and undergoing an inspection by the JCAH or CAP is one of the most valuable experiences in which a laboratory manager can participate. It exposes one to every aspect, both administrative and technical, of the operation of the laboratory—work load, procedure manuals, methods, report forms, personnel, continuing education, quality control, safety, and quality assurance. For the new director or administrator it is the single best way to achieve, in a relatively short time, a comprehensive understanding of the current operation, problems, and potentials of a laboratory service.

The inspection component of an accreditation process facilitates the institutional goal of excellence in patient care. The manager benefits from the help of others much more technically proficient through effective communication with those inside and outside the laboratory and through the judicious application of internal laboratory quality-control and extralaboratory quality-assurance programs. Participation in a laboratory accreditation inspection is indispensable in attaining the ultimate goal, providing excellent patient care.

REFERENCES

1. DATA ReCAP: A compilation of data from the College of American Pathologists' Clinical Laboratory Improvement Programs. Chicago, College of American Pathologists, 1981
2. Diamond I, Hamlin WB: How to prepare for an inspection. Pathologist 38:31–32, 1984
3. Laboratory Accreditation Program, Orientation Manual. Chicago, College of American Pathologists
4. Manhoff L: CAP accreditation is laboratory improvement. Pathologist 38:42–43, 1984
5. Pathology and Medical Laboratory Services, Accreditation Manual for Hospitals/87. Chicago, Joint Commissions of American Hospitals, 1986
6. Simons M: Standards for accreditation of clinical laboratories. In Snyder JR, Larsen AL (eds): Administration and Supervision in Laboratory Medicine, pp 386–393. Philadelphia, Harper & Row, 1983
7. Standards for Laboratory Accreditation, Commission on Laboratory Accreditation, Chicago, College of American Pathologists, 1987

APPENDIX 22-A. CAP STANDARDS FOR LABORATORY ACCREDITATION*

Standard I: Director and Personnel Requirements

The pathology or medical laboratory service shall be directed by a physician or doctoral scientist qualified to assume professional, scientific, consultative, organizational, administrative, and educational responsibility for the service. Generally, it is medically preferable that the director be a board-certified pathologist. The director shall have sufficient authority to implement and maintain the standards.

When a nonpathologist physician or doctoral scientist serves as director, such individual must be qualified by virtue of documented training, expertise, and experience in the areas of analytical testing offered by the laboratory. Where the functions of the laboratory so require, the services of a qualified consulting pathologist shall be retained. In all facilities where anatomic pathology services are provided, a pathologist shall perform such services.

Special function laboratories shall be directed by either a physician who is qualified to assume professional responsibility for the special function laboratory or a qualified doctoral scientist with documented training, expertise, and experience in the appropriate specific clinical discipline and area of testing.

*Reprinted with permission of the College of American Pathologists from the 1988 revision. Readers are referred to the official publication for elaboration and explanatory notes.

The location, organization, or ownership of the laboratory shall not alter the requirements of this standard, its interpretation, or its application.

Interpretation

A. *Qualifications, Responsibilities, and Role of the Director:*

To function effectively in fulfilling the duties and responsibilities as director of the pathology service, the director should possess a broad knowledge of clinical medicine, sciences basic to medicine, clinical laboratory sciences, and operations. The director should have the appropriate training and background to be able to discharge the following responsibilities:

1. Medical significance, interpretation, and correlation of data
2. Anatomic pathology
3. Consultations
4. Medical staff privileges
5. Interaction with physicians/patients/administrators/credentialing agencies
6. Standards of performance
7. Monitoring and correlation of laboratory data
8. Quality assurance responsibilities
9. Personnel
10. Strategic planning
11. Administrative and management responsibilities
12. Educational responsibilities
13. Research and development responsibilities
14. Reference laboratories
15. Safety responsibilities

B. *Delegation of Responsibilities:*

The director need not perform all responsibilities personally. Administrative functions may be delegated to qualified laboratory managers and supervisors. Medical and technical responsibilities may be delegated to physicians and other qualified laboratory personnel as appropriate. The director, however, remains responsible for the overall operation and administration of the laboratory to assure that quality patient care services are provided.

C. *Consulting Pathologist:*

When the director cannot adequately discharge all the responsibilities appropriate for the pathology or laboratory service, then the services of a qualified consulting pathologist shall be retained. Where appropriate, the consulting pathologist shall also be a member of the medical staff. A close working relationship between the laboratory director and the consulting pathologist must be established. Furthermore, the director and the consulting pathologist must establish an effective working relationship with the institution's administration; the laboratory's management and staff; the medical staff; and, where appropriate, other institutional departments and services. The consultant shall play an active role in the educational programs of the laboratory and of the institution.

When the services of the pathologist are limited to those of consultant status, these services shall be provided as often as required. A written report of the consulting pathologist's evaluation and recommendations shall be provided with each consultation visit.

D. *Personnel*

There shall be a sufficient number of qualified laboratory technologists, technicians, and other laboratory staff to perform the required tests promptly and proficiently.

The director shall assure that all procedures and tests performed by the technical staff are within the scope of education, training, and experience of the individual(s).

Qualified technical staff shall be on duty, or available, at all times that laboratory testing is being performed. Emergency laboratory testing shall be performed only by qualified medical laboratory personnel. The laboratory shall maintain documentation of the qualifications of technical personnel authorized to perform procedures.

Provision shall be made for all personnel, including physicians and supervisors, to further their knowledge and skills through on-the-job training, in-service education programs, or attendance at workshops, institutes, and/or professional meetings. In-service education programs shall be provided at defined intervals appropriate for the size and needs of the technical staff.

An orientation program shall be provided for each new laboratory employee, and the employee's participation shall be documented.

All laboratory personnel must be in compliance with applicable federal, state, and local laws and regulations. Any physician shall maintain a current medical license issued by the state in which the laboratory is located.

Standard II: Resources and Facilities

The pathology service shall have sufficient and appropriate space, equipment, facilities, and supplies for the performance of the required volume of work with accuracy, precision, efficiency, and safety. In addition, the pathology service shall have effective methods for communication to ensure prompt and reliable reporting. There shall be appropriate record storage and retrieval.

Interpretation

The scope of responsibilities and activities of the pathology service must be delineated. Once this determination has been made, sufficient and appropriate space and equipment must be provided.

The environment within the laboratory shall be conducive to effective performance of personnel and equipment. There shall be sufficient, conveniently located bench storage space for the proper handling of specimens and housing of equipment and reagents. Special areas for tests requiring a controlled environment shall be provided. Work areas shall be arranged to minimize transportation problems, and shall be adequately lighted.

Communication systems shall be appropriate for the size and complexity of the organization and institution.

Facilities, equipment, and instruments shall be appropriate for the services performed.

The laboratory must be a safe working place for the personnel and for the patients it serves. It must comply with the safety codes of the regulatory authorities. The safe collection and handling of patient specimens and of reagents shall be an integral part of the laboratory safety program. Proper disposal of hazardous wastes shall be provided.

The pathology service must have the capacity, or make provision, for the prompt performance, at any time, of those procedures necessary to aid emergency diagnosis and treatment as specified by the laboratory director with the concurrence and consultation of the medical staff.

Tests may be performed by a reference laboratory or ancillary testing program if test results are provided in an effective manner and are of acceptable quality. Reference laboratories and ancillary testing programs must meet the needs of the patients and medical staff in timeliness, quality, and safety, and the referring laboratory's needs for compliance with accrediting and peer review agencies.

If tests are to be referred to a reference laboratory, the laboratory director or consulting pathologist shall select the reference laboratory on the basis of objective evidence of acceptable quality. Except where special circumstances dictate otherwise, tests shall be referred only to laboratories that have been accredited by the College of American Pathologists or licensed under the Clinical Laboratories Improvement Act of 1967 (CLIA).

Standard III: Quality Assurance

There shall be an ongoing quality assurance program designed to monitor and evaluate objectively and systematically the quality and appropriateness of the care and treatment provided to patients by the pathology service, to pursue opportunities to improve patient care, and to identify and resolve problems.

Interpretation

The pathology service shall have a systematic process to monitor and evaluate the quality and appropriateness of its contribution to patient care and to identify and resolve problems. There shall be a written description of the program which, where applicable, shall be integrated with the institution's quality assurance program. The director of the laboratory is responsible for assuring that such program is implemented and that the pathology service participates in the institutional quality assurance programs that deal with patient care.

The effectiveness of the monitoring, evaluation, and problem solving activities must be evaluated periodically as defined by the institution's quality assurance program (where applicable).

Quality assurance applies equally to anatomic pathology, surgical pathology, autopsy pathology, and cytopathology. A written program of quality assurance surveillance designed to evaluate the accuracy of diagnoses provided may include, but is not limited to, the use of intra- and extradepartmental consultation, circulation of diagnostic material (random or by case type), archival case review, correlation of histological and cytological material, and the periodic review of completed diagnostic reports. Program design will depend upon such variables as the size of the departmental staff and volume and type of diagnostic material processed.

Standard IV: Quality Control

Each pathology service shall have a quality control system that demonstrates the reliability and medical usefulness of laboratory data.

Interpretation

A laboratory quality control system shall contain the following components: (1) The selection of test methods appropriate to the medical requirements of the patients served; (2) An internal quality control program that monitors accuracy and precision of laboratory performance on a daily basis. Such program should be clearly defined in writing, provide established limits of control, prescribe appropriate actions required before acceptance or rejection of batches or analytic "runs", and be documented with evidence of understanding and implementation by laboratory personnel; (3) An interlaboratory comparison system (proficiency testing) designed to compare laboratory performance with other laboratories; (4) An instrument maintenance program which monitors and demonstrates the proper calibration and function of equipment/instruments; (5) Appropriate feedback mechanisms to assure clinical usefulness and relevance of laboratory data; (6) An educational program for the entire laboratory staff designed to maintain or improve the quality of personnel performance; (7) An external audit or accreditation process; and (8) Appropriate documentation for the foregoing.

Procedure manuals should follow a standard format and indicate sources, dates of adoption, and evidence of periodic review as described in the National Committee on Clinical Laboratory Standards (NCCLS) *Clinical Laboratory Procedure Manuals; Approved Guideline (Vol. 4, 1984).*

Methods and instruments shall be validated when introduced and when reintroduced following correction of an "out of control" situation. A complete quality control program must include regular preventive maintenance and appropriate function checks.

Written instructions shall be available that provide, in detail, the methods for procuring, transporting, and processing appropriate specimens. There shall be a written description of the system for the timely reporting of patient data to the physician and of the safeguards taken to ensure that such data are correct.

Programs for surveillance and control of incoming material should ensure that all reagents, specimens, and materials used in the analytic process have the properties necessary for reliable performance.

The pathology service shall participate regularly in the College of American Pathologists' Interlaboratory Comparison (Surveys) Program based upon the type of testing the laboratory regularly provides.

If any Survey results are unsatisfactory according to the criteria established by the Surveys program, the cause of the unsatisfactory result shall be investigated and the problem resolved. The findings, of the investigation and the corrective measures instituted shall be recorded, dated, and signed by the responsible technologist or supervisor and the director of laboratories.

Standard V: Inspection Requirement

A pathology service which desires accreditation shall undergo periodic inspections and evaluations as determined by the Commission on Laboratory Accreditation of the College of American Pathologists.

Interpretation

The application process will be initiated by submission of a completed application containing the necessary information, evidence of enrollment in the appropriate proficiency testing programs, and payment of fees. Laboratories will be evaluated in accordance with the *Standards for Laboratory Accreditation* of the College of American Pathologists.

The pathology service must submit to a complete periodic on-site inspection. The Commission will not inspect or accredit a portion of a single cohesive laboratory except under special and/or unusual circumstances; and then only by prior arrangements with, and approval of, the Regional Commissioner. The conduct of inspections and evaluation of results shall be in accordance with the policies and procedures of the Commission on Laboratory Accreditation.

Laboratories undergoing a change in directorship, location, or ownership are subject to inspection and evaluation in accordance with applicable policy.

Laboratories enrolled in the Laboratory Accreditation Program are required to perform periodic self-evaluations. When deficiencies are noted, the laboratory shall take appropriate corrective action which shall be documented and subject to review by the Commission on Laboratory Accreditation. Uncorrected deficiencies at the next on-site inspection shall be considered recurrent. The Commissioner(s) will review deficiencies detected during self-evaluation. Corrective action responses from the laboratory director may be required.

Recurrence of the same deficiencies in consecutive inspections is considered a serious problem and is subject to review by the Commission.

APPENDIX 22-B JCAHO ACCREDITATION STANDARDS FOR PATHOLOGY AND MEDICAL LABORATORY SERVICES (PA)*

Standard

PA.1 — Pathology and medical laboratory services and consultation are regularly and conveniently available to meet the needs of patients, as determined by the medical staff.

Required Characteristics

PA.1.1 — The pathology and medical laboratory services are directed by a physician who is qualified to assume professional; organizational, and administrative responsibility for the facilities and for the services rendered.

PA.1.2 — There are sufficient qualified personnel with documented training and experience to supervise and conduct the work of the laboratory.

> PA.1.2.1 — The director of the pathology and medical laboratory services is a member of the medical staff and, whenever possible, is a pathologist, preferably one who is certified by the American Board of Pathology or has the documented equivalent education, training, and experience.

> PA.1.2.2 — The director is appointed or elected by the process outlined in the medical staff bylaws.

> PA.1.2.3 — When a pathologist is regularly available only on a part-time basis, this individual is a member of the medical staff.

> PA.1.2.4 — When the pathologist can provide services only on a consultative basis, these services are provided as often as required, but not less than monthly.

> PA.1.2.5 — The director of the pathology and medical laboratory services establishes an effective working relationship with the medical staff, the hospital administration, and other departments/services.

*Reprinted from the 1988 Accreditation Manual for Hospitals with permission from the Joint Commission on Accreditation of Healthcare Organizations. Readers are referred to the *Manual* for elaboration and interpretation.

> PA.1.2.6 — A pathologist has an active role in the in-service educational programs of the pathology services and the hospital and participates in medical staff functions as required.

> PA.1.2.7 — Within the hospital's overall quality assurance program, the director of the pathology and medical laboratory services assures that the department/service participates in the monitoring and evaluation of the quality and appropriateness of services provided.

> PA.1.2.8 — An exception to physician direction of a clinical laboratory or component thereof may occur in certain highly specialized or clinically compartmentalized hospital laboratories.

PA.1.3 — There are sufficient number of qualified laboratory technologists and supportive technical staff to perform, promptly and proficiently, the tests required of the pathology and medical laboratory services.

> PA.1.3.1 — A qualified medical technologist is a graduate of a medical technology program approved by a nationally recognized body or has documented equivalent education, training, and/or experience; meets any current legal requirements of licensure or registration; and is currently competent in the field.

> PA.1.3.2 — The director of the pathology and medical laboratory services assures that procedures and tests that are outside the scope of education, training, and experience of the individuals employed to perform technical procedures in the laboratory are not performed in the pathology and medical laboratory services.

> PA.1.3.3 — At least one qualified medical technologist is on duty or available at all times.

> PA.1.3.4 — Work assignments in the pathology and medical laboratory services are consistent with the qualifications of the employee.

> PA.1.3.5 — The director of the pathology and medical laboratory services, acting on medical staff policy, designate in writing those nonphysician laboratory personnel who are qualified and authorized to perform procedures that are associated with a potential hazard to patients, such as arterial puncture for obtaining blood samples.

PA.1.4 — There is provision for technologists and other technical personnel, including supervisors, to further their knowledge and skills through hospital-based educational opportunities, such as on-the-job training and in-service education programs, and, as feasible, at least for supervisory personnel, through attendance at outside workshops, institutes, and local regional, or national society meetings.

PA.1.4.1 — In service education programs are held at defined intervals that are reasonable for the size and needs of the technological staff.

PA.1.4.2 — Continuing education programs are based, at least in part, on the findings of the monitoring and evaluation of the quality of laboratory services provided and on the principles of laboratory safety.

PA.1.4.3 — An orientation program is provided for each new laboratory employee.

PA.1.5 — The director, supervisors, and laboratory personnel comply with applicable law and regulation.

PA.1.6 — The director of the pathology and medical laboratory services is responsible for the qualifications and performance of the staff.

PA.1.7 — A hospital that provides only psychiatric/substance abuse services may provide pathology and medical laboratory services through a contractual agreement with another health care organization that is accredited by the Joint Commission or through a contractual agreement with an independent laboratory that either is approved by the Commission on Laboratory Accreditation of the College of American Pathologists or meets equivalent standards.

PA.1.7.1 — The hospital has a description of the means of providing pathology and medical laboratory services.

PA.1.7.2 — If the hospital itself provides pathology and medical laboratory services, there is a description of the services provided and the position of those services within the organization of the hospital.

PA.1.7.3 — The hospital complies with applicable standards in this chapter of this *Manual.*

Standard

PA.2 — There are sufficient space, equipment, and supplies within the pathology and medical laboratory services to perform the required volume of work with optimal accuracy, precision, efficiency, timeliness, and safety.

Required Characteristics

PA.2.1 — Provision is made, either on the premises or in a reference laboratory, for the prompt performance of adequate examinations in the fields of anatomic pathology, hematology, chemistry, microbiology, clinical microscopy, parasitology, immunohematology, serology, virology, and, as it relates to the pathology and medical laboratory services, nuclear medicine.

PA.2.1.1 — Such examinations are performed in sufficient depth to meet the usual needs of the medical staff.

PA.2.1.2 — All laboratory testing undertaken while the patient is under the care of the hospital and of a member of the medical staff is done in the hospital laboratories or in approved reference laboratories.

PA.2.1.3 — The medical staff, through its designated mechanism, deems acceptable reference laboratories that are recommended by the director of the pathology and medical laboratory services.

PA.2.2 — The laboratory environment is conducive to the optimal performance of personnel and equipment.

PA.2.2.1 — The ventilation system provides an adequate amount of fresh air and can remove toxic and noxious fumes.

PA.2.2.2 — There is adequate, conveniently located bench space for the efficient handling of specimens and for the housing of equipment and reagents.

PA.2.2.3 — Work areas are arranged to minimize problems in transportation and communication and are adequately lighted to facilitate accuracy and precision.

PA.2.2.4 — There are a sufficient number of properly located utilities.

PA.2.3 — Equipment and instruments are appropriate for the services required.

PA.2.3.1 — There are a sufficient number of properly grounded electrical outlets with adequately stabilized voltage.

PA.2.3.2 — Voltage levels at electrical sources to which automated equipment is connected are monitored and recorded.

PA.2.3.3 — In the event of a power failure, the emergency power supply is sufficient to permit the performance of essential laboratory studies, including the use of a microscope, as well as to maintain any essential refrigerating or heating elements.

PA.2.3.4—Special precautions, including compliance with pertinent requirements of the "Infection Control" and the "Plant, Technology, and Safety Management" chapters of the *Manual,* are taken to avoid unnecessary physical, chemical, and biological hazards in the pathology and medical laboratory services.

PA.2.4—The performance of instruments and equipment is evaluated frequently enough to assure that they function properly at all times.

PA.2.4.1—Appropriate records are maintained for each piece of equipment.

PA.2.4.2—Temperatures are recorded daily for all temperature-controlled instruments.

Standard

PA.3—Channels of communication within the pathology and medical laboratory services, with other departments/services of the hospital and the medical staff, and with outside services and agencies are appropriate for the size and complexity of the hospital.

Required Characteristics

PA.3.1—All requests for laboratory tests are made in writing or through electronic means.

PA.3.1.1—Orders or requisition for inpatient and ambulatory care patient services must clearly identify the patient; the requesting individual; the tests required; any special handling required; the date and, when relevant, the time the specimen was collected; and the date and time the request and/or specimen reached the laboratory.

PA.3.1.2—Requests for examinations of surgical specimens contain a concise statement of the reason for the examination.

PA.3.1.3—The laboratory performs tests and examines specimens on the written request of the individuals authorized by the medical staff to order such evaluations and receive the results; those physicians or nonphysicians who are not members of the medical staff but have authorization from the medical staff and administration to request such support services from the hospital; and other persons, to the extent permitted by law, who are authorized by the hospital and licensed to engage in the direct treatment of patients.

PA.3.2—To assure that the specimens are satisfactory for the tests to be performed, written procedures are developed for those who collect specimens.

PA.3.2.1—There is evidence that such procedures have been approved by the director of the pathology and medical laboratory services.

PA.3.2.2—The procedures relate to at least one of the following: the ordering of tests; standard and special methods used for the preparation of patients and the collection of specimens, as well as precautions to be taken for special procedures; and proper identification, storage, and preservation of specimens.

PA.3.3—Communication systems within the pathology and medical laboratory services and between it and other departments/services efficiently accomplish both the urgent and the regular transfer of information.

PA.3.3.1—The laboratory report includes the date and time of reporting and the condition of any unsatisfactory specimen.

PA.3.3.2—A system that assures the ability to identify the individual responsible for performing or completing the procedure is used.

PA.3.3.3—Criteria are established for the immediate notification of the practitioner responsible for the care of the patient when critical limits of specified test results are exceeded.

PA.3.4—There is assurance of the direct transfer of information between the pathologist performing an operating-room consultation, with or without a "frozen-section," and the operating surgeon.

PA.3.4.1—When it is necessary to perform such a consultation at a laboratory located outside the hospital, care is taken not to subject the patient to any undue hazards, such as excessive general anesthesia, while awaiting the results of the tissue examination.

PA.3.4.2—When the operating-room consultations by a pathologist are not available within the facility, the medical staff establishes criteria for circumstances under which it is preferable to transfer the patient to a hospital where such service is provided.

Standard

PA.4—Required records and reports are maintained and, as appropriate, are filed in the patient's medical record and in the pathology and medical laboratory services.

Required Characteristics

PA.4.1—Authenticated, dated reports of all examinations performed by the pathology and medical laboratory services are made part of the patient's medical record.

PA.4.1.1—The director of the pathology and medical laboratory services is responsible for all hospital laboratory reports.

PA.4.1.2—When tests are performed in a reference laboratory, the name of the laboratory performing the test is included in the report placed in the patient's medical record.

PA.4.2—The pathologist is responsible for the preparation of a descriptive diagnostic report of gross specimens received and of necropsies performed.

PA.4.2.1—Diagnoses made from surgical specimen and necropsies are expressed in acceptable terminology of a recognized disease nomenclature and are indexed for retrieval.

PA.4.2.2—The degree of detail recorded in the microscopic evaluation is the responsibility of the examining pathologist, but in all cases when a microscopic evaluation is performed, any diagnosis rendered on the tissue is based on those findings.

PA.4.3—Reports of all anatomic and clinical laboratory tests and examinations performed are readily available to the individual ordering the tests.

PA.4.3.1—The hospital assures that the reports are filed promptly in the patient's medical record.

PA.4.3.2—Report forms are designed to facilitate comparison of each determination with pertinent reference values and sequential and related analyses.

PA.4.4—The pathology and medical laboratory services maintain a record of the daily accession of specimens and an appropriate system for the identification of each.

PA.4.4.1—The record includes at least: the laboratory and patient identification; the identification of the practitioner ordering the test or evaluation; the date and, when relevant, time of specimen collection and receipt; the reason for any unsatisfactory specimen; the test or evaluation performed; the result; and the date and time of reporting to the requesting practitioner or patient care unit.

PA.4.5—Duplicate copies of the reports of all anatomic and clinical laboratory tests and examinations performed are retained in the laboratory in a readily retrievable manner.

PA.4.5.1—Requirements for record retention are determined by applicable law and regulation and by local needs, but are in effect for at least two years.

Standard

PA.5—Quality control systems and measures of the pathology and medical laboratory services are designed to assure the medical reliability of laboratory data.

Required Characteristics

PA.5.1—The laboratory and, as appropriate, each of its components are licensed as required.

PA.5.2—There is a documented quality control program in effect for each section of the pathology and medical laboratory services.

PA.5.3—General quality controls required of and practiced by the pathology and medical laboratory services include, but need not be limited to, the following:

PA.5.3.1—Use of proficiency testing programs for each discipline offered by the clinical laboratory.

PA.5.3.2—Current descriptions of and instructions for all analytic methods and procedures.

PA.5.3.3—Validation of methods used.

PA.5.3.4—Daily surveillance of results by the director or appropriate supervisor.

PA.5.3.5—Documentation of remedial action taken for detected deficiencies/defects identified through quality control measures or authorized inspections.

PA.5.3.6—Preventive maintenance, periodic inspection, and performance testing of equipment and instruments, with the maintenance of appropriate records.

PA.5.3.7—Evaluation of analytical measuring equipment and instruments with respect to all critical operating characteristics.

PA.5.3.8—Evaluation of automated volumetric equipment.

PA.5.3.9—Performance of tests and operation of instruments within temperature and humidity required for proper performance.

PA.5.3.10—Documented monitoring of temperature-controlled spaces and equipment.

PA.5.3.11—Convenient location of essential utilities.

PA.5.3.12—Proper preparing, storing, dispensing, and periodic evaluation of all solid and liquid reagents, including water, to assure accuracy and precision of results.

PA.5.3.13—Labeling of reagents and solutions for identity, strength, cautionary/accessory information, and preparation and expiration dates, as appropriate.

PA.5.3.14—Written procedures for the preparation of patients and for the collection, preservation, transportation, and receipt of specimens to assure satisfactory specimens for the tests to be performed.

PA.5.3.15—Identification of specimens.

PA.5.3.18—Review of the performance of personnel on all laboratory work shifts on a regular basis by the pathologist or appropriate laboratory supervisor.

PA.5.4—When histocompatibility testing is performed by the pathology and medical laboratory services, appropriate control systems and validation methods are used.

PA.5.4.1—As appropriate to the study or patient procedure being carried out, the following are required: crossmatching of potential recipients and donors, using the most reactive and most recent sera, before transplantation is performed; HLA serologic typing of both donor and recipient; and characterization for antibody against histocompatibility antigens in serum from potential recipients of organ or tissue grafts.

PA.5.5—Mixed lymphocyte cultures or other recognized methods to detect cellular-defined antigens are performed in accordance with prescribed methods.

PA.5.5.1—Procedures are established for the freezing of lymphocytes and for the provision of a comprehensive panel of fresh and/or frozen lymphocytes.

PA.5.5.2—Each laboratory individual performing such tests is given, at least on a monthly basis, a previously tested specimen as an unknown to verify his ability to reproduce test results.

PA.5.5.3—The laboratory participates in at least one national or regional cell-exchange program, if available, or develops an exchange system with another laboratory to validate interlaboratory reproducibility.

PA.5.6—Quality control records are retained for at least two years.

PA.5.7—Equipment maintenance records are retained for the life of each instrument used.

PA.5.8—More specific quality controls are described under the other standards of this chapter of this *Manual.*

Standard

PA.6—Specific requirements are observed when anatomic pathology blood transfusion, and clinical pathology services are offered.

Required Characteristics

PA.6.1—Anatomical Pathology

PA.6.1.1—Surgical Pathology

PA.6.1.1.1—Specimens removed during a surgical procedure are ordinarily sent to the pathologist for evaluation.

PA.6.1.1.2—Every gross specimen sent to the laboratory is examined by a pathologist.

PA.6.1.1.3—The medical staff, in consultation with the pathologist, decides the exceptions to sending specimens removed during a surgical procedure to the laboratory.

PA.6.1.1.4—Each microscopic section is ordinarily evaluated by a pathologist.

PA.6.1.1.5—If an electron microscopy facility is present in the hospital, precautions relating to radiation and electrical hazards are established and enforced.

PA.6.1.1.6—Fluorescence and immunofluorescence procedures are available to meet indicated diagnostic requirements.

PA.6.1.1.7—Special stains are controlled for intended reactivity with positive and negative slides.

PA.6.1.2—Necropsy Service

PA.6.1.2.1—Space, equipment, and supplies for the necropsy area are adequate for the work load.

PA.6.1.2.2—Each necropsy is performed by or under the supervision of a pathologist or a physician whose credentials file documents his qualifications in anatomic pathology.

PA.6.1.2.3—When a delay occurs in performing the required necropsy, appropriate refrigeration for the cadaver is available.

PA.6.1.2.4—When observation of a necropsy is required for instructional or legal reasons, sufficient space and observational access are provided and confidentiality of patient information is emphasized.

PA.6.1.2.5—Whether a necropsy is performed within or outside the hospital, the gross and microscopic reports are made part of the patient's completed medical record.

PA.6.1.2.6—The medical staff attempts to secure necropsies in all deaths, particularly in cases of unusual deaths and cases of medicolegal and educational interest, unless otherwise provided by law.

PA.6.1.3—Cytology

PA.6.1.3.1—A cytopathology service that is adequate to meet the needs of the hospital is available.

PA.6.1.3.2—The quality of the cytopathology service is assured through direct supervision by a pathologist or other physician qualified in cytology.

PA.6.1.3.3—All abnormal smears are evaluated by a pathologist or other designated qualified physician.

PA.6.1.3.4—Abnormal smears are kept on file for as long as needed for patient care purposes and in accordance with applicable law and regulation.

PA.6.1.3.5—Normal smears are kept on file in accordance with applicable law and regulation.

PA.6.1.3.6—Reports of abnormal or suspicious smears are authenticated by a physician who is qualified in pathology or cytology.

PA.6.2—Blood Transfusion Service

PA.6.2.1—The blood transfusion service is directed by a pathologist or other physician who is qualified in immunohematology and is knowledgeable about the principles of hemotherapy and blood banking.

PA.6.2.2—Personnel in the transfusion service or blood bank have had sufficient training and/or experience to qualify as technically competent in the immunohematologic procedures performed.

PA.6.2.3—Current written policies and procedures for the blood transfusion service conform to the American Association of Blood Banks *Standards for Blood Banks and Transfusion Service* (11th edition, 1984) and are readily available, reviewed at least annually by the director of the service, and revised as necessary.

PA.6.2.3.1—Blood transfusion policies and procedures relate at least to the following: the use and selection of donors; crossmatching and compatibility testing of donor's blood with recipient's blood; instructions for the identification of the donor blood and recipient; the procedure to be followed when the blood-storage refrigerator alarm is activated; the procedure for the return to the blood bank of unused blood that was previously issued for transfusion purposes; criteria for the release of unused blood to the original organization or another organization; the reporting and investigation of adverse reactions; and testing for appropriate infectious agents, as specified by the U.S. Food and Drug Administration (which may be performed by an authorized agency outside the hospital).

PA.6.2.4—Blood or blood components are collected, stored, and handled in such a manner that they retain their maximum potency and safety, and they are properly processed, tested, and labeled.

PA.6.2.4.1—Any refrigerator used for the routine storage of blood maintains a temperature uniformly between 1°C and 6°C (34°F and 43°F), and this temperature is verified by an outside recording thermometer.

PA.6.2.4.2—Stored blood is inspected daily for evidence of hemolysis and for possible bacterial contamination.

PA.6.2.5—There is an established procedure for obtaining a supply of blood and blood components at all times.

PA.6.2.5.1—Facilities for the safekeeping and administration of blood and blood products are provided.

PA.6.2.5.1.1—Blood-storage facilities, regardless of the duration of storage required, met the requirements of this chapter of this *Manual*.

PA.6.2.5.2—For emergencies, the hospital maintains at least a minimum supply of blood; or makes arrangements by which it can obtain blood quickly from community blood sources; or maintains an up-to-date list of available donors and provides the equipment and personnel to obtain the donor blood.

PA.6.2.5.3—Outside sources of blood are

recommended by the director of the service and are approved by the medical staff and the administration.

PA.6.2.5.4 — If fresh donor blood is drawn in the hospital, an adequate history and pertinent physical examination of the donor, as well as any required laboratory screening tests, are performed to provide reasonable assurance that the safety of the donor is assured, that the individual is acceptable for donating blood, and that blood is free from infectious agents, unusual antibodies, and, as feasible, drugs.

PA.6.2.5.5 — Venesection is performed in a safe manner in accordance with a written protocol.

PA.6.2.6 — The blood sample taken from the recipient for typing and cross-matching is labeled immediately and adequately at the time it is drawn.

PA.6.2.6.1 — Identification of the sample is maintained throughout all subsequent testing.

PA.6.2.6.2 — The crossmatching and compatibility testing of the donor's blood with the recipient's blood assures maximum protection against a potentially incompatible transfusion.

PA.6.2.6.2.3 — Except for transfusion of packed red cells, a minor crossmatch is performed when donor sera are not screened for irregular antibodies.

PA.6.2.6.2.4 — All $Rh_o(D)$ negative donor cells are tested for the Rh_o variant (Du).

PA.6.2.6.2.5 — Samples of each unit of transfused blood and a sample of recipient blood are retained for at least one week following transfusion for further testing in the event of an adverse reaction.

PA.6.2.7 — Records that detail the receipt and disposition of all blood products are maintained.

PA.6.2.8 — The administration of blood is monitored to detect an adverse reaction as soon as it occurs.

PA.6.2.8.1 — Personnel who monitor blood transfusions are trained to recognize or suspect adverse reactions, have a written plan of action to follow in the event of such a reaction, and report any such reaction as soon as possible to the blood transfusion service and to the physician responsible for the patient.

PA.6.2.8.2 — Prompt investigation of the cause of an adverse reaction is instituted, including determination of whether a hemolytic reaction has occurred.

PA.6.2.8.3 — The results of all tests performed in the evaluation of an actual or suspected blood transfusion reaction are made a permanent part of the patient's medical record.

PA.6.3 — Clinical Pathology

PA.6.3.1 — Clinical laboratory services required by the medical staff are available at all times from sources internal or external to the hospital.

PA.6.3.2 — The medical staff determines which, if any, routine laboratory studies are required on admission of a patient.

PA.6.3.3 — The director of the pathology and medical laboratory services defines for the medical staff the guidelines for requesting and receiving test results on an emergency or stat basis.

PA.6.3.4 — Proficiency testing services utilized for each discipline of the clinical laboratory equal or exceed the requirements of applicable law and regulation with respect to variety and frequency of testing and to criteria for satisfactory performance.

PA.6.3.4.1 — A cumulative record of participation is maintained, including documentation of the review of each individual result that exceeds the stated limits of satisfactory performance.

PA.6.3.4.2 — When analysis of unknown samples is required by regulatory agencies, the results of such testing, as available, are considered in the overall evaluation of the clinical laboratory for accreditation purposes.

PA.6.3.5 — Clinical Chemistry

PA.6.3.5.1 — Each procedure in clinical chemistry is verified by appropriate controls at least once on each day of use.

PA.6.3.5.2 — Data are available to document the routine precision of test results and the schedule of recalibration.

PA.6.3.5.3 — At least one standard and one reference sample are included with each run of unknown specimens when such standards and reference samples are available.

PA.6.3.5.4 — Standard deviation, coefficient of variation, or other statistical estimates of precision are determined by random replicate testing of specimens.

PA.6.3.5.5—Acceptable limits for all standard and reference quality control samples are established and are available to laboratory personnel, as is the course of action to be instituted when results are outside the satisfactory control limits.

PA.6.3.5.6—Control limits on all tests are established to produce results commensurate with meaningful clinical applications.

PA.6.3.5.7—Toxicological analyses are available as necessary.

PA.6.3.6—Bacteriology and Mycology

PA.6.3.6.1—On each day of use, chemical and biological solutions, reagents, and antisera are tested to assure proper reactivity and are inspected for deterioration.

PA.6.3.6.2—All staining procedures are tested for intended reactivity by concurrent applications to smears of microorganisms with predictable staining characteristics.

PA.6.3.6.3—Before or concurrently with its use, each batch of media is tested with selected organisms to confirm the required growth characteristics, selectivity, enrichment, and biophysical and biochemical response.

PA.6.3.7—Parasitology

PA.6.3.7.1—A reference collection of slides, photographs, or gross specimens of identified parasites, as well as a calibrated measuring device for determining the size of ova or parasites, are available and are used as necessary.

PA.6.3.8—Virology

PA.6.3.8.1—Systems for the isolation of viruses and reagents for the identification of viruses are available to the hospital as necessary.

PA.6.3.8.2—Records that reflect the systems used and the reactions observed are maintained.

PA.6.3.8.3—In tests for the identification of viruses, controls that will identify erroneous results are used.

PA.6.3.8.4—If serodiagnostic tests for viral diseases are used, the requirements for quality control as specified for serology apply.

PA.6.3.9—Clinical Microscopy

PA.6.3.9.1—Urinalysis is performed only on fresh or properly preserved specimens.

PA.6.3.9.2—Qualitative tests, except microscopic examination of urine sediments, are checked daily with suitable positive and negative reference samples.

PA.6.3.10—Hematology

PA.6.3.10.1—Each instrument or other device used is calibrated/tested, as appropriate, on each day of use.

PA.6.3.10.2—Reference materials and methods are tested on each day of use against known standards or controls within the range of clinically significant values.

PA.6.3.10.3—Standard deviation, coefficient of variation, or other statistical estimates of precision are determined by random replicate testing of specimens.

PA.6.3.10.4—The accuracy and precision of blood cell counts and hematocrit and hemoglobin measurements are tested on each day of use.

PA.6.3.10.5—Reliable tests for detecting hemostatic and coagulation defects are available.

PA.6.3.10.6—Tests such as the one-stage prothrombin time are run in duplicate, unless the laboratory can demonstrate that low frequency of random error, or high precision, makes this unnecessary.

PA.6.3.11—Serology

PA.6.3.11.1—Serologic tests on unknown specimens, including those for syphilis, are run concurrently with a positive control serum of known titer or controls of graded reactivity in order to assure specificity of antigen reactivity.

PA.6.3.11.2—New lots of reagents are tested concurrently with one of known acceptable reactivity before use.

PA.6.3.11.3—Equipment, glassware, reagents, controls, and techniques for tests for syphilis conform to those recommended in the *Manual for Tests for Syphilis* (U.S. Public Health Service Publication Number 411, 1969).

PA.6.3.12—Radiobioassay

PA.6.3.12.1—When *in vivo* or *in vitro* radioisotopes are used by the laboratory, there are written quality control procedures to assure diagnostic reliability and patient and personnel safety.

PA.6.3.12.2—The requirements of the Nuclear Regulatory Commission and the recommendations of the National Council on Radiation Protection and Measurements are known and applied.

PA.6.3.12.3—Laboratories using radioisotopes comply with relevant requirements of the "Nuclear Medicine Services" chapter of this *Manual.*

Standard

PA.7—As part of the hospital's quality assurance program the quality and appropriateness of pathology and medical laboratory services are monitored and evaluated, and identified problems are resolved.

Required Characteristics

PA.7.1—The pathology and medical laboratory department/service has a planned and systematic process for the monitoring and evaluation of the quality and appropriateness of patient care services and for resolving identified problems.

PA.7.1.1—The physician director of the pathology and medical laboratory department/service is responsible for assuring that the process is implemented.

PA.7.2—The quality and appropriateness of patient care services are monitored and evaluated in all major clinical functions of the pathology and medical laboratory department/service.

PA.7.2.1—Such a monitoring and evaluation are accomplished through the following means: routine collection in the pathology and medical laboratory department/service, or through the hospital's quality assurance program, of information about important aspects of pathology and medical laboratory services; and periodic assessment by the pathology and medical laboratory department/service and the medical staff of the collected information to identify important problems in patient care services and opportunities to improve care.

PA.7.3—When important problems in patient care services or opportunities to improve care are identified, actions are taken; and the effectiveness of the actions taken is evaluated.

PA.7.4—The findings from and conclusions of monitoring, evaluation, and problem-solving activities are documented and, as appropriate, are reported.

PA.7.5—The actions taken to resolve problems and improve patient care services, and information about the impact of the actions taken, are documented and, as appropriate, are reported.

PA.7.6—As part of the annual reappraisal of the hospital's quality assurance program, the effectiveness of the monitoring, evaluation, and problem-solving activities in the pathology and medical laboratory department/service is evaluated.

PA.7.7—When an outside source(s) provides pathology and medical laboratory services, or when there is no designated pathology and medical laboratory department/service, the quality and appropriateness of patient care services provided are monitored and evaluated, and identified problems are resolved.

PA.7.7.1—The medical staff is responsible for assuring that planned and systematic process for such monitoring, evaluation, and problem-solving activities is implemented.

twenty-three

Quality Assurance and Peer Review in the Clinical Laboratory

Kathryn R. Maxwell
Thomas D. Stevenson

Measurement of health-care quality is dependent on interactive variables that influence the delivery and perception of health care. Measurement is achieved by setting standards of practice, then evaluating the actual practice for establishing whether these standards are met. If not, then corrective action is determined and implemented. Continued evaluation identifies patient-care improvement or need for further action. The expected outcome is high-quality patient care. Richard Thompson aptly defines high-quality patient care as having the following components: optimal achievable results, avoidance of iatrogenic complications, attention to the patient's needs as a person, cost-effectiveness, and documented improvement.[12] The measures are developed by setting standards to evaluate the goals of service quality and appropriateness. These goals are achieved through quality-assurance programs that incorporate the concepts of peer review and objective evaluation of care and services.

There is a natural reluctance on the part of busy professionals to take the time to develop and organize such activities. In the hospital setting, increasing patient acuity and reduced staffing have resulted in less time for management and accountability functions. However, these are the functions that ensure that care and services are provided in the efficient and effective manner demanded by our society. The health-care professional can no longer be oblivious to constraints and pressures from external factors. Certainly malpractice concerns require examination and action to prevent litigation and improve health-care quality. Cost-containment pressures from the federal government, third-party payers, and business coalitions have an impact on the amount and delivery of care and services with potential exposure concerns regarding overutilization and underutilization of services. As previously reviewed, regulatory and accrediting bodies also demand accountability and evidence of health-care quality. Consumers are also increasingly aware of the variations in utilization rates, practice patterns, and clinical outcomes. No longer is there a blind trust in the quality of health care and the mystique of medicine. In its place is a desire for information concerning the extent to which variations affect differences in quality of care.[8] As an integral part of the health-care system, the clinical laboratory is affected by these external factors.

Exposure to liability is increasing exponentially. The clinical laboratory and the professional are involved when specimen collection, accuracy of results, turnaround time on findings, and notification of abnormal findings become issues of negligence. Organized quality-assurance systems allow for effective approaches to limiting risk exposure due to professional negligence or malpractice. In order to respond to sources of liability and prevent exposure, the professional staff must have adequate information about their clinical practice and clinical decision-making. According to Joseph and associates[9]:

> The data on physician practice must cut across the entire continuum of care to examine the appropriateness of admitting practices, the completeness and timeliness of diagnostic assessments and the appropriate use of those assessments, timeliness and appropriateness of management of complications, timeliness of referrals to therapists and to discharge planners and appropriateness of patients' clinical status at discharge.

Certainly the clinical laboratory interfaces on several fronts of the above issues.

Quality assurance by the peer review process has evolved from — and, it is fair to say, received the greatest impetus from — Medicare legislation. The subsequent adoption of the prospective payment system by means of diagnosis-related groups (DRGs) has provided a further stimulus to quality assurance because critics of DRGs have alleged that patient care is compromised to contain costs. Certainly, costs of care have escalated, to nearly 11% of the gross national product in 1985 from 4.5% in 1950.[11] This escalation is attributed by various sources to availability of technology, access to care because of fee-for-service reimbursement, and the practice of defensive medicine. Two areas in the health-care setting where there is great potential for unnecessary utilization are laboratory testing and the use of x-ray filming. Some studies have shown that these tests and examinations account for 25% of health-care costs.[3] Both patients and physicians erroneously may equate more care with better care. Cost-containment incentives, based on prospective payment systems and capitated reimbursement methods, have raised concerns that necessary care and services will not be provided. However, more care does not necessarily mean better care. Sometimes more care means more tests and procedures and longer hospitalizations, which expose the patient to risks of iatrogenic complications, increased costs, unnecessary care, and inefficiency in service delivery. Myers and Schroeder[10] discuss the law of diminishing returns in relation to medical services. Whereas health is the expected outcome of care and services, and expenditures for services are the inputs, it was determined that early in the diagnostic and/or treatment process, application of certain tests, procedures, examinations may have a sizable impact on patient care. These tests, procedures, and examinations may confirm a diagnosis or provide information regarding type of treatment. When treatment is established, additional care and services add nothing to the patient's health; in fact, beyond this point additional care may be harmful, resulting in exposure to iatrogenic complications and the negation of optimal achievable results.

The Joint Commission on Accreditation of Health Care Organizations (Joint Commission) requires the establishment of effective quality assurance programs. Because of the potential for nonaccreditation, the health-care professional must participate in the review of care and services. The Joint Commission has defined the mechanism for the quality-assurance process through its standards: "As part of the hospital's quality-assurance program, the quality and appropriateness of pathology and medical laboratory services are monitored and evaluated, and identified problems are resolved."[7]

With these requirements and incentives, how can the health-care professional provide high-quality patient care in a cost-effective manner? In this chapter we will explore the quality-assurance and peer-review processes, describe current methodology in relation to the clinical laboratory, and provide a future perspective on the continued necessity for the monitoring and evaluation of care and services provided by health-care professionals.

DEFINING QUALITY ASSURANCE

Quality assurance encompasses quality assessment, peer review, and quality control. For several years, health-care service departments (radiology, pharmacy, laboratory) have confused quality control with quality assurance. In fact, these terms are often used interchangeably. Because quality assurance is elusive and difficult to define, professionals are irritated with the requirement of measuring quality. Although quality-control standards are well-known and objective, sometimes quality-assurance standards are based on "soft" variables that may not have known standards of performance. Therefore, decisions regarding the quality and appropriateness of clinical practice and decision-making are difficult. Quality assurance goes beyond the surveillance of people, tools, methods, reagents (quality control), and evaluates appropriateness of tests ordered and performed (peer review) and efficiency and efficacy of care and services.[5]

The Joint Commission has provided the initiatives and framework for the development of quality-assurance programs. These programs are to be planned and systematic/continuous and ongoing. The following definitions from the Joint Commission are important to the understanding of the quality-assurance process.

Monitoring: Monitoring is the systematic and routine process of gathering important clinical data and aggregating or displaying data so that problems or opportunities to improve care can be identified.

Evaluation: Evaluation is assessment of the meaning and import of the data, including making judgments about the quality and appropriateness of care based on comparison of observed practice and predetermined objective criteria and professional judgments of the reasons for variation from criteria.

Quality: Quality is the degree of adherence to generally recognized contemporary standards of good practice and achievement of anticipated outcomes for a particular service, procedure, diagnosis, or clinical problem.

Appropriateness: Appropriateness is the extent to which a particular procedure, treatment, test, or service is efficacious, is clearly indicated for the patient, is neither excessive nor deficient in number for the patient, and is provided in the setting (inpatient, outpatient, home) best suited to the patient's needs.

Quality assurance involves the measures taken to assure high-quality patient care. The quality-assurance process has three components: monitoring important aspects of care and outcomes, problem-solving to ensure actions are taken to improve care and outcomes, and documentation and reporting of activities.

MONITORING IMPORTANT ASPECTS OF CARE AND OUTCOMES

In the quality and appropriateness standard for pathology and medical laboratory services, the Joint Commission states: "The quality and appropriateness of patient care and services are monitored and evaluated in all major clinical functions of the pathology and medical laboratory department/service."[7]

Monitors are used to build a data base for evaluating the quality of care and services. Monitors can be defined as "mechanisms for the repeated measurement of various aspects of clinical decision-making and patient management." Joseph and associates group monitors into three types: statistical, appropriateness, and occurrence monitors. Statistical monitors provide facts about clinical practice. Such facts might include demographic characteristics, financial variables, and clinical characteristics

of patients, as well as types of treatments, procedures, or services ordered for patients. Appropriateness monitors measure the quality of clinical decision-making and compliance with established policies and procedures. Areas monitored would include

Appropriateness of the selection, frequency, duration, or timing of services

Outcomes of patients during and after treatment

Outcome, timing, and follow-up for specific conditions or diagnoses

Occurrence monitors isolate cases in which there is a strong likelihood that a patient is exposed to harm due to inappropriate clinical practice or due to misutilization of hospital resources. Categories of monitors might include complications of treatments, errors in judgment or diagnosis, therapy ordered inappropriately, and adverse reactions.[9]

Each monitor that is identified for ongoing review and evaluation must have a procedure that fully specifies how the data are to be collected. The *element* is the aspect of clinical decision-making or patient management that will be measured and evaluated. An *explanation* is provided to thoroughly define the element and to identify groups of individuals or areas covered by the monitor. The *criterion* is the yardstick against which clinical practice is measured. It is used to give objectivity to the data collection and to identify variations from accepted practice. *Data collection specifications* provide information regarding the methods and/or documents utilized to identify the monitor findings. *Responsibility* for data collection is assigned by title to those responsible for data collection and compilation.

Problem-Solving

In evaluating monitor findings, the professional observes for trends over time. Thus, past ratings or findings are compared with those of the present for determining whether care and services are acceptable. If the findings are not acceptable to the observer, then action must be taken to improve performance so that the quality of care and services falls into acceptable ranges. When the cause of unacceptable findings is known, then the corrective action can occur immediately. However, there are times when the cause and the scope of unacceptable findings are not known. Implementing a corrective action based on few facts could be compared to treating symptoms instead of the diagnosed cause of a disease or illness. Then action is palliative at best and may lead to recurrence of the problem.

Initiation of the problem-solving process to identify the cause and scope of the problem is the next component of the quality-assurance process. Problem-solving consists of five steps—identification, prioritization, assessment, corrective action, and follow-up—and may be either informal or formal.

Problem identification includes defining the topic, the frequency, the site, and practitioners involved in the problem to the extent that these are known. A clear, written statement regarding the problem allows for understanding and agreement by the professionals on the nature of the problem to be evaluated.

Prioritization of problems occurs when there is more than one problem to be addressed. Because resources are limited, problems evaluated first are those that have the greatest impact on patient safety. Other issues pertaining to clinical practice and cost containment, while affecting patient care and outcomes, should be evaluated after patient safety is improved. Issues that might influence prioritization of problems include duration; number of departments, services, or people involved; staff motivation; political environment; and interrelationship of problems.

Assessment is the process of determining the cause and the scope of the problem through evaluation of data sources based on criteria. Objectives are set to provide the reference point for the assessment activity. Criteria are established so that standards of clinical practice, decision-making, and judgment can be objectively evaluated. Enough data should be collected so that those who evaluate the findings can draw conclusions about the problem. The method of assessment is dependent upon the nature of the problem. Data can be obtained from existing hospital records/files, medical records, interviews, observations, or surveys. The assessment process ends with a listing of the findings, compared with the criteria and assessment objectives.

The findings are reviewed for determination of where there is a gap between the standards and actual practice: knowledge, performance, or systems. Corrective actions are based on the type of deficit in the practice. Knowledge deficits require education and training. Performance deficits require provision or enforcement of policies and procedures, counseling, or discipline. Systems deficits require management decisions regarding facilities, equipment, and staffing.

In order to determine whether the corrective action was appropriate, one must make a follow-up evaluation. Follow-up can be the monitoring process or a reassessment similar to the initial assessment. Patient care improvement is determined after the corrective action has been implemented.

Documentation/Reporting

Documentation to prove the effectiveness of quality-assurance activities is required by the Joint Commission. Types of reports include the trend report of monitor findings and problem-solving/corrective action activities. The monitor report should be a simple graph delineating the specific monitors in the first column and monthly findings in subsequent columns so that trends over time can be assessed. Problem-solving activities can be reported through meeting minutes and special reports. The Joint Commission will review meeting minutes and other documents to assess effectiveness of quality assurance programs. For reporting purposes the hospital may require the completion of a form documenting the problem statement, method of assessment, actions taken, and follow-up findings.

Reporting quality-assurance activities is important for assuring corrective action and accountability for care. Final reports are sent to the governing body which is ultimately accountable for the quality of care provided by the institution. Both administration and the organized medical staff need reports to assure that responsible care is being provided and actions are taken to rectify problems in the delivery of high quality patient care.

Defining Peer Review

Peer review is the process of practicing physicians evaluating the quality and efficiency of care and services by other practicing physicians. Peer review is the all-inclusive term for medical review efforts.

The Peer Review Organization

As stated earlier, the federal government through Medicare legislation has been a major influence in the development of the peer review process.[13] In 1982 the Tax Equity and Fiscal Responsibility Act provided the impetus for Prospective Payment System implementation to control Medicare healthcare cost escalation. Added to this legislation was the Peer Review Improvement Act creating the Peer Review Organizations (PROs). Peer Review Organizations are similar to their 1972 counterparts, the

Professional Standards Review Organizations (PSRO). However, changes were made to improve the cost-effectiveness and efficiency of program operations. The PSRO was based on two principles: local review and peer review. Local review became a problem for the efficient operation of the program; thus, one of the changes was to expand the responsibilities of a single review organization from several counties within a state to only one PRO per state. Another change was the funding mechanism that evolved from a 1-year grant to a bidding process for a 2-year negotiated contract. The organization could be either nonprofit or for profit. A major change occurred in review activities. Under the PSRO, hospitals were allowed to conduct and report their internal review findings and actions. With the PRO contract agreement, no delegation of review activities was allowed. The PSRO review process of concurrent review, profile-analysis and medical-care evaluation studies was described in the peer review chapter of the first edition of this book. That review process dramatically changed to incorporate contract objectives and the Joint Commission quality monitoring process.

The PSRO review goals were to determine the medical necessity, appropriateness, and quality of care provided to Medicare beneficiaries. The PRO has similar review goals plus performing validation of DRGs and providing appropriate medical determinations in connection with coverage rules.[1]

The 1986–88 Scope of Work for contracting Peer Review Organizations provided two objectives:

Reduce unnecessary or inappropriate admissions and/or procedures

Eliminate adverse outcomes (including premature discharge)

These objectives are to be achieved through certain review activities: discharge review, generic quality screens, admission review, DRG validation, and coverage review.[1]

Major general screening categories include

Adequacy of discharge planning

Medical stability of patient at discharge

Deaths

Nonsocomial infections

Unscheduled return to surgery

Trauma suffered in the hospital

These screening categories relate to laboratory operations in several respects. Under the category of "medical stability of patient at discharge," abnor-

mal results of diagnostic services that are not addressed or explained in the medical record are of concern to laboratories because of shortened length of hospitalization. Sometimes laboratory results are not reported until after patient discharge. Abnormal findings that relate to patient readmission and not documented as identified and treated can result in corrective-action plans and/or intensified review. The category of "trauma suffered in the hospital" includes physical injury such as transfusion reaction or error; a lack of diagnostic studies to confirm which drug is the correct one to administer, such as culture and sensitivity studies; and serum drug level measurements not performed as needed.[6] Hospital- and practitioner-specific findings are maintained to determine whether actions need to be taken.

The Joint Commission Medical Staff Standards

The Joint Commission, through the Medical Staff Standards, specifies that the purpose of peer review is to evaluate clinical performance in order to delineate clinical privileges. The identified review activity is the department-specific review of the quality and appropriateness of patient care provided by those with clinical privileges; review of surgical cases to ensure that surgery performed in the hospital is justified and of high quality; review of the prophylactic, therapeutic, and empiric use of drugs to ensure that they are provided appropriately, safely, and effectively; review of the quality of medical record documentation and timeliness; review of the appropriateness of the use of blood and blood products; and maintenance of the pharmacy and therapeutics function to provide policies and procedures and maintain a drug formulary.[7]

The method by which these data on the medical staff functions and the quality and appropriateness of care are linked to the credentialing process is through monitoring and evaluation (peer review). Ball[3] defines "privilege delineation" as the "process by which individual members of a hospital staff —physicians and nonphysicians—are granted the right to perform certain activities within the hospital." Training and performance form the basis of granting privileges.

Corrective Actions

The external review of physician practice conducted by the PRO provides a monitoring and sanctioning process. It is stated in the Social Security Act that health-care providers have certain responsibilities for providing services paid for by Medicare. These include (1) the provision of medically necessary services in an economical fashion; (2) the provision of quality services meeting professionally recognized standards of practice; and (3) the provision of reasonable documentation. If the PRO finds that a provider is not meeting these responsibilities, then discussion with the provider and review of additional information are conducted. A determination is made by a panel of peers whether a substantial violation of responsibilities has occurred in a significant number of cases or whether a gross and flagrant violation has occurred in one or more instances. The PRO sends a report to the Office of the Inspector General with recommendations of exclusion from Medicare participation or a monetary penalty.[4]

Internal corrective actions through peer review include various interventions of education, proctoring, second opinion, and ultimately clinical privileging through the credentialing process. The need for the active participation of peers in the decision-making process is essential in the development of fair and equitable corrective-action plans.

IMPLEMENTATION OF THE QUALITY-ASSURANCE PROGRAM

The clinical laboratory would seem at first glance to be exempt from the requirements of quality-assurance review. Inspection and certification by the College of American Pathologists are stringent and require adherence to standards of safety, accuracy, and proficiency. However, these measures do not include the review of service and care appropriateness, efficiency, and efficacy. The challenge is to design a simple system for monitoring quality and appropriateness of service and quality control; to develop a sound management-oriented database; and to demonstrate compliance with current and future requirements of this dynamic process.

Organization

A planned and organized method of monitoring and evaluation can be created by forming an interdisciplinary team of laboratory professionals who routinely evaluate monitor findings and recommend/implement corrective actions when standards of practice are not met. The team should be composed of pathologists, technologists, and administrative staff. The size of the team will vary with the size of the laboratory staff and, in general, should not include more than eight members. Members are appointed by the laboratory medical director and should be individuals dedicated to the quality-assurance process and representative of all areas of laboratory function (*i.e.,* blood bank, hematology, microbiology).

The team should meet regularly; monthly meetings are recommended. The team is convened by a chairperson appointed by the laboratory medical director. The chairperson works with an individual assigned as staff support to the team to prepare and circulate agendas prior to meetings. A worthwhile and effective meeting is convened promptly and works efficiently through the agenda. Unless there are extenuating circumstances, meetings should last no longer than an hour. It is the responsibility of the chairperson to ensure adherence to the proposed agenda.

The first responsibility of the team is to identify the requirements for a quality-assurance program within the clinical support service. Reference to the Joint Commission Standards for the Pathology and Medical Laboratories will provide the following:

A planned and systematic process for monitoring and evaluating quality and appropriateness of care

Involving all areas of clinical responsibility

Appropriate delegation of responsibility

Routine and ongoing collection of data concerning patient care

Periodic assessment of data findings to identify any problems in the provision of care and services or opportunities to improve patient care

Action taken to correct any identified problems

Effectiveness of action evaluated

Findings from monitoring, evaluating, and problem-solving activities documented and reported per requirements to the hospital-wide quality-assurance program

Yearly evaluation of effectiveness of monitors and types of problem-solving activities

Medical staff participation

Based on the team's understanding of expectations and requirements, a plan or procedure for quality monitoring and evaluation should be developed. A written hospital-wide quality-assurance plan is required by the Joint Commission, but individual departmental plans are optional. In practice, a written plan developed by the team places the work of the team in the proper perspective. A plan is also helpful in orienting new members of the team to the role and purpose of quality assurance as it relates to laboratory function.

Although plans will vary with the requirements of specific laboratories, the following areas should be addressed:

Definition of goals and objectives, to provide a well-focused program in keeping with the hospital's mission.

Delineation of authority and responsibility for re porting mechanisms not only to the hospital-wide quality-assurance committee but to the laboratory medical director and administration. Both individuals should be informed of all committee actions and recommendations. The mechanism by which the committee reports to the governing board should be described. The authority of the team is one of reviewer and advisor.

The *scope and functions* of the team with regard to the type and extent of quality-assurance activities. Monitors should be identified, and the process for evaluation and problem-solving should be detailed.

Annual evaluation of the effectiveness of monitoring and problem-solving.

Documentation of minutes, monitors, and problem-solving activity, with procedures for confidentiality identified.

Developing Monitors of Care and Services

Monitors should be developed to encompass the variety of high-risk, high-volume, problem-prone activities of the laboratories. Yet these monitors, if they are to be functional, must be simple and explicit. Only one item or variance from standard practice should be identified with each monitor; otherwise the program will generate a plethora of meaningless data. Broad categories of monitors include quality of service, quality and appropriateness, and quality control.

Categories of quality of service monitors might be as follows:

Number of stats not completed within 60 minutes

Number of corrected laboratory slips

Number of patients with greater than four blood drawings within 24 hours

Turnaround time on laboratory result—hard copy reporting within 24 hours

Physician satisfaction with service

Notification of abnormal findings

Redrawings

Patient complaints regarding venipuncture

Quality and appropriateness monitors require peer review and involvement of the physicians in evaluating the care and services. Categories of such monitors might include the following:

Repeated laboratory test when findings are within normal limits

Assays conducted at the wrong time for normal blood level monitoring

Appropriateness of orders for complete blood count (CBC), erythrocyte sedimentation rates, electrophoresis, prothrombin times, stat laboratory studies

Appropriateness of orders on specific types of patients—radioactive thyroid studies for patients with endocrine and metabolic disorders, orders of lactate dehydrogenase (LDH) and/or creatine phosphokinase (CPK) studies for patients in intensive care units

Occurrence screening for expensive, focused laboratory studies when there have been no previous orders for related routine screening tests or there have been no abnormal results—

Schilling test for pernicious anemia when B_{12} folate level and CBC are absent or normal

Thyroid stimulation test when T_4 and T_3 are normal

Urine culture when clean-catch specimen shows fewer than four white blood cells per high-power field[9]

Appropriateness and accuracy of consultations related to interpretive reports, *e.g.,* cytogenetics, electrophoresis, blood work evaluation.

Categories of quality control monitors include

Number of quality-control entries falling beyond the expected parameters

Scores for proficiency samples

Reliability checks ensuring that assays correlate with health-care needs

Number of misinterpreted orders

Identifying Areas for In-depth Review

In-depth review and action are not limited to monitor findings. Reports from staff regarding concerns, complaints from physicians, staff, and patients, and referrals from other areas within the hospital are further examples of methods for identifying areas for patient-care quality improvement. Data collection on identified problems is based on preestablished criteria to promote objectivity in the assessment process.

The following will serve as an example of a process of in-depth review and evaluation for corrective actions.

Problem: Ten percent of the digoxin assay findings were recorded as too low to measure.

Assessment: A review of the patient's records revealed:
x% patients were not on digoxin.
x% of the assays were drawn at the incorrect time.
x% routine orders for assays.
x% were on the general surgery service.

Findings: No guidelines for ordering of assays.
No concensus for timing of blood drawing.
No monitoring and intervention when laboratory ordered inappropriately.
No controls for routine orders.

Action: Develop guidelines for assay ordering; incorporate concensus decision *re* timing of blood drawing.
Utilize pharmacokineticist to intervene on selected assays which are misused.
Do not allow routine orders for assay levels.
Provide continuing education *re* guidelines for assays to the general surgery physicians.

Follow-up: Continue to monitor the percentage of too-low-to-measure findings.

The next is an example of an occurrence monitor that has significant quality-of-care concern and risk.

Problem: Lab findings are added to the medical record after patient discharge, resulting in several instances in which premature discharge due to abnormal laboratory values was identified.

Assessment: The number of times abnormal laboratory values were reported after discharge were compared with patient readmission for complications of unmet discharge screens.
Mechanism for reporting abnormal laboratory findings after discharge was evaluated.

Findings: x% patients were discharged with unrecognized abnormal laboratory values.
x% patients were readmitted for complications relating to the abnormal finding.
Inadequate mechanisms for notifying the attending physician after patient discharge of abnormal laboratory findings.
Shorter patient lengths of stay contribute to earlier discharges before all laboratory data are available.

Action: Mechanisms are to be put into place to allow for timely notification of all laboratory findings provided after discharge.

Follow-up: Continue to monitor the patients readmitted for complications relating to abnormal laboratory findings on first admission.

FUTURE PERSPECTIVES

This chapter has explored the mechanisms and processes for providing high-quality care and services in the clinical laboratory. Some might believe the emphasis on peer review and quality assurance is excessive. However, in this era of cost containment, evolving reimbursement incentives, professional liability, and health-care competition, professionals must be able to prove that quality care is provided. To meet demands of the consumers of health-care services, systems that assure high-quality care and services must be implemented.

Through its "Agenda for Change," the Joint Commission is placing renewed emphasis on continuous, ongoing monitoring and intervention to provide health-care quality by routine evaluation of outcomes. The burden of proof is on the health-care provider to demonstrate that high-quality care *can be* and *is* provided. The PRO is adding its pressures to ensure that patient care is optimal and that good value is received for Medicare dollars. Private review programs (fourth-party payers, HMOs, PPOs) are adding their voice to the emphasis on health-care quality. Health-care providers have a choice and must exert the effort and energy to become involved in the quality-assurance process so that a true peer-review process occurs.

Quality assurance is the single most important aspect of health care. The process for monitoring quality has been described in the chapter. Many aspects of health care are not exact and do not yield readily to measurement. Judgment is difficult to quantify, and problems with developing standards of practice persist. It should be abundantly clear, however, that the process of quality assurance will not go away. Data will be used to direct the choices of health-care providers, including medical laboratories, of the payers of health-care services. These choices will be based on outcome, with high-quality care and services as the standard of performance.

REFERENCES

1. American Hospital Association: PRO scope of work. Washington Memo, Washington, DC, 1986
2. Ball JR: Credentialing versus performance: A new look at old problems. Quality Review Bulletin, December 1984
3. Carels EJ, Tabatabai C: Increased utilization of laboratory tests and x-rays: Effect on quality and cost of health care. Quality Review Bulletin, June 1980: 5–6
4. Champion PR: OIG's role in the PRO sanctioning process. QRC Advisor 3:1, 6–8, 1987
5. Diamond I: Quality assurance and/or quality control. Arch Pathol Lab Med 110:875–876
6. Generic screens required by new PRO scope of work. Journal of AMRA, April 1986:5–6
7. Joint Commission on Accreditation of Health Care Organizations: Accreditation Manual for Hospitals, pp 125–129, 1972, 1988
8. Joint Commission on Accreditation of Health Care Organizations: Agenda for Change. August 1987:18
9. Joseph E, Devet C, Dehn TG: The Monitoring Sourcebook, Vol 3, p. 9. Chicago, Care Communications, Inc., 1986
10. Myers LP, Schroeder SA: Physician use of services for the hospitalized patient: A review, with implications for cost containment. Milbank Memorial Fund Quarterly/Health and Society 59:483–485, 1981
11. Paris J, Drake III W: Allocation of scarce resources: A challenge for American medicine. Prim Care 13:343, 1986
12. Thompson R: The Nuts and Bolts of Hospital Quality Assurance. Chicago, Thompson, Mohr and Assoc., 1985
13. US Department of Health and Human Services, Health Care Financing Administration. Review activities. Federal Register 49:282, 1987

BIBLIOGRAPHY

Ball JR: Prospective payment: Implications for medical technology. Ann Intern Med 100(4):606–607, 1984

Borger ID: Quality for surgical pathology 101. Pathologist 40(12):10–13, 1986

Belyus S, Burgess TE, Walsh PR: Quality assurance in a large reference laboratory. Clin Lab Med 6(4):745–754, 1986

Bernstein LH, Kleinman GM, Davis GL, Chiga M: Part A reimbursement: What is your role in medical quality assurance? Pathologist 40(4):24–29, 1986

Dunham WG, Quinlan A, Krolikowski FJ, Reuter K: Quality assurance programs cope with today's demands. Pathologist 40(6):24–28, 1986

Friedman E: Doctors and rationing: The end of the honor system. Primary Care 13(2):349–364, 1986

Gary JP: Coping with the Joint Commission: The New Quality Assurance—Third Generation. Irving, Dallas-Fort Worth Hospital Council, 1985

Greeley H: Continuous monitoring and Data-Based Quality Assessment. Salem, Wisconsin, Greeley Associates, 1983

Kilshaw D: Quality assurance: I Philosophy and basic principles. Medical Laboratory Science 43:377–381, 1986

O'Leary DS: The Joint Commission looks to the future. JAMA 258(7):951–952, 1987

Pennock M: Quality assurance. Canadian Journal of Medical Technology 48:120–121, 1986

Reinhardt UE: Future trends in the economics of medical practice and care. Am J Cardiol 56:50C–59C, 1985

Schacter Y: Keeping on top of quality assurance. MLO 19(5):48, 55, 1987

Thompson JS: Diagnosis related groups and quality assurance. Topics in Health Care Financing 8(4):43–49, 1982

US Department of Health and Human Services, Health Care Financing Administration: Review activities. Federal Register 48(171):September 1, 1983

twenty-four

Medicolegal Concerns in Laboratory Medicine

Daniel I. Labowitz

Laws govern the relationships among individuals and between an individual and society itself. The proper management of a clinical laboratory requires that the supervisor and the technologist be aware of the laws affecting that laboratory and its operation. This chapter is concerned with the controls upon the operation of the laboratory and will discuss the responsibilities and liabilities of the laboratory technologist within society. Specific coverage will be given to possible areas of negligence liability, how to recognize problems before they give rise to a lawsuit, and how best to handle a problem that may have already occurred. As society becomes more involved with lawsuits for various reasons, the technologist may be called upon as a witness in court. This chapter will discuss how to respond to a subpoena, how to prepare for the court appearance, either as a fact witness or as an expert, and how best to present testimony. One of the most important areas of laboratory management, both from a medical as well as from a legal viewpoint, is the keeping of proper and accurate records. The legal problems of record-keeping will be developed to allow proper planning by the supervisor. The material presented in this chapter is intended as a guide and cannot be considered to be legal advice, because of the constantly changing laws on this subject and the diversity among the many jurisdictions in the United States. If the administrator or supervisor has a specific problem, legal counsel should always be sought to ensure proper action.

LEGAL LIABILITY

A proper understanding of why a laboratory may become liable for the actions of its personnel requires a basic knowledge of the law involved. This area is known as tort law and involves three types of wrongful conduct: intentional acts, strict liability, and negligence. Intentional acts are those that a person intends to commit and also intends to result in harm to someone else. Intentional acts, such as the willful falsification of laboratory records, would leave an individual, but not the laboratory, liable and will not be covered here.

Also, those areas covered by the doctrine of strict liability are not applicable to the clinical laboratory, because the doctrine applies to product liability and not to the performance of a service. This doctrine does become involved with the blood bank and is discussed in that section. A *tort* can be defined as a civil wrong or injury, not arising from a contract, and *negligent acts* are defined as the failure to do something that a reasonable man, guided by the considerations that ordinarily regulate human affairs, would do, or the doing of something that a reasonable and prudent man would not do. The standard against which all action must be measured is this mythical "reasonable man," or in the case of the laboratory, the "reasonable, trained technologist." It is wise to remember that bad results sometimes occur when the proper procedures have been followed and that the mythical standard person would have acted in the same manner. Not all bad results make the technologist or the laboratory liable.

To prove that a negligent act has been committed and to prove liability, the injured party, known as the plaintiff, must prove to the court each of the following elements:

The laboratory had a specific duty to which to conform. The injured party must prove that a duty of care existed and that the laboratory was obligated under that duty to the plaintiff to perform under a set standard of care. In the case of *Lauro v. Travelers Insurance Company,* 261 So. 2d 261 (1972), a pathologist, on examining a frozen section cut on a freezing microtome, diagnosed the tissue sample as scirrhous carcinoma, and surgeon performed a radical mastectomy. When a paraffin section was examined the following day, the diagnosis was changed to granular cell blastoma, not a malignancy. In reviewing a jury verdict for the pathologist, the court said a pathologist was not to be held to the highest degree of skill but to the ordinary level of skill employed by other pathologists in good standing. The trial evidence supported the procedure followed by the defendant and found that he did not vary from the duty to conform to a specific standard of care. In addition, the court held that a freezing microtome, although not as advanced as a cryostat, was scientifically acceptable and that the standard of care did not require the use of a cryostat. If the laboratory procedure followed is acceptable to the scientific community, an element of negligence cannot be proven, and no liability will result against the technologist or laboratory.

The accepted standard of care must be followed. Once the plaintiff establishes a standard of care, the fact that the laboratory fails to conform to that standard is the next element of proof. It must be shown that the laboratory did not follow the established, accepted scientific practice or performed it in an erroneous manner. As an example, in the *Lauro* case cited above, if the testimony had been such that a freezing microtome was an acceptable procedure but an ordinarily skilled pathologist would not have made the same diagnosis as the defendant, an element of proof of negligence would exist. In some instances, a plaintiff would be able to prove this element by establishing the standard of care and claiming that the result obtained by the laboratory was not possible if the procedure

had been performed properly. The legal doctrine applicable here is called *res ipsa loquitur,* which means "the thing speaks for itself." Under this doctrine, the plaintiff alleges that because the procedures were under the total control of the laboratory and because the results obtained were in error, the procedures could not have been followed, and, therefore, the laboratory was negligent. This doctrine has been barred in many states from being raised in medical negligence cases. If this doctrine is unavailable, the plaintiff must prove by the use of evidence and expert testimony exactly what was done and why that failed to conform to the scientifically acceptable standard of care. This may be accomplished by testimony of the technologist as to what was done and by an expert witness that the procedure was not acceptable in a similar scientific community. If the technologist performed according to accepted standards, there is no liability. Perhaps technology should be mentioned at this point, because an often-raised issue is that the laboratory failed to use the most up-to-date or state-of-the-art equipment to perform the procedures. Do not fall into the trap of "newest is best," which does not apply in a legal setting. Concern in a court of law is that a procedure is acceptable, accurate, and reliable, not necessarily the newest or fastest means of obtaining the same results. If either procedure is acceptable, reliable, and accurate, then either will be a valid standard of care for the court to apply in the case before it. The technologist has cause for concern if the procedure used is not accurate or reliable, for the question of liability will arise.

The failure to conform to the standard of care must be the direct cause of the injury. The legal concept called *proximate cause* means that a causal chain must exist from the breach of duty by the laboratory to the injury suffered by the plaintiff. Even if the technologist failed to follow an accepted procedure, no liability may exist if that error does not have a direct link to an injury to another person. This chain from laboratory to plaintiff may be broken by another party or by an intervening act of negligence. Courts have generally held that a treating physician who should have realized the laboratory results were in error, owing to his own standard of care, becomes such an intervening factor to break the causal chain. However, in determining proximate cause, the court is not limited as to time or number of intervening factors. In the case of *Renslow v. Mennonite Hospital,* 367

N.E. 2d 1250 (1978), the Supreme Court of Illinois allowed a child born in 1974 to sue a hospital for a negligent blood transfer in 1965. The negligence consisted of failing to notify the mother that she had been sensitized with Rh-positive blood, which caused a hemolytic disease process in the child. As remote as this may seem and with 9 years intervening between the negligent act and the injury, the court found proximate cause to exist. A federal court in Florida in *Givens v. Lederle,* 556 F.2d 1341 (1977), allowed a mother to recover from the manufacturer of an oral polio vaccine given her child because the child contracted the disease and the mother had not been warned of that possibility. The opposite situation, where no proximate cause was held to exist, may be exemplified by the Georgia case of *Lankford v. Trust Co. Bank,* 234 S.E. 2d 179 (1977), which is not medically based but illustrates the point. The plaintiff had lost his charge card and notified the bank of the loss; yet the bank paid a hotel bill charged by a person who had obtained the card and then billed the plaintiff. Plaintiff's wife saw the hotel bill; and despite her husband's explanations, a divorce resulted in which she was awarded alimony and child support. Plaintiff sued the bank for the loss resulting from his divorce, but the court held the divorce was not in the relationship of having been proximately caused by the bank's negligent billing. This is a bit farfetched, perhaps, but it is an actual case that exemplifies how far some people will go to attempt to recover on a lawsuit. When the question of laboratory liability exists, proximate cause is always involved because of the frequency with which the laboratory deals indirectly with the patient and because the results of its procedures are interpreted by a physician.

The plaintiff must have damages. The term *damages* does not refer to the specific injuries suffered by a person, but rather to a probable amount of money to pay for the value of those physical injuries. Because no possibility exists to return the plaintiff to a physical or mental condition that existed prior to the wrong done, some measure of reparation must be found. Damages have two categories: special and general. The easier to determine are the special damages, which include such items as medical and hospital bills and related expenses. Little question exists as to these amounts because they have been billed to the plaintiff and are a known amount. General damages raise a differ-

ent question, because they encompass the pain and suffering of the plaintiff, future loss of income, and future expenses necessitated by the physical or mental loss. Any injury to the plaintiff must be converted into a sum of money either for amounts due in the past or which may be due in the future. Any future amounts must be based upon current injuries and not on possible future injuries that are speculated upon the plaintiff. If no monetary damages can be proven—and this possibility has occurred—then even if the three other elements are proven, the laboratory will not be held liable.

When considering the possible liability of the clinical laboratory, the technologist must consider the elements of proof required to establish that liability before a court of law. An error by the technologist may not give rise to automatic liability, because of the many variables to be considered and proven by an injured party. The most important factor is that the procedures followed were accurate, reliable, and acceptable to the scientific community and that all ancillary functions were performed as a reasonable and prudent technologist would perform them. One additional factor in the question of laboratory liability is the legal doctrine of *respondent superior,* which is concerned with the liability of the employer for acts of the employee. The employer, whether the laboratory director or the hospital (usually both), is generally held liable for negligent acts of the employee that are performed while the employee is performing the duties for which he was hired or is reasonably expected to perform. The technologist is not relieved of personal responsibility; rather, the supervisory chain to the employer will be made responsible in addition because a supervisor is responsible for the work of those persons under him. The Texas Court of Civil Appeal in *Wilson N. Jones Memorial Hospital v. Davis,* 553 S.W. 2d 180 (1977), held a hospital liable for the negligent acts of an employee on the basis that the employee had lied on his employment application as to his qualifications and the hospital had failed to check out the history. The hospital could not claim the employee was performing outside of his training when they failed to confirm the extent of that training and assigned the tasks to be done by him. The manager, therefore, should be certain of the background and training of persons employed in the laboratory, because he will be responsible for their actions. This doctrine provides sufficient basis for managers to consider the possible liabilities of their laboratory operations and act to prevent the

Problem Areas

Direct exposure to the patient raises the possibility of a liability suit. Laboratory personnel involved in obtaining the specimen from the patient must be aware of the problems involved in patient contact and liability. An incident that in itself is not negligence, yet causes panic among most technologists is the breaking of a syringe needle during the collection of the specimen. Needles do break for various reasons, many of which do not result in the liability of the technologist; however, liability may result if the technologist fails to react properly. Preventing the broken part from traveling in the vein is the first concern. The second is obtaining assistance. Remaining calm and professional is the best method of avoiding liability. Another common problem in venipuncture is not being able to find a vein from which to draw the specimen. It is more difficult to do this with some persons than with others; so failure is not negligence. What may cause the patient to bring a lawsuit is what I call the "patient pincushion syndrome," where the technologist, upon failing to obtain a vein, continues to probe and probe until one is obtained. The patient is outraged and injured because of apparent ineptitude. Again, reasoned thinking and seeking assistance would possibly avoid a lawsuit, whether negligence existed or not. In *Leiman v. Long Island Jewish Hillside Medical Center-South Shore Division,* 401 N.Y.S. 2d 562 (1978), the New York Court held that expert testimony was required to prove negligence when a patient claimed damage to a median nerve from numerous venipuncture attempts during which the patient suffered extreme pain. The Louisiana Court of Appeals in *Sugulas v. St. Paul Insurance Company,* 347 So. 2d 855 (1977), held that a large hematoma and false aneurysm caused by a punctured artery during an intravenous pyelogram was not due to the negligence of the physician. The court, relying on expert testimony, said that even the most skillful practitioner may have results such as this and that it is a risk of the procedure.

Although not thought of as relating to venipuncture, the problems associated with the fainting patient are easily prevented, yet if not anticipated, may expose the laboratory to liability. The technologists should assume that all persons are subject to fainting when the specimen is being drawn and should take precautions, including using a patient chair with arms or having the side rails up on a patient-transfer cart. The negligence is not in the fainting; it is in allowing the patient to fall and become injured when basic precautions have not been taken. The same can be said of any other patient reactions, which, by asking the patient or reviewing the chart, can be avoided. This brings us to the question of consent. Normally, this is not a problem for the laboratory, but it may become so with patient contact. The treating physician should have informed the patient that a specimen would be drawn and obtained consent prior to the request to the laboratory. The simple precautionary measure of reminding the patient of the physician's request and explaining what is going to occur should solve this problem. If, however, the patient objects to the sample being drawn, it is advisable to proceed no further before clarifying the issue with the treating physician. Remember, an annoyed patient is more likely to bring a lawsuit than one who is treated with kindness and concern.

Before we leave the subject of consent, the questions of blood samples drawn at the request of a police officer should be considered. Under implied-consent laws enacted in each state, a person is deemed to have given consent to a blood-alcohol test by operating a motor vehicle upon the highways of that state. A police officer, after arresting a person for driving while intoxicated or under the influence, whatever the offense is called, may request a blood test to determine a blood-alcohol level. Some states allow a conscious person to refuse the test and suffer the loss of driving privileges. However, if the person consents or is unconscious, then the specimen may be drawn for analysis. The United States Supreme Court in the landmark case of *Schmerber v. California,* 384 U.S. 757 (1966), allowed a blood sample to be taken from a person who was conscious and protesting on the grounds that the sample was evidence that could cease to exist if not taken then and that therefore a search warrant was not necessary. The court did hold that removal of a blood sample was a search and seizure subject to the protections of the Fourth Amendment to the United States Constitution and would be valid if certain provisions were met. These provisions are

The blood must be drawn by medical personnel.

Standard medical procedures must be followed.

No physical force may be used if the person gives physical resistance.

Laboratory personnel, when requested to obtain a blood sample by a police officer, should be concerned with the last provision, because the first two are only good medical practice. If the person gives physical resistance, do not get involved. Let the police handle the matter, and then the laboratory will not face a possible liability suit. Remember, local laws vary, and the laboratory should have a policy developed after consultation with an attorney.

'ed to notify the laboratory of a
ᆟure, then the manufacturer,
ᆞry, is the negligent party.
ᆞmplified by the case of
2d 385 (1977), where
's upheld a verdict
ᄀod-sugar test. The
ᆞed ribs and sub-
ᆞism, for which
ᄀhysician or-
ᆞhe dextran
2000 mg
ᆞeen 65
ᆞ pa-
ᆞng
ᆞg
ᆞe-
ᆞ was
ᆞory, the
ᆞy held the
ᆞᵴs on the evi-
ᆞde available as to
ᆞᵤ by recent doses of
ᆞcose test. The results
ᆞrror was not due to any
ᆞatory, which was absolved of

ᆞvery of an instrument failure, the
ᆞshould document what occurred, de-
ᆞnether any analysis results were released
ᆞre possibly in error, and determine why the
ᆞument failed. If results have been given to a
ᄀnysician, he must be notified immediately of the
error and given possible corrective measures, if any.
If it is determined after examination of the malfunctioning instrument that the error was due to a manufacturing fault or a component failure, this should
be documented by an independent source, not
laboratory maintenance or the manufacturer. The
independent evaluation should assist the laboratory
in avoiding liability and possibly shifting it to where
it may belong: with the reagent or equipment manufacturer. I should emphasize that the instrument
should not be used until a complete check has been
made and it is again certified as performing
properly.

When the increased use of electronic calculators and computers in the laboratory, as well as for
personal use, mathematical errors have decreased.
The ever present decimal ᵖᵒⁱⁿᵗ will

to provide for a clear, readable numeral printout are the best means of avoiding liability for simple computation errors. I have mentioned the requirement for test reliability earlier and believe it should be re-emphasized now. If you are scientifically satisfied that your method of analysis is reliable and accurate, then by all means continue to use it. Remember that you must document reliability should you ever need to prove it to a court of law. When performing any test, document the method of analysis used and the accuracy of the equipment. This is best done by daily or weekly logs showing when blanks and knowns were run and the result obtained. If done on a regular basis, these logs are admissible as evidence of the reliability and accuracy of test procedures and equipment.

One legal doctrine that must be followed if any specimens are retained at the laboratory that are known to be evidence is called the *chain of custody*. This means that the evidence must be accounted for from the time it is obtained by the laboratory until it is delivered to the court or its agent. If these specimens are kept frequently, then a locked refrigerator and a limited-access policy should satisfy the requirements of the chain of custody. If the situation is unique, a locked container in the normal specimen refrigerator should suffice. The purpose of being able to account for the sample is to assure the court that the correct specimen was analyzed and to allow its identity to remain out of question. Whether dealing with an evidence sample or a normal specimen for analysis, the laboratory manager should establish standard procedures for the handling of all biologic materials brought into the laboratory to assure anyone as to exactly what chain of events occurs from acceptance of the sample, through analysis, to disposal or storage. A well-established procedure will aid in avoiding liability as well as providing for an efficiently run laboratory.

After the analysis has been performed, the next step is reporting the results, which also has problem areas to be aware of in the attempt to avoid liability. The case of *Jones v. French Drug Company*, decided by the Massachusetts Court of Appeals in 1977, exemplifies what can occur when documents are illegible or unclear in their meaning. The plaintiff was given a prescription for the circulatory drug Ethatab, and the pharmacist filled it will Estratab, a female hormone. The injuries suffered by the male, 51-year-old plaintiff included memory lapse, en-

Warvel v. Michigan Community Blood Center, 253 N.W. 2d 791 (1977), in which evidence was presented that laboratory tests for hepatitis in blood were only 45% to 60% effective. State law was such that if no valid test existed to test the fitness of whole blood, the furnishing of blood became a service and not the sale of a product. It must be noted that without statutory protection, most courts would hold that the furnishing of blood was a sale and subject to strict liability. This was laid down by the Florida Court of Appeals in *Lewis v. Associated Medical Institutions, Inc.,* 345 So. 2d 852 (1977), where the transfusions were made before the status holding transfusions a service became effective and hepatitis was discovered afterwards. The court held that the discovery of the disease was made after the law changed and that therefore it would not allow the lawsuit based on strict liability. This situation does not absolve a laboratory from bad results in the furnishing of blood for a transfusion, because a plaintiff can still allege negligence in the testing of the blood, in obtaining data as to the donor's health, or in storage procedures in the blood bank. Following proper scientific and laboratory procedures should avoid a holding of liability in this area. The procedure of requesting an emergency supply of blood that has not been crossmatched to a patient may open up the blood bank for liability. If the request is truly for an emergency and plasma will not suffice until a crossmatch has been done, then as a general rule no court will hold a laboratory liable in providing whole blood. There have been occasions, however, where the request was not an emergency, but the result of the surgeon or nurse having neglected to request a crossmatch in sufficient time or having requested an insufficient supply be set aside. The best procedure to establish to cut down on the number of "emergency" requests for other than true emergencies is to require the requestor to sign a request form that states that the need is truly an emergency and that the laboratory is absolved of all responsibility in providing blood that has not been crossmatched to the patient. While this may not remove the laboratory's responsibility to the patient, it should reduce the number of "emergency" requests and also would be looked upon favorably by a court of law should a question arise.

THE SUBPOENA

If a laboratory becomes a defendant in a negligence case or a technologist has become so knowledgeable in the field that his testimony is needed at another trial, the first knowledge of involvement may be the delivery of a legal document known as a *subpoena.* This document may be in any one of numerous forms and says that the person subpoenaed must appear at a specified place and time to provide testimony on a case of which he has knowledge. A subpoena may be one or both of two types: one calls for personal appearance for giving testimony, and the other asks for records to be delivered to the proper party. Most frequently both are called for in cases where the clinical laboratory is involved. A request for records is called a *subpoena duces tecum.*

Upon receipt of any subpoena, the first thing you should do is notify the laboratory director and the attorney for the laboratory. Time is normally short on the response to a subpoena, and your attorney will need all the time he can get to prepare for the court proceedings or to make arrangements if you cannot be available at the time and place requested. A subpoena is a *command* by a court, which must not be taken lightly. Failure to obey the command of the court (or of a grand jury, which also has subpoena power) could put a person in contempt of that court. In contempt-of-court proceedings a judge may order the person he holds in contempt to go to jail or to pay a fine. Although this rarely occurs in civil cases, there is no excuse for not answering a subpoena or making arrangements with all parties to appear at a different time or date, if necessary. On rare occasions a subpoena may arrive with little or no time left before the court appearance date. At such times contact with your attorney is essential in avoiding the anger of the court and being allowed to fully present your case. Where the laboratory is a party to a lawsuit, you should be told in advance what is happening and when you will be required to testify. You should still check with your attorney upon receipt of the subpoena to confirm what it is for and what you are to do. If the subpoena is for a criminal action—for example, a case in which a blood sample has been analyzed for blood-alcohol content—you should contact the person who sent the subpoena as well as your attorney. In criminal cases your attorney will have little to do with the prosecutor who will be presenting the case. Above all, when you receive a subpoena, do not file it away to be looked into tomorrow or in the future, but look into it immediately. Receipt of a subpoena is not cause for panic, but it does require actions not within most technologists' normal operational habits and should be a cause for concern. Remember to call your attorney, check to see whether you have the materials requested, refer to your notes or log books on the case, and approach the subject of testimony with scientific caution, and no problems need arise.

THE TECHNOLOGIST AS WITNESS

If a person makes an observation of an occurrence that later becomes important in a civil or criminal court proceeding, that person is subject to being called as a witness to testify in court. Any person who has knowledge of an event that was gained by that person's own observations is called an *ordinary* or *fact witness.* Such a witness is limited in the testimony given to the facts so obtained and may not venture an opinion except in limited circumstances. An ordinary witness may give an opinion only if formed upon his own experience. A common example is observation of intoxication, if the witness has a basis upon which to make that conclusion. A technologist would be a factual witness if he were to testify regarding facts obtained from observations made in the laboratory. These could include the procedure for a specific analysis in question or the operating procedure for handling reports in the laboratory. There is no limit to what such a witness may testify to as long as the information sought is relevant to the issue at the trial; however, such a witness may not give an opinion as to whether the analysis was done within acceptable scientific guidelines or whether the procedure was proper. This opinion calls for the testimony of an *expert witness.* A technologist may be very well qualified as an expert in the laboratory; but until that person qualifies as an expert before the court, an opinion on the science or procedure involved may not be given. Why do courts require expert testimony? Where the knowledge involved is outside the common understanding of the finder of fact, whether the jury or the judge, an expert witness is necessary to establish that fact or knowledge. The field of medicine and laboratory science is outside such a common understanding and requires that an expert form an opinion and testify as to that opinion, which may not be based on personal knowledge gained by the witness. An expert witness is allowed to form an opinion based on "reasonable scientific certainty" from facts or information provided from another source. The case of *Todd v. Eitel Hospital,* 237 N.W. 2d 357 (1977), illustrates the need for expert testimony in medical cases. The court stated "where the conduct of the physician involves complexities of pathological diagnosis, we are not persuaded that non-medically trained jurors are competent to pass judgment." Expert witnesses were held to be necessary to establish the standard of care; the jury could not establish one without such assistance. Expert testimony is the only time such testimony is admissible as evidence in a court of law. This opinion is just that, an opinion, but it must not act as a determination of guilt or liability, since that is the sole prerogative of the finder of fact. An expert opinion may be based upon a hypothetical question, formulated for the jury and requiring an opinion upon facts alleged in that, sometimes lengthy, question. Facts in evidence must be used in such a question, and the opinion must be based upon those facts to be allowed. A question such as this is most often used by the opposition attorney in an attempt to get the expert to change the opinion based upon a slight change of fact in his client's favor. That is an acceptable form of examination of an expert in most jurisdictions and should be expected by an expert witness.

An expert witness is distinguished from a fact witness in that the expert is arranged for beforehand by the attorney and is paid for his expertise and time, rather than receiving a set witness fee for the court appearance. The amount the expert charges will vary among communities and among experts of various levels of experience and knowledge. Determination of a fee based upon an hourly rate should include research time, preparation time, and time in court and should be discussed with the attorney at the time the expert is hired. Remember that the expert is being paid for his time and experience and that the testimony is not being bought. Another point that was made by the United States Court of Appeals for New York in 1977 should be kept in mind. That court approved a local rule barring the payment of contingent fees to expert witnesses. A contingent fee is one of which the expert would receive a percentage of the award if the party on behalf of whom he testified won the lawsuit. If that party (usually the plaintiff) did not win, the expert would receive nothing. Such arrangements are common in negligence suits where the plaintiff shares his proceeds with the attorney, because this allows a person to obtain a lawyer without having to produce a fee and allows less wealthy persons to bring a lawsuit. However, when the expert witness has an economic interest in the outcome of the lawsuit, he loses all scientific objectivity, becomes an advocate for that party, and ceases to be a proper scientific expert. Whether barred by your jurisdiction or not, do not become an expert on a contingency-fee basis.

Trial Preparation

Whether a technologist is testifying as a fact or as an expert witness, he should always prepare for that testimony even if he has testified numerous times before. The first step is to meet with the attorney who will be presenting the testimony, not just to establish fees for the expert but to discuss the entire case and learn the part the witness plays in the attorney's presentation. Determine from the attorney who is to obtain records and other necessary materials upon which an expert opinion will be formed. Also determine whether the attorney is aware of whatever laboratory records you have that are pertinent to the case. If unaware of what the attorney is attempting to prove with expert testimony, do not be afraid to ask and to provide advice to help him understand the science and laboratory procedures involved. Treat the relationship as a partnership in the effort to present the complete case to the jury, and you will have the proper attitude. Upon obtaining all of the records and reports, review them thoroughly, even if you are already familiar with them. Your testimony will be based upon the record, and you must be as knowledgeable of it as possible to do your best as a witness. If further records are needed, obtain them so that you will have a complete understanding of the case and all of the possible issues involved.

In your review of the case materials it is not advisable to discuss them with other technologists unless they have been involved in the case also. The testimony you will give must be your own, and if others have been consulted, you must be prepared to explain why and what assistance they provided. This may appear to the jury as a means of reassuring yourself as to your testimony, or, even worse, an attempt to develop a better story for the witness stand. These problems may easily be avoided by limiting your consultations with nonwitnesses and other experts who have not been retained to testify. While reviewing the case material, also review the literature on whatever science or procedure is involved to become as current as possible on the subject. The opposing attorney and his experts will do this, and your preparedness will enable you both to advise the attorney with whom you are working and to respond to questions on cross-examination. This review is especially helpful if some new technique has been reported and you are able to discuss it and its effect, if any, on the case at hand. Frequently, these issues are raised in an attempt to have the jury believe that the procedures followed were not the latest or best. This is usually a smokescreen, and your preparation with all of the latest literature will avoid problems at trial.

After your initial review of all of the records and all of the literature with the attorney, another review is necessary. The first review is to assist you; the second is to allow you to educate the attorney about what he must know to properly question you and to

rebut any claims by the opposition's attorney. Your assistance is invaluable in the attorney's preparation of a cross-examination if any experts testify for the opposition. It is at this stage that you can best provide that assistance.

Because you must qualify as an expert at the trial to be allowed to give an opinion on a scientific matter, frequently your training and experience will be in issue as a fact witness if the question of proper procedure and analysis is raised. For this reason you should thoroughly review your *curriculum vitae* and be prepared to explain what your duties were at various places of employment or your course of study at school or continuing education courses. The opposition attorney may waive your qualifications, and your attorney may still put them in to show the jury that you are an expert and impress tham with your education and experience. Thorough familiarity with your *curriculum vitae* as well as what went into it is an important asset for your attorney in establishing either your expertise or as a good basis for your knowledge of how a specific analysis is performed. The important factor here is not to allow the opposing attorney to raise any doubt about your qualifications or your knowledge. If your attorney approves, and never without his approval, bring all the records to the trial. This will speed the procedure if you have to refer to them and will allow for a more professional presentation. However, in some jurisdictions, the records may not be available to the opposition, and they should not be brought to court without the attorney's approval.

As an expert witness, the technologist has agreed to review the records, advise the attorney, and present testimony in court if the need should arise. Not all lawsuits result in a court trial. Rather, the minority do; and therefore, many attorneys will rely upon an expert's advice on the validity of the allegations about the scientific aspects of the case. As an expert, if you believe that the case as portrayed by the attorney is not coordinated with the science and is therefore difficult to prove, let him know. If the science is either nonprovable or not supportable from a legal viewpoint, then the attorney should attempt to obtain an out-of-court settlement of the case, rather than expending time, effort, and the hopes of his clients on a weak or nonexistent case. The sooner he knows this the easier it is for him to work out an amicable settlement.

The only other obligation of the expert witness is to fulfill the agreement and appear to give testimony when called. The New Jersey Superior Court in the 1976 case of *Lapham v. Dingwall* allowed a plaintiff to recover a monetary award from an expert witness who failed to come to the trial and thereby caused the plaintiff to receive a lower award at trial. If you fulfill your agreements, there is no cause for worry. After a thorough preparation and evaluation of the records, the next step is to present the testimony if the case goes to trial.

Presentation of Testimony

As a general rule, witnesses are not allowed in the courtroom while other witnesses are testifying; so you will not be able to observe the trial at which you are to testify before your turn arrives. If you are unfamiliar with the courtroom, ask your attorney if you can see it when a case is not being presented so you can sit in the witness chair and become acquainted with your surroundings. If possible, observe another trial in which your attorney is involved to see how questioning is done. This pretestimonial familiarization will help to alleviate any fear or nervousness you may have as a new witness. A witness who is comfortable in the courtroom will present a more relaxed and professional appearance and will be able to concentrate on the questions and answers. The technologist should strive to present a professional appearance, both in clothing and demeanor. Do not try to act out a preconceived notion of what a professional looks like. Rather, be yourself; and seek your attorney's advice if you have any problems. Casual clothes are usually not the proper attire for testifying, but neither is a three-piece suit if you are not accustomed to it. Self-assuredness will allow you to keep mentally alert, the most important item to remember when testifying.

After you are called and take the witness chair, listen carefully to each question before you respond. Do not anticipate questions and thereby shut your mind down while you give a prepared answer. Wait until the question has been completed before answering. Especially on cross-examination, attorneys may hesitate in their questioning, hoping to get a response to an incomplete question, and thereby throw the witness off the issue concerned and cause him to worry about what was done or said. If you wait and listen until the question is complete, you should have no problem. Always speak clearly, distinctly, and with understandable language. Avoid the use of technical slang or abbreviations, which confuse a jury composed of persons with no knowledge of the laboratory. Explain terms you must use in your testimony. If the witness were to think of himself as a teacher and the jury as students, the relationship would be easier to comprehend. Do not talk down to the jury, and do not

present an attitude of preacher expressing dogma, but explain the science in clear, understandable language, and they will appreciate it. Do not go far afield in responding to a question, and do not volunteer information not requested. Confine your response to the question asked, unless you do not believe that you will be able to do so. If you must explain further, tell the judge that this is the case and seek permission before you begin your response. In addition, if you do not understand a question, say so and ask for clarification. Do not appear argumentative or uncooperative, but professional and unwilling to respond incorrectly to question you believe cannot be answered properly. If you cannot answer a question because you do not know the answer, do not be afraid to say "I don't know," which is a valid and aceptable response. This does not weaken your expertise or knowledge in the eyes of the jury; rather, it makes you appear human and more believable. You should keep in mind why the testimony is being given, keep alert mentally and physically, and remain professional in all ways to be an effective witness in a court of law.

RECORDS

One area of the clinical laboratory that causes many questions to be asked is that of records-keeping and the quality of those records, and a brief discussion of the legal aspects of medical records will be made here to enable the technologist to better understand the responsibilities and liability involved.

The prime consideration is the ethical, and in many jurisdictions legal, requirement of confidentiality of medical records. Either by agreement between the patient and the laboratory or by stature, confidentiality requires that these records not be released to anyone outside the laboratory except the treating physicians without the patient's consent. There are a few exceptions, such as in response to a valid subpoena, to the next of kin of a deceased patient, or to an attorney of the patient. The exceptions vary between jurisdictions and should be listed in any statutory "privacy act." A laboratory would be liable if it released information to a person without authority. This liability could be just to the patient, if injury could be proven, or in the form of a fine to the state if the statute so provides. Therefore, access to laboratory medical records should be limited and controlled to avoid the unauthorized release of analysis results and other patient information. As was stated earlier in this chapter, a telephone request is the easiest way for information to be released to a person without authority to be obtaining it. A single authorized person responsible for telephone requests who also maintains a log book for such requests will eliminate much of the problem. In addition, a system of call-backs, whereby the laboratory will call back the requestor at a valid number, rather than giving the data at the requestor's call, will cut down appreciably on the frequency of the giving of data to unauthorized persons. Do not let so-called freedom of information statutes confuse you as to which takes precedence, privacy or freedom of information. In the federal act (US Code Svc. Tit. 5 §552), as in many state acts, medical records held by a governmental agency are exempt from disclosure and protected by the privacy act (US Code Svc. Tit.5 §552a). Remember, when in doubt as to whether or not records should be released, consult your laboratory administrator and legal counsel before releasing them.

A phrase heard frequently regarding records is that they are privileged and therefore not releasable. This term relates solely to the use of medical and laboratory information at a trial and is a legal principle that would ban its admissibility as evidence if the information fell within this classification. In order to be so classified, records must have the following four elements:

1. *A patient–physician relationship must exist.* This relationship includes the entire healthcare team, not just the treating physician. The laboratory qualifies here whether the analysis has been run at the request of the treating physician or another outside medical source. A test requested by a police officer does not qualify for the privilege because no physician–patient relationship exists.
2. *The information was obtained during treatment.*
3. *The information was necessary for diagnosis and treatment.* Therefore, even if a patient–physician relationship existed, if the information given by the patient was irrelevant to the treatment, no privilege exists. The laboratory would rarely come under this exception, since by the very nature of its function, any information it receives and any reports generated are necessary for diagnosis and treatment of a patient. The only exception here would be if the laboratory accepted specimens from nonmedical sources for analysis for reasons not needed or outside a physician–patient relationship.
4. *The interest of society in keeping information privileged outweighs any instant interest to*

release it. The privilege is one that has been established by statute passed by the legislature, speaking for society, saying that the need to have a free flow of information from patient to physician for treatment is superior to anyone else's interest in knowing what was said. All privileges (except for attorney–client) are established by statute and may be eliminated by statute. It should be noted that no physician–patient privilege is recognized in the federal courts. The privilege belongs to the patient, and it is the patient who must waive the privilege and allow the other party to release the information at trial. The patient cannot use the privilege to the disadvantage of others, such as by claiming certain medical status and barring the release of his medical information. In such cases where the laboratory is the subject of a lawsuit brought by the patient, the privilege is waived by the patient's actions and the information may be testified to in court. Therefore, if you are called to testify regarding patient information and the patient or his representative is not bringing the lawsuit, check to determine whether a waiver has been made; if not, you are barred from testifying about that information. This is another reason you should consult an attorney upon receipt of a subpoena for laboratory records.

Finally, who owns medical records? This question has given some cause for concern when patients want to transfer records to another physician or a laboratory consolidates with another and the question of patient files is considered. The general legal proposition is that a practitioner owns the files he has maintained regarding his patients. He may do as he would with them, keeping within any restraints set up by statute and ethical considerations. The major consideration is that upon request of a patient he must transfer these records to another physician with the promise that the patient is not in debt to that physician. Also, hospital records are the property of the hospital when an agreement between a physician and the hospital modifies that general rule. Laboratory records, therefore, generally are the property of the laboratory or of the hospital if the laboratory is owned by the hospital. Frequently, clinical laboratories are operated on a contractual basis for one or more hospitals; the contract should cover who has control over laboratory records. It must be noted that the ownership of the records is to be contrasted with the ever-expanding right of the patient to have access to the information in his records.

The legal aspects of laboratory administration and practice are not intended to confuse the practitioner nor difficult to understand if common sense is applied to a problem and an objective viewpoint is taken. It must be remembered that the practices and procedures of the laboratory, whether scientific or record-keeping, are subject to the ultimate review of a panel of jurors who are not scientists and must be instructed by experts about what the correct procedure is. This perspective should help any laboratory administrator or supervisor avoid liability, both personally and on behalf of the laboratory.

ANNOTATED BIBLIOGRAPHY

The Citation. Chicago, American Medical Association (semimonthly)
  This text is a compilation with synopses of court decisions affecting medical practice with an interpretation of the meaning of the decisions. It is an excellent means for updating the legal aspects of laboratory medicine with actual court decisions.
Feegel J: Legal Aspects of Laboratory Medicine. Boston, Little, Brown, 1973

Of interest to the pathologist, in particular, coverage of the areas of records keeping, consent, blood banking, and testimony in court would be of general interest to the laboratory supervisor. A general guidebook for the pathologist is those areas of practice concerned with legal matters.
Hoyt E: Medicolegal Aspects of Hospital Records. Berwyn, H: Physician's Record, 1977
  This book is intended for persons who deal in the maintenance and release of hospital records. It is an excellent text for laboratory supervisors who are more and more becoming concerned with records keeping problems. Specific coverage of the legal system, evidence, trial practice, and the right to privacy should be helpful to the laboratory technologist.
Laboratory Regulation Manual. Germantown, Aspen Publications
  An extensive resource for the laboratory director or supervisor which is updated on a regular basis. Although its prime interest is in government regulatory rules, three chapters of its three volumes deal with business conduct, laboratory employees, and malpractice.
Warren DG: Problems in Hospital Law, 3rd ed. Germantown, Aspen Publications, 1978
  This book is a general treatise on the legal problems applicable to all aspects of hospital operation. Although it is not concerned with laboratory operation, Chapter 7, "Principles of Liability," and Chapter 9, "Collection and Disclosure of Patient Information," should be of interest to the laboratory supervisor.

twenty-five

Marketing Clinical Laboratory Services

Carolyn C. Hart
Sharon S. Gutterman

Until the 1980s, the word "marketing" was not used to describe business-building activities in health care. Many hospitals had a public relations department whose job was to disseminate information about special events and procedures in the hospital, but marketing as a strategic planning tool was virtually unknown. In fact, to many health-care professionals the word *marketing* was synonymous with *advertising* and, therefore, considered unethical. Codes of ethical conduct, established by professional associations, prevented professionals from engaging in any active solicitation of new patients. To hospital boards, the thought of marketing smacked of crass commercialism. Attitudes changed as decision-makers began to understand the meaning of marketing, the changes in health care economics, and the potential benefits to the hospital.

In recent years, competition in delivering health-care services has increased sharply. Providers of medical services now see themselves as serious business people and recognize the need to use the same tools that other businesses use. Hospitals are looking for profit centers, and laboratory services present a revenue-producing opportunity. Administrators understand that marketing activities are necessary to provide people with satisfying goods and services.

As you will see, the basic constructs that define marketing are quite compatible with the goal of offering excellent service to consumers. In fact, chances are that you already perform marketing activities, but never think about them as such. Posting signs to help outpatients find the laboratory, extending hours of service to accommodate both patients and physicians, and telephoning results are outcomes of marketing planning.

DEFINING THE MARKETING CONCEPT

"Professional services marketing consists of organized activities and programs designed to retain present clients and to attract new clients . . . by sensing, serving, and satisfying needs through delivery of appropriate services, on a paid basis, in a manner consistent with credible professional goals and norms."[5] The marketing concept can be summarized in three patient-oriented words: *sensing, serving,* and *satisfying*. Marketing plans begin with sensing what needs in the marketplace are not currently being met.

Sensing market needs can be achieved by using sophisticated market research methods or more informally by listening to people's questions and requests. The business that is attuned to what its audience needs and wants has a greater chance of succeeding in a competitive environment. Data are gathered, processed, and interpreted to improve managerial decision-making.

Serving refers to developing and implementing the marketing program. Decisions concerning personnel tasks and which laboratory service to promote must be addressed.

Satisfying involves ensuring that purchasers of the laboratory service have their expectations met. A satisfied customer is the goal.

Marketing, then, focuses the health-care provider's attention to the needs and desires of the potential buyer as the starting point for planning. The range of activities that brings the buyer and seller together for their mutual benefit is the marketing function.

An organization must try to identify and satisfy the needs of customers, clients, or patients by coordinating a set of activities that concurrently allows the organization to achieve its own goals. When the business learns what will satisfy customers and creates products and services accordingly, then the business must continually monitor the environment in order to adapt its services to changing desires and preferences.

It should be clear by now that marketing refers to much more than the words *selling* or *advertising*. There is a strong research component necessary to identify customer needs, competitors' offerings, and environmental trends. In general, more research and program development have been done on how to market *goods*. As the dollars spent by Americans continue to increase—for health care, entertainment, repair services, airlines, and so forth—there is an accompanying need to learn whether the approach to marketing *services* parallels the approach to marketing *products*. In other words, is services marketing different?

According to Leonard L. Berry[2]:

A good is an object, a device, a thing; a service is a deed, a performance, an effort. When a good is purchased, something tangible is acquired, something than can be seen, touched, perhaps smelled or worn or placed on a mantel. When a service is purchased, there is generally nothing tangible to show for it. . . . Services are consumed but not possessed.

Berry continues by discussing how service delivery is perceived as an intrinsic part of the "product." For example, clinical laboratories have an ongoing internal process to control the quality of the results; the patient, however, may evaluate the quality of the laboratory on the basis of the pleasantness

and skill of the phlebotomist. Physicians may evaluate the laboratory on the basis of the turnaround time. Clearly the performance is part of the laboratory "product."

The communication component of marketing comprises the techniques a business uses to tell potential buyers what it has for them. Human beings constantly scan their environment looking for reliable ways to satisfy needs. Promotional communication methods attempt to inform and persuade customers to choose their company's products and services. Market research methods can reveal buyers' television show preferences, magazines they read, radio programs they listen to, and newspapers they buy.

MARKET RESEARCH

Market research methods provide vital information to assist in making marketing decisions. Research and information storage systems provide feedback to the organization. Strategic planning is influenced by the opinions expressed by members of the target market. Consider the hospital laboratory, for example, that wants to market routine chemistry tests and blood counts to physician offices. The market research indicates that the physicians are very satisfied with the commercial service. The hospital laboratory cannot compete with the price the physicians are getting from the commercial laboratory. To compete on strictly business terms, the hospital laboratory would have to provide the physicians equivalent service at a lower price or additional needed services for the same price. The decision not to enter the market when the chance for success is borderline can result from market research.

Although marketing managers rely on gathering systematic, objective data, intuition also plays a role. Marketing managers may make decisions because "it feels right." Experience and personal judgment are valuable inputs. Scientific research and intuition meld in reaching a decision.

A number of research techniques and resources are available: surveys, direct questioning and observation, reviewing records, and using sources of stored data. Survey methods include questioning people by mail, in person, and by telephone. The market researcher carefully designs a research problem based on what he or she wants to find out, designates the population to be reached, and recommends the methods to be employed. In a mail survey, questionnaires are sent to representatives of the target market, who are encouraged to complete and return the survey instrument. For telephone surveys, respondents answer questions posed by the telephone interviewer, and their answers are recorded. Personal surveys conducted face-to-face are highly favored but may be difficult to obtain because people's schedules and lifestyles are so varied. A variation of the personal survey is the focus group interview, which consists of approximately 10 persons who share characteristics of the market one wants to reach. The group is given an incentive to meet with a trained moderator and answer questions and express opinions about the product or service undergoing scrutiny.

Observation methods include quietly observing what is occurring in the setting by recording information from an unobtrusive spot. If the presence of an observer might bias behavior, then devices such as cameras, recorders, counting machines, and other mechanical equipment may be used.

Sources of stored data include reviewing records in the hospital, studying census tract information, and identifying other public records resources in the community. In addition, companies sell data about people and their buying habits. Many insights can be gleaned from going to these sources, and the cost of "secondary data" is far less than if one had to generate information by developing one's own study.

Selecting the appropriate market research instrument and developing, administering, and evaluating it require skills that are usually not part of the medical technology curriculum. Laboratories in larger hospitals may get help from the professional marketing staff employed by the hospital. When that support is not available, contracting for consulting services with an independent marketing firm can be worthwhile.

MARKET SEGMENTATION

Marketing experts recognize that the general population is composed of groups of people, i.e., "segments" who share certain similar characteristics. These segments become "target markets" for business planning. Groups of people can be segmented according to any variable that has relevance for the business.

Health-care services are segmented into specialty areas. People sharing certain medical needs go to physicians who specialize in a particular area. A laboratory may segment the market in the same way, for example, by developing a set of services to meet the special needs of a group of patients such as oncology patients. A laboratory may also segment the market on the basis of the requirement for spe-

cialized skills or equipment. Virology and toxicology are examples of this kind of segmentation.

Two major ways of segmenting a market are by grouping people according to demographic variables and by psychographic variables.

Demographic Variables

Consumer buying habits correlate with characteristics such as age, sex, address, income, occupation, and education. Women over the age of 40 having regular mammograms are an example of market segmentation using demographic data.

Psychographic Variables

Behavioral and psychologic attributes can be used to segment the population. Psychographic variables include identifying lifestyle activities, interests, values, attitudes, and opinions. Although it would be difficult for a hospital laboratory to segment the market using psychographic variables, laboratory participation would be important for some hospital programs that segment the market this way. Sports medicine, weight reduction, and wellness programs would fit this category. A hospital's affiliation with a religious group would also tend to segment the population by psychographic variables.

THE MARKETING ENVIRONMENT

Although a need for services may have been identified, forces in the environment also influence business decisions. External environmental forces are referred to as "uncontrollables" because the individual business cannot immediately change what is occurring. Uncontrollables are trends, and to change these trends in one's favor requires time and support from many groups of people. The decision to market laboratory services is complex and must take into account pressure from environmental forces beyond the control of the individual hospital.

Economic Forces

The economic condition of the marketplace affects the size and strength of demand for goods and services. The state of the nation's economy has bearing on the buyer's ability and willingness to make purchases. During times of prosperity, buying power is increased. During recessionary periods, buyers are cautious about their limited buying power.

Technologic Forces

New technology has a direct impact on consumer buying behavior. Technologic developments affect our standard of living as thousands of new products and services are introduced each year. The speed at which new laboratory procedures are introduced can make previous methods appear slow and even obsolete. Consider, for example, that the time-consuming isolation and identification of some microorganisms are no longer performed because new immunologic techniques take only a few minutes. In addition, some laboratory services that were only performed in hospitals are now being performed routinely in outpatient service centers or even by the patient at home.

Legal Forces

Marketing decisions must be sensitive to laws that restrain and control certain business activities. Laws are enacted to preserve a competitive marketplace or to protect consumers.

Regulatory Political Forces

Regulatory units at the local, state, and federal levels affect marketing decisions. Trade commissions and special-interest associations exert pressure on businesses to inhibit undesirable behaviors.

Societal Forces

Shifts in population, dual career families, and lifestyle and life-cycle preferences are some of the forces to which marketing must be attuned. Increased spending for services continues in the United States economy. In their book *The Service Society,* Gersuny and Rosengren[4] comment on social change and the growth of services.

> Our society is marked by the emergence of secularized services rendered outside the family. A service revolution has, in fact, followed on the heels of the industrial revolution. This service revolution brings with it not only great new markets for the distribution of intangibles, but a new and highly significant dimension in the division of labor—the active participation of the consumer in the production of many services.

THE MARKETING MIX: THE CONTROLLABLES

What variables are available to the marketing planner? Over which factors does he or she have more direct control? The marketing mix consists of five major components, which, although affected by the general marketing environment at large, can be modified to fit business goals. The marketing-mix variables include: product, distribution, place, promotion, price, and people. It quickly becomes obvious that there are limits to how controllable these variables really are. For example, a laboratory is not free to adjust prices whimsically on a daily basis because of economic conditions or government regulations. In addition, promotional campaigns must adhere to certain guidelines and cannot be changed overnight. Although the hospital can control the hiring and firing of staff, the marketing manager cannot always control workers' behavior or productivity. A major goal is to adjust marketing-mix variables to create and maintain satisfying goods and services.

Product refers to goods, services, and ideas an organization provides. Naturally, one's decision about which laboratory services to market is tempered by what one's competition is doing as well as other broader environmental forces; however, the final decision is ultimately one's own. New products are introduced in the marketplace all the time. It is the marketing department's responsibility to monitor their success and to decide when it is necessary to eliminate them. Market researchers attempt to discover wants and needs so that they can modify goods and services to meet the desired characteristics. For example, a laboratory may alter the format of the requisition form or the written reports to make them more convenient for the physician to use.

Place refers to the site of the physical facilities. It may be the hospital, a satellite laboratory, or perhaps a remote blood-drawing station.

Distribution involves the logistic arrangements required physically to get the goods from the manufacturer to the point at which they are sold. Laboratory equipment and supplies pass through many distribution points before ultimately reaching a hospital laboratory. Selecting wholesalers, developing and maintaining inventory, and managing transportation and storage systems are within the realm of the marketing manager. The logistics of marketing laboratory services, picking up specimens, and delivering reports in an efficient and timely manner may be the most difficult part of the service process.

Promotion is the variable that usually comes to mind when one thinks about marketing. The goals of promotion are to inform, to persuade, and to remind buyers about a business and its services. The word *promote* is derived from the Latin word meaning "to move forward."

Personal selling, advertising, sales promotion, publicity, and packaging design compose the "promotional mix." A major decision for service businesses is determining which vehicle in the promotion mix should be emphasized. Someone within the hospital or an outside agency assumes overall responsibility for coordinating the promotional mix. Too frequently, promotional activities involve different goals and vague personal accountability. A promotion program must be integrated into the organization. For example, assume the laboratory develops a direct-mail campaign. The people working in the laboratory and any sales staff must be aware of the advertising message so that they can reinforce the message when they come in contact with potential clients.

Advertising is a paid form of communication, and the sponsor of the message is clearly identified. Advertising messages are presented to large numbers of people via television, radio, direct mail, billboards, newspapers, and magazines.

Personal selling is a closer interpersonal interaction. It may be accomplished face-to-face or by telephone (telemarketing).

Public relations activities attempt to create awareness and a positive image for the company with its constituent groups. Although a public relations agency may be hired to represent the business to the media, the publicity message itself is free. Newspaper stories about newsworthy events, tours of facilities, and even thank-you letters are included in the realm of "good" public relations.

Sales promotion techniques include incentives to directly influence consumer action. Contests, trading stamps, premiums, and trial-size displays are examples.

People are an important variable in the marketing mix. They must be trained to communicate the image of the hospital, they need to understand the rules and regulations and have a general knowledge of the tests and services the hospital wants to sell.

THE MARKETING PLAN

The successful marketing of clinical laboratory services requires the same careful, thorough planning as the development of any kind of business, especially in light of today's competitive health-care environment. There is a series of logical steps in developing a marketing plan: developing a mission statement, formulating goals and objectives, conducting a study of internal strengths and weaknesses, analyzing the competition, and finally preparing a plan. A football game analogy is helpful in defining these terms. The mission statement describes the general task, to win the game. Goals are steps necessary to accomplish the task, getting the ball over the goal line as frequently as possible. Objectives are even smaller steps, stated in measurable terms, that are designed to help meet the goal. In football, an objective would be keeping possession of the ball by moving it at least ten yards in four tries. In football, as in business, studying the competition is important. The final plan is the amalgamation of all of the information that describes who is going to do each task and when it is going to be done—in other words, the game plan.

The first step is the development of a mission statement. It encompasses the criteria against which one will measure the appropriateness of proposed activities and should be worded so that it gives guidance without being too limiting. The mission statement does not need to be a lengthy, complicated treatise, but should clearly spell out the nature of the business and the reason for that business. One way to start developing this is to examine the mission statement or philosophy of the parent organization. The chances of success will be greater if the statement developed is congruent with the written mission of the institution and if it is also consistent with the mission of the institution as perceived by those associated with it, such as physicians, other health professionals, patients, the community, and the administrative or governing boards. Without the support of any one of these groups, it may be difficult to grow.

The goals and objectives of one's enterprise should also be part of one's mission statement. These describe what one is going to do to accomplish the mission. They may be stated in terms of revenue or may reflect where that revenue will be beneficial. The following is an example of a mission statement and goals.

The mission of this venture is to create the most efficient, profitable and progressive clinical laboratory possible.

Goal 1: Acquire two major instruments per year.

Objective: To increase test volume by 10% to justify the acquisition of new equipment.

Goal 2: Increase market share to 40%.

Objective: To achieve competitive prices by selecting instruments that increase productivity and take advantage of the economics of batch testing.

The mission is general, but the goals and objectives are more specific and can be measured.

The next step in the marketing process is the research component. The major questions that need to be answered can be divided into several general areas: the internal strengths and weaknesses, the market's wants and needs, the competition's ability to satisfy the market, and other factors in the market environment that may affect business activity. These areas will be addressed in a stepwise manner, but the information for all areas can be collected simultaneously.

Internal Strengths and Weaknesses

Conducting an objective study of one's own institution can be both satisfying and painful. Traditionally, laboratories have evaluated themselves on the speed and accuracy of their work within a well-defined internal system of receiving a specimen, producing the requested result, communicating that result to the appropriate person, and doing whatever is necessary to be financially compensated for the service. The same steps are necessary in the commercial environment, but there are more potential complications, because the laboratory does not have the same degree of control over the external part of the process. The evaluation of the internal operation of the laboratory should answer questions about services that one has to offer. The following questions address broad major areas. Each institution will have a unique set of questions.

What does it cost to perform the tests that are currently being done in the laboratory?
Other chapters of this text deal with laboratory finance and how to determine these costs. Remember that one will have some costs in addition to the cost of performing the test. These costs cannot be calculated until the extent of services to be provided is actually determined. For example, printing special forms or providing courier service would be additional expenses. This information is crucial in pricing services.

Are the testing methods currently being used cost-effective and efficient?
The instrumentation in some laboratories was selected to serve a hospital population whose needs may be different than the needs of the external market. The hospitalized patient may need rapid results, whereas the outpatient may be more concerned about low-priced testing. For example, the instrument that provides rapid turnaround time for an individual test may not be able to provide the efficiency of an instrument designed for high-volume batch testing. Obviously, if one is using inefficient testing methods, it will be difficult to compete in the marketplace on the basis of price.

Does the laboratory have excess capacity in terms of personnel and instrumentation? Is there adequate backup capability? Can you get additional people, equipment, or space when needed?
These are critical questions for any laboratory considering marketing its services. A service cannot be produced and stored in a warehouse like goods, but is produced when the customer needs it. This presents a major difficulty in planning.[1] Excess capacity and backup capability enable one to provide consistent service. If one has gone to considerable effort to market one's services and then cannot consistently provide those services, the customer may look for another provider. Not only is it difficult to get customers back once they have become dissatisfied, but they may tell potential customers about the problem.

What is the attitude of the laboratory staff toward marketing laboratory services?
Laboratories may have to change staffing patterns to satisfy customers' needs—for example, increasing the evening shift to process a larger volume of work arriving late in the afternoon. Demands made on the staff will increase, and a laboratory is truly fortunate if the staff sees this venture as an opportunity to expand services, increase job security, or benefit in other ways. An internal program to communicate the plans for the venture and the importance of the staff's involvement may increase the morale and job satisfaction in those who will be affected by this effort.[1]

What is the reputation of your laboratory within the target area?
Are there areas of the laboratory that are recognized by the users in the community for their excellence? Conversely, are there areas that need to be improved? These questions help to determine one's market position or what attributes the marketplace ascribe to one's organization.[6] The answers to these questions will be more objective if they are compiled from information from a variety of sources. It is important to separate perception from actuality. If the perception is inaccurate, it may be necessary to develop a strategy to change that belief.

Does the marketing effort of the laboratory have the full support of the administration of the hospital?

Ideally, the marketing process is a part of the overall strategic planning and budgeting process of the organization. Even though written plans and budgets for the implementation of the new venture may be in place, it is important to be sure that the people who have control of the finances understand the potential changes that may occur if one's efforts are successful. They may have to make special arrangements to increase orders for supplies and reagents. Additional people may need to be hired, or equipment may need to be replaced sooner than planned. The revenues from the marketing effort should justify increases, but institutions generally budget once a year, and it could be difficult to make one's requests heard in the middle of a budget cycle. The ability to respond quickly to customer needs will be important in maintaining customer satisfaction.

Is the internal system for handling the clerical work adequate to handle an increased work load?

The paper flow is extremely important because it is the interface with the customer. Delays and confusion in this area can be a major cause of customer dissatisfaction. It is crucial to ensure that clerical work affecting the work load of other departments be well planned. Patient billing frequently falls into this category.

The Market

Sensing the market needs is done by using a multifaceted study designed to answer a variety of questions about potential customers themselves, their current needs, and possible future needs. Unclear or incomplete information about the needs and wants of prospective customers is the reason many plans fail during implementation.[8]

Who is the customer?

This question may seem to have an obvious answer, but in reality there are many choices: the patient, the physician, another laboratory, industry, or third-party payers such as insurance companies and government agencies. It is equally important to identify the decision-makers, the decision-influencers, and the criteria used to make the decision. For example, a physician may select a laboratory on the basis of the convenience to his staff. The staff would be decision-influencers, and it would be important for one to talk with them to determine their needs.

What range of service is required for the laboratory to compete?

The services required will, of course, vary with the size and nature of the customer. Some services may not be feasible now but could be areas for future development. Consider a large nursing home that now has phlebotomy service, courier service, "stat" service, and printer on site. These services are costly and would require a large testing volume to justify them. Most businesses cannot be all things to all customers; rather, they try to find their niche. O'Donnell defines *niche* as the set of needs that the hospital chooses to fill.[6] Finding an unsatisfied need or detecting a new trend can help one find a unique place in the market.

What is the market potential?

Several other questions need to be answered before determining the probability of a profitable venture. First, what is the volume of testing in the target market? Second, what percentage or share of the market would have to be captured for a profit to be made? Is it realistic to expect to get that share of the market? In general, laboratory services provided by one organization increase at the expense of another similar organization because the market is shrinking.

The Competition

Who is the competition?

The list of those trying to capture the dollars spent on laboratory testing includes not only commercial laboratories and hospitals but also physicians. Even patients are trying to avoid the cost of laboratory services by doing some tests at home. The competition is also a potential market if they have testing needs that are currently unmet.

What are they charging for their services?

In general, businesses charge whatever the market will pay. Most laboratories have a published list price and discount from that for larger accounts according to their volume. The price of any given test, therefore, may vary considerably. A more key question is how much they can lower the price and remain profitable. Cutting prices is a strategy used in some industries to discourage new competitors. That is one reason for considering factors in addition to price in the marketing mix when planning the strategy for a new venture.

Does the competition have any problems providing service to the target area?

Laboratories may produce very accurate test results and may still not be able to serve customers adequately. For example, if the location is remote, they may not be able to provide "stat" service, or the area may not fit into the courier schedule at a time that is desirable for the customer. The market survey should help to uncover information that will help the company or laboratory be more competitive in variables other than price.

Other Important Factors

How will current Medicare and other regulations affect the marketing effort?

In his article "Independent Laboratory or Hospital Laboratory: What Difference Does it Make?" Barry[2] discusses the Medicare treatment of both kinds of laboratories. He states . . . "there is wide disparity in the way carriers and intermediaries apply Medicare rules. Before deciding on a particular course of action it is advisable to consult with knowledgeable carrier and intermediary personnel." State laws, tax laws, and anti-trust statutes should be reviewed before implementing any marketing activity. The more creative your efforts, the more carefully anti-trust statutes should be examined. According to Polk,[7] such practices as joining with competitors to divide markets or to allocate customers, controlling market prices, boycotting third parties, "tying" the sale of one product to the separate purchase of another, and forming group purchasing agreements that unreasonably restrain trade have generated controversy.

The information gathered in the above process is used to answer the primary question: Can the institution profitably satisfy the needs of the target market? The marketing process is summarized in Figure 25-1. This overview emphasizes that marketing is a process that is constantly being reviewed and evaluated to detect changes in the marketplace. Change implies not only challenge but opportunity. It is through the marketing process that laboratories prepare to meet the challenges and take advantage of the opportunities.

FIGURE 25-1. Marketing process overview. (Copyright Gutterman Associates, 1987)

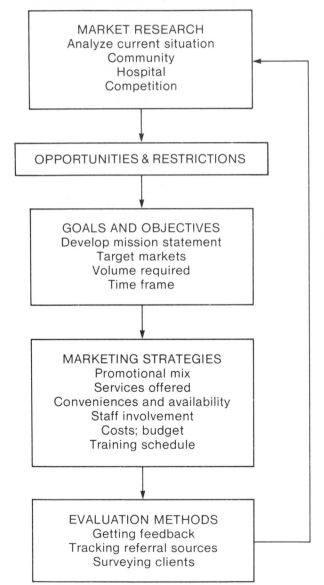

MARKET RESEARCH
Analyze current situation
Community
Hospital
Competition

OPPORTUNITIES & RESTRICTIONS

GOALS AND OBJECTIVES
Develop mission statement
Target markets
Volume required
Time frame

MARKETING STRATEGIES
Promotional mix
Services offered
Conveniences and availability
Staff involvement
Costs; budget
Training schedule

EVALUATION METHODS
Getting feedback
Tracking referral sources
Surveying clients

REFERENCES

1. Albers J, Vice JL: Strategic planning. American Journal of Medical Technology 49(6):411–414, June 1983
2. Barry DM: Independent laboratory or hospital laboratory: What difference does it make? Pathologist, pp 31–36, February 1985
3. Berry LL: Services marketing is different. Business Magazine, May–June 1980
4. Gersuny C, Rosengren WR: The Service Society. Cambridge, Schenkman Publishing Company, 1974
5. Kotler P, Conner P: Marketing professional services. Journal of Marketing, January 1977
6. O'Donnell M: Finding you niche in the marketplace. Optimal Health, pp 20–24, September/October, 1985
7. Polk LT: Avoid conflict: Know the legal complications. Pathologist, pp 546–548, August 1983

8. Portugal B: Strategic planning for outreach laboratory services. Pathologist, pp 537–540, August 1983

BIBLIOGRAPHY

Hillestad SG, Berkowitz EN: Health Care Marketing Plans: From Strategy to Action. Homewood, Dow Jones–Irwin, 1984

This book identifies and applies marketing techniques for improving the effectiveness and profitability of health-care organizations. The focus is on integrating planning with marketing, and a step-by-step approach to setting and achieving objectives is presented.

part five

Principles of Laboratory Finance

twenty-six

Basic Elements of Laboratory Financial Management

David J. Fine

Rohn J. Butterfield

Justin E. Doheny

FINANCING HEALTH CARE

Medicare, Medicaid, prospective payment, DRGs, PPOs, HMOs, managed care systems, payback, fiscal intermediary, return on investment, not for profit — the financial side of the health-care industry possesses a vocabulary that is, for the most part, unknown to the medical technologist, and the financing of hospitals and laboratories is as strange to the laboratorian as a type and crossmatch is to the hospital financial officer. However, in order to succeed as a laboratory manager, one must be able to speak both languages, to understand both sides of the many complex issues, and to be as concerned about positive cash flow and controlling the laboratory's costs as one is about quality-assurance and procedure controls.

The objective of this chapter is to provide the reader with a general understanding of hospital finance, an appreciation of how the laboratory fits into the overall picture, and an introduction to the tools of the financial manager. It is not expected that readers will be able to master each of these subjects, but it is hoped that they will become knowledgeable enough to use certain of the techniques and gain sufficient insight into the world of

financial management to serve as an interface between the laboratory and the financial stewards of the hospital.

Industry Overview

The health-care industry is among the largest in the country, and it is second only to defense in its share of the gross national product (GNP). In 1984, health-care expenditures accounted for 10.6% of the GNP, although this level of resource utilization was actually a reduction from 1983's historical zenith of 10.7%.[3]

Historically, hospitals have been a growing segment of the health-care sector and have also been a major driving force in the expansion of overall health-care costs. In 1965, 33.3% of national health expenditures were for hospital services; by 1984 this had grown to 40.8%, although, as with GNP, this figure represents a downturn from the peak of 41.9% attained in 1983. Expressed on a per capita basis, $1580 was spent on health care in 1984, of which $645 was for hospital services.[3]

These figures demonstrate that hospitals are big business. There are, however, several unusual characteristics of hospitals that affect their performance and behavior. First, while many people consume health-care services, few pay the bills directly. Most people in the United States are beneficiaries of health or hospital insurance of some sort, and it is the insurers, including the federal government, who pay most of the health bill. Second, in many cases within the industry, especially in the laboratory, the patient does not choose whether or not to purchase a service. Nor do patients typically choose from which service or vendor to buy. These choices are all made for patients by their physicians. Third, most hospitals in this country are *not-for-profit,* meaning that no profits or earnings are distributed to owners of the hospital. Thus, hospitals have not historically been as profit-conscious as typical corporations, and their success or failure has been judged not so much on profitability as on a number of other considerations.

In the past, these factors significantly modified the traditional free-market competition concept governing most United States industries. While profitability may not have been a prime concern for hospitals in the past, the unique characteristics of the hospital industry cited above have been modified or eliminated by massive changes in the financial incentives created for hospitals, physicians, and their patients by the public and private health insurance industry. These changes are described in some detail below and represent the most dramatic alteration of the nation's health delivery system since the Medicare and Medicaid legislation of 1966. With some assurance, one may point to these changes as the major causal factors for the retardation of the rate of health-care expenditure growth noted for 1984 as opposed to the inexorable rise in costs experienced before 1984.

Medicare and Medicaid

Prior to 1983, the single event having the greatest impact on the health-care marketplace was the enactment and implementation of Medicare and Medicaid in July 1966.

This legislation, also known as Title XVIII and Title XIX of the Social Security Act, was perhaps the most significant piece of social legislation since the original Social Security Act of the 1930s, because it established a mechanism for financing the health care of the elderly and poor.[2]

Medicare eligibility is limited to those 65 and over or to those who meet other criteria related to disability or chronic renal disease. Medicaid eligibility is based upon a number of criteria established by the individual states within a framework established by the federal government. It is the intent of the Medicaid program to pay the health-care costs of the poor or medically indigent.

The Medicare program is split into two parts: Part A provides payment for inpatient services in a hospital or skilled nursing facility, or to a home health agency after discharge from a hospital or skilled nursing facility. Medicare Part A will pay for laboratory tests along with a long list of other covered services. Medicare Part B helps to pay the bills from physicians, hospital outpatient visits, and certain other medical services and supplies not included in Part A coverage.

Figure 26-1 indicates the dramatic increase in federal financing of health care, owing largely to the advent of Medicare and Medicaid. One can also see a concomitant drop in direct payments and payments from philanthropic sources. There has also been a significant increase in private health insurance payments.

Before 1983, all Part A payments to hospitals by Medicare were based on the hospital's actual and imputed costs. Under such a reimbursement system, there were strong economic incentives for hospitals to sacrifice cost-containment efforts in order to provide the highest quality patient care and technology possible. This incentive, along with absolute growth in the amount of services provided to the newly enfranchised elderly population, were the primary factors driving the tremendous growth in federal expenditures for health care. Also during this era, Part B payments to physicians were made on the basis of reasonable charges. Among other services, Part B paid professional fees charged by a pathologist for laboratory and pathology procedures.

In October 1983, based on a growing national concern over health-care costs in general and hospital expenditures in particular, Medicare began implementation of a completely new method of payment to hospitals called the prospective payment system (PPS) for covered inpatient Part A services. Essentially, the thrust of the PPS was to ensure that hospitals assumed financial risk for their cost in exchange for Medicare payments.[6]

Medicare established 468 diagnosis-related groups (DRGs); that is, patient diagnoses were grouped according to the diseases affecting specific organ systems of the body. The basis of payment was the discharge, which was classified into one of the DRGs. Payments per discharge in a specific DRG were set prospectively based on average historical Medicare costs for discharges in that DRG.

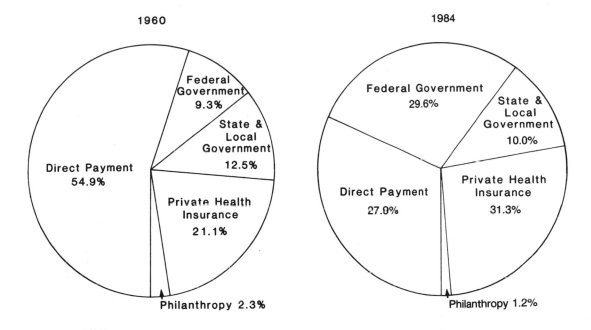

1960

1984

Federal Government 9.3%

State & Local Government 12.5%

Direct Payment 54.9%

Private Health Insurance 21.1%

Philanthropy 2.3%

Federal Government 29.6%

State & Local Government 10.0%

Direct Payment 27.0%

Private Health Insurance 31.3%

Philanthropy 1.2%

TOTAL: $23,700,000,000   TOTAL: $341,800,000,000

FIGURE 26-1. A comparison between personal health-care expenditures in the United States in 1960 and 1984 (excludes prepayment and administration expenses and government public health activities). (From Health United States 1985. Hyattsville, Department of Health and Human Services, 1985)

The changeover from the cost-based system to the DRG-based PPS was to be completely phased in by 1988.[6]

The effects of the change from a retrospective cost-based *reimbursement* system to a prospective price-based *payment* system (PPS) were immediate. The federal government had, for the first time since Medicare was enacted, introduced competitive principles into the quasi-monopolistic health-care marketplace. For example, prior to the PPS, if a hospital's cost for a particular Medicare discharge was $5000, this cost would have been reimbursed in full by Medicare. Under the PPS, by contrast, Medicare may have set the DRG price for that discharge at $4000, regardless of the hospital's actual cost. In this example, the hospital would lose $1000 for every discharge in that DRG unless the cost of delivering care to patients in that DRG could be reduced. Conversely, of course, if the hospital's cost were $3000, the hospital would realize a $1000 surplus. In short, the risk for health-care costs under the PPS shifted from Medicare to the hospital and established Medicare as a "prudent buyer" of health-care

services, as opposed to the government's formerly passive funding role.[5]

Under the PPS, then, hospitals are attempting to define and control the costs of delivering services to an extent unknown just a few years ago. As a result, the laboratory, for Medicare purposes at least, becomes a true cost center and just one of the variables whose cost must be controlled for realization of a net surplus from the patient's stay in the hospital.

Part B changes affecting pathologist professional fees were also enacted in the early 1980s, before PPS. On the basis of Medicare's contention that certain payments to hospital-based physicians (including pathologists) under Part B should more properly be paid to hospitals under Part A (for activities such as supervision of laboratory personnel, hospital administrative duties, and so forth) and that Part B payments should be related only to those physician services requiring clinical judgment for which the physician had been uniquely trained, reasonable charges paid under Part B were limited only to those clinical activities deemed appropriate by

Medicare (*e.g.,* written laboratory and pathology consultations), and the balance of Part B payments were to be factored into Part A DRG discharge payments upon full implementation of the PPS.

Although this change had little net effect on most hospital-based physicians, pathologists were greatly affected, because professional fee charges rendered to Medicare for most clinical laboratory tests would no longer be paid under Part B but would be paid to the hospitals under Part A. Because the amount of Part B dollars to be incorporated into Part A DRG payments by 1988 has as yet to be specified, additional cost pressures on the hospital laboratory are a distinct possibility.

It is difficult to make generalizations about payments under the Medicaid program because the specific eligibility requirements and services covered are defined by the various states. In most cases, charges by pathologists and hospitals related to laboratory tests are included.

It should be noted, however, that many states have taken Medicare's lead and have adopted pro-competitive models of Medicaid payment, including contracts for discounted charges, DRG-based payments, contracts with health maintenance organizations (HMOs), and so forth.

Private Health Insurance

Although local, state, and federal governments account for nearly 40% of all health-care expenditures, private insurance policies and plans account for the balance of insured health care and comprise over 30% of all health-care costs. Included among the list of nongovernmental health insurers are Blue Cross and Blue Shield. These insurance plans have grown significantly since the establishment of the First Blue Cross plan in 1929. Today there are some 80 separate Blue Cross corporations providing hospitalization insurance benefits to their subscribers. Blue Cross was established to pay hospital bills, and Blue Shield was established to pay physician fees. Commonly thought of together, they are generally separate corporations, although in certain areas they are one legal entity. Until recently, Blue Cross usually paid hospitals on a negotiated cost basis, whereas Blue Shield paid physicians on some basis related to charges.

Although slow to respond to the competitive forces initiated by Medicare, both Blue Cross and Blue Shield have established a number of alternative payment and delivery systems in the past few years. These include negotiated discounted price contracts with hospitals and physicians alike; the creation of preferred provider organizations (PPOs), which contract on a discounted basis with low-cost providers and include certain utilization restrictions; and HMOs, which are really health-care membership organizations that pay a set price from member "dues" to providers on a per member (capitation) basis, utilizing primary-care physicians to monitor and control the patient's use of downstream and generally more expensive providers of care such as hospitals and physician specialists. In addition to these newer systems, of course, most of us have witnessed the rise in deductions and co-insurance percentages in traditional indemnity policies and increased coverage for outpatient medical and surgical care, both of which are intended to guide and control consumer choice regarding cost and utilization patterns.

In contrast to Blue Cross and Blue Shield, which are not-for-profit organizations, the private, for-profit insurers have diversified rapidly. In addition to the alternative delivery systems and other changes noted above, these firms have merged or joint-ventured with for-profit hospital chains and voluntary hospital groups in an attempt to create total health-care systems on a national or regional basis to include all forms of insurance plans, wide-ranging availability of services, and centralized management of resources. Although the jury is still out on the success of these more global health delivery systems, the lesson is quite clear: consolidation of health-care providers and insurers will continue as competitors scramble to maintain and improve upon their traditional share of the market through enhancement of economic clout.

The Future

What is the effect of the changes in health-care financing for hospitals and their laboratories? With the passing of the "quality at any cost" philosophy that dominated previous decades, the challenge for hospitals in the 1980s and beyond is to provide lower prices and easy access to services while reducing per capita cost and maintaining high standards of quality. Central to this strategy is the redefinition of the hospital's business and, where possible, diversification away from high-cost inpatient care.

As more of the decisions regarding the cost and volume of health services to be delivered move from the physician and hospital to the purchasers of care, and the growth of managed care systems accelerates, hospitals have focused increasing energy on accounting for and managing inpatient costs, as well as diversifying into a heavier commitment to outpatient care as a lower-cost method for ensuring market share. In either case, the economic mission of the hospital laboratory has shifted from revenue generation *per se* to both the revenue and cost sides of the equation. Mirroring the larger health-care industry, hospital laboratories have increasingly replaced labor with technology; creatively dealt with productivity issues; merged, consolidated, regionalized, and joint-ventured to achieve economies of scale and market share improvements; and generally become more complete participants in the marketplace.

These trends, of course, make the laboratory's responsibilities considerably more challenging than in the past. The financial techniques, strategies, and approaches discussed in this chapter and the next are now more important than ever, since the laboratory, along with all other hospital departments, is required to be considerably more discerning in its consumption of ever scarcer resources. Price competition is a reality, and the laboratory must of necessity become more productive by producing more with the same or fewer material and human resources. Familiarity with the types and interrelationships of production costs will be essential to the achievement of higher productivity through cost containment.

COST, VOLUME, AND REVENUE RELATIONSHIPS

Fixed and Variable Costs

Operating expenditures in a laboratory may be divided into the broad categories of fixed and variable costs. This classification reflects the sensitivity of costs to increases or decreases in clinical volume. If a cost changes in more or less direct proportion to volume, it is *variable*. If a cost remains unchanged in total for a set time period, despite fluctuations in volume, it is *fixed*. Examples of fixed costs include supervisory and custodial wages and benefits required regardless of volume, as well as depreciation of plant and equipment. Variable costs include technologist wages and benefits, reagents, glassware, disposable supplies, and forms. Figures 26-2 and 26-3 graphically display the behavior of variable and fixed costs.

It must be noted that these costs are often difficult to classify definitively. Clerical staff can be reduced given a decrease in clinical activity, but a certain number of such persons are required regardless of volume. These are referred to as *mixed costs* and compose a third, more subtle, classification of cost. In addition, fixed costs hold constant only over a *relevant range* of activity. If volume increases or decreases dramatically, all fixed costs become vari-

FIGURE 26-2.   Behavior of variable costs. In this figure, a simplifying assumption is made that total variable cost varies directly with the number of tests. For example, as volume increases from X_1 to X_2, total variable cost also increases by the same percentage amount. Thus, $\dfrac{X_2}{X_1} = \dfrac{Y_2}{Y_1}$

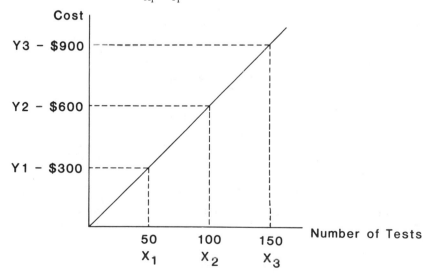

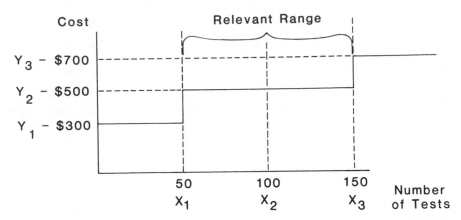

FIGURE 26-3. Behavior of fixed costs. Total fixed cost remains constant at \$500 (Y_2) over all three levels of volume (50, 100, 150 tests) within the relevant range (see Table 26-1). However, should volume drop below X_1 or increase above X_3, associated total fixed cost may decline to Y_1 or rise to Y_3 respectively. The step phenomenon reflects the fact that certain costs remain fixed over large ranges of volume but ultimately become variable to some extent.

able to some extent. For instance, even supervisors may be laid off in the event a hospital is compelled to close a substantial number of its beds because of a downturn in business fortunes, a fire, and/or other extraordinary events.

For the purposes of this discussion, all costs are assumed to be either fixed or variable, and variable costs are assumed to vary in a direct linear relationship with volume. Given these assumptions, Figure 26-4 displays how fixed and variable components compose total cost. Many factors may affect their behavior; and if the cost of labor, supplies, and other variable operating expenses rise, then total costs will rise, regardless of volume changes. If the diagnostic composition of the patient population changes, costs may rise or fall accordingly. Seasonality may affect volume levels, since there are certain periods when the census is higher or lower than the average.

Direct and Indirect Costs

Direct and indirect costs are still another discrete categorization of total costs. All costs that can be specifically linked to a test are *direct costs*. Those costs not directly traceable to the test but included in total laboratory expense are termed *indirect costs,* or *overhead.* Examples of direct costs include technicians, supervisory and clerical personnel, overtime, on-call payments, and chemicals and sup-

plies related to the test. Examples of indirect costs include depreciation, building and equipment maintenance, insurance, utilities, housekeeping, purchasing, and billing services.

Unit Costs

For many of the laboratory manager's financial decisions, *unit costs* are crucial. Their analysis helps to identify fluctuations in the cost to produce a given unit of service, thereby permitting measurement of productivity. The first step in calculation is to identify the unit of measurement, usually an individual laboratory test. Many laboratories also use relative value units, discussed in the next two chapters, as the unit of measure.

Next, unit costs are classified into fixed and variable components. Variable costs per unit generally remain the same regardless of volume. Fixed costs per unit, on the other hand, are reduced as the total fixed cost is spread over more tests (Fig. 26-5). Graphically, these illustrations are quite different from those describing fixed, variable, and total costs. This is because there is a conceptual difference between total costs and total cost per unit. Table 26-1 demonstrates how costs behave as total costs and total costs per unit.[1] Note that as volume increases, variable cost increases by the same percentage; yet on a per-unit basis, variable cost remains unchanged. Likewise, fixed costs remain the

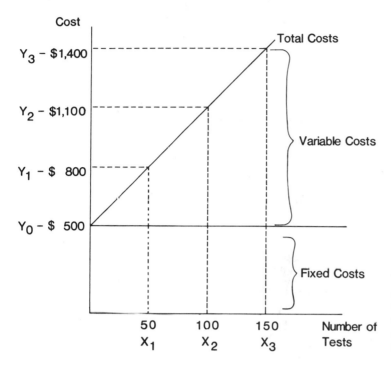

FIGURE 26-4. Total cost curve. In constructing a total cost curve, total fixed cost is assumed to remain at Y_0 ($500) over all levels of volume, forming the base to which the total variable cost curve is added. For example, if volume increases from X_1 to X_2, total cost will increase from Y_1 to Y_2, and $\dfrac{X_2}{X_1} = \dfrac{Y_2 - Y_0}{Y_1 - Y_0}$ Notice that the same variable cost and volume relationship exists in the total cost curve as in Fig. 26-2, except that the constant, Y_0, is subtracted from each cost level. This can be verified by referring to the data in Table 26-1.

same regardless of volume increases; whereas on a per-unit basis they decline. As can be inferred from Table 26-1, the higher the volume of tests, the lower the total unit cost. This, of course, illustrates the economies of scale available in the active laboratory.

Interaction and Control of Types of Costs

As demonstrated, total variable and fixed costs may be recast to form unit costs. In addition, direct and indirect costs interact with fixed and variable costs. For instance, supervisory personnel are considered as both a fixed and direct cost of operation. Thus, there are fixed and variable direct costs and fixed and variable indirect costs. Generally, however, direct costs are coincident with variable costs, and indirect costs are consonant with fixed costs. The reader is cautioned not to apply this rule-of-thumb blithely.

Costs are subject to varying degrees of management control. In general, variable and direct costs are controllable by the manager, and fixed and indirect costs are uncontrollable. However, as noted earlier, in unusual circumstances fixed costs may become variable. The laboratory manager must be continually sensitive to opportunities to control any and all costs, regardless of formal classification.

Accumulation of Direct and Indirect Costs

There are two basic methods for accumulating direct and indirect costs in the laboratory.[4] The first method, *direct costing,* assigns all direct costs to the laboratory. Generally, a *chart of accounts* is used to delineate the appropriate categories within which costs are to be assigned. These natural classifications may be detailed or very broad. For instance,

Table 26-1
Behavior of Total Costs and Unit Costs

	Number of Tests		
	50	*100*	*150*
Total Cost			
Variable cost	$300	$ 600	$ 900
Fixed cost	500	500	500
Total cost	$800	$1,100	$1,400
Unit Cost			
Variable cost per unit	$ 6	$ 6	$ 6
	10	5	3.33
Total cost per unit	$ 16	$ 11	$ 9.33

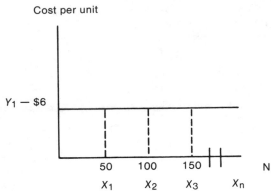

A

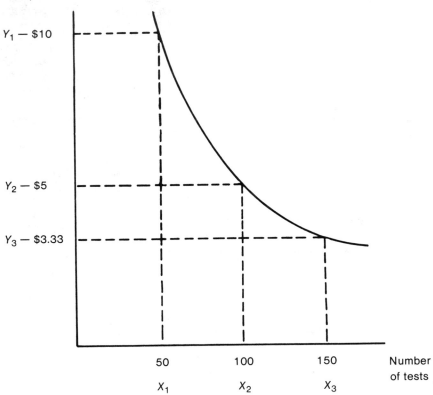

B

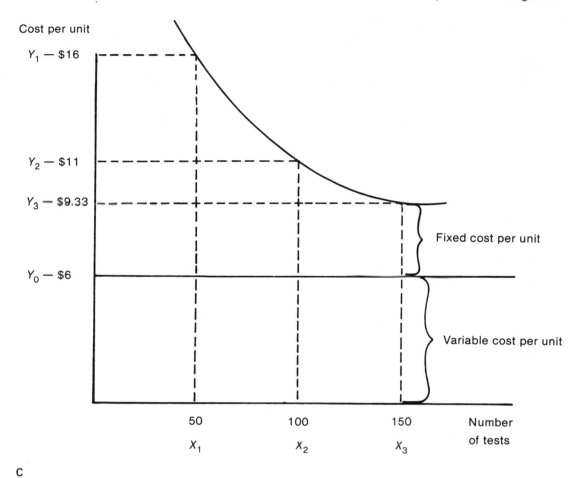

C

FIGURE 26-5. Graphic representation of unit costs. (*A*) Variable cost per unit, Y_1, holds for all levels of activity (Table 26-1). Thus, for X_1, X_2, X_3, ... , X_n, Y_1 is the variable cost per unit. As volume increases from X_1 to X_3 (*B*), fixed cost per unit decreases from Y_1 to Y_3 (Table 26-1). This is the component of total unit cost that yields economies of scale at higher levels of production. Since variable unit cost remains constant at Y_0 (*C*) over all levels of activity, this cost forms the base upon which fixed costs are added. The result of this addition is the total cost per unit curve. Note that as volume increases, total cost per unit declines (Table 26-1).

the major direct expense categories are labor and supplies. However, many subdivisions of these broad categories are possible and, indeed, desirable for analytic purposes. These categories are discussed in greater detail in the next chapter.

The second method, *full costing*, attempts to allocate indirect costs to the hospital laboratory to achieve accumulation of total operating costs. In industry, indirect expenses are transferred to the affected department or are allocated on some rea-

sonable basis when the service performed cannot be directly linked to a specific department. Once full costing is completed, *standard costs* are developed that reflect what an efficient department should cost in total, and this costing system is compared with actual costs through *variance analysis*. As such, the cost-accumulation system also serves as a measure of cost effectiveness. In hospitals the industry norm has been traditionally eschewed for various cost-finding methods. The literature, however, has emphasized the benefits of standard costing and variance analysis for controlling costs.[4] The reader is encouraged to become familiar with this approach, even though it may not be feasible currently. Although complicated to implement, this system will become more popular as cost-containment pressures increase.

Indeed, several cost-accounting systems utilized in private industry have been adapted for hospitals and are currently being incorporated into hospital automated accounting systems. Once implemented, such improvements should help to mitigate a major weakness of current hospital ledger systems: the inability to identify specific unit costs and the concomitant inability to price units of service on a precise costing basis.

Assuming the hospital has not yet attained improved identification of costs through more sophisticated accounting systems, there are generally four methods of cost-finding: *direct apportionment, the step-down method, double step-down,* and *algebraic apportionment.* Application of these methods is a task for the hospital finance officer. Should the reader wish to explore cost-finding in more detail, he should refer to Berman and Weeks.[2]

Although the laboratory manager may not be involved in the apportionment of indirect costs to cost centers, to the extent that the manager is responsible for setting prices for services provided in the laboratory, a working knowledge of cost-accounting techniques is quite helpful, because fixed and variable costs of direct and indirect expenses are often identified in the more sophisticated systems.

The Break-Even Point

The *break-even point* is that point of laboratory test volume where total revenues equal total costs and where there is neither a profit nor a loss. This point serves as the baseline for evaluation of changes in revenue, costs, and/or volume.

In an accounting sense, *net income* equals total revenue less bad debts and allowances minus all variable and fixed costs. Because of the peculiarities of the hospital field, gross charges rarely yield a 100% return in revenue. Reimbursement based on cost, reductions in payments based on discounted charges, and charity care result in deductions from gross charges and are often termed *allowances.* The resulting revenue actually received, then, is gross charges less allowances and bad debts. Any rate-set-

ting based on required revenue must take these circumstances into account in order to ensure that prices are realistic. The subject of price-setting is discussed in some detail in the next chapter. The following equation formally defines net income:

Net income =
Revenue (gross charges less allowances and bad debts) − Variable costs − Fixed costs

Revenue, then, may be stated as follows:

Revenue =
Variable costs + Fixed costs + Net income

If net income is set at zero (*i.e.,* no profit or loss), equality between revenue and costs is attained, and the break-even point can be calculated:

Let x = The break-even point in number of tests

r = Revenue per unit

v = Variable cost per unit

f = Total fixed cost

c = Net income contribution

Then the general formula for the break-even point is

$$rx = vx + f + c$$
$$rx - vx = f + c$$
$$x(r - v) = f + c$$
$$x = \frac{f + c}{r - v}$$

With the example presented in Table 26-1, v = \$6 and f = \$500. If we set the unit revenue(r) at \$10 and c at zero, then

$$x = \frac{500 + 0}{10 - 6} = \frac{500}{4} = 125 \text{ tests}$$

Thus, 125 tests must be performed in order to break even. Graphically, the break-even point just calculated is illustrated in Figure 26-6. Note that the break-even point is the intersection of the total cost line and the total revenue line where total cost equals total revenue. The shaded area below the break-even point is the area of net loss; the area above the break-even point is the area of net income.

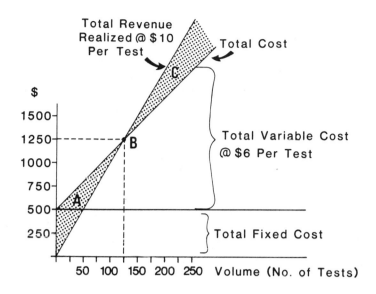

FIGURE 26-6. The break-even point. Break-even occurs at point B where 125 tests are performed. In zone A the test is losing money, and in zone C it is showing a profit.

As stated earlier, one must be cautioned that total revenue is not a 100% reflection of total charges. For instance, if a hospital receives as revenue 80% of total charges, then the hospital must charge 25% more per test, or a total of $12.50, in order to ensure recovery of the $1250 required to cover the total fixed and variable costs of producing 125 tests.

Sensitivity Analysis

Assume for the moment that a hypothetical laboratory is currently operating at the break-even point determined in Figure 26-6. What about next year? What happens if volume, cost, and/or revenue increases or decreases? The method most often used for exploration of future outcome questions is *sensitivity analysis.* This is a "what if" technique that uses data provided from the break-even point analysis and informs the manager about the effects of changes in costs, revenues, volumes, and/or net income. Several specific examples should help to illustrate the usefulness of this technique for the laboratory manager.

I. Assume that a 20% increase in volume is predicted.

Since variable costs are assumed to vary directly with volume, variable costs will also increase by 20%. Fixed costs may realistically increase by a small percentage but in this

example can be assumed to remain constant. Since total revenue also varies directly with volume, total revenue will increase by 20%.

Component	Current	+20% Volume
Volume	125	150
Total revenue @ $10/test	$1250	$1500
Variable cost @ $6/test	$750	$900
Fixed cost	$500	$500
Net income	$-0-	$100

Thus, the volume increase contributes $100 to the hospital's operating surplus. If management does not require these funds, assuming no bad debts or allowances, the test price may be reduced from $10 to $9.33. In a price-competitive market, this reduction could result in a significant marketing advantage and help to ensure the predicted volume increase. As a practical matter, some midpoint price would probably be selected, illustratively $9.75.

II. Assume a price increase that produces a 20% increase in revenue, again assuming no bad debts or allowances. In this case, volume and all costs are assumed to remain at the current level.

Component	Current	+20% Revenue
Volume	125	125
Total revenue	$1250 (@ $10/test)	$1500 (@ $12/test)
Total Cost	$1250	$1250
Net income	$-0-	$250

The net income contribution can either be added to hospital surplus or it can be a reserve against misestimated volume levels or an unexpected increase in costs.

III. Assume that it is possible to produce the same number of tests with 20% less variable labor, unit revenue remaining the same.

Component	Current	+20% Labor
Volume	125	125
Total revenue @ $10/test	$1250	$1250
Variable cost	$750 (@ $6/test)	$600 (@ $4.80 test)
Fixed cost	$500	$500
Net income	$-0-	$150

Hence, by virtue of productivity improvement, the laboratory realizes net income in the amount of $150.

IV. Finally, assume that management requires a $400 net income, that total costs can be increased a maximum of 18%, and that volume will increase 8%. What price must be charged per test if the laboratory recovers 80% of charges in actual revenue?

Component	Current	Future
Volume	125	135 (+8%)
Total revenue	$1250	?
Total cost	$1250	$1475 (+18%)
Net income	$-0-	$400

Total revenue required = Total cost + Net income
$$= \$1475 + \$400$$
$$= \$1875$$

$$\text{Unit revenue required} = \frac{\text{Total revenue}}{\text{Volume}}$$
$$= \frac{\$1875}{135}$$
$$= \$13.89$$

Price per test that must be charged at 80% recovery =
$$\frac{\$13.89}{0.8} = \underline{\$17.36}$$

As can be seen, almost any future situation may be analyzed with the use of current data. Generally, all laboratories are required to produce a net contribution to help cover losses experienced in other revenue-producing departments and to provide for future economic growth of the institution.

Although sensitivity analysis is appealing because of its simplicity, caution must be exercised for the same reason. Remember that before the analysis, all costs were categorized as either variable or fixed (*i.e.,* no mixed costs), variable costs were defined as *directly* proportioned to volume, and a relevant range was assumed to exist for all levels of activity. These simplifications make the analysis possible, but they should also temper the manager's interpretation of analytical results. A realistic attitude toward the analysis of costs, especially as they pertain to the unknowns of the future, will serve the prudent manager well.

Generally, the easiest variable to affect positively is the containment of costs. Many laboratories now experience strong price competition, and hospital utilization review can produce a downward trend in the number of tests ordered. Of course, sensitivity analysis is also useful for evaluating negative trends in operations, including increased costs and volume reductions.

THE CLINICAL LABORATORY IN HOSPITAL CONTEXT

Role of the Laboratory Manager

The role and responsibility of the laboratory manager will vary depending upon the placement of the laboratory and the laboratory manager within the hospital organization structure. Normally the clinical laboratories will, as a whole, be considered one department of the hospital. The person responsible for the management of the laboratory will then report to a member of the hospital administrative staff. Although usually a pathologist, the manager can be an administrative technologist or trained business administrator.

The laboratory manager often will be caught between the competing goals of quality and cost: he will be held responsible by the hospital to operate within budget and professionally obligated to achieve the highest possible level of quality. In the real world, a compromise of cost and quality must be achieved, and this is the province of the laboratory manager

It is imperative that laboratory managers understand what responsibilities they hold for the financial performance of the laboratory, as well as the many other aspects of laboratory management. Who proposes and approves price changes? Who approves adding or deleting a procedure, and what criteria are used to make this decision? Is the revenue budget as much the responsibility of the laboratory manager as is the expense budget? Is the laboratory manager to determine the staffing pattern of the clinical laboratories? These questions and others must be answered before one can comprehend the role of the laboratory manager in a particular setting and fully understand the manager's financial responsibility.

Planned Service Capacity

It is often said that there are distinctions as well as similarities between the hospital-based clinical laboratory and its free-standing counterpart. However, there is perhaps no single distinction that so affects the operating cost of the laboratory as its planned service capacity. *Planned service capacity* can be defined as the anticipated volume, time distribution, and array of procedures the laboratory will perform. It is the level to which the laboratory is designed and staffed.

Planned service capacity is often outside the control and influence of the hospital laboratory manager but instead is determined by such parameters as the parent hospital's goals and objectives, the spectrum of medical and surgical specialties the hospital provides to its community, and/or its operation as a teaching institution. The clinical laboratory is asked to be all things to all people and to provide each medical discipline with the laboratory diagnostic capabilities it requires and to do so at a moment's notice.

The freestanding laboratory can generally reject such demands on economic grounds alone, but the hospital-based laboratory must come up with a different answer, one that requires all the analytic and political skills the laboratory manager can muster.

Physician demands for service further exacerbate these issues in the laboratory given the advent of DRGs, because any costs assignable to the laboratory, beyond the minimum necessary to adequately care for a patient, expose the hospital to potential operating losses. While the portfolio of tests to be offered to physicians is the one factor most controllable by the laboratory, active education of the hospital's medical staff regarding diagnostic and therapeutic laboratory testing requirements may also be helpful in controlling utilization. In addition, levels of service beyond the test itself may also be negotiable. For instance, is 24-hour phlebotomy necessary? What tests can and should be batched that were formerly produced on a stat basis? While change in these areas is far more problematic in the hospital environment, the laboratory manager should be alert to all opportunities to reduce costs while still providing effective service at an acceptable quality level.

It is through establishing new procedures in house only when there is a sufficient cost/benefit justification that the laboratory can maximize its use of resources. New services must be added in a way that maximizes the diagnostic ability of the attending physician and minimizes additions to planned service capacity. Any procedure that cannot achieve its break-even point is a new cost burden to be carried by other procedures. The laboratory manager must always evaluate whether a test can be done more economically. Should a contract with a reference laboratory be undertaken? Is there another laboratory that has or can develop this expertise and with which a reciprocal relationship can be developed?

These and other questions should be asked and answered as the proposal for establishing a new test is prepared. It is in this process of judicious addition of new or deletion of old procedures that staffing can best be controlled, that capital equipment can best be utilized, and that operating expenses can best be contained. It is through this financial and clinical decision-making process that laboratory managers can make their contribution to the health of the clinical laboratory.

REFERENCES

1. Anthony RN, Reece JS: Accounting Text and Cases, 7th ed. Homewood, Richard D. Irwin, 1983
2. Berman HJ, Weeks LE: The Financial Management of Hospitals, 5th ed. Ann Arbor, Health Administration Press, 1982

3. Health United States, 1985. Hyattsville, U.S. Department of Health and Human Services, 1985
4. Managerial Cost Accounting for Hospitals. Chicago, American Hospital Association, 1980
5. Managing Under Medicare Prospective Pricing. Chicago, American Hospital Association, 1983
6. The Medicare Prospective Payment System (E & W No. J58475). Chicago, Ernst and Whinney, 1983

ANNOTATED BIBLIOGRAPHY

Berman HJ, Weeks LE: The Financial Management of Hospitals, 5th ed. Ann Arbor, Health Administration Press, 1982

This source presents a complete overview of the major topics confronting health-care financial managers. The discussion includes sources of revenue, budgeting, financial planning, and the management of working capital. See Chapter 5 on cost analysis and Chapter 7 on Medicare and Medicaid. A new sixth edition (1986) of this standard text is now available and may be quite helpful in understanding recent health-care financing changes. At this time, however, the authors have not yet reviewed the latest revision.

Cleverley WO: Essentials of Health Care Finance. Rockville, Aspen Publishers, Inc., 1986

This is a "how-to" book for those who wish to have a better understanding of hospital finance.

Health United States, 1985. Hyattsville, U.S. Department of Health and Human Services, 1985

This report, prepared annually, presents a wealth of statistical information regarding the status of health care in the United States.

Managerial Cost Accounting for Hospitals. Chicago, American Hospital Association, 1980

This publication introduces modern cost accounting principles for the management of today's more complex institutions. Major topics include cost classification and behavior, cost analysis, standard costs, variance analysis, and flexible financial reporting.

twenty-seven

Budgeting Laboratory Financial Resources

David J. Fine
Rohn J. Butterfield
Justin E. Doheny

THE OPERATING EXPENSE BUDGET

Why Have a Budget?

Twenty years ago it was not uncommon for hospitals to operate through an informal process of matching revenues and expenditures without a specific budget. This simple approach to management would seem amazingly primitive for today's health-care executive. Budgeting in businesses of all kinds has matured rapidly in sophistication in recent decades and is now one of the most fundamental building blocks of the well-managed organization. There are many factors contributing to the prominence of the budget. Principal among them is the planning and control capability that the carefully formulated budget represents. As an instrument through which the manager projects the near term or longer term revenues and expenses of the entire business entity, or any of its departments, the budget serves as a guidepost against which actual performance can be measured. A budget agreed to by department manager, administration, and, as appropriate, the governing board, is considered to be the principal tool through which the various levels of an organization achieve financial accountability to one another.[8]

In recent years, as health-care organizations have been called upon to be increasingly cost-effective, the expense associated with services rendered has come to receive as high a profile in public policy debates as their quality. Because of this, the budget, which is, after all, a systematic expression of the institution's operational plan, is used by external regulatory and reimbursement agencies as well as by internal management.

It was, in fact, the Medicare-enabling legislation that first required participating institutions to have a budget. Section 234 of Public Law 92-603 required

An annual operating budget, including income and expenses

A 3-year capital expenditure plan

Annual review and revision

Governing board, medical staff, and administrative participation in the budgeting process

In this context, our discussion shall focus on the planning, organizational, and control characteristics of the laboratory budget.

The Budget Forecast and Narrative

The development of a sound budget is highly dependent upon clearly stated institutional goals and objectives within which the laboratory has a known role and upon which it can base its own specific objectives.

The budget is also dependent upon historical data and projections of future activity. For the laboratory, a desirable data base would include a weighted procedure volume report for the most recent 5 years or more. Such a weighting sets forth the relative value of each procedure through a process more fully discussed in Chapter 29. Set forth in graphic format (Fig. 27-1), the data permit trend analysis by the manager.

In addition, the laboratory manager should expect to receive budget guide-lines from the institution's financial officer that would include expected inpatient and outpatient census for the budget year, demographics of the patient population, and a concise statement of any anticipated changes in the total service program of the organization. Illustrative of this point might be installation of a new linear accelerator in the radiology department, which would result in a significantly expanded load of oncology patients who would require frequent laboratory monitoring.

The laboratory manager should expect to provide the financial officer with a brief statement of program changes that should be expected as a result of changes in laboratory science. Examples of such changes would include procedures that will be diminishing in volume because of obsolescence or physician education, volume estimates for newly implemented procedures, and a technology forecast underlining any predictable changes in laboratory practice for the coming year.

Once these matters have been established, the laboratory manager is in a good position to state the expected volume of activity in terms of procedures per patient day in the least complicated budget approaches, or as a specific enumeration of the expected number of procedures by type in each laboratory section in the more advanced methodologies. Although physical counts of procedures may be the practical limit for some organizations, those who are making use of relative value units can avail themselves of a far more useful tool.

Inasmuch as the budget presentation is often the only time of year the laboratory manager enjoys a thorough review of operations by the senior management team, preparation of a budget narrative outlining in a candid way the operational successes and failures of the concluding budget year, and a statement of the principal goals and objectives of the coming year are often in order.

Once this basic information has been compiled, the more advanced budget program will often incorporate volume projections specifically by

FIGURE 27-1. Procedure volume trend analysis. Here the manager can visualize the growth in relative value units produced from 180,000 in 1980 to 500,000 in 1985. Although steady growth has been experienced, the rate of increase has declined markedly. The conditions contributing to a drop in volume in 1983 should be reviewed to assist in the accurate projection of 1986 volume.

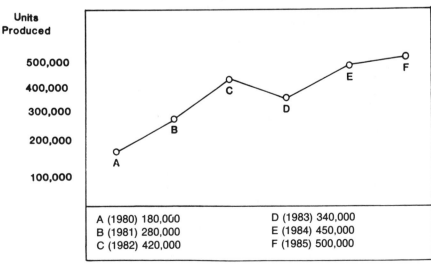

A (1980) 180,000	D (1983) 340,000
B (1981) 280,000	E (1984) 450,000
C (1982) 420,000	F (1985) 500,000

month and day of the week. This ultimately permits far greater sophistication in laboratory staffing and cost analysis.

TYPES OF BUDGET

Broadly speaking, institutions select their budgeting approach from among three general systems: the appropriation budget, the fixed forecast budget, or the variable or flexible budget.

Appropriation Budget

This budget is most common to government institutions dependent upon periodic appropriations from central authorities. Typically, this form of budget will assign a fixed sum to each department. Often expressed in terms of expenditure authority, the appropriation-oriented budget is characterized by inflexibility as a function of clinical volume and poor incentive or reward for the manager.

In the event that expenses run below appropriated levels, the laboratory may have little incentive to return funds to the central authority, because this can often lead to lower appropriations in subsequent years. In the unhappy circumstance of expenses that are higher than budget, any number of authoritarian controls may be imposed.

Fixed Forecast Budget

This budget is probably the most common form in use today and differs in concept from the appropriation budget only in the ease of making programmatic adjustments without resort to approval from external authorities. In this approach, there is typically an annual negotiation of expenditure levels that is subject to recasting in the event operating assumptions change.

Variable or Flexible Budget

This budget is a more creative tool than either of the traditional approaches mentioned heretofore. Such a budget is developed with the assumption that certain operating expenses are relatively fixed for a given range of clinical activity, whereas others vary directly with the level of activity. Identification of cost elements associated with each component of the budget is often difficult and therefore requires greater data management sophistication.

Once established, and given the fine tuning of experience, this approach is an excellent way to set realistic expenditure expectations for the laboratory that obviate the need for frequent renegotiation as the fiscal year progresses. Once the variable and fixed components of cost are negotiated by the laboratory manager, the variable elements will be expressed in terms of expense per unit of output, and the fixed elements will be budgeted in the traditional fashion.[7]

In recent years the *limited-term budget,* generally cast for a single fiscal year, has been replaced by the *continuous budget* in a relatively small number of organizations. In this approach, the manager is continuously updating his budget, replacing the concluding month with a new one so that there is always a 12-month expense forecast. Although the broad applicability of this approach has not yet been established, it is possible to predict that its combination with the variable budget will become increasingly popular with the wider dissemination of computerized financial reporting systems.

The budget is typically segmented into categories of expense called *natural classifications.* Although considerable latitude exists in most instances, some states with significant health-care regulatory activity have mandated classification systems. The objective of the natural classification is to group like expenditures together, with the end-result that the departmental budget is neither too detailed nor too summarized. Table 27-1 provides a sample natural classification system. Some institutions will use even more detailed breakdowns, and others may simply divide expenses into the two broad zones of personnel and supplies and materials.

In addition, the total budget is divided into cost centers to permit the accounting process to follow responsibility lines within the organization. For hospitals with over 250 beds, this usually results in separate cost centers for chemistry, hematology, the blood bank, microbiology, immunology, anatomic pathology, and perhaps others.

Budgeting for Personnel Expenses

Having established the staffing levels required for efficient laboratory operation (see Chap. 12), the budget preparation cycle requires the translation of full-time equivalents (FTEs) into dollars and cents. A necessary first step will be to compare expected laboratory work load for the coming fiscal year as developed in the budget forecast with current staffing levels, making upward or downward adjustments as necessary.[5] This process yields a staffing plan. Although the marginal capacity of laboratories to absorb increased volume without staffing changes in heavily automated areas is high, in man-

Table 27-1
Natural Classification of Expense

Salaries and Wages

Professional personnel
  Regular pay
  Supplemental pay
Technical personnel
  Regular pay
  Overtime pay
  Shift differential
  Supplemental pay
Office and service personnel
  Regular pay
  Overtime pay
  Shift differential
  Supplemental pay

Employee Benefits

FICA
Retirement plan
Health insurance
Life insurance
Workmen's compensation

Operating Expenses

Postage
Communication
Freight and cartage
Data processing
Publishing, printing, photography
Insurance
Awards
Dues, subscriptions
Conference registration
Employee relocation
Job-applicant expense
Gas and heating fuels

Operating Expenses (continued)

Electricity
Water
Heating and cooling
Building rental
Office equipment rental
Data-processing equipment rental
Other rentals
Building repair and maintenance
Medical equipment repairs and
  rentals
Other equipment repairs and
  rentals
Travel expense
Legal services
Medical and clinical contracts
Accounting and auditing services
Other consultants
Laboratory fees
Custodial contracts
Office supplies
Household and institutional
  supplies
Food
X-ray film
X-ray tubes
Sutures
Cylinder gas
Chemicals and reagents
Instruments
Drugs
Disposable packs and instruments
Reusable sterile service items
Prostheses and implants
Other supplies
Research and laboratory supplies

ually oriented sections this is often not the case. Because the effects of understaffing and overstaffing are equally bad for the employee and for the organization, great care must be taken in casting the personnel requirements.

In a typical hospital, personnel expenses constitute almost 60% of total expenditures (Fig 27-2), and therefore control of this area is fundamental to the efficiency and resulting cost-effectiveness of the organization. In addition, assembly of the proper mix of appropriately certified personnel is essential to the assurance of a quality product.

It is important to note that development of the staffing plan for budgeting purposes is a process entirely separate from scheduling. As a result, it is not appropriate to base the new fiscal year budget on current work schedules. Rather, the reverse is true, and the schedule would be derived from the staffing plan.

Having determined the numbers and types of personnel required, the next step in budgeting is to identify the wage level that will be required to attract qualified individuals in the marketplace. In most instances, the laboratory manager can depend upon the personnel department to conduct timely compensation surveys for this purpose. It should be noted, however, that the laboratorian may more

readily sense shifts in the labor market as a result of wage increases at competing institutions and should communicate this to those charged with administering these matters.

As illustrated in Table 27-1, the personnel budget is divided into several categories. Projection of salaries and wages is an arithmetical process derived from the number of workers in a given category and their hourly, weekly, or monthly wages. It is usually appropriate to budget technicians and technologists, phlebotomists and messengers, and doctorally prepared staff separately.

Employee benefits in most organizations are derived by formulas linked to a percentage of basic wages. As a result, social security insurance, health and life insurance, pension funds, workmen's compensation, and other fringes will often be calculated by the financial officer on the basis of departmental wage and salary budgets. The treatment of vacation, holiday, and sick leave for budget purposes will vary from organization to organization as a function of the policies governing their accrual and payment. Where employees have no limitations on accrual and are eligible to be paid for unused time off, it is often necessary to budget these benefits specifically. Table 27-1 does not take this approach.

Because of their particular characteristics, most

FIGURE 27-2.   Typical distribution of hospital income.

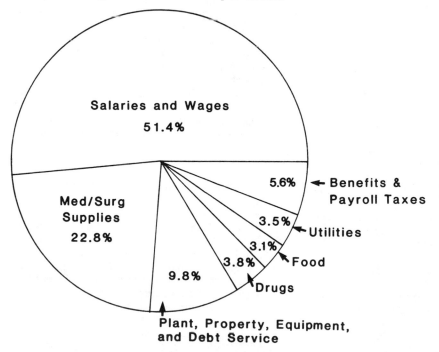

Salaries and Wages
51.4%

Med/Surg
Supplies
22.8%

5.6% ◄ Benefits &
Payroll Taxes

3.5% ◄ Utilities

3.1% ◄ Food

3.8%

9.8% ◄ Drugs

Plant, Property, Equipment,
and Debt Service

departments are asked to budget overtime and shift differentials separately from regular pay. Shift differentials are reasonably straightforward and are usually a function of the institution's personnel policies. Overtime, however, is often a sensitive matter, and highlighting it in the budget typically results in lengthy management debate.

The obligation to pay overtime wages is defined in the Fair Labor Practices Act and is administered by the Federal Department of Labor. Although the cost premium involved in this payroll category is desirable to avoid, it is in actuality unlikely that the laboratory can function efficiently without some scheduled overtime. In many instances, modest amounts of scheduled overtime are a less costly alternative to adding another employee with attendant training, supervision, and benefit costs. Unscheduled overtime is also a reality in the laboratory, since peak work-load levels must be staffed and illnesses covered, and compensatory time off is not always available. These issues notwithstanding, the effective manager schedules in a fashion to minimize the number of these high-cost hours.

A word should be said about part-time employees. As a rule, fractional FTEs are budgeted according to their normal payroll category. The administrative costs associated with part-time workers is slightly higher because of supervision, training, and miscellaneous paperwork. However, their judicious use is one of the manager's creative opportunities to staff for average levels of work load and still meet anticipated peaks on high hospital admission and surgery days, cover vacations, and provide for on-call technologists to cover for sick employees. Obviously, the great advantage of this approach is the avoidance of premium overtime pay for the full-time staff who might otherwise be called upon to work in addition to their normal shifts.

Budgeting for Supplies, Materials, and Other Operating Expenses

Table 27-1 suggests the array of expenditure classifications that may be found in a typical health-care institution where detailed budgeting is being emphasized. While the laboratory will not have budget entries in every category, many of them will be used.

Successful budgeting for operating expenses is dependent upon the laboratory manager's detailed knowledge of the material ingredient costs of each procedure (see Chap. 31), his accurate estimates of repair and maintenance costs (see Chap. 19), and his determination of employee development standards, including attendance at outside seminars, travel, and other factors.

Probably most significant in the difficult projections required to predict operating expenses is the estimate of price changes that will occur in chemicals; petroleum-derivative products, including syringes; gases; and laboratory glassware. The former two items, in particular, are subject to tremendous inflationary and market-price shifts, and the prudent manager must plan to provide sufficient funds for such eventualities. Although the purchasing agent may be called in for support, the laboratory manager's role in negotiating with vendors cannot be overstated. This is particularly true when product evaluation may permit the substitution of lesser-cost items or when decisions concerning reusables versus disposables must be made.

There are a number of techniques used to estimate price escalation of supplies; most common among them is the consumer price index (CPI) to laboratory operating expense ratio.[5] As illustrated in Figure 27-3, operating expenses in the laboratory for supplies and material are plotted against the CPI. Once derived, the ratio can be applied to the CPI forecast issued quarterly by the federal government.

Perhaps the best means of taking the uncertainty out of supply prices is the fixed price contract through which the laboratory manager can set prices of high-use items for a given length of time, usually a year. Although most hospitals still undertake contracting on their own, many are entering into consortia for group purchasing, which permits even greater buying leverage and often results in fractional-cent savings on every item used.

The budgeting approach for operating expenses usually begins by projecting the actual expenses of the current year to a full 12 months. From this baseline, the next fiscal year is budgeted by adjusting for anticipated volume and estimated price changes.

Assessing Performance Relative to Budget

As previously mentioned, the budget serves both as a planning document and as a control document. To maximize its use as a tool through which control is exercised, it is important to have a financial reporting system that will track actual expenditures against budgeted figures. The financial officer of the organization should be expected to produce a variety of timely reports at the close of each operating period, usually a calendar month.[2,10] The most common reports are discussed below:

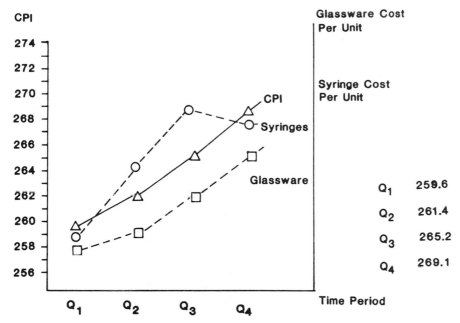

FIGURE 27-3. Ratio of consumer price index (CPI) to laboratory operating expenses. The CPI (base year = 1967 = 100) can be plotted by calendar quarter ($Q_1 \ldots Q_4$) and then compared with the unit cost trend line of a given supply item over the same period. For example, by simultaneously plotting the unit cost of glassware, a manager can establish the historical relationship of the CPI and laboratory glassware. If the two are synchronous, federal government projection of the CPI can be used to project future glassware expenditures at constant levels of volume. Certain supply items, including petroleum derivatives such as syringes, often do not lend themselves to such a predictive formulation.

The *departmental trend summary* (Table 27-2) displays the month's expenditures relative to budget and year-to-date totals. In advanced budgeting systems, departments can divide their annual expenses in ways other than 1/12 each month to more accurately reflect anticipated clinical activity differences from month to month or an uneven pattern of expense disbursement. Also included in this report are work-load measures. Sometimes called a general ledger, this report is often presented with monthly columns totaled for the year-to-date with calculation of percent variation from budget.

The *work-force analysis* shows the number of FTEs employed in the cost center, along with an analysis of productive time and overtime. The data in Table 27-3 illustrate a laboratory's chemistry section now at full staffing following a year of below-budget salary expenses. The productivity coefficient, 0.82 for the full year, is a manager's index to the percentage of paid time consumed by training, illness, vacation, and other non-production-oriented functions. For obvious reasons it would be unusual to see a figure above 0.90.

Perhaps the most important report for the cost conscious manager is the *profit and loss statement* (P&L). As more fully set forth later in this chapter, revenue is budgeted and actual collections can be plotted against actual expense to yield the profit-or-loss position of the laboratory. As in any business, a certain profit margin is necessary to provide for capital improvements and program development, and the P&L is the acid test of the manager's performance in this regard. Income and expenses that are out of synchrony are the inevitable alarm signal for the department head. An example of a P&L for a pathology department is shown in Table 27-4.

Although administrative practices vary a good deal from organization to organization, today's laboratory manager should seek accountability for what is known as bottom-line performance, another term for profitability or net income. In far too many organizations, the laboratory manager is held account-

Table 27-2
An Abbreviated Departmental Trend Summary for a Clinical Laboratory

Natural Classification	September Budget	September Actual	August Actual	July Actual	YTD Actual	YTD Budget	Variance $	Variance %
Salaries and Wages								
Technical personnel								
Regular pay	29,500.00	26,686.42	25,923.41	25,761.38	78,371.21	88,500.00	(10,128.79)*	(11.4)†
Overtime pay	1,700.00	2,602.38	2,200.67	1,906.41	6,709.46	5,100.00	1,609.46	31.5
Total	31,200.00	29,288.80	28,124.08	27,667.79	85,080.67	93,600.00	(8,519.33)	(9.1)
Employee Benefits								
Retirement	2,360.00	2,134.91	2,073.87	2,060.91	6,269.69	7,080.00	(810.31)	(11.4)
Health insurance	875.00	807.32	723.22	706.41	2,236.95	2,625.00	(388.05)	(14.8)
Total	3,235.00	2,942.23	2,797.09	2,767.32	8,506.64	9,705.00	(1,198.36)	(12.3)
Operating Expenses								
Repair and maintenance	2,100.00	2,383.46	1,680.44	2,707.39	6,771.29	6,300.00	471.29	7.5
Medical contracts	800.00	627.91	627.91	627.91	1,883.73	2,400.00	(516.27)	(21.5)
Cylinder gas	200.00	198.37	177.62	163.69	539.68	600.00	(60.32)	(10.0)
Other supplies	14,900.00	16,575.64	15,982.21	15,631.13	48,188.98	44,700.00	3,488.98	7.8
Total	18,000.00	19,785.38	18,468.18	19,130.12	57,383.68	54,000.00	3,383.68	6.3‡
Total	52,435.00	52,016.41	49,389.35	49,565.23	150,970.99	157,305.00	6,334.01)	(4.0)
Work-load units	41,650	43,621	40,790	41,000	125,411	124,950	(461)	(0.4)

*Parentheses denotes favorable variance.

†This department is 11.4% below budget in technical personnel. The strong clinical volume supports the 31.5% higher than budgeted overtime and suggests the manager may be facing some technician recruitment difficulty.

‡Operating expenses are running 6.3% above budget, owing primarily to supplies. This figure is not consistent with work load and suggests either unusually high purchasing levels in the current period, price increases that have not been properly planned for in a budgeting sense, or extraordinary utilization. Management intervention is indicated to establish the cause and to take appropriate corrective action.

Table 27-3
Work-force Analysis — Chemistry Section

Period	Full Time Equivalents		$		Overtime			Productivity
	Budget	Actual	Budget	Actual	Hours	$ Budget	$ Actual	
June	14.9	14.9	20,179	19,920	0	800	0	0.85
YTD	14.9	12.4	242,148	205,826	973.8	9600	11,245	0.82

Table 27-4
Profit and Loss Statement — Pathology — For the Nine Months Ending March 31

	This Month			Year to Date		
	Budget	Actual	Variance	Budget	Actual	Variance
Gross revenue	395,000	407,058	+12,058*	3,400,000	3,630,044	+230,044
Allowances	15,000	28,494	−13,494†	136,000	181,502	−45,502
Net revenue	380,000	378,564	−1436	3,264,000	3,448,542	+184,542
Salaries and benefits	159,316	148,000	+11,316	1,433,844	1,375,422	+58,422
Operating expenses	76,596	85,000	−8404	703,872	758,733	−54,861
Total direct expenses	235,912	233,000	+2912	2,137,716	2,134,155	+3561
Overhead (0.32)	74,761	74,560	+201	684,069	682,930	+1139
Surplus (deficit)	69,327	71,004	+1677	442,215	631,457	+189,242

*The + denotes favorable variance.
†The − denotes unfavorable variance.

able only for adequate control of expense. It is the authors' opinion that this traditional approach fails to offer the department head sufficient understanding of the contribution he is making to the hospital as a whole.

There are many other financial reports produced regularly, including balance sheets, fund-balance statements, and cost reports. Because these have less direct applicability to the laboratory manager, they are not discussed here. For further information, consult the sources listed in the chapter bibliography.

CAPITAL DECISION-MAKING

Preliminary Considerations

In addition to the need for careful operational budgeting, some method must be developed to allocate resources for major investments in buildings and equipment. This process is referred to as capital budgeting. There is a dependent relationship between the operating and capital budgets, since efficiency of operations may largely depend upon the wisdom of capital-acquisition decisions.

The capital-budgeting decision is important for another, more obvious reason. As Berman and Weeks have noted, "If an error in judgment is made, the costs of the decision error can be expected to be incurred over a considerable length of time."[3] Thus, for instance, if the purchased equipment does not

operate efficiently or is underutilized, a high cost may be incurred over time in lost revenue and increased expenses.

In accounting terms, a capital item is generally referred to as a fixed asset expected to provide service for more than one year.[1] This very general definition of a capital item can lead to confusion about what should properly be classified as capital, and some additional guidelines may be helpful:

Repair and maintenance costs should be differentiated from improvements. Maintenance and repair work keeps the equipment in good condition and is treated as an expense in the operating budget. Improvements make equipment better than when it was purchased and are treated as a capital expenditure.

Generally, the replacement of an entire fixed asset is a capital expenditure; the replacement of a component part is an operating expense.

There are subtleties in types of leasing arrangements that define an expense as either a capital or an operating item.

Relatively low-cost items that meet the one-year criterion are often classified as capital expenditures initially but are treated as operating expenses when replaced (*e.g.,* furniture and items under $500 or some other set dollar figure).

Given the critical nature of capital decisions for laboratories and, indeed, for any business enterprise using high-cost equipment, it is incumbent upon the laboratory manager to be fully cognizant of the methodologies employed in analyzing capital-investment alternatives.

Before applying precise decision techniques, the hospital clinical laboratory should first determine a budgeting period. In the case of capital equipment, there are usually two periods: a short-term, or 1-year, horizon; and a long-term, or three-to five-year, horizon.

As in operational budgeting, it is also necessary to clearly identify the goals and objectives of the laboratory. Goals should be specific and based upon planned new programs and projections of future work load. Objectives of the laboratory should be consonant with hospital goals and objectives. Laboratory capital decisions are then examined in light of the needs specified in the department's goals and objectives. A word of caution must be interjected here. The viability of a long-range set of goals is largely dependent upon the accuracy of prediction. The longer the time horizon, the more likely it is that predictions will fall prey to the risks inherent in the basic uncertainty of the future. Therefore, a flexible attitude toward the capital plan must be assumed, and at least annual review of the plan must take place.

Another major intervening factor in the capital-budgeting process is the inevitable political reality of prioritization of competing demands. A prioritized departmental capital-acquisition list, which has already weathered departmental and sectional politics, must then be cast in with other departmental lists for prioritization at the institutional level. While the ideal situation would be a simple matching of institutional goals with departmental requests and available funds, projects of influential departments may often appear as non sequiturs on the capital plan of the hospital. This does not necessarily imply that projects have been considered capriciously; there are usually solid reasons for the ultimate decision. The point is made primarily to emphasize the enormous complexity involved in making such important determinations.

Finally, it must be stated that development of a detailed hospital long-range plan involves significant expense and may include extensive marketing studies. Because not all organizations are able to afford such research, hospital long-range plans are quite variable in their relative sophistication. These cautionary notes should not dissuade laboratory managers from attempting to develop a worthwhile long-range plan for the laboratory. On the contrary, reduction of risk associated with capital decisions is, to a great extent, a function of the rigor with which the capital budget is developed.

Capital Budget Categories

The capital budget is generally divided into two categories. The first is composed of relatively low-cost items, perhaps under $5000, for which the level of analysis is normally minimal. All that is normally required is a simple outline of the costs involved; classification of the request as a replacement, new item, renovation, or improvement; and a brief narrative justification. Items in this category may be given simple numeric priority rankings or classified into groups in the following manner[3]:

1. Capital expenditures necessary for continuance of present service or new equipment required for volume growth
2. Capital items that represent a cost savings or profit with the present service volume and mix
3. Capital items that represent an improvement in the quality or effectiveness of present services
4. Capital items related to new programs or improvement of existing programs

In this manner, decisions may be made either sequentially through priority rankings or categorically. Some consideration might be given to both methods to assure greater flexibility.

The other major category of the capital budget is for all items over $5000. This category usually is split into yearly purchase requests over a 3- to-5-year period. It is at this point that the level of analysis must increase significantly. While the basic classification format for high-cost items remains the same as for low-cast items, support documentation becomes more detailed and specific. In general, the following is necessary for each item[3]:

A statement of the general purpose of the item

A statement of the importance of the item

Some measure of expected utilization of the item

A description of availability of the same or similar items or services available elsewhere

An estimate of patient-care benefits, the number who will benefit, and the basic characteristics of the population served by the item

An estimate of the expected life of the item

An estimate of all costs associated with the acquisition of the item

An estimate of yearly cash outflows associated with the item

An estimate of yearly cash inflows or savings associated with the item

The last two elements are often quite difficult to estimate. Data on expected cash inflows and outflows, however, are crucial to the analytic techniques to be used in the evaluation of capital alternatives, and a few guidelines should aid in their identification[11]:

Consider only incremental amounts. The question to ask is, What additional cash outflows and inflows will occur as the direct result of this project above and beyond those that would occur anyway?

Only *cash* inflows and outflows should be counted. Accounting statements of revenue and expense are generally unreliable as estimates of actual cash generated or spent, unless accounting is on a cash basis. The ideal to be sought here is the actual change in cash that occurs because of the project, not what the accountant will report as expenses and revenues.

Data Analysis Techniques

After the major capital list has been prioritized on the basis of perceived need, supporting data must be gathered for further refinement of priorities. Because capital items are so important in providing for the financial strength of the hospital laboratory and in helping to ensure the viability of future growth, an attempt must be made to assure a reasonable return on the investment. Generally, the hospital's financial officer will provide the laboratory with a return percentage, referred to as a *required rate of return*. In the following discussion, a 15% rate will be used.

The actual required rate of return on a project may be based on a number of single factors or be a combination of all factors. Elements generally considered are the following:

The cost of borrowing new funds (*i.e.,* the interest rate at which the hospital can borrow money)

The return realized on investments of hospital profits in short-term liquid money markets such as government securities or certificates of deposit

In a for-profit environment, the return on investment expected by stockholders

A "fudge factor" to account for misestimates or relative risk of a given project

Depreciation is another datum required for the analysis of capital alternatives. Depreciation recognizes the fact that fixed assets have a limited useful life. Therefore, depreciation is an accounting method whereby "a fraction of the cost of a fixed asset is properly (charged) as an expense in each of the accounting periods in which the asset is used. . . ."[1] Because useful lives of assets are difficult to establish accurately, the fraction expensed each year is generally an estimate.

Standard accounting practices sanction several methods for determining the size of the fraction expensed. *Straight-line depreciation* is the most commonly recognized means of expensing fixed assets. In this method, the estimated useful life in years is divided into the total acquisition cost of the item, expensing the result in each period:

$$\frac{\text{Item's acquisition price} = \$10,000}{\text{Estimated useful life} = 10 \text{ years}}$$
$$= \$1,000 \text{ per year expensed as depreciation}$$

A case example demonstrating the evaluation of a capital purchase follows. As noted earlier, cash inflows must be incremental. In the case of the hypothetic automated differential counter year 1 cash inflows and outflows are estimated to be $75,000 and $25,000, respectively. The inflow figure reflects cash that would not be realized if the counter were not purchased. Likewise, the outflow figure represents cash that would not be spent if the counter were not purchased. Outflows are then subtracted from inflows to yield a net cash-flow figure to be used for future decision analysis. This same calculation is performed for all remaining years of the equipment's useful life, yielding a complete net cash-flow schedule.

Finally, it should be noted that, in the case of the counter, cash outflows increase over time, and cash inflows decrease over time. While this need not be the case for all projects considered, it is a fairly typical pattern for capital investments. For instance, as the counter gets older, repair and maintenance costs can be expected to rise. Resulting downtime from this activity will generally yield some loss in revenue. In addition, equipment purchased in future years may replace or negatively affect procedure volume performed on the counter, rendering the counter underutilized or obsolete.

Case Example—Purchase of an Automated Differential Counter

An automated differential counter is purchased for $125,000. The equipment's useful life is estimated to be 5 years. Yearly depreciation is established at $25,000 with the straight-line method. Estimated yearly cash inflow generated by the machine is hypothetically as follows:

Year 1 = $75,000
Year 2 = $75,000
Year 3 = $67,000
Year 4 = $60,000
Year 5 ± $50,000
Total = $327,000

Estimated yearly cash outflows related to the machine are estimated to be

Year 1 = $25,000
Year 2 = $25,000
Year 3 = $30,000
Year 4 = $35,000
Year 5 = $40,000
Total = $155,000

Calculated net cash flow for each year is then

Year 1 = $50,000 ($75,000 – 25,000)
Year 2 = $50,000 ($75,000 – 25,000)
Year 3 = $37,000 ($67,000 – 30,000)
Year 4 = $25,000 ($60,000 – 35,000)
Year 5 = $10,000 ($50,000 – 40,000)
Total = $172,000

PURCHASE PRICE

$125,000

CASH FLOWS

Year 1 = $50,000
Year 2 =   50,000
Year 3 =   37,000
            $137,000

PAYBACK

$50,000 + $50,000 + $25,000

Year 1 + Year 2 + 0.68 years = 2.68 years

Payback Analysis

The *payback method* will be examined first because it is the simplest approach and has retained some value over time. This method calculates the point in the useful life of the counter when the original investment is recovered from cash flows. Alternative capital projects can be ranked, and the shortest payback is the most desirable financially.

This method has received much criticism because it does not recognize the time value of money (discussed in succeeding paragraphs) and ignores cash flows beyond the payback period. While these are certainly valid points, there are significant benefits to the method as well.[9] The method is useful for comparing projects having roughly the same benefits and economic life and is valuable as a crude measure of risk, because it favors projects with a short time horizon for payback. Specifically, this reduces the impact of uncertainty inherent in longer time horizons.

Average Rate of Return

A second method has been termed *average rate of return* (ARR).[11] In this approach, an attempt is made to average the initial investment over the useful life of the project and compare this with the average investment return over the same period. Average annual investment return divided by average annual investment yields the ARR.

The concept of average annual investment may be somewhat confusing, because it does not represent an actual cash flow in each year, as does the average annual investment return. For purposes of analysis, average annual investment means the average amount of the original investment still tied up in the counter each year.

It should also be noted that conservative calculations of ARR use the initial investment as the denominator. Thus

$$\text{ARR} = \frac{\text{Average annual investment return}}{\text{Initial investment}} = $$

$$\frac{\$\ 34,400}{\$125,000} = 27.5\%$$

If cash flows in this example had actually been equal for each year of the useful life (i.e., $34,400 for years 1 through 5), payback would have been 3.63 years. ARR would then simply have been the reciprocal of payback, or 1/3.63 = 27.5%.

Regardless of the ARR approach used, alternative projects considered are ranked, the highest ARR being most desirable. Although this method does make an attempt to account for all cash flows, its major weakness is, again, a lack of recognition for the impact of time. Thus, taking an extreme example, two proposals may be calculated to have the same average rate of return, but one project may return all of its investment in the first year and the other in the last year. In such a case, the former project would be more desirable because funds would be freed sooner for other investments. Averaging blurs this important decision criterion.

The Concept of Present Value

The time factor has been demonstrated to be of importance when one is considering investment proposals. The time value of money is sometimes difficult to understand intuitively and is worthy of some exploration prior to discussing analytic techniques using the concept.[1]

In growing up, many people were taught to save money in their piggybanks. They were congratulated when the bank was opened and the coins counted. At that time, they learned implicitly that it was better to have money in the future than in the present, that the value of money in the present is less than its value in the future.[1]

In business, however, the values are different. The expectation in this arena is that money invested today should *increase* in value in the future, that a return on today's investment must be realized. Thus, money that is available for investment today is more valuable than an equal amount of money that will not be available until some point in the future. As a result, the manager values an amount of money in the present more than the same amount in the future.

The concept of present value is so important to capital investment analysis that it deserves precise definition. Anthony and Reese[1] provide the following: "The present value of an amount that is expected to be received at a specified time in the future is the amount which, if invested today at a designated rate of return, would cumulate to the specified amount." The formula for calculating the present value of $1.00 to be received n years in the future at a required rate of return i is

$$\frac{\$1.00}{(1 + i)^n}$$

The numerator is generally referred to as the *future value,* since it is the amount to be received in the future, in this example $1.00.

Since, in the example of the counter, cash flows will be received at the end of a number of periods, the additive effect of multiple periods must be calculated. For equal yearly cash flows, the general formula for present value is

$$PV = CF \left[\frac{1 - (1 + i)^{-n}}{i} \right]$$

where PV = present value of all cash flows and CF = yearly cash flow. For unequal yearly cash

---

CALCULATION OF AVERAGE ANNUAL INVESTMENT RETURN

Sum of cash flows = $172,000

Useful life = 5 years

Average annual investment return =

$$\frac{\text{Sum of cash flows}}{\text{Useful life}} = \frac{\$172,000}{5 \text{ yr}} = \$34,400$$

CALCULATION OF AVERAGE ANNUAL INVESTMENT

Initial investment = $125,000

Annual depreciation (straight line) = $25,000

Investment in counter over six years =

Year 1 = $125,000
Year 2 = $100,000

Year 3 = $75,000
Year 4 = $50,000
Year 5 = $25,000
Year 6 = $-0-

Sum of years 1 though 6 = $375,000

Average annual investment =

$$\frac{\text{Sum of years 1 through 6}}{6} = \frac{\$375,000}{6} = \$62,500$$

CALCULATION OF AVERAGE RATE OF RETURN

$$ARR = \frac{\text{Average annual investment return}}{\text{Average annual investment}} =$$

$$\frac{\$34,400}{\$62,500} = 55\%$$

flows, as in the counter, the general formula is

$$PV = \frac{CF_1}{(1+i)^1} + \frac{CF_2}{(1+i)^2} + \frac{CF_3}{(1+i)^3} + \cdots + \frac{CF_n}{(1+i)^n}$$

where $CF_1 \ldots _n$ = cash flows in years 1 to n.

The reader should note that it is not necessary to manually undertake this calculation since present value tables exist for this purpose, and modern financial calculators are preprogrammed for this use.

Net Present Value

The first method using the time value of money is the technique of *net present value* (NPV). NPV is the present value of all cash flows minus the initial investment. If the NPV is positive or zero, then the project is generally considered financially acceptable. This is because all future cash flows have been converted into current dollars, with the use of a preestablished required rate of return and then have been compared with the initial investment. However, small negative NPVs should also be examined for possible inclusion in the list of acceptable projects, since other factors may influence acceptability, including risk inherent in the project, size of initial investment, and benefits to patients.

Returning to the case of the automated differential counter, we see that NPV is calculated as follows:

Calculation of Net Present Value

Initial investment = $125,000 Required rate of return, $i = 15\% n = 5$ years Cash flows Year 1 = $50,000
Year 2 = $50,000
Year 3 = $37,000
Year 4 = $25,000
Year 5 = $10,000
$PV -$ Initial investment = $PV -$ $125,000
Where $PV = $124,879
$NPV = $124,879 - $125,000 = \underline{-\$121}$

Given the decision rule, the project could be rejected. In practice, given the small negative result and the large investment cost, the project might usefully be accepted as financially viable given a 15% required rate of return. Aside from this subtlety, the manager must also evaluate investment size with

respect to competing alternatives. A large investment ranking the same as a small investment in terms of NPV may not be as wise as the smaller project, since it involves the commitment of considerably more absolute dollars for the same return. This may be rectified by constructing *profitability indexes*[1] and ranking projects accordingly. This is done by dividing present value by initial investment, the highest index being most desirable.

Also, given varying useful lives of alternative projects, some method must be found for equating useful lives to assure proper comparison. There are several sophisticated methods for approximating equal useful lives, but a crude technique[1] is to take the shortest useful life, say 5 years, and use only the first 5 years of longer-lived projects for comparative purposes. Cash flows beyond year 5 would be treated as part of the cash flow in year five.

Time-Adjusted Return Method

Another method using the time value of money may be termed the *time-adjusted return* (TAR) method. This technique does not require the selection of a required rate of return. Instead, it "computes the rate of return which equates the present value of the cash flows with the amount of the investment; that is, that rate which makes the net present value equal zero."[1] The resulting rate is termed the *internal rate of return* (IRR). Alternative project proposals are then ranked from highest to lowest IRR, highest being most desirable. Those projects not meeting management's preset required rate of return, in this case 15%, may be discarded after review.

Calculation of the IRR for a project is relatively simple for even yearly cash flows, since present value tables may be used. For uneven cash flows, however, the rate must be determined through a time-consuming iterative mathematic process. Many current financial calculators quickly compute IRR, and this has simplified the process enormously.

With the use of a calculator, the IRR for the counter under consideration can be determined as 14.949%. The accuracy of this figure can be verified by referring to the discussion of NPV, where NPV nearly equaled zero at the 15% required rate of return.

The major potential weakness of this method is that an implicit assumption is made that all cash flows are reinvested for the rest of the project's useful life at the same IRR.[9] This is not a problem if the laboratory realizes a 14.949% return on all of its other investments. However, if the average return is only 10%, the reinvestment assumption of 14.949%

Table 27-5
Data Analysis Techniques — Alternative Project Evaluations

Method	Calculation	Ranking System	Decision Rule	Benefits	Deficiencies
Payback	Years until original investment recovered from cash flows	Shortest to longest payback in years	Shortest payback best	Useful for comparing projects with similar useful lives A crude measure of risk	No recognition of time value of money Ignores cash flows beyond payback
ARR	Average yearly return as percentage of average yearly investment	Highest positive to lowest positive ARR	Highest ARR best	Accounts for all cash flows	No recognition of time value of moeny Blurs differences in timing of cash flows
NPV	PV minus initial investment	Highest positive to lowest positive NPV	Highest NPV best	Accounts for time value of money Evaluates projects at same required rate of return	Ignores differences in investment size Comparison of projects with different useful lives difficult
TAR	Rate of return at which NPV equals zero is calculated; result is internal rate of return (IRR)	Highest to lowest IRR; reject if below required rate of return	Highest IRR best	Accounts for time value of money	Usefulness questionable if IRR is substantially different from actual expected return on reinvestment

is unrealistic. Because the NPV method uses a common required rate of return, it is not subject to the same criticism and is therefore generally the method of choice.

Table 27-5 presents a comparison of each of the analytic techniques discussed and may help to put the four methods into perspective.

Capital Budgeting — The Decision Process

While all of these techniques are useful in the financial evaluation of proposed projects, final prioritiza-

tion of projects for the capital budget must address other factors as well. Each of the classifications in the section on capital budget categories may be examined. Projects in the first category generally do not require any financial analysis, since they are required to maintain the existing level of service. On the other hand, projects in the second category, those that increase profit or produce a cash saving given present service levels and patient mix, are particularly well-suited to financial evaluation. Those projects improving the quality or effectiveness of present services and those relating to new programs should generally be subject to both financial and benefit analysis. Benefit analysis, not considered here, is often highly problematic and subjective, but efforts have been made to quantify the evaluation and link it with the financial analysis to achieve an overall ranking of such projects. The reader is referred to Berman and Weeks[3] for a good discussion of this technique.

Once all four categories have been adequately ranked, the stage is set for final determination of items to be included in the capital budget. Generally, projects in the first category should be funded first, followed by second, third, and fourth category projects. However, the laboratory manager or the capital planning committee of the hospital may wish to pick some projects from each category, depending upon the overall needs of the laboratory or hospital and the available funding resources.

While it again must be emphasized that the decision phase of capital budgeting is subject to considerable adjustment of priorities, the decision-makers will have the best available objective data if one of the above formulations is employed. A schematic representation of the capital budgeting process is shown in Figure 27-4.

Alternative Choice Financing Decisions

Once the decision to acquire capital items has been made, financial analysis techniques may be used again to evaluate the least costly financing alternative.[4] A common decision of this type for the laboratory manager is the lease-or-buy decision, which is an example of present value analysis. Basically, there are two kinds of leases: cancelable and noncancelable. If the laboratory can cancel the lease and stop making payments at any time, the lease is treated as an operating expense according to generally accepted accounting principles. This is termed an operating lease. If a lease is noncancelable for the period of the lease and there is an option to purchase, it is viewed as a form of borrowing for a purchase and is treated as an asset, or capital acquisition, for accounting purposes. Such leases are termed capital leases and are included in the capital budget.

While this distinction has important implications for operating and capital budgets, it does not affect the basic lease-or-buy decision. Generally, the three choices open to the laboratory manager are to purchase from internal funds, to borrow funds, and to obtain a lease. With the present value technique, costs associated with each alternative need to be analyzed. A general example follows:

PURCHASE FROM HOSPITAL FUNDS

Present Value = Initial Investment

FIVE-YEAR LEASE

Present Value = Annual lease payments discounted at the hospital's required rate of return for period of the lease

BORROW FUNDS

Present Value = Annual loan payments and associated interest, discounted at the hospital's required rate of return for period of the loan

---

With this general example in mind, the automated differential counter will now be examined.

Case Example — Financing of Automated Differential Counter Acquisition

PURCHASE WITH HOSPITAL FUNDS

Cash outflow = $125,000

FIVE-YEAR LEASE

Required rate of return = 15%

Annual lease payment = $30,000

Present value of five-year lease discounted at 15% = $100,565

FIVE-YEAR LOAN AT 12%

Required rate of return = 15%

Annual loan payment at 12% interest = $30,961

Present value of loan payments discounted at 15% = $103,786

Given the above results, the five-year lease is the best method of financing the counter's acquisition since it is the lowest cost financing alternative.

At this level of analysis, the alternative with the *lowest* present value is the best method of financing the acquisition.[4]

Assuming the hospital has decided on a noncancelable lease and does not have access to a salvage market at the end of the lease, the analysis ends at the level described in the example. If the hospital does have a salvage market, there is a simple method by which one can further analyze the viability of the lease or purchase.

First, the manager subtracts the present value of the lease from the present value of the purchase. Given that the lease was chosen, the resulting number will be positive and represents the present value of the amount that must be provided from future resale. Then the required future resale price is calculated and compared with the manager's best estimate of future market conditions. If the manager believes the item can be sold for more than the required future resale price, then purchase is the correct decision; if the item cannot be sold at the required future resale price, leasing is the best alternative. The same procedure may be employed in lease-or-loan decisions. An example of this analysis in the case of the differential counter is shown on this page.

REVENUE BUDGET AND RATE-SETTING

Revenue Budget

As will be recalled from the discussion of the break-even point and sensitivity analysis in Chapter 26, there is a crucial relationship among volume, cost, and revenue. While the expense budget outlined in this chapter incorporates the volume and cost factors to yield an operating plan, some mechanism must be developed for forecasting the revenue required to ensure institutional viability.

The *revenue budget* is a forecast of expected gross charges, deductions from gross charges, and resulting revenue. The forecast revenue requirements may take many forms given the goals and objectives of the institution.

In many institutions, the expense budget is completed prior to the revenue budget. However, it is often more logical to project revenue first. Most hospitals find there are always more requests than can be reasonably supported from available revenue. Given a preliminary revenue projection, expenses can be budgeted hospital-wide to meet that projection. This permits the overall budgeting process to be iterative, giving a target for the expense budget. In point of fact, many prospective reimbursement plans are just that; hospitals negotiate a fixed level of revenue from a given third-party payer and then must perform their service within that previously negotiated limit. This, of course, is also true

---

Case Example—Financing of Automated Differential Counter Acquisition with Availability of a Salvage Market

LEASE OR PURCHASE

Present value of purchase = $125,000

Present value of lease = $100,565

Present value of resale = Present value of purchase − Present value of lease = $125,000 − 100,565 = $24,435

Required future value of resale to provide for present value of resale = $PV (1 + i)^n$

Where PV = Present value of resale = $24,435
$\quad i$ = Required rate of return = 15%
$\quad n = 5$

Required future
value of resale = $24,435 $(1 + 0.15)^5$
$\quad\quad\quad$ = $24,435 $(1.15)^5$
$\quad\quad\quad$ = $24,435 (2.01)
$\quad\quad\quad$ = $49,148 The required resale price at end of period 5

LEASE OR LOAN

Present value of loan = $103,786

Present value of lease = $100,565

Present value of resale = $103,786 − 100,565
$\quad\quad\quad\quad\quad\quad\quad\quad\quad$ = $3,221

Required future
value of resale = $3,221 $(1 + 0.15)^5$
$\quad\quad\quad$ = $3,221 (2.01)
$\quad\quad\quad$ = $6,479 The required resale price at end of period 5.

FINANCING DECISIONS BASED ON RESIDUAL MARKET ANALYSIS

Resale Price Assumption	Appropriate Decision
$0 – $6,478	Lease
$6,479	Indifferent to lease or loan
$6,480 – $49,147	Loan
$49,148	Indifferent to lease or purchase
$49,149 +	Purchase

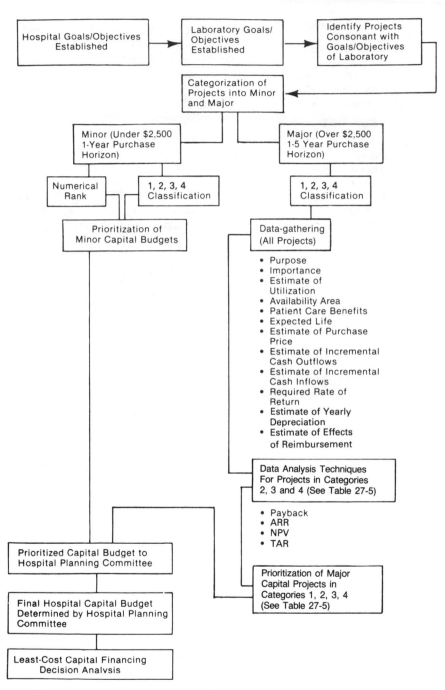

FIGURE 27-4. Capital decision-making flow chart.

of Medicare's prospective payment system (PPS), except that the established price is not negotiable.

Regardless of whether the expense or revenue budget is prepared first, they both must be matched to produce a positive net income. If the expense budget is so large that it cannot be supported by expected revenue, and revenue cannot be further increased, then reductions must be made in the expense budget. This may necessitate two or more cycles in preparation of the expense and revenue budgets. In many institutions, the successive budgeting cycles will be completed by senior management without the involvement of the laboratory manager; however, a number of hospitals now include their managers in the later stages of budgeting to ensure a sense of ownership for the budget by the departmental executive.

Rate-Setting

Rate-setting in the health-care field is the subject of much study and recent progress. There are certain basic principles that are generally accepted, and there are a limited number of approaches to determining rates in the laboratory. The basic philosophy underlying rate-setting is that there should be equity among all patients. This means that the charge for a given service should reasonably reflect the cost of providing the service.[6]

The second principle is that aggregate rates must cover all costs. Expressed in another way, rates must be structured so as to meet the full financial requirements of the institution. In the previous chapter, the various components of cost were defined. These components include direct costs, such as personnel, supplies, and reagents; and indirect costs, such as heat, light, administration, and others. In addition to these costs, a variety of other expenses must be covered by revenue, including bad debts, charity care, and the cost of capital acquisition. The laboratory will usually be allocated a specific dollar amount of these expense items to support from its revenue. In the for-profit sector of the health care field, return to the investors must also be taken into account.

The third principle is that profit centers, those departments that generate income over and above their level of direct and indirect expense, must support those departments that do not cover the full costs of delivering their services. It is commonplace for hospital administrators to require that the laboratory and other service areas, such as pharmacy, radiology, central supply, and the operating rooms, operate at a profit to offset losses in other areas,

such as labor and delivery and the emergency room. This required contribution will vary, depending upon the financial requirements of the individual hospital. However, it can be expected that the surcharge would fall in the range of 10% to 90% of direct and indirect cost, although a higher percentage may be required.

Although these principles hold true in the main, there is a corollary to the third principle that should be kept in mind by the reader: where payment to the hospital for laboratory services is not based on a test as the unit of service, test prices set by the hospital are diminished in importance. For instance, under the PPS, Medicare payments are based upon the discharge as the unit of service, and all hospital services become costs centers in relation to the single discharge profit center. In some cases, health maintenance organizations pay hospital expenses on a *per diem* or per stay basis, again focusing one's attention on the cost of producing a day's care or a patient stay in relation to the overall negotiated price. In such cases, all the rate-setting principles are still applicable to the specified unit of service; however, laboratory tests are but one of the costs of producing that unit, and the tests are not priced units *per se*.

Although alternative payment systems by no means represent the majority of admissions at most hospitals, these systems are growing rapidly in importance. Regardless of the method of payment for laboratory tests, however, the incentives to effectively identify and control costs to ensure market competitiveness are pervasive.

Rate-Setting Techniques

There are three rate-setting mechanisms recommended by the American Hospital Association for use in ancillary service areas. They are hourly rates, surcharge, and the weighted-value basis.[6] The weighted-value method is the technique most frequently used in laboratories, but the other approaches are worthy of comment and brief description.

The hourly-rate method is useful in those departments where the service provided to the patient can be reasonably correlated to the time required for the procedure. This method is commonly employed in the operating room and may also be used in labor and delivery. This method requires the calculation of the total cost of the department, including direct and indirect costs. A projection of the hours the facility is used is then made, and the charges are billed on the basis of cost per hour.

The cost-plus, or surcharge, approach is useful in departments such as pharmacy and central supply, where the supply cost is high compared with the labor cost involved in providing a service. This method requires the identification of the cost of supplies to be sold to patients, other costs in the department, and determination of a ratio between the two (*i.e.,* other costs to billable supplies). The cost of an item is then increased by the calculated percentage. This method can be further modified by introducing a variable surcharge based upon variability in costs associated with handling different classes of supplies.

It should be pointed out that it is not uncommon to find these two methods combined and used together in single departments. A prime example is the operating room. While the department may use an hourly rate to charge for time in the room, use of manpower, and routine supplies, it may also use a surcharge method for unusual supplies such as pacemakers or artificial joints. This helps to equitably allocate the burden of these costly devices to the people who benefit from them, rather than distributing their costs to all patients.

Weighted-Value Basis

Of most interest to the laboratory manager is the weighted-value, or relative-value, basis of rate-setting. This method is also useful in other areas where different types of procedures are done, including radiology, cardiography, and encephalography. In this approach, each procedure is assigned a relative weight based upon the direct costs of performing the procedure. This value is multipled by the number of times the procedure is performed, and one arrives at a total number of weighted units produced in an accounting period. Weighted units for all procedures are added together, and the total is then divided into the total financial requirements of the laboratory for a cost per weighted unit. The cost per weighted unit is then reapplied to the specific procedures based upon the relative weight assigned in the first step of the method to yield a price. A brief example is shown on the opposite page. A more detailed explanation of this subject is provided in Chapter 29.

In the laboratory it is tempting to use the College of American Pathologists' (CAP) relative values as published in their *Laboratory Workload Recording Method* as the basis for establishing the relative weight. However, this method is not intended to be used for establishing rates and provides relative values based only on the productive time required to perform a given procedure. It does not account for differences in cost of equipment or supplies. Admittedly, salary expense can comprise 60% to 70% of the total laboratory budget; however, this still leaves the remaining 40% to be allocated. One need only consider the vast difference in supply expense between a complete blood count and an immunoglobulin E test performed by radioimmune assay to understand the problems with assuming supply expense is equally distributed among procedures.

The weighted-value basis of rate-setting is recommended for the laboratory because it provides a mechanism of apportioning the financial requirements of the laboratory equitably across the consumers of its services. Additionally, this method provides the basis for beginning to measure the productivity of the laboratory to determine how effectively the laboratory manager is using the resources at his disposal. Although the method is relatively difficult to implement because of the great variety of procedures completed in today's clinical laboratory, it is preferred because of the logical, cost-oriented foundation it establishes for rate-setting.

The Realities of Rate-Setting

This section has addressed the rationale and theory of rate-setting in the ideal world. Unfortunately, the practice of rate-setting requires that theoretically ideal rates be adjusted to fit reality. Earlier in this section, the need to adjust rates to cover hospital costs not paid from other departments was discussed. This is, however, but one of the realities that confront the hospital.

Now that health-care costs are no longer simply passed on to businesses, individuals, and the government without scrutiny by these constituencies, virtually all purchasers of care have become prudent buyers searching for the best price for equivalent services. As a result of this phenomenon, laboratory prices have become increasingly more sensitive to competition for market share among numerous suppliers. Nowhere is this competition more highlighted than in the market for outpatient testing, where consumer choice is more likely than in the inpatient setting and out-of-pocket costs to the consumer are still significant as compared with hospital care. To illustrate, if a routine urinalysis costs $12.50 in the hospital outpatient department, why should local physicians refer their patients to the hospital instead of the local private laboratory, which perhaps charges only $8.00? For procedures sensitive to the marketplace, it may well be a good strategy to set a price below the ideal and make up the revenue

Weighted-Value Basis of Rate-Setting

Test	Number Performed	Relative Weight	Weighted Units
Irregular antibody screen	300	1.2	360
Complete blood count	750	0.8	600
.	.	.	.
.	.	.	.
.	.	.	.
.	.	.	.
Chemistry, profile	1,000	2.3	2,300
Luteinizing hormone and follicle-stimulating hormone	325	4.5	1,462.5
Total number of weighted units produced			47,220.0

FINANCIAL REQUIREMENTS

Direct costs	$435,000	
Indirect costs (28%)	121,800	
Required contribution (10%)	55,680	
		$612,480

COST PER WEIGHTED UNIT

($612,480/47,220)	$12.97

Test	Relative Weight	Cost/ Weighted Unit	Price
Irregular antibody screen	1.2	$12.97	$15.56
Complete blood count	0.8	12.97	10.38
.	.	.	.
.	.	.	.
.	.	.	.
.	.	.	.
Chemistry, profile	2.3	12.97	29.83
Luteinizing hormore and follicle-stimulating hormone	4.5	12.97	58.37

difference by charging above the idea level for a less price-sensitive procedure. A basic rule of thumb, however, should be to set the price no lower than the direct cost level, because on a per test basis the institution will lose money for every unit priced below direct costs. Where this is not possible, cost shifting, cost reduction, or deletion of the test from the price list are generally the alternatives of choice, all other factors being equal.

Alternatively, the laboratory manager may give consideration to establishing a separate outpatient laboratory to compete with the private laboratory. Under this scenario, the outpatient laboratory would offer a limited array of procedures priced to compete successfully, while the inpatient laboratory would establish prices at a level sufficient to recover its full financial requirements. Such a device permits the laboratory to compete on a price basis in the outpatient setting and to set its inpatient rates recognizing that they are not as price-sensitive nor as subject to direct competition. In a similar vein, third-party payers who base their payments on area-wide norms may stimulate upward or downward price adjustments by hospitals who attempt to maximize their reimbursement from these sources.

As can be seen from the foregoing, rate-setting

is an extremely complex process requiring certain inputs from the financial officer and certain inputs from the laboratory manager. Although it is always desirable to properly relate relative value and the rate schedule, marketplace realities will often require strategic readjustments. The laboratory manager should be an active participant in this process and should expect to be the hospital's expert in the pricing practices of the competition.

REFERENCES

1. Anthony RN, Reese JS: Accounting Text and Cases, 7th ed. Homewood, Richard D. Irwin, 1983
2. Beck DF: Basic Hospital Finance Management. Germantown, Aspen Systems Corporation, 1980
3. Berman HJ, Weeks LE: The Financial Management of Hospitals, 5th ed. Ann Arbor, Health Administration Press, 1982
4. Boer GB: Analysis of equipment leases. In Bennington JL, Boer GB, Louvau GE, Westlake GE (eds): Management and Cost Control Techniques for the Clinical Laboratory, pp 199–208. Baltimore, University Park Press, 1977
5. Budgeting Manual. Sacramento, California Hospital Association, 1974
6. Cost Finding and Rate Setting for Hospitals. Chicago, American Hospital Association, 1968.
7. Deason JM (ed): Flexible budgeting. Topics in Health Care Financing 5, No. 4, 1979
8. Griffith JR, Hancock WM, Munson FC (eds): Cost Control in Hospitals. Ann Arbor, Health Administration Press, 1976
9. Hunt P, Williams CM, Donaldson G: Basic Business Finance, 4th ed. Homewood, Richard D. Irwin, 1971
10. Lusk EJ, Lusk JG: Financial and Managerial Control: A Health Care Perspective. Germantown, Aspen Systems Corporation, 1979
11. Silvers JB, Prahalad CK: Financial Management of Health Institutions. Flushing, Spectrum Publications, 1974

ANNOTATED BIBLIOGRAPHY

American Hospital Association: Cost Finding and Rate Setting for Hospitals, 1968
This manual describes the basic logic and concepts for establishing charges in hospitals. See Chapters 2 and 3 for a treatment of cost finding.

Berman HJ, Weeks LE: The Financial Management of Hospitals, 5th ed. Ann Arbor, Health Administration Press, 1982
This source presents a complete overview of the major topics confronting health care financial managers. The discussion includes sources of revenue, budgeting, financial planning, and the management of working capital.

Boer GB: Analysis of equipment leases. In Bennington JL, Boer GB, Louvau GE, Westlake GE (eds): Management and Cost Control Techniques for the Clinical Laboratory, pp 199–208. Baltimore, University Park Press, 1977
This source presents a detailed analysis of the lease-or-buy decision. Other chapters contain good material on cost analysis, price analysis, forecasting, and capital and operational budgeting.

Griffith, JR, Hancock WM, Munson FC (eds): Cost Control in Hospitals. Ann Arbor, Health Administration Press, 1976
This is a now classic work that still has a number of pertinent chapters for the laboratory manager.

Lusk EJ, Lusk JG: Financial and Managerial Control: A Health Care Perspective, Germantown, Aspen Systems Corporation, 1979
This is a good single volume sourcebook for hospital department heads being introduced to financial management.

Silvers JB, Prahalad CK: Financial Management of Health Institutions. Flushing, Spectrum Publications, 1974
While not as comprehensive as other books of this nature, this text has many chapters containing cases that require the reader to analyze data and recommend decisions. Coverage on the effects of internal hospital politics and external forces is excellent and integrated well with the technical material. Specific topics covered are basic accounting concepts, forecasting and analysis, control systems, capital budgeting, capital and short-term financing, and the external environment.

twenty-eight

Wage and Salary Administration

John R. Snyder

Despite the large expenditures for capital equipment and supplies to operate a clinical laboratory, the wage and salary component of the budget represents approximately 50% to 70% of the department's total operating costs.[15,22] Although many of the functions of compensation management are the responsibility of an institution's fiscal officer for human resources, it is helpful for the laboratory manager to be familiar with the terminology, processes, and procedures used in wage and salary administration.

THE REWARD SYSTEM: COMPENSATION AND NONCOMPENSATION DIMENSIONS

From a department administrator's or supervisor's perspective, it is important to recognize that pay is only one part of the laboratory's reward system. No doubt appropriate financial compensation is necessary to attract and retain personnel who have the necessary knowledge and skills for laboratory operations and are willing to put forth the effort needed to help the laboratory function. Recall, however, that pay has been identified as a satisfier in some situations, a dissatisfier in other situations, but seldom an effective long-term motivator.

The reward system in the laboratory includes anything that an employer is willing and able to offer and an employee values sufficiently to accept in exchange for performance. The reward process is composed of both compensation components and noncompensation components, as illustrated in Figure 28-1.[15]

Compensation Dimensions

All rewards classified as monetary and in-kind payments constitute the eight compensation dimensions of the reward system.[13] These include both the amount of money paid for work and performance in a specified job and money paid for time not worked, for example, holidays, paid vacations, and paid time off for various personal reasons. Other dimensions address continued compensation or job security in the form of loss-of-job income; disability income; spouse or family income continuation after an employee's total and permanent disability or death; and health, accident, and liability protection. Two remaining dimensions include deferred compensation to continue income after retirement and income equivalent payments or perquisites ("perks").

Noncompensation Dimensions

Noncompensation rewards are the work situation-related factors that relate to the employee's emotional and psychologic well-being.[13] Many of these are similar to the motivational factors that behavioral scientists suggest for improving work performance. Henderson[13] identified seven dimensions of the noncompensation reward system: dignity and satisfaction from work performed; physiologic health, psychologic well-being, and emotional maturity; constructive social relationships with coworkers; jobs designed to require adequate atten-

439

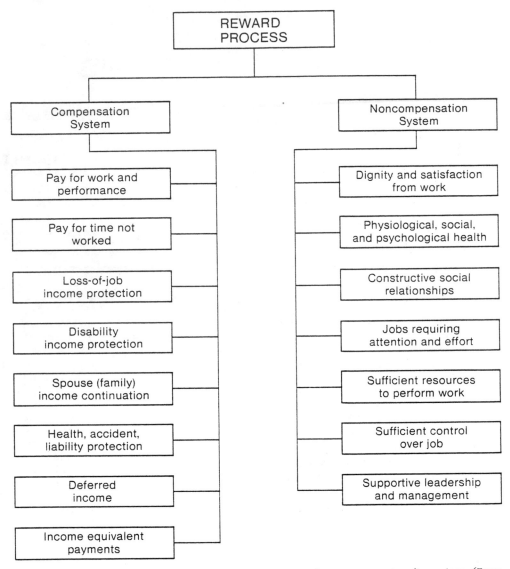

FIGURE 28-1. The reward system: compensation and noncompensation dimensions. (From Henderson RI: Compensation Management: Rewarding Performance, 4th ed, pp xiii, xiv, xx. Reston, VA, Reston Publishing, 1985. Adapted with permission)

tion and effort; sufficient resources to perform work assignments; sufficient control over the job to meet personal demands; and supportive leadership and management.

The purpose of this chapter is to introduce the complex area of wage and salary administration as applicable to the clinical laboratory. The chapter begins with a historic perspective of health-care wage determination with citations of significant legislation. Attention is then focused broadly on the accounting of human resources, followed by more specific information about personnel budgeting, financial compensation for laboratory staff and managers, employee incentive systems based on merit, payroll accounting, and benefit plans. The final section addresses arrangements for compensating physician services in the clinical laboratory.

LEGISLATION GOVERNING COMPENSATION ADMINISTRATION

Wage and salary administration programs in health-care institutions followed a fairly simplistic approach before 1967.[17] The majority of workers were women, and wages were therefore viewed as "supplemental income," because women were viewed as secondary breadwinners. This perception was complicated by a belief that health-care institutions, in general, and hospitals, in particular, were charitable institutions having limited resources available for improving wages. In hospitals, nurses represented a norm group of "professionals"; and wages for allied health professionals, including laboratory workers, tended to fluctuate with nursing salaries.

In the early 1950s, unions entered the health-care fields, which resulted in third-party negotiating through collective bargaining for salary adjustments. The American Nurses Association in 1966 also influenced wage structures in hospitals by establishing a national minimum wage for nurses.

The inclusion of hospitals under the Fair Labor Standards Act in 1967 called attention to the need for both upward adjustment of health-care wages and study of jobs and job content to guard against problems under the Equal Pay for Equal Work Provisions of the Act. Further modifications resulted from guidelines established in the Economic Stabilization Program under the Johnson Administration in 1971. These guidelines determined poverty wage rate levels, and hospitals realized that a large percentage of employees were below or only slightly above the federal guidelines.

Specific legislation influencing compensation practices can be put into four major categories: (1) wage and hour legislation, (2) income protection legislation, (3) antidiscrimination legislation, and (4) wage and price control legislation.[13] The intent of select laws under each of these categories follows.

Wage and Hour Legislation

Laws in this category were established to restrict hours worked and set basic rates of pay.

1935: National Labor Relations Act

This act provided employees the right to bargain collectively for wages and benefits. Nonprofit health-care institutions were excluded from the act until the enactment of Public Law 93-360 in 1974 (see Chap. 15).

1938: Fair Labor Standards Act (FLSA)

After earlier unsuccessful attempts at establishing a regulated minimum wage, the FLSA established minimum wages for all employees engaged in interstate or foreign commerce or the production of goods for foreign commerce and employees of certain other enterprises. Although specific occupations are exempt, revisions of the act from 1938 have enlarged the number of work groups covered and steadily increased the minimum age. The act also requires employers in covered enterprises to define a fixed workweek and pay time-and-a-half for all hours worked in excess of 40 hours a week. Child labor provisions of the act call for (1) a minimum hiring age of 14 to 16, depending on the kind of work performed and whether the employer is the child's parent; and (2) a minimum age of 18 for work in hazardous occupations.

State Laws on Minimum Wages

Some states have passed their own minimum-wage legislation, and if the state labor laws are more rigorous than Federal laws, they supersede the federal statute.

Income Protection Legislation

During the last century, a number of laws have been enacted to provide economic protection for employees who, due to circumstances beyond their control, cannot continue to work.

1911: Workers' Compensation

This enduring piece of legislation is now handled by state compensation laws to (1) provide prompt and reasonable income and medical benefits to victims of work-related accidents or income benefits to their dependents, regardless of fault; (2) provide speedy resolution to disputes arising out of personal injury litigation; (3) relieve public and private charities of financial drains from uncompensated industrial accidents; (4) minimize costs associated with time-consuming trials and appeals; (5) encourage employer involvement in safety and rehabilitation; and (6) promote the study of causes of accidents to prevent future occurrence.[3,13]

1935: The Social Security Act

This law requires employers and employees to contribute equally to guard against loss of income due to termination of employment beyond the employees' control. Although primarily a retirement program, the law also established Federal Old-Age, Survivors, Disability and Health Insurance Systems. Amendments to this act established Medicaid and Medicare programs. Significant changes in the act were made in 1983 with the Social Security Reform Bill. Under Title IX of the Social Security Act, unemployment compensation is provided for, but each state establishes amounts of weekly benefits, total number of eligible weeks, the qualifying employer/employee relationship, and waiting time after employment ceases before benefits are received.

Pension Plans

Several pieces of legislation enable private retirement protection programs, including the Welfare and Pension Plan Disclosure Act of 1959, the Employee Retirement Income Security Act of 1974, and the Multiemployer Pension Plan Amendment Act of 1980. These acts attempt to improve the operation and financial viability of private pension plans.

1973: The Health Maintenance Organization (HMO) Act

Most employers provide health and welfare benefits, including life insurance and death benefits, sickness and accident benefits, hospitalization, and medical care. Under the HMO Act, employers covered under FLSA and having 25 or more employees for whom health benefits are provided are required to offer an HMO if available in the area where the employees reside.

Antidiscrimination Legislation

Equal protection under the law is afforded in both the Thirteenth and Fourteenth Amendments to the Constitution of the United States and the Civil Rights Acts of 1866, 1870 and 1871.

1963: Equal Pay Act

This act requires equal pay for equal work for men and women. Equal work is defined as work requiring equal skill, effort, and responsibility under similar working conditions. Similar working conditions are dependent on surroundings and hazards. Under the Equal Pay Act, employers can establish different pay rates based on (1) a seniority system; (2) a merit system; (3) a system that measures earnings by quantity or quality of production; and (4) a differential based on any factor other than sex. Additional protection against discrimination is afforded in Title VII of the Civil Rights Act of 1964. (Other applicable legislation prohibiting discrimination are listed in Chapter 13).

Tax Investment Legislation

Most tax legislation relates to the deferral or sheltering of income tax payments. Legislation such as the Revenue Act of 1978 and Tax Equity and Fiscal Responsibility Act (TEFRA) of 1982 have impacted the take-home pay of employees.

Wage and Price Control Legislation

Wage and price controls attempt to reduce rapid inflation during low levels of unemployment. For example, the Economic Stabilization Act of 1970 allowed identical pay increases to all employees, across-the-board raises irrespective of high-performing employees.

Although this discussion of the legislation governing compensation is an overview at best, it does lay the groundwork for job analysis and design of a pay structure for clinical laboratory personnel.

HUMAN RESOURCE COST ACCOUNTING

Before beginning a discussion about the mechanics of personnel budgeting, compensation, and payroll accounting, it is helpful to gain a perspective on the costs associated with the human resources entrusted to the laboratory manager's care. This human resource accounting (HRA) process attempts to quantify the value of the "human assets" to the laboratory. Flamholz[9] states:

> A major purpose of human resources accounting is to help managers to use an organization's human resources effectively and efficiently. HRA is intended to provide managers with information needed to ac-

quire, develop, allocate, conserve, utilize, evaluate, and reward human resources.

Human resource costs, like other costs accounted for in the clinical laboratory, have asset and expense components.[7] As an asset, human resources are expected to provide a return on the financial investment in the form of productivity, during future accounting periods. As an expense, human resources will consume some portion of the total financial and physical resources allocated the laboratory during the current accounting period.

Flamholz proposed a model for identifying and classifying relevant human resource costs (Fig. 28-2).[9] For an individual already employed in the laboratory, the appropriate categories for historic analysis of human resource costs are acquisition costs and development costs. If employee turnover occurs, separation costs are incurred and added to the acquisition and development costs.

Acquisition Costs

Human resource acquisition costs include recruitment, interview and selection, and hiring costs. Recruitment costs are incurred in advertising, identifying and attracting a potential employee. Expenditures include personnel department and recruiter salaries, advertising costs, agency fees if used, possible travel and entertainment costs for investigation of leads for possible applicants, and other administrative expenses such as telephone, postage, and printed recruitment materials. These costs are pro-

rated for the employees netted. If, for example, a single advertisement listing multiple positions, placed in several issues of a professional journal, costs $1200 and nets two employees, the allocated cost would be $600 per person independent of the number of interviews generated.

Interview selection costs are those incurred in evaluating and selecting the final candidate. These costs include laboratory administration and personnel department salaries for time spent reviewing resumes, checking references, and interviewing. Also, travel and entertainment costs for each candidate become part of the net acquisition cost.

Hiring costs are incurred in bringing the successful candidate into the laboratory and placing the individual in the job. Relocation expenses are an example of actual hiring costs.

Development Costs

Development costs stem from orientation, possible off-the-job training, and on-the-job training until the new employee is prepared to handle a work volume normally expected of an individual in the position. Orientation costs are incurred in lost productive time for both the employee and immediate supervisor in ensuring that the new employee is familiar with institutional and laboratory policies and procedures.

Should the new employee need to learn a new skill that cannot be taught in the laboratory by existing technical staff, off-the-job education costs might

FIGURE 28-2. Model for measurement of human resource cost accounting. (From Flamholz EG: Human resource accounting. In Davidson S, Weil R (eds): Handbook of Cost Accounting, pp 12, 26. New York, McGraw-Hill, 1978. Adapted with permission)

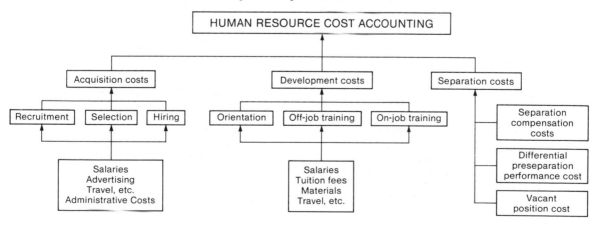

be incurred. Perhaps the new employee needs to attend a week-long course on how to operate an analyzer in the new employment setting. Costs for this experience would include the employee's salary, course tuition, travel, meals, and lodging.

On-the-job training costs are those largely associated with the employee's salary during the period that he is not to a level of expected productivity. This cost obviously is dependent on the breadth and depth of skills of the new employee. For example, an employee with prior experience in general hematology may require a short training period of 1 to 3 weeks in a new hematology laboratory, whereas a general chemistry technologist may require 1 to 3 months to prepare for a position in a special chemistry laboratory.

Separation Costs

If a currently employed laboratorian leaves the institution, additional costs are incurred. Separation costs include separation compensation, differential preseparation performance costs, and vacant position costs. Separation costs may include severance pay for some positions if the separation is at the employer's option. Separation costs probably also include payment for accrued vacation and possibly sick time.

Differential preseparation performance costs reflect a loss in productivity prior to the employee's leaving. Preoccupation with getting ready to leave or a "short-timer" attitude tends to diminish the employee's work output despite the fact that there are no changes in the resources consumed.

Vacant position costs may be direct or indirect costs resulting from an unfilled position. If other technical staff are expected to pick up the responsibilities of the vacant position, their own productivity may suffer. This may necessitate overtime and will certainly take its toll on the long-term psychologic and perhaps physical well-being of the remaining staff.

To illustrate this model of human resource cost accounting, consider a situation in which a general chemistry technologist is hired to fill a 3 to 11 PM vacancy for a general technologist to work in the chemistry, hematology, and body fluids sections. Assume that acquisition costs, including advertising, travel, appropriately allocated portions of salaries, administrative costs, and relocation total $3200. A 3-week orientation on the day shift for the employee to become fully familiar with the procedures used primarily in hematology and body fluids preceded the actual start on the assigned 3 to 11 PM

shift. Allocated costs associated with this on-the-job training period are $1600 (3 weeks of someone else covering the 3 to 11 shift at $10.00 per hour plus the equivalent of 1 additional week's salary of nonproductive work while learning). Also, orientation costs allocated to the preservice experience total $150. Because the new employee will be required to troubleshoot problems in the hematology analyzer, a single-day workshop at a local meeting is planned as off-the-job training. Total costs, including an additional day's salary, are $230. Adding the acquisition costs of $3200 to the total development costs of $1980, the total invested "hook value" of the employee is $5180—and he has not yet begun the shift for which he was hired!

While there are obviously a number of cost estimates included when calculating an employee's human resource value, these costs are often overlooked. The human resource cost accounting model is helpful in gaining a perspective of the monetary investment represented by employees in the laboratory.

PERSONNEL BUDGETING

The personnel budget can be defined as a definite financial plan for personnel expenditures that imposes goals and limitations on staffing in the laboratory. The number of personnel needed for a given laboratory can be determined with the use of the College of American Pathology (CAP) work-load units and forecast test volume, as will be described in Chapter 29. Esmond[8] recommends that line managers be responsible for preparing the personnel budget, because they are ultimately responsible for implementing the plan.

The personnel budget for a laboratory includes the wage and salary calculation for each position and each worker, including anticipated raises and adjustments from a change of employment status.[19] Personnel budgets, prepared by laboratory managers, typically include justification statements regarding overtime pay, vacation relief, and temporary help. Support information may detail calculation of personnel hours required but not immediately perceptually justified by work-load calculations. These may be hours to ensure 24-hour coverage or hours not available to the laboratory if the formula for staffing has not included non-revenue-producing activities or vacation time and holidays. Historic information about turnover rate and absenteeism may also be useful in the budget justification.

Two figures illustrate the categories and detail typically included in a budget. Figure 28-3 is an

General Hospital

Approved Responsibility Center Manpower

Date: _____   Page no.: _____

Responsibility center no.: _____   Responsibility center name: _____

Labor Grade Class	Classification	Approved Full-Time Equivalents	Approved Wage. Salary Range[a]	Additional Data

Wage-earning (hourly) full-time equivalents _____
Administrative (salaried) full-time equivalents _____
Total full-time equivalents _____

[a]This column required only if wage or salary ranges are not built into the labor grade classification structure.

FIGURE 28-3. Position control document for a responsibility center.

example of a position control document for a responsibility center.[8] Personnel on this form are expressed in full-time equivalents as defined by personnel policy. Each entry line includes a labor grade classification code and description designating wage and salary ranges matched with skill requirements. The American Hospital Association's Chart of Accounts for Hospitals[1] suggests using a decimal system for coding in which 0.01 represents laboratory supervisors; 0.02, technical specialists; 0.03, technologists; 0.04, technicians; and so on.

Figure 28-4 displays an example of a laboratory section personnel budget that lists each employee

separately.[19] This sample budget worksheet also includes a position or grade code, abbreviated job title or category, number of personnel hours per position, rate of pay, projected annual base salary, and projected annual increase.

FINANCIAL COMPENSATION FOR LABORATORY STAFF

While the process for identifying job content and determining pay structures usually is the responsibility of an institution's fiscal officer, knowledge of

FIGURE 28-4. Example of laboratory section personnel budget for fiscal year.

Grade Code	Position Title	PT/FT Day Eve	Incumbent	Current Bi-weekly	Projected Annual Base	Anniv. Date	Projected Annual Increase	Projected Total Salary	Hours Per Pay Period Bi-weekly
.01	Dept. Head	FT-D	M. Smith	$1350.77	$35,120	1/2/89	$1756	$36,876	80
.02	Section Supv.	FT-D	J. Wilson	$1200.00	$31,200	3/1/89	$1560	$32,760	80
.03	Technologist	PT-D	F. Bard	$1007.69	$26,200	9/15/89	$1310	$27,510	80
.03	Technologist	FT-N	K. Lewis	$1057.69	$27,500	7/1/89	$1375	$28,875	80
.04	Technician	FT-D	G. Upton	$ 646.14	$16,800	1/2/89	$840	$17,640	80

the components of the process will help laboratory managers participate in the process, rather than having the end result "handed" to them. Figure 28-5 displays the components of the job analysis process, the foundation for a fair and just salary system.

Job Analysis

The first step in designing a compensation system is to define the work content of each job and the worker characteristics (knowledge and skills) required for successful performance of the job. Data for analyzing job activity can be collected by interviews with workers doing the job, observation of the work being done, questionnaires completed by either the person doing the job or his immediate supervisor, or completed journals or logs detailing activities performed.[13]

Job analysis is accomplished following seven steps[13]:

1. Determine the use of the data and information. This focuses the job analysis questions. Information is useful for developing job descriptions and specifications, compensable factors, job evaluations, and job classifications.
2. Select methods and procedures for securing job data and information. In addition to departmental goals and objectives and existing position descriptions, the organizational chart and a work process chart can be extremely helpful.
3. Schedule the necessary and logical work steps. Use of CAP workload data and the personnel budget are helpful in this step.

4. Identify desired job performance requirements. This step helps focus the analysis on what should happen as opposed to what is.
5. Assess the present situation. An assessment must be made of the current job-holder's work performed.
6. Clarify any deviation between identified or observed activities and activities that should be performed.
7. Review the data and the information with the participants. This review offers an opportunity to correct misconceptions, ensure factual information, and ensure that information describing the job is complete.

Compensable Factor-Based Job Evaluation

Key to the establishment of a compensation system is identification of compensable factors.[13] These factors distinguish between jobs by establishing degrees of difficulty. The distinction between a career-entry technologist and a senior technologist in a chemistry section might be the ability to solve a problem with a procedure that is out of control due to an interfering substance. Likewise, a distinction may be made between two technical staff members in hematology regarding the judgment used in evaluating an abnormal leukocyte count.

Universal compensable factors as defined by the United States Department of Labor include *skill* —experience, education, and ability; *effort*— physical or mental exertion required; *responsibility* —dependence on the employee to do the job as expected; and *working conditions*—physical surroundings and hazards of a job. These factors are

FIGURE 28-5. An example of a laboratory payroll journal.

Section: Hemostasis Laboratory　　　　　　　　　　　　　　　　　　　　　　　　　　　　**Month: November**

Grade Code	Employee	Regular Hours	Regular Salary	Overtime Hours	Overtime Salary	Sick Hours	Sick Salary	Vacation Hours	Vacation Salary	Holiday/Other Hours	Holiday/Other Salary	Total Hours	Total Salary
.01	M. Smith	163	$2,752	0	$ 0	0	$ 0	0	$ 0	8	$ 135	171	$2,887
.02	J. Wilson	147	$2,205	0	$ 0	16	$ 240	0	$ 0	8	$ 120	171	$2,565
.03	F. Bard	163	$2,054	4	$ 50	0	$ 0	0	$ 0	8	$ 100	175	$2,204
.03	K. Lewis	155	$2,049	0	$ 0	0	$ 0	8	$ 106	8	$ 106	171	$2,261
.04	G. Upton	163	$1,317	4	$ 33	0	$ 0	0	$ 0	8	$ 65	175	$1,414

relatively abstract and too general for use in the clinical laboratory.

A more appropriate cost system was developed by the Office of Personnel Management, called the Factor Evaluation System (FES).[13] This method has been used successfully to classify jobs on the basis of the following factors: knowledge required in the position, supervisory controls, guidelines, complexity, scope and effect, personal contacts, purpose of contacts, physical demands, and work environment. Each of these factors can be described for a given job and weighted; and the job can then be placed in a continuum of jobs, or a hierarchy.

Designing a Pay Structure

Once a job hierarchy has been established, a pay system needs to be decided upon.[14,18] Heneman and associates[14] define four basic types of conventional pay systems: (1) job-based systems, rewarding the employee for the complexity of task in the job hierarchy; (2) seniority systems, based on length of service; (3) merit systems, which reward performance; and (4) a mixture of the previous three. Heneman and colleagues then defined four decision points to consider in pricing (setting wages) within the systematic hierarchy:

> 1) whether to establish a single rate or rate range; 2) whether to establish a rate or rage range for each job or for a lesser number of pay grades; 3) what the actual rates, or the minima and maxima of the rate ranges will be; and 4) how to handle current wages or salaries that are out of line.

There obviously needs to be internal consistency in the pay structure, and pay should reflect the laboratory's goals and competitive levels for comparable jobs in the marketplace.

Principles for a Compensation System

Laliberty and Christopher[17] provide the following principles as guidelines for establishing a compensation system:

- Wages should purchase performance, rather than buy time and talent. Differences in educational degrees and laboratory certifications (generalist versus specialist) reflect talent. Although differential talent should lead to differential tasks, different jobs, and thus a differential wage, many laboratorians are performing similar tasks

with the same degree of responsibility despite differential talent.
- A wage should be viewed as an investment; the greater the wage, the greater the rate of performance.
- Wages respond to the supply-and-demand factor. In some instances, this depresses the wage scale; in other instances, it unjustifiably inflates the scale.
- Management essentially controls the work to be performed but does not control the price paid to the worker.
- There is no concept of usage that is absolute. A correct wage justly compensates the employer for the level of performance rendered.
- Wages must be correct in their relationship both within the institution and between the institution and outside sources of competitive employment.
- Fringe benefits are classified as collateral wages and must be specifically defined as payment by unit of work.
- Recruitment is based on money; retention is based on fringe benefits.
- Wages have a low priority when the basic wage is adequate.
- The complexity of wage and salary administration requires a formal system.

Compensation Survey

Several of the preceding principles and earlier citations noted the need for compensation systems to be competitive in the marketplace. Many laboratory managers conduct informal compensation surveys. The key is selecting institutions of approximately the same size, in a comparable geographic location, with a comparable complexity of laboratory analysis.

A number of professional organizations and other groups conduct periodic national surveys of laboratory personnel salaries. While these data offer a "snapshot" view of salaries, observation of trends is possible. One national study recently reported increases ranging from 17% for technicians to 25% for supervisors.[6] Table 28-1 displays starting salaries for six levels of laboratory personnel subdivided by bed size and type of institution and geographic location.[6]

When comparing laboratory manager's salaries with other managers of patient care services in 1987, Santos found that only pharmacy directors received higher salaries.[21] This study also subdivided respondents by institution size, but used the total number

Table 28-1.
Starting Salaries in Clinical Laboratories in 1986

	All Laboratories	Independent/ Group Practice Laboratories	All Hospital Laboratories	Bed Size			Geographic Location			
				Under 200	200– 399	400+	East	South	Midwest	West
Technician	$15,140	$14,515	$15,311	$14,318	$15,931	$15,493	$15,802	$14,340	$14,950	$15,813
Technologist	$19,344	$18,828	$19,499	$18,811	$20,101	$19,589	$18,693	$18,273	$18,977	$22,355
Supervisor	$23,667	$23,833	$23,663	$21,241	$23,798	$25,487	$24,596	$22,037	$22,933	$25,561
Chief technologist	$26,972	$25,785	$27,389	$24,956	$27,674	$29,499	$26,406	$24,773	$27,083	$30,055
Laboratory manager	$31,722	$30,596	$31,946	$27,949	$32,491	$34,432	$32,533	$29,238	$30,922	$35,220
Laboratory director	$49,923	$44,383	$51,529	$45,400	$53,160	$52,991	$53,500	$44,732	$48,809	$52,712

(From Benezra N: Lab salaries and benefits: Are they keeping pace? MLO 19, No. 1:30–34, 1987. Reprinted by permission of the publishers.)

of hospital FTEs. As expected, the larger the institution, the higher the laboratory manager's salary.

Equal Pay and Comparable Worth

The difference in pay received by men and women is at the heart of controversy over comparable worth. From a global perspective, it is true that women earn substantially less than men. Some argue that this situation is largely a reflection of wage discrimination. The fundamental problem, as identified by Henderson,[13] is "that when women dominate an occupational field, the rates of pay for jobs within those occupations appear to be unfairly depressed when compared with the pay men receive in jobs where they are the dominant incumbents within the occupational field." The workforce in clinical laboratories, composed predominantly of women, is a reasonable example.

The Equal Employment Act cited earlier addresses this specific issue by enforcing *equal* (not comparable) pay for comparable *work* (not worth).[13] If charged with wage discrimination under the Act, a defendant must demonstrate that pay differences result from seniority, merit, or quality or quantity of work.

A number of studies have attempted to unravel the comparable worth and wage discrimination issues. Muller and colleagues examined the effect of the concentration of female employees within select hospital jobs on wage rates while statistically controlling for differences in the "comparable worth" of various jobs.[20] Medical technologist and laboratory aide were among the 40 hospital positions selected for study. They concluded that hospitals do systematically apply job evaluation criteria in establishing salary levels for job categories, and that small but significant pay inequities exist between jobs held predominantly by men and those held predominantly by women. They report that a wage discrimination interpretation is consistent with their findings and encourage continued work with compensation systems to eliminate pay inequities.

EMPLOYEE BENEFITS AND SERVICES

In 1982, the Chamber of Commerce of the United States of America calculated that total employee benefits as a percentage of payroll were 36.7%. These benefits are a popular form of compensation because they are not currently subject to income tax. Based on the percentage of payroll represented by benefits and the popularity of this portion of the compensation package, laboratory managers are encouraged to study options available in their institution. The reader will note that many of the benefits are mandated by legislation cited earlier. The purpose of this section is to display the range of benefits and services in categories.[13]

Disability Income Protection

Insurance coverage is frequently provided by the employer to ensure continued income in the event of an accident or health-related problem. Major components of this category include the following:

Short-term disability or sickness and accident plans

Long-term disability

Workers' compensation in the form of occupational disability insurance

Nonoccupational disability (temporary disability resulting from injury or illness that is not job related

Social security

Travel accident insurance

Sick leave when an employee is unable to work because of illness

Supplemental disability insurance

Accidental death and dismemberment

Group life insurance with total permanent disability

Disability retirement option

Benezra[6] found that 91% of clinical laboratory employers offered paid life insurance, and 99% offered paid sick leave. Pension plans were offered by 89% of laboratory employers.

Loss-of-Job Income Continuation

Benefits in this category are designed to assist employees during short-term periods of unemployment resulting from layoffs or termination,[13] for example:

Unemployment insurance

Supplemental unemployment benefit insurance

Guaranteed annual income (usually in unionized laboratories)

Individual account plan to set aside a portion of income

Severance pay

Job contract for senior-level management

Short-term compensation program

Spouse and Family Income Protection

Many of the components identified under the disability income protection category have provisions for caring for dependents and survivors of the employee in case of his death.

Health and Accident Protection

Health-care insurance benefits cover medical, surgical, and hospital bills resulting from illness or an accident. These may include the following[13]:

Basic medical, hospital, and surgical insurance

Major medical coverage

Comprehensive physical examinations

In-house medical services

Post-retirement medical services

Comprehensive health plan or HMO

Workers' compensation medical benefits

Dental care benefits

Vision care

Hearing aid plan

Medicare in the Social Security program

For this category of benefits, Benezra found 98% of employers offering paid medical insurance and 71% offering a dental plan.[6]

Property and Liability Protection

Only recently have employers begun to provide employees with personal property and liability protection, including[13] group auto, group home, group legal, group umbrella liability, employee liability, and fidelity bond insurance. In clinical laboratories, many employers provide group umbrella liability insurance.

Pay for Time Not Worked

One of the less recognized benefits is time off with pay. The more common time-off opportunities during which employees continue to receive their daily base rate pay include holidays, vacations, jury duty, maternity leave, witness in court, military duty, funeral leave, time off to vote, and time off for blood donation.[13] Although virtually all laboratories afford full-time, regularly scheduled employees paid holidays and vacation, only 84% in Benezra's survey provided paid maternity leave.[6]

Income Equivalent Payments/Reimbursements for Incurred Expenses

Some employers offer education subsidies, child-care services, subsidized food service, physical awareness and fitness programs, social and recreational opportunities, parking, clothing allowances, emergency loans, and credit unions.[13] Under current cost-containment efforts, education subsidies appear to be declining, although in 1987 employers were still paying 84% of seminar and workshop expenses and 72% of paid employee tuition.[6] Other types of compensation in this category were less frequently paid: parking, 39%; uniforms, 27%; professional membership dues, 26%; child day care, 13%; laundry allowance, 12%; and meal allowance, 10%.[6]

Deferred Compensation

Deferred compensation plans have become increasingly popular in recent years. Such plans allow temporary exclusion of a portion of gross income from taxation until it is paid out in the retirement years. Because not all deferred compensation arrangements are tax exempt, employers and managers must carefully analyze the attributes of qualified, nonqualified, and Section 403(b) plans (tax-sheltered annuities).[13]

EMPLOYEE INCENTIVE SYSTEMS BASED ON MERIT

Employee incentive systems are pay plans that reward individuals or work groups for outstanding productivity.[18] Basically, with this approach, technologists or managers are compensated above the normal rate for specific activities such as cost control, improved output, or creativity in handling a particular situation.[29] Five aspects of incentive programs are essential[12]: (1) incentive plans require a total organization commitment; (2) such plans do not substitute for employee supervision; (3) employees must have faith in their employers; (4) cost-consciousness must be a top priority of the organization; and (5) incentive plans need to be carefully implemented.

For an employee incentive system to be implemented, performance must be based on appraisals with measurable performance standards directly linked to responsibilities in each employee's job description. Barrows[4] offers the following steps in developing an employee incentive system based on merit:

1. *Define the system.* The merit system must be first completely conceptualized, published, and then explained to employees, probably in group meetings. The anticipated objectives of the system must be clearly spelled out so that its accomplishments are measurable. Employees will need to understand the benefits of such a system to both themselves and management.

2. *Build a foundation.* Since the system relies heavily on job related responsibilities, it is likely that position descriptions will need careful review and even adjustment. A job analysis or reanalysis may be necessary.

3. *Establish performance standards.* While the position description states what is to be done, the performance standards include criteria for how it is to be done.[5,10] Standards should include such terminology as "consistently uses," "not more than two occurrences," or "80% of the time" to specify expectations on such activities as turnaround time and equality and quantity of work.

4. *Be consistent with institution's job classifications.* It is important that the revised position descriptions and performance standards adhere to the job classification system as described in this chapter, and that the system does not violate the institution's job classification system.

5. *Set up a scale for performance appraisal.* A scale for evaluation of work needs to differentiate among unacceptable performance—"consistently has not met expectations in all major areas of responsibility," marginal performance needing significant improvement—"not fully met expectations in areas of responsibility," expected average performance—"has consistently met and occasionally exceeded expectations in all major areas," above-average performance—"has consistently exceeded expectations in most areas," and outstanding performance—"has far exceeded expectations in all major areas."

6. *Determine salary increases.* The final step is determining how much merit pay is to be added beyond the usual increase (cost-of-living increases or other adjustments). Barrows suggests using a point system for each of the job responsibilities evaluated in step 5 to provide a quantitative basis for calculating salary increases.

Although salary adjustments are calculated at the time of performance appraisal in a merit plan, it is advisable to hold separate meetings between the supervisor and employee to discuss the performance review and the pay adjustment.[27] If a discussion of both of these elements occurs simultaneously, some employees will listen only to the part about their salaries at the expense of the performance review comments; others will tend to become argumentative about the appraisal rating because it is tied to the salary adjustment. In the same situation, managers tend to inflate ratings to avoid a confrontation about why an employee's performance does not warrant a merit adjustment. Also, managers may tend to rush through the process to "get it over with" or focus on employee weaknesses, rather than accomplishments. All of these characteristics negate the goal of employee development in the performance appraisal process.

The literature reports more than a dozen hospitals that have successfully implemented incentive plans.[24] Benefits to these institutions include decreased turnover, increased productivity, decreased overtime, decreased sick time, decreased work hours, increased communication with employees, improved management control systems, increased cash, and above-area average employee compensation.[24] Problems have also been reported: objective performance data is difficult to compile for some positions; aggressive and assertive staff are more likely to be rewarded than more passive co-workers; and evaluators may overrate performance to sidestep an unpleasant confrontation.[28]

One final observation by Umiker on the value of seniority raises is worthy of note.[26] When studying the question of when a laboratory employee reaches his peak job performance, he found that job performance usually improved during the first 5 years of employment before reaching a plateau. This plateau often lasted until the tenth year of employment, followed by another gradual upward swing. Upon further investigation, he found this latter improvement was based on the employee being assigned some additional challenge, promoted, or put in charge of a new procedure. He concludes that raises during the first years of employment based on a seniority system are justified.

PAYROLL ACCOUNTING

The purpose of a payroll accounting system is to document compensation costs incurred in providing laboratory services. Payroll records are also maintained by personnel departments for federal, state and local tax purposes and to maintain employment history and service files. For the latter, a W-4 form must be filed by all new employees for calculation of income tax withholding exemptions. A payroll accounting system must have a clear-cut procedure for recording and reporting time worked, including attendance, scheduled work hours, and overtime authorization.[23] Managers are typically involved in the timekeeping function of hourly employees; payroll deduction activities for Social Security tax, income tax, and other deductions are handled by the personnel department.

Recording the Payroll

A payroll journal or register maintained by the laboratory manager is a helpful accounting tool.[22] Figure 28-5 illustrates a department payroll journal that documents for each employee the hours worked, salary paid, overtime approved, sick days used, vacation days taken, and holidays and other days used for a given month. The journal shows that for the maximum 171 hours worked in November, all employees were paid a holiday, one employee took 2 days of sick time, one employee took 1 day of vacation, and two employees were paid time-and-a-half (overtime) for working the holiday. This journal helps managers keep abreast of salary expenses incurred.

Payroll-Related Costs

As evident in Figure 28-5, a number of payroll-related cost elements enter into the labor cost calculations beyond the basic earnings of hourly and salaried employees. These include overtime, vacation and sick pay, and holiday pay. Overtime premium pay, as provided for under the Fair Labor Standards Act of 1938, is earned at time-and-a-half for hours worked in a given week in excess of 40 hours. While the figure shows vacation and sick pay as an expense during the actual month it was paid out, Seawall[23] recommends charging the expense over the entire year, the period during which the pay is earned. Not evident in Figure 28-5 are other payroll-related costs that would normally be included in a journal kept in the personnel department, such as payroll taxes, workmen's compensation, life and hospitalization insurance, and pension and retirement plans.[23]

Donated Services

For institutions operated by or affiliated with a religious group, it may be necessary to record donated services.[23] Volunteers who transport laboratory specimens or reports are, for example, providing donated services. These services, work without monetary compensation, are recorded at fair market value if there is an equivalent employer/employee relationship and there is an objective basis for calculating the amount that might otherwise be paid for this service.

ARRANGEMENTS FOR COMPENSATING PHYSICIANS

Recent legislation, written to regulate and monitor the financial activity of the health-care industry, has attempted to influence arrangements for compensating physicians, primarily in hospital settings. The American Hospital Association has determined that hospital-based physician remuneration as a percent of total hospital operating costs ranges from 5.45% in hospitals of less than 50 beds to 9.22% in teaching hospitals of less than 400 beds.[2]

The key factor governing all compensation arrangements with hospital-based physicians is whether the Internal Revenue Service views the arrangement as creating employee status or independent contractor status for the physician. Tax ratings set forth four criteria for determining physicians' employee status[25]: (1) the degree to which the physician is integrated into the operating organization of the hospital for which the services are performed; (2) the substantial nature, regularity, and continuity of the individual's work for such hospital; (3) the authority vested in or reserved by the hospital to require compliance with its general policies; and (4) the degree to which the physician is accorded the rights and privileges the hospital provides its employees. These criteria are met if the physician is on a fixed salary or salary range and hospital policy prevents the physician from employing associate physicians or substitutes and prevents the physician from engaging in private practice.

Basic Arrangements

While fixed salaries or percentage contracts are the foundation for most physician compensation arrangements, various other components such as fringe benefits packages and retirement plans are often included. Remuneration modes can be classified as follows[16,25]:

1. *Fixed compensation salary.* As described above, this arrangement treats the physician as an employee, and a physician is compensated for administrative and teaching services for patient-care services.
2. *Percentage of income.* An arrangement may be made that compensates the physician with a predetermined percentage of other gross receipts minus adjustments (uncollectible accounts, and so forth) or net income (revenue after deductions for direct and indirect expenses). These arrangements typically specify minimum and maximum compensation limits.
3. *Fee for service.* This arrangement compensates the physician for each unit of service rendered. Billing may be either by the institution from which the physician receives a portion or by the physician directly.
4. *Department leasing.* A physician may lease equipment and/or space from the institution while providing a service. In this case, the patient is billed directly by the physician. Lease fees are then paid from revenues received by the physician.
5. *Combination arrangements.* Other arrangements incorporate a minimum guaranteed income plus some form of incentive compensation.

When reimbursement for different types of services are provided from different sources, accountability becomes a key issue.

Setting Physicians' Fees

While many institutions have historically set fees for services based on a local community average, consideration currently must be given to the demand for services and inputs required in providing those sources.[16] Glaser[11] suggests that the following areas need addressing when one is setting physicians' fees:

Cost of services rendered
  Expenses incurred (office expense, capital equipment, and so forth)
  Time involved
Patient demand
  Number of patients
  Each patient's ability to pay
Value of service rendered
  Success or failure
  Severity of disease
  Complexity of treatment
Customary fees in the community

Third-Party Reimbursement Aspects of Physician Compensation

Third-party reimbursement concepts are of significant importance to both the laboratory manager and physician provider. Third parties are agencies such as insurance companies or Medicare that pay for services consumed by their constituents. The current Medicare system has marked similarity to various other cost payers like Blue Cross and Blue Shield plans. Under Medicare, physician compensation arrangements include "fixed" and "variable" types.[16]

Fixed methods. Most fixed methods require that the provider bill for the physician's services. This billing includes both the provider and professional service components.

Variable methods. By this method, the physician may bill through the provider or bill the patient directly.

Compensation components are divided into two parts: A, administration and supervision of professional services rendered; and B, direct professional service rendered in patient care.

Physicians' Reasonable and Customary Charges

Provider-based physicians, those whose practice allows for the physician to be compensated for services from billings by the provider, are compensated upon reasonable and customary charges under Part B, professional service. The schedule of charges for Part B must approximate the actual net payments to physicians for their professional service. Three possible methods exist for establishing a schedule of charges: optimal, item-by-item, and *per diem*.[16]

Optimal. By this method, the provider determines the professional component for all services rendered to patients. This is accomplished by applying a uniform percentage to the providers' total charges. This method is particularly well suited for clinical laboratories and pathologist remuneration, because most of the pathologist's services cannot be directly traced to specific patients; service is therefore classified as Part A. The percentage of gross or net charges constitute Part A remuneration, and Part B is calculated separately (Fig. 28-6).

Item-by-item. This method identifies a separate professional charge for each service rendered. Figure 28-7 illustrates how each specific charge relates to the type of procedure. This method obtains a charge rate for Part B service similar to that used when a physician charges separately from charges by the provider.

Per diem. This third method is used when a schedule of charges has all-inclusive rate structures. A fixed compensation arrangement can be made for all inpatient and outpatient services.

SUMMARY

This chapter has introduced the terminology, processes, and procedures in wage and salary administration of importance to laboratory managers. The reward system was globally described in terms of compensation and noncompensation dimensions. Select legislation governing compensation administration was identified. Costs associated with selecting and developing employees were delineated, as well as costs incurred in employee turnover. Two financial strategies, personnel budgeting and payroll accounting, were described as methods for planning for and controlling costs associated with

The Uniform Optional Percentage

1	2	3	4	5	
		Estimated Gross	*Uniform*	*Approved*	
	Part B	*Department*	*Optional*		
Department	Amount	Charges	Percentage	Carrier	Intermediary
Pathology	$14,800	$200,000	7.5[1]		

Divide Column 2 by Column 3 to obtain the uniform optional percentage. This percentage is applied to all departmental billings and will yield in the aggregate an amount equal to the Part B amount (Column 2).
[1]Rounded to nearest ½ percent.
Source: Medicare Carriers Manual, HIM-14, §8099, Exh. 4; *Provider Reimbursement Manual,* Part I, HIM-15, §2108.11.

FIGURE 28-6. Optimal method for establishing physicians' charges.

Alternate Item-by-Item Method

					Pathology Department		
1	2	3	4	5	6		
Procedure	Professional Component Percentage	Part B Compensation	Estimated Procedures (Annual)	Part B Component Charges	Approved		
						Carrier	Intermediary
M	15%	$2,220	1,100	$ 2.00			
N	10	1,480	200	7.50			
O	5	740	55	13.50			
P	20	2,960	300	10.00			
Q	25	3,700	1,700	2.00			
R	5	740	100	7.50			
S	10	1,480	150	10.00			
T	10	1,480	200	7.50			
	(100%)						
	Total	$14,800					

Column 2: Professional Component Percentage—Show the percentage of time which the physicians collectively spend performing each procedure. (The total time spent should equal 100 percent of the time devoted to direct patient services.)
Column 3: Part B Compensation—Multiply the total amount ($14,800) by each percentage in Column 2.
Column 4: Estimated Annual Procedures—Estimate the number of times each procedure will be performed in the coming year.
Column 5: Part B Component Charges—The physician Part B charge is derived by dividing Column 3 by Column 4 rounded to nearest 50 cents.
Source: *Medicare Carriers Manual*, HIM-14, §8099, Exh. 6; *Provider Reimbursement Manual*, Part I, HIM-15, §2108.11.

FIGURE 28-7. Item-by-item method for establishing physicians' charges.

the human resource in the clinical laboratory. The process for developing a financial compensation system was described stepwise from job analysis to design of a pay structure. The range of employee benefits and services, 30% to 40% of payroll costs, was detailed. Managers are challenged to investigate positive outcomes possible by implementing an incentive-based rewards system. Finally, arrangements for compensating physicians were described.

REFERENCES

1. American Hospital Association: Chart of Accounts for Hospitals. Chicago, American Hospital Association, 1976
2. American Hospital Association: Physician remuneration has impact on hospital costs. Hospitals 51, No. 15:34, 1977
3. Analysis of Workers' Compensation Laws, p vii. Washington, DC: U.S. Chamber of Commerce, January 1980
4. Barros A: Setting up a system of pay for performance. MLO 18, No.11:40–45, 1986
5. Bachert LB: Performance standards for the transfusion service. MLO 19, No. 11:33–39, 1987
6. Benezra N: Lab salaries and benefits: Are they keeping pace? MLO 19, No. 1:30–34, 1987
7. Dillard JF: Human resource accounting, In Cleverly WO (ed): Handbook of Health Care Accounting and Finance, pp 223–236. Rockville, Aspen Systems Corporation, 1982
8. Esmond TH: Budgeting Procedures for Hospitals, pp 55–65. Chicago, American Hospital Association, 1982
9. Flamholtz EG: Human Resource Accounting, p 21. Encino, Dickensen, 1974
10. Garcia LS: Creating job standards for a merit pay plan. MLO 18, No. 10:30–36, 1986
11. Glaser WA: Paying the Doctor, p 7. Baltimore, Johns Hopkins Press, 1970
12. Groner DN: Employee incentives. Topics in Health Care Finance 3:63–86, 1977
13. Henderson RI: Compensation Management: Rewarding Performance, 4th ed, Reston, Reston Publishing Company, 1985
14. Heneman HG, Schwab DP, Fossum JA, et al: Managing Personnel and Human Resources: Strategies and Programs, pp 280–282. Homewood, Dow-Jones-Irwin, 1981
15. Herkimer AG: Understanding Hospital Financial Management, Germantown, Aspen Systems Corporation, 1978
16. Kaskiw EA, King PH, Morell JC, et al: Physician compensation. In Cleverly WO: Handbook of Health Care Accounting and Finance, pp 757–792. Rockville, Aspen Systems Corporation, 1982
17. Laliberty R, Christopher WI: Enhancing Productivity in Health Care Facilities, pp 109–121. Owings Mills, National Health Publishing, 1984
18. Levey S, Loomba NP: Health Care Administration: A Managerial Perspective, 2nd ed, pp 448–451. Philadelphia, JB Lippincott, 1984.
19. Liebler JG, Levine RE, Hyman HL: Management Principles for Health Professionals, pp 234–238. Rockville, Aspen Systems Corporation, 1984
20. Muller A, Vitali JJ, Brannon D: Wage differences and the concentration of women in hospital occupations. Health Care Management Review 12, No. 1:61–70, 1987
21. Santos A: Annual salaries of top managers to rise 4.7% in 1987. Hospitals 61, No. 9:52–57, 1987
22. Sattler J: A Practical Guide to Financial Management of the

Clinical Laboratory, pp 30–35. Oradell, Medical Economics Company, 1980

23. Seawall LV: Hospital Financial Accounting: Theory and Practice, 2nd ed, pp 193–202. Dubuque, Kendall/Hunt Publishing Company, 1987

24. Shyavitz L, Rosenbloom D, Conover L: Financial incentives for middle managers: Pilot program in an inner city, municipal teaching hospital. Health Care Management Review, 10, No. 3:37–44, 1985

25. Stevenson DK: Compensation of hospital-based physicians and key administrative employees. In Cleverly WO: Handbook of Health Care Accounting and Finance, pp 577–591. Rockville, Aspen Systems Corporation, 1982

26. Umiker WO: Pay raises: Merit or seniority? MLO 15, No. 9:63–68, 1983

27. Umiker WO: Salary talk: When and how? MLO 18, No. 4:43–44, 1986

28. Umiker WO, Yohe SM: How to make certain you get your merit increase. MLO 17, No. 1:77–80, 1985

29. Williams F: Employee incentive systems. In Cleverly WO: Handbook of Health Care Accounting and Finance, pp 395–412. Rockville, Aspen Systems Corporation, 1982

ANNOTATED BIBLIOGRAPHY

Cleverly WO (ed): Handbook of Health Care Accounting and Finance, Vol 1. Rockville, Aspen Systems Corporation, 1982

This handbook is a classic tome, rich in information regarding financial management in health-care institutions. Four specific chapters offer valuable insight regarding wage and salary administration, including: Chapter 12, "Human Resource Accounting"; Chapter 20, "Employee Incentive Systems"; Chapter 28, "Compensation of Hospital-Based Physicians and Key Administrative Employees"; and Chapter 36, "Physician Compensation."

Famularo JJ (ed): Handbook of Human Resources Administration, 2nd ed. New York, McGraw-Hill Book Company, 1986

This handbook contains eight chapters addressing wage and salary administration covering topics related to job evaluation and pay plans, compensation plans for executives, and establishing and maintaining a wage and salary program. An additional five chapters describe employee benefits.

Henderson RI: Compensation Management: Rewarding Performance, 4th ed. Reston, Reston Publishing Company, 1985

This resource provides a comprehensive discussion of work and rewards, identifying job content and determining pay, the compensation package, and managerial and professional compensation. Readers will find the following chapters useful: Chapter 3, "Government Influences"; Chapter 5, "Job Analysis"; Chapter 7, "Job Evaluation"; Chapter 8, "Compensable Factor Based Job Evaluation Methods"; Chapter 10, "Designing a Pay Structure"; and Chapter 11, "Employee Benefits and Services."

Metzger N: Personnel Administration in the Health Services Industry, 2nd ed. New York, Spectrum Publications, 1979

In this resource, Chapter 3, entitled "Job Evaluation and Wage and Salary Administration," offers a step-by-step approach to job evaluation using ranking, classification, and point methods. Guidance is provided for determining relative value of job factors and degrees.

Sattler J: A Practical Guide to Financial Management of the Clinical Laboratory, 2nd ed. Oradell, Medical Economics Company, 1986

Using a commonsense approach to financial management of the clinical laboratory, this resource provides practical guidance for setting up a system of accounting and record-keeping of personnel hours worked and salary. The author describes the application of basic accounting principles to the CAP work-load units system.

Seawell LV: Hospital Financial Accounting: Theory and Practice, 2nd ed. Dubuque, Kendall/Hunt Publishing Company, 1987

Written under the auspices of the Health Care Financial Management Association, this comprehensive text provides in-depth coverage of financial accounting as well as related management considerations. Chapter 8, entitled "Accounting for Hospital Expenses," includes valuable information regarding compilation of gross payrolls, payroll deduction, denoted services, payroll-related costs, and internal control documents.

twenty-nine

Laboratory Cost Accounting and Work-load Analysis

David W. Glenn

WORK-LOAD RECORDING

Purpose, Use, and History

A laboratory manager has many tools available to help him make decisions affecting the future existence and growth of the laboratory. As a staff medical technologist, he has quality-control statistics to help him assess the acceptability of patient results. Similarly, as a laboratory manager, he can use work-load statistics to measure laboratory productivity and forecast future needs. The College of American Pathologists (CAP) provides a work-load recording program that has received wide acceptance. Much of the information included in this chapter is based upon the CAP program and its laboratory work-load recording method, the definitive resource for work-load recording.

The CAP method is based on the approach used by Statistics Canada, developed by the Canadian Association of Pathologists in collaboration with other professional organizations. In 1970, CAP published the first edition of *A Workload Recording Method for Clinical Laboratories,* based largely on Canadian data. As CAP continued to increase and revised their data, refinements of their laboratory work-load recording method were published.

CAP work-load time studies use classic time-engineering techniques and a standard format for all procedures.

As procedures continue to change in the laboratory, CAP continues its testing. The assigning of new or changed work-load values has an inherent lag period, which must be tolerated by those using the method. As updates are published annually, the laboratory manager should obtain each new manual. This enables data to be revised to provide the most current and fair assessment of the laboratory's operation.

Terminology, time studies, and the use of work-load statistics are explained in detail in the CAP manual. The reader is instructed to consult the manual if more information than is presented here is required.

Terminology

CAP has assigned each test procedure a five-digit number. A three-digit suffix code is used following the basic five-digit code number to designate the analytic method or automated instrument.

Normally, the laboratory is divided into sections for the purpose of accumulating data for work-load analysis and cost accounting. The small laboratory may wish to count all the work load of the laboratory as one total. The large laboratory will usually assign sections based on work areas, such as chemistry, hematology, microbiology, and the other departments within the laboratory. Smaller sections, such as automated chemistry, electrophoresis, stat lab, and so forth, may be assigned according to specific needs.

Item for count defines for each procedure the entities to be counted. The counting method is standardized to eliminate ambiguity in deciding what constitutes one procedure. Most chemistry and hematology procedures are simply counted by test, such as glucose or hemoglobin. The microbiology procedures are not as easily counted. For example, a request for culture may signify very little work performed if there is no growth, or considerable work if numerous pathogens require identification. In cases such as this, individual test components (*e.g.,* plate, tube, specimen or slide) are counted. The manual lists all of the items for counting alphabetically and by laboratory section. *Raw count* is the tally of the items for count.

Unit value per procedure represents the mean number of laboratory work-load units (WLUs) required to perform the procedure once. Each unit is equivalent to 1 minute of technical, clerical, and aide time as defined by the time studies.

Unit values are based on the time required for the following:

Initial handling of the specimen includes receipt of the specimen by the laboratory, time-stamping the requisition, sorting specimens, logging the patient's name, assigning a laboratory number, preparing the work sheet, labeling the sample, loading the sample into and unloading the sample from a centrifuge, separating the serum/plasma, and delivering the sample to the work area. The time the specimen is spinning in the centrifuge or is being incubated is not included. The specimen collection time is not included, since this procedure has its own unit value.

Specimen testing time generally represents the least amount of time of all the areas measured. Specimen testing includes diluting the specimen, adding reagents, adjusting the analytical instrument, introducing the test into the instrument, taking readings, and removing the test from the instrument.

Recording and reporting time includes calculation of results, recording of results on report and laboratory record forms, checking, sorting, and filing of completed reports. Also included is time for telephone calls (incoming and outgoing) related to the initial report. This area of the time studies often represents the greater portion of the time studied.

Daily or routine preparation time includes only those activities that are routinely required but not repeated for each sample. This includes time for reconstitution of lyophilized controls, standards, or samples, and the dilution of stock standards. When an instrument is used, time required for cleaning, warm-up, calibration, and shut-down is included.

Maintenance and repair time includes scheduled and minor nonscheduled maintenance performed by laboratory staff. Major repairs and maintenance performed by nonlaboratory personnel are not included.

Solution preparation time includes reagent, solution, and quality-control material preparations that are required for the procedure.

Glassware wash-up time includes washing, drying, and sterilization of nondisposable supplies used in the procedure.

Technical supervision time includes technologist time for evaluating quality-control results and approving the reporting of results.

The time studies do not include the performance of standards or quality controls. These samples are counted separately in the raw count and are given the same unit value as a patient procedure. Serum/reagent blanks were included in the time studies and must not be counted as separate procedures.

Repeat and replicate are terms that must be understood by personnel using work-load recording. When a procedure must be performed a second time to solve a problem, it is counted as a *repeat.* A repeat is equivalent to one raw count and is customarily recorded in the QC column of the work-load recording work sheet. A repeat procedure has had all of the analytical, data handling, and recording steps repeated.

Some procedures (*e.g.,* radioimmunoassays) require duplicate performance of certain steps. When a procedure requires the multiple analysis of each specimen, it is considered a *replicate* analysis and part of the procedure. Replicates are not counted individually. Time for replicate analysis is included in the unit value time studies.

Collecting Data

The actual process of performing the work-load recording method can be broken down into four stages:

1. Divide the laboratory into function sections. The CAP work-load recording manual is based on nine laboratory sections. The laboratory manager is not locked into using these divisions. Rather, sections in the laboratory for work-load recording purposes should be defined to best meet the needs for assessing staffing and productivity.
2. Set up the user procedure file. List each of the procedures performed according to the sections designated in the above step. The unit value for each procedure is assigned on the basis of the lists in the CAP manual.
3. Choose a method for tallying raw counts. A computer can assist in tallying the work load, but the tally must be examined to see that it includes all standard, quality-control, and repeat tests performed. If the computer can give only the number of billed tests, this data must be augmented. The blood bank and microbiology sections are difficult to count for work-load recording, because these areas are not always counted per test but per specimen, bottle, plate, slide, and so forth. The more sophisticated computer programs allow entry of this data. Many systems do not, necessitating manual recording of this information. The work-load recording work sheet illustrated below may be very simple and record only "inpatient," "outpatient," and "other" tests; or it may be expanded to help monitor quality control, standard,

WORKLOAD RECORDING WORK SHEET

Laboratory Section _____ Month ____ Year _____

DAY	PROCEDURE / UNIT VALUE — IP	OP	OTH	PROCEDURE / UNIT VALUE — IP	OP	OTH	PROCEDURE / UNIT VALUE — IP	OP	OTH
1									
2									
3									
4									
5									
6									
7									
8									
9									
10									
11									
12									
13									
14									
15									
16									
17									

DAY	PROCEDURE / UNIT VALUE — IP	OP	OTH	PROCEDURE / UNIT VALUE — IP	OP	OTH	PROCEDURE / UNIT VALUE — IP	OP	OTH
18									
19									
20									
21									
22									
23									
24									
25									
26									
27									
28									
29									
30									
31									
RAW COUNT									
TOTAL									
WORKLOAD									

IP = Inpatient
OP = Outpatient
OTH = Other

repeat, emergency room, referral, interstate, and any other categories that may aid the laboratory management process. The most accurate method of manually recording work-load data is "as-you-go." Work-load recording forms are placed in each work area. When time allows during the day, the previous day's work load is recorded on a work-load recording work sheet.

4. Tally the data. Data are usually tallied at monthly intervals. However, if there exists a need for more frequent information, this step may be performed on a daily, weekly, or biweekly basis. The data are first collected by procedure. Then tallies for each section and the total laboratory are made. This allows the laboratory manager to evaluate productivity of a certain instrument or shift, since these data are easy to retrieve.

Some computer programs allow the manager to monitor and evaluate productivity of employees on an ongoing, daily basis. This information may be used in determining employee performance and may be useful in preparing job descriptions or setting individual productivity goals.

COST ACCOUNTING AND WORK-LOAD STATISTICS

The purpose of cost accounting is to identify the costs involved in a specific set of activities. This information is invaluable for budgeting, planning, fee-schedule construction, cost containment, and resource efficiency. Another important purpose of cost accounting is to provide the information necessary for third-party reimbursement. The intent of the CAP work-load recording method is to provide a standard, simple, and credible means of measuring laboratory activity. These data then provide the information needed for evaluating productivity and staffing needs.

Relative Value Units

The laboratory usually considers the laboratory test as its main product. The fee for tests must cover all of the direct and indirect costs assigned to the laboratory. One method for assigning costs in the laboratory is by test. Because of the great variation of costs associated with the different tests performed in the laboratory, a more equitable method is the use of relative value units (RVUs).

An RVU represents a standard for assigning costs. The RVU has a monetary value apportioned to it based on the costs associated with providing one RVU of product. If the only cost in the laboratory were for labor, one could simply accept time as the basis for the RVU. Assuming the cost for this labor was $1.00 per minute, we could define 1 RVU as 1 minute and equal to $1.00 cost. A laboratory test that required 15 RVU (15 min) would then cost $15.00. Laboratory costs contain many other costs in addition to labor; however, labor represents 60% to 70% of the direct costs in most laboratories.

Because of the need for a standardized method of determining and allocating costs in the laboratory, many hospital controllers have accepted the CAP work-load program and used the patient-charged WLUs as RVUs. There are several problems associated with the use of CAP WLUs as RVUs:

The CAP program was not designed for this purpose.

The CAP time studies do not include the professional time component and many other untimed activities. (See the section on specified productivity in this chapter.)

Some tests require more standards and controls per patient specimen than do other tests.

A wide variation of instrument and reagent costs per labor costs exists among the various laboratory procedures.

However, as this practice continues to grow in acceptance, it is expected that CAP will work more closely with the American Hospital Association and others to provide a more standardized and equitable means of using work-load data for accounting purposes.

Hospital Administrative Services MONITREND Report

The Hospital Administrative Services (HAS) is the division of the American Hospital Association that provides participating hospitals with computerized monthly reports of the hospital's activities and their relation to costs. The report generated by the HAS computer service is called MONITREND. The MONITREND report includes a section entitled "Laboratory-Blood Bank," of value to the laboratory supervisor in a hospital using the MONITREND statistics.

The MONITREND report uses CAP WLUs and finances provided by each participating hospital to provide individual institutions with their own monthly average of the following:

WLUs/adjusted patient day
Percent charged WLU/total WLUs
Revenue/100 WLUs
Direct expenses/adjusted patient day
Direct expense/100 WLUs
Salary expense/100 WLUs
Physician remuneration/100 WLUs
Ratio total direct expenses to revenue
Direct expense percent
Outpatient revenue percent
Paid hours/100 WLUs

The MONITREND report also provides group medians and averages of other participating hospitals for comparative purposes with regional, state, and national statistics. For these statistics to be meaningful and useful, each participant must use the CAP work-load recording method correctly. Because the MONITREND service is widely used and demonstrates the relationship between work-load recording and cost accounting, a brief example and description of the report follows. A more detailed presentation of this information is available.*

MONITREND Input

The hospital must submit total WLUs, broken down into two specific components: (1) WLUs for tests charged to patients and (2) all other WLUs. The hospital submitting data must be certain the charged WLUs do not represent charged *tests*. This could happen if a person were submitting data from billing activities and not using the work-load recording method. If the hospital does not bill for the collection of tests separately, the charged WLUs should not contain these work-load values. Other WLUs are all other procedures performed that were not charged to the patients. Other WLUs include quality controls, standards, repeats, noncharged specimen collection, hospital employee health tests, hospital environment infection-control tests, and research and development tests.

MONITREND Output

A laboratory ratio of charges to charges (RCC) may be calculated with

*The Laboratory Workload Recording Method MONITREND Focus, Vol I, No. 9. Chicago, Hospital Administrative Services, American Hospital Association, 1980.

Example of Hospital MONITREND Monthly Input for a Laboratory Blood Bank	
PAID HOURS	6800 hr
Direct expenses	
Salaries	$44,000
Other	$36,000
Physician remuneration	$17,000
REVENUE	
Inpatient revenue	$140,000
Outpatient revenue	$30,000
WLUs	
Charged WLUs	330,000 WLUs
Other WLUs	90,000 WLUs
TOTAL PATIENT DAYS	7000 days

$$RCC = \frac{\text{Lab inpatient revenues}}{\text{Lab inpatient revenues} + \text{Outpatient revenues}}$$

If the inpatient revenues are $140,000 and the outpatient revenues are $30,000, the RCC is

$$\frac{140,000}{140,000 + 30,000} = 0.8235$$

Thus, 82.35% of revenue is from inpatients. The next step is to determine the costs (direct and indirect) of the laboratory. (An example of the step-down analysis for assigning these costs is provided later in the chapter.) If total costs for the laboratory are determined to be $150,000, only $123,525 (82.35%) is associated with inpatient work.

The percent charged WLUs of total WLUs is calculated as

$$\frac{\text{Charged WLU}}{\text{Charged WLU} + \text{Other WLU}} \times 100$$

Using our example input, we can calculate

$$\frac{330,000 \text{ WLU}}{330,000 \text{ WLU} + 90,000 \text{ WLU}} \times 100 = 78.57\%$$

Charged WLUs represent 70% to 80% of total WLUs in many short-term, acute-care general hospitals. If a laboratory has a "stat" section, the percentage may be much lower. Stat tests often require that a standard and quality-control sample be run with only one patient sample. When batching is not possible, productivity falls.

The overall productivity of the laboratory can be followed by using paid hours per 100 WLUs.

$$\frac{\text{Lab paid hours}}{\text{Total WLUs} \div 100} = \frac{6,800 \text{ hr}}{4200} = 1.62 \text{ hr}/100 \text{ WLUs}$$

The paid hours per 100 WLUs value should be closely monitored. If the figure increases (productivity falls), the laboratory manager should evaluate the following possible reasons for the decreasing productivity:

Change in paid time off for employees

Old equipment requiring more maintenance time

Increased turnover of employees requiring greater orientation time

New regulations or requirements affecting staff time

Construction or other physical plant changes that impede productivity

Increase in stat work

Addition of new laboratory section, instrument, or testing, requiring a learning period before peak productivity is achieved

Lower laboratory work load without proper staff cutback

Independent Laboratories

The MONITREND report is available for hospital laboratories only. Independent laboratories must generate their own statistics and cost-accounting techniques. One major difference between hospital laboratory costs and independent laboratory costs is the advantage the independent laboratory realizes by not having a high percentage of indirect hospital-allocated costs. This reflects the independent laboratory's decreased need for costs associated with tissue analysis and pathologist consultations. Independent laboratories do not have to absorb the high cost of providing stat procedures and are able to take advantage of larger batches. Since the independent laboratories receive specimens collected by the submitting party, the cost of specimen collection is reduced or avoided. Hospital laboratories must provide special services such as environmental cultures for infection control and cumulative record-keeping for tests performed on all patients. Again, the independent laboratory avoids or minimizes these additional costs.

Step-down Accounting Method

Regardless of the type of laboratory situation, the step-down accounting method is appropriate. In the hospital laboratory the manager will not be responsible for determining overhead (hospital-allocated) costs. The hospital controller will provide that data. However, the laboratory manager may be required to help provide information regarding the assignment of direct costs to the proper cost centers in the laboratory. If you are a manager of an independent laboratory, you may have responsibility for performing many of the duties performed by hospital controllers in determining and apportioning direct and overhead costs.

The following list provides a basic picture of the step-down accounting method.

Have at hand the laboratory's cost and revenue figures, including all direct and indirect costs the laboratory must recover. Traditionally, the laboratory supervisor has not always been privy to the total expense and revenue figures for the laboratory. The laboratory supervisor was expected to control costs only. The survival of a laboratory is dependent not on how much it saves, but on how well it can produce a profit. Today, the laboratory manager must be prepared to deal with greater fiscal responsibility in the laboratory. Without access to the total expense and revenue figures for the laboratory, only limited efforts can be made to manage cost effectively.

Define cost centers. There are two types of cost centers in the laboratory: revenue-producing cost centers and non-revenue-producing cost centers. Revenue-producing cost centers in the laboratory have charged WLUs associated with the work produced by that center. In the example shown in Table 29-1, the major sections of the laboratory, including chemistry, hematology, microbiology, blood bank, and anatomic pathology, represent the revenue-producing cost centers. The non-revenue-producing cost centers are laboratory administration, glassware wash-up, media preparation, and physician remuneration.

Consider salaries. Salaries often represent 60% to 70% of the direct costs in a laboratory. The fringe benefits must also be considered a cost for labor. In some hospital laboratories, the cost of fringe benefits is included in the hospital allocation of overhead costs to the laboratory. The cost of fringe benefits such as FICA, retirement plan, health insurance, life insurance, and workman's compensation is very high (often equal to 15% to 20% of the salary).

Consider equipment costs. Equipment costs include the cost of purchase, lease or rental, depreciation, and costs for maintenance and repair. The

Table 29-1
Example of Laboratory Direct Costs

| | Revenue-Producing Cost Centers | | | | |
	Chem	Hema	Micro	Blood Bank	Path
Salaries	$180,000	$116,000	$ 86,000	$58,000	$70,000
Equipment	30,000	15,000	8000	4000	9000
Supplies	38,000	21,000	18,000	12,000	13,000
Other	6000	4000	2000	2000	6000
Subtotal	$254,000	$156,000	$114,000	$76,000	$98,000

| | Nonrevenue-Producing Cost Centers | | | |
	Lab Admin	Glassware	Media	Physicians
Salaries	$ 80,000	$ 8000	$14,000	$220,000
Equipment	30,000	3000	1000	
Supplies	20,000	2000	3000	
Other expenses	6000			
Subtotal	$136,000	$13,000	$18,000	$220,000

higher a hospital presents its costs to third-party reimbursers, the better are its chances of receiving the highest allowable reimbursement. To prevent a rapid depreciation of equipment, resulting in very high equipment costs, Medicare has established a conservative schedule for the depreciation of equipment that must be used by those seeking Medicare reimbursement. When projecting the cost of maintaining analytical equipment not covered by a service contract, a rule-of-thumb estimate commonly used is 10% of the original purchase price per year. Recently, several major instrument manufacturers have begun to use 15%.

Consider supplies. Supply costs include office supplies, reagents, pipettes, tubes, slides, laboratory report and request forms, and all other consumables used in the laboratory; other expenses are for continuing education, library, or any other items that are directly related to the laboratory and not included in one of the above groups.

Consider laboratory administration costs, which include the salaries of the laboratory manager, secretaries, clerks, and other personnel not directly associated with the performance of charged work-load units within a specific revenue-producing cost center. The cost of appro-

priate office equipment, supplies, and the laboratory computer are included in this section. Glassware wash-up and medium preparation costs include salaries, supplies, and equipment costs associated with providing these services.

Consider physician remuneration costs. At this time, the system of hospital-based pathologist remuneration is being examined by the federal government. Currently, some hospitals hire the pathologist, others work out contractual agreements, and some hospitals pay on a fee-for-service basis.

Accumulate direct costs. This is a very difficult task and represents the bulk of work in performing cost accounting.

Apportion nonrevenue costs to the revenue-producing cost centers. Table 29-2 shows laboratory administration costs apportioned to each department based on its percentage of the total costs of the revenue-producing centers. The apportionment of glassware, medium, and physician costs is done according to use of these services by each revenue center. One should strive to apportion these costs as fairly as possible to provide a true representation of where costs actually belong. This information becomes vital when one is establishing test fees.

Table 29-2
Example of Laboratory Nonrevenue Cost-Center Apportionment

		Revenue-Producing Cost Centers				
		Chem	Hema	Micro	Blood Bank	Path
Revenue center direct costs		$254,000	$156,000	$114,000	$ 76,000	$ 98,000
Nonrevenue center direct costs						
Lab administration	$136,000	50,000	30,000	22,000	15,000	19,000
Glassware	13,000	9000	1500	1500		1000
Media	18,000	2000		14,000	2000	
Physician	220,000	24,000	14,000	10,000	7000	165,000
Total apportioned direct costs		$339,000	$201,000	$161,500	$100,000	$283,000

Allocate overhead (hospital) costs. The costs of housekeeping, maintenance, building depreciation, and utilities, among other overhead costs, are commonly allocated to the laboratory on the basis of the amount of square footage the laboratory occupies. For this reason, hospitals occasionally try to give the laboratory large amounts of storage space to increase the allocation of allowable costs for reimbursement purposes. Table 29-3 is an example of the allocation of these expenses to each of the revenue centers.

Consider personnel department and food service costs, which are often allocated to the laboratory on the basis of the number of employees in the laboratory. Purchasing department costs are normally allocated on the basis of the percentage of the total purchases handled by the purchasing department made by the laboratory. The costs of the medical records department, hospital computer service, and other central administration costs may be allocated according to the percentage of the laboratory direct costs as compared with the total hospital direct costs. The method for allocation of these costs is often determined by third-party reimbursers. Table 29-3 also shows the allocation of overhead costs and the basis of their allocation.

Fee-Setting by the Macro-Approach

Once the step-down allocation of costs is completed, the patient-charged CAP WLUs can be applied to the costs and used as RVUs (Table 29-4). In the example of the MONITREND statistics given earlier in this chapter, one could calculate the cost/RVU based on total laboratory costs and patient-charged WLUs. By performing the step-down allocation for each department in the laboratory, the laboratory manager has a more equitable basis for setting fees by RVU. This macro-approach can be refined by defining more revenue-producing cost centers for the laboratory. There comes a point, however, when the time spent defining and allocating costs to a multitude of laboratory revenue-producing cost centers becomes counterproductive. Thus, one should establish the minimum number of cost centers in the laboratory that are essential for equitable fee-setting.

Fee-Setting by the Micro-Approach

Today's laboratory manager receives a plethora of computer data concerning labor hours, labor costs, and material costs. A systematic approach to cost analysis is made easier with this information. Many very good cost-analysis computer programs exist. They are most helpful in providing rapid, easy calculations regarding projections based on instrument, labor, and other cost changes or revenue changes the laboratory manager may be considering.

The total cost per test can be determined by adding together the cost per test of direct and indirect labor and direct and indirect materials, equipment costs, and overhead expenses. (See page 466 and the summary on page 467.)

Direct labor costs include the costs of technical personnel who actually perform the testing. By di-

Table 29-3
Example of Allocation of Overhead Costs

Indirect Costs — Amount		Allocation Basis	Lab Revenue-Producing Centers				
			Chem	Hema	Micro	Blood Bank	Path
Building maintenance and depreciation housekeeping and utilities	$340,000	Square footage	$120,000	$ 50,000	$ 68,000	$ 34,000	$ 68,000
Personnel department; food services	65,000	Personnel	26,000	14,500	10,500	5500	8500
Purchasing	45,000	% Purchases	18,000	10,000	7000	4000	6000
Central administration	280,000	% Direct cost	87,500	52,000	42,000	26,000	72,500
Total overhead costs			251,500	126,500	127,500	69,500	155,000
Total direct costs			339,000	201,500	161,500	100,000	283,000
Total allocated costs			$590,500	$328,000	$289,000	$169,500	$438,000

viding the annual cost of technical labor by the annual total of WLUs performed, one derives the direct labor cost per WLU. If a new test is being evaluated, the direct labor cost per test is computed by multiplying the WLUs for the new test by the direct labor cost per WLU.

Indirect labor costs represent the cost of all other lab support and supervisory personnel costs. The indirect labor costs are calculated by dividing the total cost of support and supervisory

personnel by the total WLUs and then multiplying the result by the number of WLUs for the individual test.

Indirect materials costs encompass the costs of shared equipment and supplies that cannot be directly allocated to individual tests. The costs of the laboratory computer system, centrifuges, refrigerators, and office equipment and supplies are included in this area. The cost per test is calculated by dividing the annual cost of indi-

Table 29-4
The Relationship Between Total Cost and Patient Work-load Units

	Revenue-Producing Centers				
	Chem	Hema	Micro	Blood Bank	Path
Total costs	$590,000	$328,000	$289,000	$169,500	$438,000
Charged WLUs	480,000	340,000	320,000	200,000	310,000
Cost per RVU	$1.23	$0.96	$0.90	$0.85	$1.41

Equipment Costs

Equipment Description	a Replacement Value	b Useful Life	c Annual PM Contract	d Annual Tests	Cost [(a/b)+c]/d
Analyzer	$11,900	7 yr	$1,200	840	$3.45
Pipettor	$ 950	7 yr	—	840	$ .16
Total Equipment Cost					$3.61

rect materials by the laboratory's annual WLU volume and then multiplying this by the number of WLUs for the individual test.

Overhead costs include the hospital's allocation for utilities, housekeeping, administration, and other costs, including profit if it is an invester-owned facility. Some hospitals require that the laboratory multiply the total laboratory-related costs by an overhead factor to calculate the allowance for overhead costs when pricing new tests. Other hospitals will assign a fixed cost to be recovered by the laboratory. In this case, the overhead costs can be allocated by dividing the total overhead costs by the total WLU volume and assigning the cost per WLU.

A simplified example of this micro-approach follows:

A laboratory has been sending the XYZ test to a reference laboratory. The test volume has reached a point where the laboratory manager decides to evaluate the cost-effectiveness of performing the test in his own laboratory. The laboratory anticipates performing 528 patient tests and 312 other tests (standards, controls, repeats), for an annual total of 840. The XYZ analyzer has been assigned 2 WLUs per test.

The hospital controller provides the following data:

Chemistry Section: Annual Costs

Direct labor	$0.38/WLU
Indirect labor	$80,000
Indirect materials	$56,000
Annual overhead	$251,000
Annual WLU volume	480,000

Using the calculations explained above and the Equipment Costs and Materials Costs forms, the laboratory manager is able to derive the costs in the following Test Cost Analysis Summary:

Materials Costs

Item Description	a Unit Cost	b Items/Unit	c Items/Test	Cost (a/b) x c
Reagents	$33.67	100	1	$ .34
Calibrator	$21.00	1,000	1	$ .02
Sample Cups	$17.50	1,000	1	$ .02
Pipette Tips	$31.00	1,000	1	$ .03
Disposable Cuvettes	$ 9.75	100	1	$ .10
Total Materials Costs				$ .51

Test Cost Analysis Summary

Direct labor	$0.76
Indirect labor	0.34
Direct materials	0.51
Indirect materials	0.24
Equipment	3.61
Overhead	1.05
Total costs	$6.51
Cost/patient test*	$10.33

Because only 528 (63%) of the total 840 tests can be billed to patients, the actual test cost per patient billable test is $10.33. If the hospital had not built its profit or contribution into the overhead allotment of costs, this would have to be added. Before pricing the test, the laboratory manager must also consider fixed third-party reimbursement, his bad-debt rate for laboratory fees, competitive pressures, and whether it would be more cost-effective to continue sending the test to a reference laboratory.

If the lab manager had only calculated costs based on the macro-approach, 2 RVUs × $1.23, a test cost of only $2.46 would have been established. However, the XYZ test requires dedicated equipment at a higher cost per test than most tests performed in the laboratory. The test volume is rather low, and a high ratio of nonpatient to patient tests exists. Thus the micro-approach is most useful in evaluating new procedure costs prior to committing to performing them in-house.

REVENUE. If revenue falls short of costs because of a high bad-debt rate or a low reimbursement rate, fees would have to be adjusted upward to recover loss.

OTHER USES OF WORK-LOAD ANALYSIS

The purpose of the CAP work-load recording program is not to provide a mechanism for cost accounting. The original objective was to provide a standard, credible, and simple means for measuring laboratory activity. The data collected from the CAP work-load recording method can be used in evaluating productivity, determining staffing needs, computing the labor component of test costs, comparing the costs of the two methods, determining cost-ef-

$$*\text{Cost/patient test} = \frac{\text{Cost/test} = \text{Total test volume}}{\text{Patient test volume}}$$

fective instrument operation, assessing space needs, and identifying problem areas.

Evaluating Productivity

Each laboratory manager must define acceptable productivity. No two laboratories are exactly alike. Thus, it is very difficult to state an ideal productivity rate. The laboratory manager must first determine the current productivity rate for the laboratory. Then this rate must be monitored, and action taken to prevent a lowering in productivity. There are three ways to view productivity: (1) as related to paid man-hours, (2) as related to worked man-hours, and (3) as related to specified man-hours.

Paid Productivity

Even though 1 CAP unit is equivalent to 1 minute of time, no person is able to achieve 60 WLUs/hr paid (100% productivity). Paid absentee time is usually 10% to 20% of total paid time. This is dependent on the employee's benefits, including paid vacations and holidays, paid sick time, paid time away from the laboratory (e.g., continuing education, jury duty, personal leave), and overtime hours actually worked. Each laboratory's benefits and employee use of sick leave will vary. The amount of overtime must be controlled. When overtime is paid at the customary time-and-a-half rate, every paid hour of overtime includes pay for 30 minutes of time not worked.

Paid hours represent the entire personnel burden in the laboratory, excluding only the laboratory physicians, doctoral-level clinical scientists, and students. All paid time, productive or nonproductive, must be included. The institution's payroll clerk can provide the number of paid hours needed for this calculation:

$$\text{Paid productivity} = \frac{\text{Total WLUs}}{\text{Total paid hours}}$$

Paid productivity is the most commonly used measure to determine cost-effective use of personnel. To calculate the paid productivity of each section in the laboratory, the manager needs to apportion the time of department-shared supervisors and clerks by allocating their time to the various departments (similar to the step-down method used for allocating costs). An example of paid-productivity calculation follows.

Paid Productivity Example

If a laboratory section employs five full-time equivalents (FTEs) and produces a total of 460,000 WLUs annually, the paid productivity rate is 73.7%.

Total paid time
$$= (8 \text{ hr/day} \times 5 \text{ days/wk}) \times 52 \text{ wk/yr} = 2080 \text{ hr}$$

$$\text{Paid productivity} = \frac{\text{WLUs/yr}}{\text{Total paid hr/yr}}$$

Paid productivity
$$= \frac{460{,}000 \text{ WLUs}}{2080 \text{ hr/FTE} \times 5 \text{ FTE}} = 44.2 \text{ WLUs/ paid hr}$$

$$\frac{44.2 \text{ WLUs/paid hr}}{60 \text{ min/paid hr}} \times 100 = 73.7\% \text{ paid productivity}$$

At the time of this printing, the CAP reported the median paid productivity ranged from 34 to 36 units per paid hour for community hospitals and from 31 to 35 units per paid hour in university and other teaching hospitals.

Because of the wide discrepancy of laboratory situations, it is often useful for the laboratory supervisor to present productivity to administration as worked and specified productivity as well as paid productivity. This will help justify what may at first appear to be an unacceptable paid productivity. On the other hand, the calculation of paid, worked, and specified productivity may objectively show the need to reduce personnel.

Worked Productivity

Total worked hours are the total paid hours minus the total paid hours not worked (*e.g.,* paid vacations, holidays, sick leave, continuing education leave). These figures should also be available from the payroll clerk.

$$\text{Worked productivity} = \frac{\text{Total WLUs/yr}}{\text{Total worked hr/yr}}$$

Worked productivity will naturally be higher than paid productivity. However, worked productivity will never reach 100%. If it does, either (1) the work-load data is incorrect, or (2) the staff is overproducing at a rate considered hazardous to quality. Many laboratorians set a goal of 50–52 units per worked hour. The worked productivity is often the best way for management to evaluate the laboratory's labor productivity. See the Worked Productivity Example that follows.

Worked Productivity Example

IF the five FTEs in a laboratory section each annually average 15 days vacation, 10 holidays, and 6 sick-leave days, worked productivity is 83.7%.

Total paid time/FTE/yr	2080 hr
Minus nonworked paid hr/FTE/yr	
Vacation (15 days $\times$ 8 hr/day)	120 hr
Holidays (10 days $\times$ 8 hr/day)	80 hr
Sick leave (6 days $\times$ 8 hr/day)	48 hr
Nonworked paid time/FTE/yr	248 hr
Total worked hr/FTE (2080 − 248)	1832 hr

$$\text{Worked productivity} = \frac{\text{Total WLUs}}{\text{Total worked hours}}$$

$$\text{Worked productivity} = \frac{460{,}000 \text{ WLUs}}{9160 \text{ hr } (1832 \times 5 \text{ FTEs})}$$

$$\text{Worked productivity} = 50.2 \text{ WLU/hr}$$

$$\text{Worked productivity} = \frac{50.2 \text{ WLU/hr}}{60 \text{ min}} \times 100 = 83.7\%$$

Specified Productivity

A list of the items included in the CAP time studies was presented earlier in this chapter. There are many other activities performed by the laboratory personnel that are not part of the CAP work-load unit time. These activities include:

Laboratory administrative duties, such as compiling work-load statistics, budgeting, recruiting, orientation, discipline, performance evaluation, and employee scheduling

Lunch and coffee breaks mandated by law or contract

Education of others in formal programs, such as residency or medical technology schools

Accounting, billing, and related activities

Purchasing and procurement time, including sales visits, demonstrations, and the inventory of supplies

Computer activities

Clerical support, mail handling, photocopying, typing letters, courier activities

Clearly identified research and development

Grouped in-service education, bench training, lecture

Laboratory staff meetings and other meetings including safety committee, infection control committee, and consultations with pathologists and other specialists

Preparation of reports such as a tumor registry, transfusion reactions for utilization review, and similar activities

Morgue activities and decedent affairs

Laboratory procedures that do not have a unit value assigned

Any other activities not included in the CAP time studies

The CAP manual includes a "Non-Specified Hours Weekly Worksheet" and a "Laboratory Staffing Analysis Employee Diary," which are valuable in collecting data for studying specified productivity.

Total specified hours are total worked hours less all paid hours for untimed activities.

$$\text{Specified productivity} = \frac{\text{Total WLUs}}{\text{Total specified hours}}$$

If specified productivity is over 100% and no work-load recording errors are evident, more personnel are indicated. Demanding 100% or higher productivity forces employees to take shortcuts, and the quality of patient care will suffer.

Determining Staffing Needs

One of the most common uses of work-load recording is in determining the number of FTEs required to perform the laboratory's work load. The easiest way is to use last year's work-load figures and change them by the percentage of change forecast. For example, if one anticipates a 5% increase in work, the current total of FTEs is multiplied by 1.05 for determining the FTEs required to undertake the increased work load. This approach is valid only if (1) the work-load recording method has been used for several years and the data obtained is acceptable, (2) the laboratory's present rate of productivity is satisfactory, and (3) the forecast change in work load is reasonably accurate.

If one wishes to increase paid productivity by 5%, it will be necessary to either reduce paid hours by 5% or increase volume by 5% without allowing a concurrent increase in paid hours beyond the present level. By performing worked- and specified-productivity studies, the laboratory manager can identify areas in the laboratory where change is needed. By studying productivity of various work shifts, he may discover ways to reorganize work load or personnel in such a manner as to allow a reduction in paid hours. The work-load recording program and productivity studies provide an objective approach for determining staffing needs. Otherwise, the manager has only a subjective feeling about whether the lab is understaffed or overstaffed.

Computing the Labor Component of Test Costs

The cost of labor in the laboratory is often 60% to 70% of total direct costs. Before performing a cost-effectiveness study, the manager must know the labor cost of performing a WLU in the laboratory.

Specified Productivity Example

Assume the five FTEs each average 30 minutes of breaks per day, 30 minutes of staff meeting time per month, and 1 hour of inservice education per month. In addition, the administrative time included in the five FTEs time totals 10 hours per week. Purchasing functions require an extra 4 hours per month.

SPECIFIED TIME

Breaks
(0.5 hr/day × 229 days/yr × 5 FTEs)
572.5 hr/yr

Meetings
(0.5 hr/mo × 12 mo × 5 FTEs)   30 hr/yr

In-service
(1 hr/mo × 12 mo × 5 FTEs)   60 hr/yr

Administrative
(10 hr/wk × 49 wk)   490 hr/yr
1152.5 hr/yr

TOTAL UNTIMED HOURS

Total worked hours   9160 hr/yr
Total untimed hours   152.5 hr/yr
Total specified hours   8007.5 hr/yr

$$\text{Specified productivity} = \frac{\text{Total WLUs/yr}}{\text{Total specified hr/yr}}$$

$$\text{Specified productivity} = \frac{460{,}000 \text{ WLUs}}{8007.5 \text{ hr}} = 57.4 \text{ WLUs/hr}$$

$$\text{Specified productivity} = \frac{57.4 \text{ WLU/hr}}{60 \text{ min/hr}} = 95.7\%$$

Cost accounting by the macro-approach and the micro-approach demonstrate how each laboratory procedure is unique. The macro-approach compares patient-charged WLUs with total costs. The macro-approach does not appreciate the relationship of a procedure's work-load time to its individual reagent, instrument, or nonpatient (standard and controls) requirements.

When performing a cost-effectiveness study, it is necessary to know the labor cost of the WLU in the laboratory. If the laboratory participates in the MONITREND service, the cost of salary expense/100 WLUs is supplied. If this figure is $14.20, divide by 100 to obtain the WLU cost of $0.142.

Laboratories that are not using MONITREND can divide the total WLUs for a time period into the cost of laboratory technical, clerical, aide, and appropriate laboratory administrative (excluding physicians) pay for the same period. Because of the variation of productivity from month to month in many laboratories, a calculation should usually not be based on less than 3 months' data. If the laboratory performed 412,500 WLUs in 3 months, and the cost for laboratory salaries (excluding physicians) for that period was $58,575, the laboratory labor cost per WLU is $58,575 divided by 412,500 WLUs, or $0.142/WLU.

Comparing the Cost-Effectiveness of Two Methods

When justifying the acquisition of new equipment to administration, the manager should be aware that the speed, accuracy, and precision of the new equipment does not carry as much weight as does the bottom-line figure of how much the new method will cost and how much revenue it will generate.

Automated equipment is able to reduce the cost of labor in the laboratory (Table 29-5). However, before the cost of automated equipment can be justified, one must perform a sufficiently large work load to reach the break-even point and surpass it to show a profit. Naturally, the instrument manufacturer's sales personnel will be eager to share this information with you. Unfortunately, the sales representative's figures often suggest that unreasonably small work loads are adequate to justify the equipment purchase. Thus, the ultimate responsibility for realistically evaluating the cost falls to the laboratory manager.

You will find the following formula useful when comparing two methods to determine the volume of tests to reach break-even. Break-even occurs when

$$A_1(X) + B_1 = A_2(X) + B_2$$

where A_1 = Variable costs per test of method 1, X = Break-even volume, B_1 = Total fixed costs of method 1, A_2 = Variable costs per test method 2, B_2 = Total fixed costs of method 2.

To perform this comparison, you must know the annual fixed and variable costs associated with each method. The institution-allocated indirect costs and the laboratory cost center's indirect costs are fixed. These indirect costs are the same for each method being compared.

The fixed direct costs for each method will not be the same. They include the cost of equipment depreciation and maintenance for that particular method. The variable costs for each method will depend upon the method's direct costs for labor, reagents, and disposable supplies.

As an example of how this cost comparison method can be used, consider a laboratory situation where 6300 12-test chemistry profiles are being performed annually. This laboratory wishes to purchase a semiautomated analyzer. A cost study and determination of break-even volume are needed.

Table 29-5

Unit Values for 12 Commonly Performed Chemistry Tests with Manual and Semiautomated Equipment

Test	Manual Unit Value	Semiautomated Unit Value
Glucose	8	4
Urea	8	4
Uric acid	10	4
Calcium	14	4
Phosphorus	10	4
T. bilirubin	15	6
T. protein	12	4
Albumin	12	4
Cholesterol	8	6
SGOT	10	4
LDH	10	4
CPK	13	4
Total	130	52

Work Sheet for Comparing Cost-Effectiveness of Two Methods

PROCEDURE <u>Chem. 12-Test Profile</u>

METHOD 1 <u>Manual</u>

VARIABLE COSTS PER TEST

Direct labor	$18.46	
Reagents and Supplies	7.04	
Total variable costs per test........	A$_1$ $25.50	

FIXED COSTS

Institution-allocated indirect	$22,000	
Cost center indirect	6,800	
Equipment depreciation	860	
Equipment maintenance	400	
Total fixed costs	B$_1$ $30,060	

METHOD 2   <u>Semi-Automated</u>

VARIABLE COSTS PER TEST

Direct labor	$7.38	
Reagents and supplies	4.55	
Total variable costs per test........	A$_2$ $11.93	

FIXED COSTS

Institution-allocated indirect	$22,000	
Cost center indirect	6,800	
Equipment depreciation	3,571	
Equipment maintenance	2,500	
Total fixed costs	B$_2$ $34,871	

The laboratory's institution-allocated costs for this cost center total $22,000, the laboratory cost center's indirect costs $6800. The direct labor cost of each WLU in this laboratory is $0.142. Thus, the direct labor cost for performing a manual profile is $18.46 (130 × $0.142). The direct labor cost for performing the same profile on semiautomated equipment is $7.38 (52 × $0.142). The purchase price of the new semiautomated equipment is $25,000, depreciated over 7 years at an annual cost of $3571. The maintenance cost per year is $2500.

The reagent and disposable supplies cost is $2.55 per profile. Using the break-even formula

$$A_1(X) + B_1 = A_2(X) + B_2$$

we find

$$25.50(X) + 30,060 = 11.93(X) + 34,871$$
$$13.57(X) = 4811$$
$$(X) = 355$$

Thus, 355 profiles must be performed annually to reach the break-even point. Since this laboratory is currently performing 6300 profiles annually, the semiautomated equipment is justified.

Determining Cost-Effective Instrument Operation

The break-even formula is useful for performing cost studies when the purchase of new equipment is questioned. But often a laboratory has more than one instrument available for performing the same test. One of the most cost-effective means of controlling costs in the laboratory is using the proper procedures and instruments for testing at the proper times. The cost of performing stat tests will always be unproductive when compared with batching of samples. However, serving the acutely ill patient often requires immediate performance of a test. If one determines the most cost-effective means of performing such a test, it is possible to make the best of a bad economic situation without lowering the quality of patient care or wasting money.

By comparing the variable direct costs of labor, reagents, supplies, and equipment for the different instruments used in the laboratory that are capable of performing the same tests, the manager can determine the most cost-effective use of the alternatives available.

In the following discussion, the labor, reagent, supply, and instrument costs of performing a stat glucose on a semiautomated analyzer are compared with the respective costs on a discrete automated analyzer. Because the instruments are already in the laboratory and being used for many different tests, instrument depreciation and maintenance costs per test are based on current volume. The instrument costs for depreciation and maintenance are calculated per test by dividing the total of these two costs by the number of tests performed on the instrument annually.

Assume the semiautomated equipment requires a minimum of one zero calibrater, one standard, and one control per test run. Thus, if only one stat patient test is performed, an additional three nonpatient tests must also be performed. The discrete analyzer needs to be calibrated only once every 90 days (manufacturer- and government-approved). In addition, the discrete analyzer requires only two control determinations each 8-hour shift. The WLU value for the semiautomated procedure is 4, and the WLU value for the discrete analyzer is 3. The cost per WLU in this laboratory is $0.142. These data, as well as the reagent and disposable supply costs per test, are summarized in Table 29-6.

The summary indicates that the semiautomated instrument is the most cost-effective for stat glucose assays. However, this is deceiving. The most cost-effective method is dependent on how many stat glucose tests are performed per 8-hour shift. For instance, if another stat glucose test were performed within the 8-hour shift, the semiautomated cost ($3.37) would remain the same, since all the work would be repeated. With the discrete analyzer, which requires that only the single patient test be performed, the cost is $2.64 for the second stat glu-

cose assay (Table 29-7). Batching of samples brings a different conclusion. Table 29-8 shows the cost of performing different volumes of glucose runs with the same data.

Identifying Problem Areas

By calculating work-load productivity for each department, work station, instrument, or procedure, one can monitor efficiency and identify areas needing improvement. Without work-load statistics, the

Table 29-7
Cost Comparison of Performing Each Additional Glucose Assay

	Semiautomated	Discrete Analyzer
Labor	$0.57	$0.43
Reagents	.39	.85
Instrument	.31	1.36
Total	$1.27	$2.64

Table 29-6
Cost Comparison of Stat Glucose Assays Done on Semiautomated Equipment and Discrete Analyzer

	Semiautomated	Discrete Analyzer
WLU	4	3
Work load per run		
Zeroes	1	0
Standards	1	0.1*
Controls	1	2
Patient	1	1
Total	4	3.1
Labor cost ($0.142/WLU)	$0.57	$0.43
Reagent and supply cost/test	0.39	0.85
Total reagent and supply cost	1.56	2.64
Instrument cost/test	0.31	1.36
Total instrument cost	1.24	4.22
Cost per stat run	$3.37	$7.29

*Nine standards are used to calibrate every 90 days: $9 \div 90 = 0.1$/day.

Table 29-8

Labor, Supply, and Instrument Cost of Glucose Assays

Patient/Run	Semiautomated	Discrete Analyzer
1	$3.37	$ 7.29
2	4.64	9.93
3	5.91	12.57
5	8.45	17.85

manager might devote time and effort to areas that seem inefficient but actually are not. One should collect several months' data to avoid seasonal variation.

It is possible to carry work-load recording even farther by keeping track of repeats separately as a measure of efficiency in the automated chemistry department. Table 29-9 shows that increased numbers of repeat analyses occurred in the period February through April. Failure to perform necessary preventive maintenance was identified as the cause. Resumption of adequate preventive maintenance by the end of April resulted in a return of repeats to expected levels.

The many uses of work-load analysis are continually growing. CAP presents workshops concerning the work-load recording method and laboratory management. These workshops are valuable to those who are initially instituting the method or to those already using the method who wish to obtain updated information.

ANNOTATED BIBLIOGRAPHY

American Hospital Association: The laboratory workload recording method. MONITREND Focus, Vol 1, No. 9., 1980

Balkonis BJ: How to perform CAP workload recording method time studies. Pathologist 34:10, 1980

The CAP time studies editor describes the time studies and gives examples of the flow charts and work sheets used in the studies.

Bean K: Marketing and Managing the Clinical Laboratory Workshop. AMST Region IV Meeting, Columbus, Ohio, October 1985

This presentation focused on the information found in Fee-Setting by the Micro-Approach. The Department of Management Planning and Analysis division of The Ohio State University Hospitals developed this format.

Bennington JL (ed): Financial Management of the Clinical Laboratory. Baltimore, University Park Press, 1974

This source begins with an overview of cost analysis and proceeds to give examples of test price analysis, equipment purchase decisions, budgeting, and forecasting.

Bennington JL (ed): Management and Cost Control Techniques for the Clinical Laboratory. Baltimore, University Park Press, 1977

This book is especially good at relating fiscal management with the overall management of the laboratory. Chapter 9 gives good examples of cost analysis and discusses the problems with third-party reimbursement.

College of American Pathologists: Manual for Laboratory Workload Recording Method. Skokie, College of American Pathologists, 1987

The lists of workload unit values, description of terms, and the directions for use of the method make this manual essential to the student and user.

Hannon GT, Koger SE: Developing a cost accounting system for a group practice lab. MLO 11:43, October 1979

This source provides an example of one method used to allocate costs in a nonhospital laboratory.

Johnson JL: Reimbursement: The paradox of federal policy. MLO 12:55, February 1980

This article clearly describes the differences in costs between hospital and independent laboratories. Examples of these costs are presented. An excellent graphic presentation of the cost comparisons is especially interesting.

Krieg AF, Israel M, Gink R, et al: An approach to cost analysis of clinical laboratory services. Am J Clin Pathol 69:525, 1978

A detailed presentation of data acquisition and allocation. Elaborate formulas are offered for the allocation of costs within the laboratory.

McCutchen G: Space Allocation Guidelines for the Clinical Laboratory. J Med Technol 2:12, 1985

This article discusses the use of work-load recording data for determining space needs in the laboratory.

Table 29-9

Breakdown of Analyses in Automated Chemistry Department

Month	% Patient Tests	% Controls	% Standards	% Repeats
January	72.5	12.9	9.6	4.8
February	70.1	13.2	9.8	6.9
March	67.4	14.1	10.3	8.2
April	62.3	16.2	11.7	9.8
May	71.9	13.1	9.7	5.3
June	72.1	13.0	9.6	5.3

Reed LB: Assessing productivity and staffing through workload recording. MLO 11:147, September 1979
> This source discusses productivity calculations using an efficiency adjustment formula. A useful article for those having difficulty determining staffing based on workload data.

Robinson TC: Cost Analysis Module—Management in the Clinical Laboratory. Manual for Cost Accounting and Cost Benefit Analysis Workshop, University of Kentucky at Lexington, 1981
> This workshop and manual present a detailed example of the step-down allocation method and work-load data used to calculate cost by relative value units.

Templin JL Jr: Specified hours: A new approach to calculating productivity. MLO 12, No. 6:83–92, 1980
> This article presents a brief description and example of specified productivity.

thirty

Financial Ratios for Laboratory Management Decision-making

James W. Sharp

NEW GOALS AND CHALLENGES

The Tax Equity Fiscal Responsibility Act (TEFRA), passed in 1982, ushered in a new operating environment for hospital clinical laboratories. Before TEFRA, the goal of the clinical laboratory was to provide quality laboratory services in a timely fashion. Now the goal is to provide quality, timely laboratory services in a cost-effective manner.[6]

The shift in emphasis has created new challenges. And new challenges require new resources. Today's laboratory decision-makers need a thorough understanding of laboratory economics, as well as access to detailed quantitative cost data. The purposes of this chapter are twofold: first, to present an overview of an effective laboratory information management system; second, to demonstrate how this system provides the essential data necessary to make critical operational and functional management decisions.

Most businesses are split into marketing and sales, production and manufacturing, and accounting and finances.[3] The marketing and sales division identifies the need for a product and its likely markets; the manufacturing people are responsible for efficiently producing the product; and the financial division sees that the products are produced, marketed, and sold at a profit.

Similarly, a clinical laboratory has three functional divisions (Fig. 30-1). In the laboratory, the marketing and sales function is called utilization and is controlled by the physicians on the medical staff. By ordering laboratory tests to diagnose disease and monitor therapy, for example, physicians ultimately determine the number and types of tests processed and performed in the laboratory.

The type of clinical tests performed by the laboratory range from the simple, highly automated, routine chemistry tests, to the complex, esoteric, labor intensive, low-volume hormone assays. The physician sets the service-level requirements for each test. For example, a test may be ordered in a "stat" mode with a 2-hour turnaround-time require-

FIGURE 30-1. Interrelationships among three laboratory divisions.

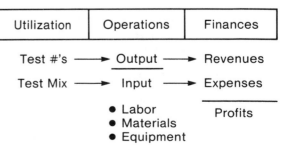

Hospital Clinical Laboratory

Utilization	Operations	Finances

Test #'s ——→ Output ——→ Revenues

Test Mix ——→ Input ——→ Expenses

- Labor
- Materials
- Equipment

Profits

ment, or it may be ordered in a "routine" mode with a 24-hour turnaround time. Because it is more expensive for the laboratory to provide the rapid service, physicians control, to a large extent, laboratory costs.

The operations, or production, division of the laboratory processes and produces the test results. This division is under the control of the laboratory director or the laboratory manager. These individuals are charged to produce the physician-requested output (laboratory tests), using an efficient combination of input factors (labor materials, and equipment).

The hospital administrator controls the financial side of the laboratory. Decisions about test prices affect laboratory revenues, and decisions about employee pay policies affect laboratory expenses. Therefore, the hospital administrator determines the laboratory's profit or gross margin (excess of revenues over expenses).

Figure 30-1 shows the interrelationships between the three laboratory divisions. Decisions made in one sphere have an impact on the other two. For example, a financial decision to raise test prices made by the administrator might cause a decrease in the number of tests physicians order and lead to an overall decrease, rather than an increase, in revenues. In addition, the "productivity" of the laboratory would suffer because it would be doing fewer tests.

THE THREE-STEP PROCESS

Managing a clinical laboratory is a three-step process. The manager first sets appropriate and realistic goals, then develops a system for evaluating and measuring progress toward those goals, and finally takes corrective action when necessary.

Laboratory goals and objectives are arrived at through a strategic planning process. In strategic planning, certain external, environmental factors and internal, laboratory factors are examined and analyzed.[3] A thorough analysis of the external factors uncovers the opportunities and constraints in the current economic climate. Internal factor analysis identifies the strengths and weaknesses of the laboratory. The strengths and weaknesses are matched with the opportunities and constraints, and appropriate goals and objectives are determined.

Some of the environmental factors examined are the impact of recent legislation on laboratory activities, current economic trends, projected industry growth rates, impact of new technologies, local competition, and community expectations.[2]

For example, an analysis of recent legislative activity might reveal that an increasing number of hospital patients are covered by fixed-rate insurance, such as diagnosis-related groups (DRGs), health maintenance organizations (HMOs), or prospective payment organizations, (PPOs). This means that a significant percentage of laboratory tests are reimbursed at a set rate regardless of the laboratory's charges for these services. This severely limits the effectiveness of the strategy of increasing test prices to raise revenues.

An analysis of economic trends and industry growth rates suggests that the population is growing older. Older patients are usually "sicker," and sicker patients require more laboratory tests. This suggests that laboratory test volume should continue to increase. However, the business community complains about the high cost of health insurance premiums it pays for its employees. This is a powerful downward force tending to negate the upward pull of an aging population of health-care resources and laboratory test volume.

Another trend is the shift of patient care from the hospital environment to home health-care centers and outpatient surgery units. There is a parallel shift of laboratory testing from the hospital laboratory to physician's offices.[5] What percentage of hospital laboratory tests will eventually be affected by these shifts? What are the long-range effects of these trends on laboratory revenues?

Every day new and less expensive method of performing laboratory tests are introduced by various manufacturers. Physicians—and even patients—are encouraged by these manufacturers to perform more and more diagnostic testing themselves. This trend in technology will probably continue and serve to further erode the test bases of the large hospital laboratories.

The large commercial laboratories see much opportunity in the changing times. These giants are actively competing with hospital and physicians' office laboratories for a shrinking number of laboratory tests. This intense competition is causing a downward trend in test prices, further squeezing already tight operating margins. In addition, the commercial laboratories are offering to manage entire laboratories for hospital clients.[4] This raises questions regarding the adequacy of the quality and service of laboratory testing.

The feelings and expectations of the local community also affect laboratory decision-making. For example, does the community expect its hospital to provide complete medical coverage because it is the only hospital in town? If this is so, then the laboratory will be forced to provide a wider variety of tests and services than is economically prudent.

Internal factor analysis involves studying the

laboratory's management and organizational structure, its type and use of labor, and its financial condition. For example, an analysis of the organizational and management structure may reveal that the laboratory lacks the ability to respond to the demands and provide the levels of service requested by the medical staff. Or the analysis might reveal that because there is no method of calculating data on resource utilization and distributing it to the appropriate section supervisors, labor and supply costs are higher than expected.

It is important to analyze the work force, because labor costs are the largest budget item. An analysis of the work force may reveal that the majority of the technolgists are specialized and capable of working only in certain areas of the laboratory. This lack of flexibility means that it takes more full-time equivalents (FTEs) to adequately staff the laboratory. If, because of unionism or other outside forces, laboratory salaries are artificially inflated, cost-reduction strategies will be only marginally successful.

The financial condition of the hospital and laboratory is important in formulating short- and long-term goals. Although a particular strategy may make sense, capital is needed for implementation. The options available to a cash-poor laboratory are limited.

After the external and internal analyses are concluded, goals and objectives are set. What are reasonable laboratory goals and objectives? Since TEFRA, the survival strategy of most hospitals is clear—increase revenues or decrease costs. For the laboratory, increasing revenues means marketing laboratory tests to new, previously untapped sources. Decreasing costs involves lowering laboratory operating expenses. The two strategies are mutually incompatible. That is, a hospital or laboratory must choose one or the other—not both.

For example, marketing laboratory tests to physician offices, nursing homes, and local HMOs should increase revenues. If successful, this strategy will also increase laboratory costs. Costs rise because new resources are needed to implement the strategy. A marketing and sales person is needed to approach potential customers. Computer equipment is needed to streamline test ordering and billing. Automated analyzers may be required to speed test processing. All these items increase costs. It is hoped that the increase in revenues will outstrip the increase in costs.

The point is, it is not possible for the laboratory to compete for the outside business unless it is given the resources to carry out the job. In this case, the laboratory goals of increasing test volume while lowering costs are clearly incompatible.

It would not be realistic for a laboratory to define as a goal increasing test volume if the external analysis revealed that the surrounding commercial laboratory competition was great and the internal analysis revealed that the laboratory lacked the equipment to process large volumes of tests efficiently. Similarly, it makes no sense to set as a goal a reduction in the ordering by physicians of esoteric, expensive tests if the hospital is a teaching or research center. In this case, the hospital's mission directly conflicts with the cost-reduction strategy. It is very important that all three laboratory divisions communicate clearly and decide upon mutually compatible goals and objectives.

Once the laboratory's goals and objectives are defined, a system should be developed that helps the laboratory manager measure and evaluate progress toward the goals. This management system should accomplish several tasks, including tracking the flow of laboratory revenues and expenses, providing useful data to the proper management person in a timely fashion, and comparing the laboratory's performance against some accepted standards of productivity and efficiency.[7]

From an operational viewpoint, the system should be easy to implement, be inexpensive to operate, and have the flexibility of expanding or contracting to meet the needs of a large or small laboratory. The management system presented here provides a series of ratios that measure laboratory performance over time. Charting and watching the ratios enables the laboratory manager to detect trends and potential trouble spots that need correction or improvement.

Calculating the ratios involves cost-accounting the basic units of laboratory output. But what are the basic units of laboratory output? If the function of the laboratory is to provide physicians with medical information concerning their patients, then the output is an intangible measurement of a physiologic or pathologic parameter in a patient's body fluids or tissues. These intangible measurements or units of information are the laboratory "tests." Therefore, the finished product or output is the test result or billable procedure. A billable procedure is a "finished" test result charged or billed to a patient or third-party payer.

After the output is defined, all laboratory costs and expenses are related to this unit. For example, labor expense is described as labor cost per billable procedure, and supply expenses are described as supply cost per billable procedure. The ratios are charted or graphed on a monthly basis and provide a means of tracking laboratory performance.

Similarly, utilization data are described in terms of the billable procedure. For example, billable tests per patient day, or billable procedure per patient admission are ratios for evaluating the medical staff's laboratory utilization patterns.

Before we set out to develop the system, we need to collect the appropriate statistics and financial data. All needed data are collected from the hospital admitting office, business office, or laboratory department management reports. Once the data are gathered, the laboratory is "modeled."

Modeling the laboratory means breaking down the laboratory into its component parts. Most clinical laboratories can be viewed at the level of the total laboratory, the laboratory subsection, or the individual cost centers within each subsection (Fig. 30-2). The object of the game is to trace all laboratory revenues and expenses through each of the three levels. Ultimately a portion of these expenses is allocated to each unit of laboratory output—the billable procedure.

This may seem an overwhelming task, but it can be accomplished with a few hours' work with a calculator or computer spreadsheet. Figure 30-2 shows that our sample hospital is organized along traditional lines into six major subsections or production centers. These subsections are chemistry, hematology, microbiology, blood banking, serology, and anatomic. The cost centers within each subsection are also listed.

Tables 30-1, 30-2, and 30-3 are examples of budgets or operating statements for each of the three levels. It is easy to figure the direct labor costs or technical personnel costs for each department. One simply counts the number of technical staff members in each department and lists their total

Table 30-1
Example of Hospital Laboratory Budget (Level-1)

Revenues	$9,172,526
Expenses	
Salaries	
Technical labor	$1,668,365
Nontechnical labor	
Lab receptionists	$197,680
Administrative	$114,525
Nites	$119,873
Phlebotomists	$314,490
Path secretaries	$128,804
Professional fees	$1,286,906
Supplies	$1,498,399
Equipment	
Depreciation	$147,506
Service contracts	$105,643
Repairs	$40,842
Other	$115,475
Direct costs	$5,738,508
Indirect costs	$2,215,221
Total costs	$7,953,729
Net income	$1,218,797

FIGURE 30-2. Laboratory organization with six major production and cost centers.

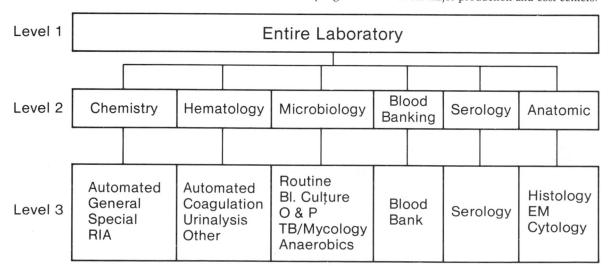

Level 1	Entire Laboratory					
Level 2	Chemistry	Hematology	Microbiology	Blood Banking	Serology	Anatomic
Level 3	Automated General Special RIA	Automated Coagulation Urinalysis Other	Routine Bl. Culture O & P TB/Mycology Anaerobics	Blood Bank	Serology	Histology EM Cytology

Table 30-2
Example of Hospital Laboratory Budget (Level-2)

	Microbiology	Blood Bank	Chemistry	Hematology	Anatomic	Serology
Revenues	$1,006,444	$1,002,114	$4,106,062	$1,457,584	$1,262,867	$337,455
Expenses						
Salaries						
Technical labor	$245,674	$237,429	$557,584	$352,500	$193,455	$81,723
Nontechnical labor						
Lab receptionists	$19,217	$13,440	$84,595	$61,845	$8,961	$9,622
Administrative	$11,133	$7,787	$49,011	$35,829	$5,190	$5,575
Nites	$0	$41,955	$35,962	$41,956	$0	$0
Phlebotomists	$46,002	$14,748	$131,439	$98,531	$4,453	$19,317
Path. secretaries	$12,932	$1,006	$6,333	$4,630	$103,183	$720
Professional fees	$98,215	$98,214	$210,636	$98,214	$683,413	$98,214
Supplies	$144,979	$332,708	$760,486	$140,793	$47,035	$72,398
Equipment						
Depreciation	$13,084	$9,768	$50,804	$45,802	$23,658	$4,390
Service contracts	$9,516	$2,088	$52,313	$32,459	$7,732	$1,535
Repairs	$2,375	$1,661	$10,452	$24,058	$1,107	$1,189
Other	$11,947	$7,796	$49,069	$35,883	$5,198	$5,582
Direct costs	$615,074	$768,600	$1,998,684	$972,500	$1,083,385	$300,265
Indirect costs	$298,183	$312,921	$740,798	$400,102	$340,721	$122,496
Total costs	$913,257	$1,081,521	$2,739,482	$1,372,602	$1,424,106	$422,761
Net income	$93,187	($79,407)	$1,366,580	$84,982	($161,239)	($85,306)

salaries. But what about the nontechnical salaries or indirect labor such as those for pathology secretaries, laboratory receptionists, and phlebotomists? They are not usually assigned to a particular area, but their work benefits the entire laboratory. How should their salaries be allocated?

To handle this step, we devise an allocation schedule. This schedule uses a formula for assigning the costs of the nontechnical personnel or indirect labor, the equipment expenses, professional fees to each subsection and cost center. The formula may differ for each group or item allocated; the only requirement is that it realistically reflect the department's use of that item. Following is a description of the budget line items and the formula used to allocate costs for the laboratory subsections and cost centers.

Revenues: The revenues were calculated by multiplying the procedure price by the number of procedures. The hospital business office supplied the current price list.

Technical labor: Technical labor includes the salary costs of the technologists and supervisors working in each laboratory department. Data were collected from the department time cards.

Laboratory receptionists: The salary costs for the laboratory receptionists were distributed on the basis of the procedure volume of each cost center. For example, if a cost center performed 6% of the laboratory's billable procedures, then 6% of the laboratory receptionists' salaries were distributed to that cost center.

Administration: This category includes the salaries of the laboratory manager, quality control officer, and research technologist. These costs were allocated in the same fashion as the laboratory receptionists costs.

Nites: This category includes the salaries of the night-time personnel. These costs were allocated on the basis of assignments of the night personnel in the specific cost centers.

(text continues on p 483)

Table 30-3
Example of Hospital Laboratory Budget (Level-3)

	Routine	Blood Culture	O & P	TB/Mycology	Anaerobic	Blood Bank
Revenues	$500,477	$276,144	$76,837	$53,435	$99,551	$1,002,114
Expenses						
Salaries						
Technical labor	$110,339	$50,571	$53,262	$12,180	$19,322	$237,429
Nontechnical labor						
Lab receptionists	$10,956	$3,577	$3,041	$944	$699	$13,440
Administrative	$6,347	$2,072	$1,762	$547	$405	$7,787
Nites	$0	$0	$0	$0	$0	$41,955
Phlebotomists	$23,324	$12,706	$6,481	$2,011	$1,480	$14,748
Path. secretaries	$7,621	$2,488	$2,115	$656	$52	$1,006
Professional fees	$55,995	$18,281	$15,542	$4,823	$3,574	$98,214
Supplies	$68,836	$54,514	$14,447	$3,887	$3,295	$332,708
Equipment						
Depreciation	$10,152	$1,907	$495	$371	$159	$9,768
Service contracts	$8,152	$556	$512	$187	$109	$2,088
Repairs	$1,354	$442	$376	$117	$86	$1,661
Other	$6,355	$2,075	$1,764	$347	$1,406	$7,796
Direct costs	$309,431	$149,189	$99,797	$26,070	$30,587	$768,600
Indirect costs	$146,707	$50,364	$46,228	$33,339	$21,545	$312,921
Total costs	$456,138	$199,553	$146,025	$59,409	$52,132	$1,081,521
Net income	$44,339	$76,591	($69,188)	($5,974)	$47,419	($79,407)

Table 30-3 (Continued)

	Automated-Chem	General	RIAP	Special	Send Out
Revenues	$2,208,366	$907,008	$474,800	$237,368	$278,520
Expenses					
Salaries					
Technical labor	$202,072	$178,547	$69,863	$69,853	$37,249
Nontechnical labor					
Lab receptionists	$51,387	$18,555	$7,534	$2,495	$4,624
Administrative	$29,771	$10,750	$4,365	$1,446	$2,679
Nites	$35,962	$0	$0	$0	$0
Phlebotomists	$74,655	$29,115	$10,705	$3,620	$13,344
Path. secretaries	$3,847	$1,389	$564	$187	$346
Professional fees	$127,950	$46,201	$18,760	$6,213	$11,512
Supplies	$207,653	$198,851	$52,707	$24,474	$276,801
Equipment					
Depreciation	$23,144	$17,719	$3,068	$6,404	$469
Service contracts	$20,577	$23,165	$1,171	$6,682	$718
Repairs	$6,350	$2,293	$930	$308	$571
Other	$29,807	$10,763	$4,370	$1,447	$2,682
Direct costs	$813,175	$537,348	$174,037	$123,129	$350,995
Indirect costs	$289,980	$214,749	$80,638	$64,507	$90,924
Total costs	$1,103,155	$752,097	$254,675	$187,636	$441,919
Net income	$1,105,211	$154,911	$220,125	$49,732	($163,399)

(continued on page 482)

Table 30-3 (Continued)

	Automated-Hem.	Coagulation	Urinalysis	Other	Histology	Cytology	EM	Serology
Revenues	$791,497	$282,885	$281,229	$101,973	$1,115,168	$137,739	$30	$337,455
Expenses								
Salaries								
Technical labor	$157,859	$84,531	$87,592	$22,518	$130,589	$52,249	$10,617	$81,723
Nontechnical labor								
Lab receptionists	$34,355	$9,113	$14,370	$4,007	$7,117	$1,829	$15	$9,622
Administrative	$19,903	$5,280	$8,325	$2,321	$4,123	$1,059	$8	$5,575
Nites	$24,921	$6,611	$10,424	$0	$0	$0	$0	$0
Phlebotomists	$48,813	$13,242	$30,627	$5,849	$854	$3,547	$52	$19,317
Path. secretaries	$2,572	$682	$1,076	$300	$103,045	$137	$1	$720
Professional fees	$53,940	$14,308	$22,562	$7,404	$649,239	$34,174	$0	$98,214
Supplies	$62,021	$35,077	$33,815	$9,880	$39,134	$4,759	$3,142	$72,398
Equipment								
Depreciation	$34,267	$9,219	$1,457	$859	$10,254	$1,818	$11,586	$4,390
Service contracts	$23,427	$5,776	$2,233	$1,023	$3,141	$839	$3,752	$1,535
Repairs	$20,661	$1,126	$1,776	$495	$879	$226	$2	$1,189
Other	$19,928	$5,287	$8,344	$2,324	$4,129	$1,060	$9	$5,582
Direct costs	$502,667	$190,252	$222,601	$56,980	$952,504	$101,697	$29,184	$300,265
Indirect costs	$196,910	$76,399	$94,134	$32,659	$267,188	$46,245	$27,288	$122,496
Total costs	$699,577	$266,651	$316,735	$89,639	$1,219,692	$147,942	$56,472	$422,761
Net income	$91,920	$16,234	($35,506)	$12,334	($104,524)	($10,203)	($56,442)	($85,306)

Phlebotomists: This category includes the salaries of the individuals responsible for drawing blood and collecting the laboratory specimens. These costs were distributed by multiplying procedure volume by the estimated collection time per procedure in each cost center.

Path secretaries: This category includes the salaries of the individuals responsible for typing departmental reports. These costs were allocated on the basis of the percentage of time the secretaries type reports for each cost center.

Equipment depreciation: These costs were distributed on a specific basis for all major equipment items. For example, the depreciation cost of a chemistry analyzer was allocated to the chemistry department. All minor depreciation costs were distributed to the cost centers on the basis of procedure volume. Depreciation was calculated on a 5-year, straight-line basis.

Service contracts: These costs include the maintenance contracts for laboratory instruments. The costs were allocated to the specific cost center on the basis of department records. All general instrument maintenance contracts (*e.g.,* centrifuges) were distributed across all cost centers on a procedure volume basis.

Repairs: These costs are the costs of repairing specific instruments not covered by the maintenance contracts. The costs were allocated into the appropriate departments.

Other: This category includes the costs associated with travel, education, office supplies, dues, and fees. They were distributed on the basis of the procedure volume.

Supplies: These costs were distributed to the cost centers on the basis of data obtained from the laboratory cost ledgers.

Professional fees: This category includes the salaries of the pathologist and the clinical scientists. The costs were allocated to the costs centers on the basis of the amount of time the professionals spent in each center.

Indirect costs: This category includes employee benefits, building depreciation, operation of the plant, administration and general, housekeeping, cafeteria, and medical records. These costs were allocated on the basis of standard formulas provided by the hospital business office.

There is no standard allocation formula that applies to all laboratories. But each laboratory manager should be able to create accurate formulas for each item and department based on his knowledge of laboratory operations.

Next, the costs are tracked to the individual cost centers (Table 30-3). This is important because at this level the laboratory manager exerts control. That is, even if the manager cannot influence the physicians' patterns of test ordering, he can make sure that the tests, once ordered, are performed as efficiently and economically as possible.

In our sample hospital, the chemistry department is divided into five cost centers. Each cost center performs only certain types of procedures. For example, the automated cost center performs only electrolyte studies and automated chemical tests. When all the costs are allocated, it is possible to calculate the total cost of each type of test.

Operating ratios are tools that help in analyzing laboratory operations. These formulas highlight the relationships among laboratory variables. The ratios provide quantitative information about test ordering patterns, productivity, efficiency, resource utilization, and financial margins—data that help the manager control costs and improve service.

Figure 30-3 shows how the operating ratios are calculated. Table 30-4 shows how the ratios are applied to the chemistry department cost centers. The same format can be applied to the other laboratory cost centers.

The test utilization ratios are designed to track physician utilization of the laboratory. The billable procedures per patient day and billable procedures per patient admission may rise or fall if the physicians alter their test ordering patterns. For example, the ratios increase if the physicians "feel pressure" to rapidly diagnose, treat, and discharge patients and order more laboratory tests.

The resource utilization ratios monitor the monthly consumption of labor, materials, equipment, and overhead by the cost center. Most of these parameters are under the direct control of the laboratory director and laboratory manager. A rise in the technical labor per procedure, for example, may signal a scheduling problem in a cost center involving the use of expensive overtime labor.

If the supply cost per billable procedure rises at a cost center, the manager should ask why. Are supplies being wasted? Are too many controls or small batches being run? Are ordering patterns resulting in lost discounts? The ratios pinpoint the troubled cost center and allow for early corrective action.

The most important utilization ratio is the total cost per billable procedure. In a prospective payment environment, it is vital to determine an accurate total cost per procedure for each hospital product and service. Comprehensive cost data provide valuable ammunition when the hospital competes for patients with HMOs and PPOs. Like DRGs, these prepaid health plans reimburse the hospital on a set

(text continues on p 486)

Utilization Ratios

$$\text{Billable Procedure per Patient Day} = \frac{\text{Billable Procedures}}{\text{Patient Days}}$$

$$\text{Billable Procedure per Patient Admission} = \frac{\text{Billable Procedures}}{\text{\# Patient Admissions}}$$

Resource Utilization Ratios

$$\text{Total Cost per Billable Procedure} = \frac{\text{Total Costs}}{\text{Billable Procedures}}$$

$$\text{Direct Cost per Billable Procedure} = \frac{\text{Direct Costs}}{\text{Billable Procedures}}$$

$$\text{Nontechnical Labor Cost per Billable Procedure} = \frac{\text{Nontechnical Labor}}{\text{Billable Procedures}}$$

$$\text{Technical Labor Cost per Billable Procedure} = \frac{\text{Technical Labor Cost}}{\text{Billable Procedures}}$$

$$\text{Supply Cost per Billable Procedure} = \frac{\text{Supply Costs}}{\text{Billable Procedures}}$$

$$\text{Equipment Cost per Billable Procedure} = \frac{\text{Equipment Costs}}{\text{Billable Procedures}}$$

Productivity Ratios

$$\text{Professional Fee Cost per Billable Procedure} = \frac{\text{Professional Fee Cost}}{\text{Billable Procedures}}$$

$$\text{Billable Procedure per \$ of Labor} = \frac{\text{Billable Procedures}}{\text{\$ Labor}}$$

$$\text{Billable Procedure per \$ of Supply} = \frac{\text{Billable Procedures}}{\text{\$ Supply}}$$

$$\text{Billable Procedure per \$ of Equipment} = \frac{\text{Billable Procedures}}{\text{\$ Equipment}}$$

Financial Ratios

$$\text{Revenue per Billable Procedure} = \frac{\text{Revenue}}{\text{Billable Procedures}}$$

$$\text{Margin per Billable Procedure} = \frac{\text{Margin}}{\text{Billable Procedures}}$$

$$\text{Revenue per Patient Admission} = \frac{\text{Revenue}}{\text{Patient Admission}}$$

FIGURE 30-3.   Laboratory ratios.

Table 30-4
Example of Cost Center Operating Ratios

	Automated-Chem	General	RIA	Special
Revenues	$2,208,366	$907,008	$474,800	$237,368
Expenses				
Salaries				
Technical labor	$202,072	$178,547	$69,863	$69,853
Nontechnical labor				
Lab receptionists	$51,387	$18,555	$7,534	$2,495
Administrative	$29,771	$10,750	$4,365	$1,446
Nites	$35,962	$0	$0	$0
Phlebotomists	$74,655	$29,115	$10,705	$3,620
Path. secretaries	$3,847	$1,389	$564	$187
Professional fees	$127,950	$46,201	$18,760	$6,213
Supplies	$207,653	$198,851	$52,707	$24,474
Equipment				
Depreciation	$23,144	$17,719	$3,068	$6,404
Service contracts	$20,577	$23,165	$1,171	$6,682
Repairs	$6,350	$2,293	$930	$308
Other	$29,807	$10,763	$4,370	$1,447
Direct costs	$813,175	$537,348	$174,037	$123,129
Indirect costs	$289,980	$214,749	$80,638	$64,507
Total costs	$1,103,155	$752,097	$254,675	$187,636
Net income	$1,105,211	$154,911	$220,125	$49,732
Procedures	105,750	38,185	15,505	5,135
Patient Admissions	25,935	25,935	25,935	25,935
Patient Days	161,056	161,056	161,056	161,056
Procedure / patient day	0.7	0.2	0.1	0.0
Procedure / patient admission	4.1	1.5	0.6	0.2
Total Cost / procedure	$10.43	$19.70	$16.43	$36.54
Direct Cost / procedure	$7.69	$14.07	$11.22	$23.98
Nontechnical labor / procedure	$1.85	$1.57	$1.49	$1.51
Technical labor / procedure	$1.91	$4.68	$4.51	$13.60
Supply Cost / procedure	$1.96	$5.21	$3.40	$4.77
Equipment Cost / procedure	$0.47	$1.13	$0.33	$2.61
Professional Fee / procedure	$1.21	$1.21	$1.21	$1.21
Procedure / $ labor	0.5	0.2	0.2	0.1
Procedure / $ supply	0.5	0.2	0.3	0.2
Procedure / $ equipment	2.1	0.9	3.0	0.4
Revenue / procedure	$20.88	$23.75	$30.62	$46.23
Margin / procedure	$10.45	$4.06	$14.20	$9.68
Revenue / patient admission	$85.15	$34.97	$18.31	$9.15

fee scale. The hospital that underestimates costs risks bidding too low and locking itself into unfavorable and unprofitable contracts. Accurate cost-per-billable-procedure data enable the laboratory manager to put the correct price tag on laboratory services.

The ratios also monitor productivity. Laboratory productivity is measured in many ways, such as the minutes per hour a technologist works on a particular test or procedure or as the output of tests from an automated instrument over a period of time. Both of these methods of measuring productivity have a major shortcoming—they fail to define productivity in terms of cost.

In the DRG environment, productivity is defined as output per unit of input. For the laboratory, the output is the billable procedure, and the input is the labor, materials, equipment, and overhead measured in dollars. Productivity is increased by performing more billable procedures or by decreasing input expenses.

The billable procedure/dollar of technical labor ratio measures productivity in terms of labor utilization. The billable procedure/dollar of equipment cost ratio allows the manager to compare the productivity of two different instruments or analyzers.

The financial ratios allow the hospital administrator to track the laboratory's financial condition over time.[1] A decrease in the margin (profit) per billable procedure may signal a shift in the laboratory's case-mix patterns. That is, a higher percentage of less profitable (lower margin) tests may have been ordered. If the billable procedures/patient admission ratio decreases, the administrator may wish to compensate for the decreased revenues by increasing the prices of all procedures.

The revenue per billable procedure is the income the laboratory receives from performing and selling one billable procedure. Table 30-3 shows that several of the cost centers operate at a loss. That is, total cost per billable procedure exceeds revenue. This happens because many laboratory managers base prices on estimates of total costs. Unfortunately, these estimates are often low.

If competitive forces allow it, it is better to adopt a pricing policy that yields a constant margin on all tests, for instance, 10% to 15% per procedure. Setting the prices of all tests 10% to 15% above costs protects the laboratory from revenue shortfalls caused by changing test-mix patterns.

This management system is flexible. Many ratios or only a few ratios may be calculated for all or only a few cost centers. Once the laboratory costs are categorized and allocated and the ratios calculated, the only factors that change significantly are the number of billable procedures and the labor and supply utilization. Most other budget items remain relatively constant from month to month.

This system, which may appear complex, is not difficult to put into practice. Data-gathering is the biggest hurdle. It is worthwhile to establish a good relationship with the admissions and business office personnel to obtain better access to the data.

Now that cost efficiency is a watchword in the health-care industry, a comprehensive laboratory management system is a necessity, rather than an option. Quite simply, those managers who develop a system to set goals, measure progress, and point out trouble spots will utilize their limited resources more intelligently than those managers who do not.

REFERENCES

1. Cleverly WO. Financial ratios: Summary indications for management decision making. Hosp Health Serv Admin 26, No. 3, Special Issue 1:26–47, 1981
2. Greiner LE, Metzger RO. Consulting to Management. Englewood Cliffs, Prentice-Hall, 1983
3. Kotler P. Marketing Management. 5th ed. Englewood Cliffs, Prentice-Hall, 1984
4. Sharp JW. The cluster lab: A model for the DRG era? MLO 15(11):40–44, 1983
5. Sharp JW. A DRG survival guide for the laboratory budget. MLO 16(9):38–43, 1984
6. Sharp JW: Directing the post-TEFRA laboratory. Pathologist 39, No. 2: 1985
7. Sharp JW. A cost accounting system targeted to DRG's. MLO 17(9):34–38, 1985

ANNOTATED BIBLIOGRAPHY

Horgren CT: Cost Accounting: A Managerial Emphasis, 5th ed. Englewood Cliffs, Prentice-Hall, 1982
> This source is generally considered the bible of cost accounting. Chapter 14 nicely demonstrates the mechanics of allocating costs to output. This is a very useful book for learning how to perform cost accounting a clinical laboratory.

Kotler P: Marketing Management, Analysis, Planning, and Control, 5th ed. Englewood Cliffs, Prentice-Hall, 1984
> This book is an excellent source of marketing information. Chapter 2 presents an excellent summary of the strategic planning process and its relationship to the overall goals and objectives of the institution.

Viscone JA: Financial Analysis, Principles and Procedures. Boston, Houghton Mifflin, 1977
> This is an excellent short source for understanding financial ratio analysis. The financial planning process is explained in detail. The theoretic concepts of financial planning are supplemented with practical problems and solutions. Many useful productivity and utilization ratios are presented and explained.

Greiner LE, Metzger RO: Consulting to Management. Englewood Cliffs, Prentice-Hall, 1983
> This book is another good source for understanding the strategic planning process. It is written in a lively, easy-to-read fashion. Chapter 8 presents a good synopsis of the problems associated with data-gathering in the institutional setting.

thirty-one

Inventory Management and Cost Containment

Robert V. Lucchetti
John R. Snyder

The concept of matériel, or inventory, management is not new. It was first recognized in industry around the turn of the century. It took an external force, World War II, to initiate matériel management as a practical entity in industry. Another external force, cost containment, has brought inventory management to the health-care industry. Health care has come to the forefront of public scrutiny within the last 5 to 8 years. The rising costs of quality health care have brought pressures to bear upon health-care institutions from the general public as well as the government. Inventory management is viewed as an opportunity to reduce what seem to be spiraling cost increases. In order to understand clearly the potential for reducing costs, let us first look at the cause of cost increases.

Three broad areas can be identified as contributing to increasing health-care costs. First, government regulation with respect to product quality and integrity and other regulations imposed upon manufacturers have contributed greatly to the increased cost of medical supplies and equipment. Additional government regulations relative to quality assurance within the field of medical testing have contributed to the increased cost of medical care at the level of the health-care institution. Government regulations relative to personnel and third-party reimbursements have additionally affected the cost of medical care. Second, hospitals are labor-intensive. The increased cost of labor has contributed significantly to

rising health-care costs. High-technology equipment and high-technology testing procedures have created a demand for a greater level of expertise within the labor force. Expanding technology has created a need for an even more diverse, yet highly specialized labor force. The availability of quality care is the third cause of rising health-care costs. New technology offers quality care that did not exist in years past. Additionally, as the population grows, it is necessary to provide these new services to an even greater population base. The cost of significantly expanding high technology delivered to an increasing population base is dramatic.

As will be demonstrated later, the matériel management department is responsible for approximately 30% to 40% of the total operating budget of a hospital. Matériel management is directly responsible for all supplies—the unit cost of the supplies themselves and the logistical support costs necessary to order, receive, inventory, distribute, and dispose of or reprocess them. It seems only natural that pressure for reducing costs would come to bear ultimately on matériel management.

SCIENTIFIC INVENTORY MANAGEMENT

Today many inventory management and control systems are computerized; but the same basic principles apply to a sophisticated computer system or to an effective manual system that uses ordering charts, economic order quantity (EOQ) wheels, or other devices. There are some advantages to computer systems, because manual systems require the interpretation and implementation of inventory directives by numerous individuals involved in the inventory replenishment cycle. This situation perpetuates inconsistencies between stocking units: several items may be seriously overstocked while many other items are in short supply. Manual systems hinder the reaction to shifts in the management of inventory conflict and permit poor decisions by some individuals involved in inventory replenishment to go undetected. As a result, investment in inventories is often greater than required to produce a desired supply service objective. This excess investment in inventory generally represents potential savings that could be realized from the use of computerized inventory systems.

This does not mean that manual inventory management systems cannot work efficiently. Given trained individuals with sufficient time to consider relevant variables, there is little doubt that manual systems are superior. Unfortunately, time is a luxury that health-care institutions with broad supply lines can rarely afford.

When to Order — Replenishment

The most important operating consideration of an inventory management system is *when* to reorder a particular item. This decision (the reorder point) will determine the supply service attained for a given item. The order quantity is of secondary importance in the determination of supply service.

The relationship between the reorder point (ROP) and supply service stresses the importance of promptly issuing purchase orders for stock that has fallen below the ROP. Using valid data to arrive at the ROP is crucial. If purchase orders are not issued at the appropriate time, supply service will suffer adversely. Furthermore, if the data used in arriving at the ROP are not accurate, the computation of the ROP becomes a futile exercise in mathematics. The lead time, the expected demand, and the errors in forecasting expected demand are the important elements in determining the ROP. These elements and their roles will be discussed in greater detail later in this chapter.

How Much to Order — Order Quantity

Once a decision has been made to replenish a stock-keeping unit, order quantity is the most important operating consideration in realizing inventory investment objectives. The greater the order quantity, the higher the amount of investment required to finance inventories. Once supply service objectives have been established, the ROP becomes secondary in the determination of inventory investment. However, in establishing supply service objectives, management has its greatest impact on the amount of investment to be devoted to maintaining inventory.

The order quantity is set at a level that minimizes the total annual variable cost associated with both ordering and holding an item in stock. While a small order quantity will result in a low investment inventory (*i.e.,* a low holding cost), the cost of frequently ordering and receiving the item will be greater. In determining order quantity, the total of these costs—ordering and holding—should be held to a minimum. The elements that make up these costs and their role in influencing the order quantity will be discussed later. For the most part, minor errors in estimating these costs will have little effect on the computation of the order quantity.

Forecasting — Estimate of Expected Usage

The forecast of demand can affect both the ROP and the order quantity. The forecast is important in determining the ROP because it is necessary to anticipate demand from the time a purchase order is placed to the time it is physically received and available for use by the laboratory. The forecast is also important in determining how much to purchase.

In a computerized inventory management system, one of the most important uses of the forecast of supply demand is the measurement of inability to forecast. The forecast error, or the difference between the forecast and the actual laboratory demand, determines the buffer or *safety stock* requirement that makes up the ROP.

Purchasing

Purchasing systems translate ROP and order quantities for stock-keeping units into acceptable purchase orders and thus are concerned with the practical, everyday problems of purchasing. The system is not concerned directly with supply service, inventory investment, or order requests.

A purchasing system will modify, within defined bounds, order quantities, ROPs, and other inventory management considerations, so as to

Meet supplier purchase-order minimums
Meet supplier item minimums

Order items in standard multiples

Conform to other defined policies

TECHNICAL DESCRIPTION OF INVENTORY REPLENISHMENT SYSTEMS

There are three basic types of systems used to replenish items normally inventoried: the fixed-quantity, or trigger, replenishment system; the fixed-period, or tickler, replenishment system; and a mixed approach employing aspects common to both systems.

Fixed-Quantity System

The fixed-quantity, or trigger, system initiates (triggers) an order at the instant the balance of available stock reaches a predetermined ROP. This approach is sound in concept but in practice ignores the fact that it might be desirable to consolidate all purchase requirements for a given supplier into one purchase order for a given period of time. In addition, whether on a computer or manual system, it is highly unlikely that a purchase order would be automatically created at an instant in time.

Figure 31-1 illustrates the fixed-quantity system for known consumer demand. The graph is commonly referred to as "saw tooth." It should be noted that with known demand, the ROP equals the expected demand during the lead-time period (in this case with known demand of 40 units or 30 days'

supply). The dotted line in the chart represents an on-order quantity. Thus, when the available stock reaches 40 units, an order is automatically placed.

Figure 31-2 illustrates the fixed-quantity system for unknown demand. The element of uncertainty introduces a second component in the determination of the ROP. Rather than having a known demand of 40 units per month, the demand is now expressed as an average, assuming that the supply service objective for the item illustrated requires that during the lead-time period, demand of 60 units is reasonable. Thus, if the maximum demand materialized during the lead-time period, the item would be out of stock. To prepare for this contingency, the ROP should be increased to 60 units, 40 units of which represent an average lead-time supply and 20 units the difference between the maximum reasonable demand and the average. The 20 units designated for contingencies are usually called *safety stock*. Figure 31-3 illustrates the fixed-quantity system for unknown demand after the introduction of the safety stock.

Fixed-Period System

The fixed-period, or tickler, system initiates a purchase order at the review time regardless of the balance of available stock. The review time is usually established on the basis of the period over which the order quantity is expected to satisfy normal demand. Thus, in the example being discussed, if the order quantity is determined to be 80 units,

FIGURE 31-1. Fixed quantity replenishment system for known consumer demand.

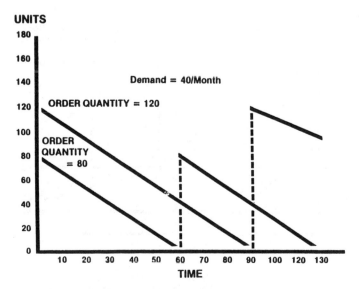

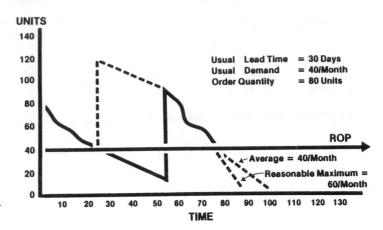

FIGURE 31-2. Fixed quantity replenishment system for unknown demand.

and the average demand is 40 units per month, the review time will usually be set at 2 months or 60 days.

It should be noted that the parameters for replenishment, order quantity, lead time, average demand, and safety stock are the same generally for both the fixed-quantity and fixed-period replenishment systems. What differs in the two approaches is the action required to initiate a purchase order. In the fixed-quantity system, the quantity ordered remains constant, and the time interval between purchases, *review time,* varies with customer demand. In the fixed-period system the review time remains constant, and the quantity ordered varies with customer demand.

The fixed-period approach is also sound in concept. However, in practice it ignores the fact that in dealing with multiple-item suppliers, varying the review time of the various items making up the vendor's line can be desirable; this approach probably comes closer to reality than the fixed-quantity system previously discussed.

Figure 31-4 illustrates the fixed-period system for unknown demand. The item illustrated is the same item previously discussed. The dotted line in the chart represents an on-order quantity. Thus, at the review time (regardless of the level of available stock), an order is placed immediately. The quantity ordered is the maximum less the amount of available stock. This maximum quantity is the total of the ROP and order quantity previously determined for the fixed quantity system.

FIGURE 31-3. Fixed quantity replenishment system, unknown demand and safety stock.

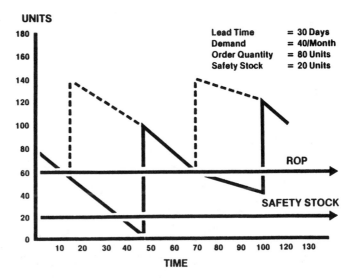

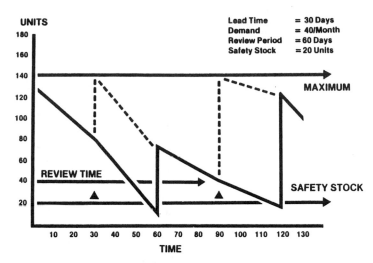

FIGURE 31-4. Fixed period replenishment system, unknown demand and order quantity.

Mixed Replenishment System

The mixed replenishment system employs aspects common to two other systems in an attempt to overcome the impractical aspects attributed to these systems when used alone. Thus, this approach will vary, depending upon specific applications. Figure 31-5 illustrates the mixed replenishment system. This mixed approach employs the safety stock and ROP common to the fixed-quantity approach, as well as a maximum and fixed review time common to the fixed-period approach. A purchase order for the item is initiated at the review time only if the amount of available inventory is less than the ROP. If a purchase is warranted, the purchase quantity becomes the maximum quantity less the amount of available inventory. Thus, the mixed replenishment approach results in the purchase of an item at irregular intervals in varying quantities.

This method more closely resembles the fixed-period approach than the fixed-quantity approach. Setting a common review period for all items in a supplier's line means that the total requirements at a review period for a particular supplier can be readily consolidated into one purchase order. Setting a frequent review period for the supplier means that the order quantities for the supplier's various items can be established independent of the period review while remaining consistent with the economics of holding and ordering costs. Ordering

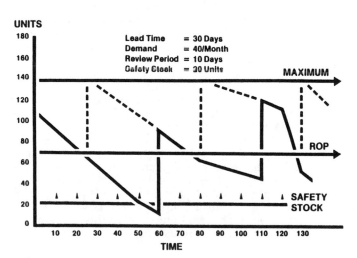

FIGURE 31-5. Mixed replenishment system when demand is unknown. Arrowheads denote maximum and fixed review time.

items from a supplier only when available inventory balances are below the ROP means that frequent purchases of small quantities, with their related ordering costs, can be minimized.

Economic Order Quantity

The initial effort of purchasing and inventory management to control costs was to attack the unit price paid for a given item. Far-reaching tactics were employed to achieve this goal. For example, the concept of group purchasing was given a great boost by purchasing agents or matériel managers. Activities such as these are quite understandable, because the unit price paid for any given item is the easiest factor to measure. Additionally, department heads, encouraged to reduce their spending, typically have only the unit price of supplies in their budget and not a fee for the logistical support services, such as inventory holding costs and purchasing expense. A true understanding of matériel management, however, shows that the unit cost is not the only or ultimate answer to reducing the overall costs. EOQ is determined so as to minimize the total annual variable cost associated with both ordering and holding an item in stock. The three relevant cost elements are (1) holding costs, (2) ordering costs, and (3) the least important consideration, the purchase price of an item.

Holding Costs. The total annual variable cost of holding or carrying inventory includes those costs incurred from the time an item is purchased and put on the shelf until that item is sold. The components of holding costs can include the following:

Personal property taxes related to inventory

Rental or depreciation of space and fixtures devoted to inventory

Maintenance of storage space (security and janitorial costs)

Real estate taxes and insurance attributed to storage space

Shrinkage and obsolescence (nonmovement and excess)

Interest costs of money tied up in inventories

Sometimes storage cost is considered not a variable cost, but a fixed or shrunken cost. However, when space is near capacity, this view is unrealistic and can lead to overcrowding. Also, the cost of money tied up on maintaining inventories is sometimes viewed not as the interest cost of money, but as the potential return on investment derived from alternative uses of the money.

Ordering Costs. The total annual cost of ordering an item for inventory includes those costs incurred from the time the item is identified as being in short supply and ordered until the time an item is received and put on the shelf. The components of ordering costs can include the following:

Stock purchase order forms, envelopes, and postage

Expediting forms, postage, telephone expense

Time related to review, purchasing, expediting, receiving, and payables

Payroll costs related to review, purchasing, expediting, receiving, inspection, warehousing, material movement, and payables.

Fringe benefits associated with payroll costs

Purchase Price. The total annual purchase price will not usually be affected by the amount purchased or the frequency of purchase. The only major exception to this is the situation in which the vendor offers item quantity discounts. Once holding costs, ordering costs, and purchase price have been determined, EOQ can be derived through trial and error. (For the purposes of our calculation, we are ignoring for the moment the possibility of item quantity discounts.) Normally the cost of holding inventory is stated as a percentage, such as 20%. This percentage is related to the unit cost of each stock-keeping unit and the annual carrying cost for that item. The cost of ordering inventory is stated as a dollar amount for each line item. This dollar amount carries the assumption that on the average a certain number of line items will be purchased on a single purchase order and accordingly includes both costs associated with ordering a line item and issuance and processing of a purchase order.

Figure 31-6 illustrates an item having a known demand of 40 units per month. In previous illustrations, the item was shown as having an order quantity of 80 units. For the purpose of determining EOQ, ROP and safety stock are ignored. Accordingly, using a known demand without consideration of the real uncertainty involved does not change the determination of EOQ. Furthermore, with a known demand, it is also possible to conclude that if an order quantity is set at 80 units, then the average amount of available inventory on hand will be half that quantity (or 40 units). With this background, the EOQ can be found through trial and error. First,

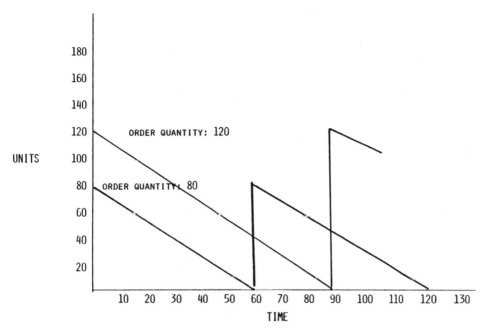

FIGURE 31-6.   Economic order quantity (EOQ).

if we start with an order quantity of 80 units and assume a purchase price of $1.50, annual variable ordering cost will be $12.00 (six purchases a year at $2.00 each). Thus, the total variable costs equal $24.00. If we use 120 units as the order quantity, total annual variable holding costs will be $26.00. If we try an order quantity of 60 units, total annual variable holding and ordering costs will be $25.00. In fact, any order quantity other than 80 units will result in a total annual expense greater than $24.00. Thus, 80 units is the EOQ.

Accuracy of EOQ

In determining the variable holding and ordering costs, it is quite possible to make an error in estimating. Furthermore, holding and ordering costs are averages and are not necessarily accurate for one item. For instance, the holding cost of an item that is bulky or must be refrigerated is greater than that of a small item kept in normal bin storage. Also, the annual usage of an item is not always known and may be subject to change as the year progresses. Fortunately, the total variable costs associated with ordering and holding inventory are not very sensitive in the range of the EOQ.

Order Quantity Sensitivity.   The example at the top of page 494 illustrates the total annual variable costs of different order quantities. As the order quantity is varied from 60 to 120 units, the total variable cost does not differ by more than $2.00. Accordingly, the necessity of estimating does not negate the EOQ concept, but rather encourages its use.

Item Quantity Discounts.   If a vendor offers an item quantity discount, sometimes referred to as a break-point algorithm, the EOQ may require adjustment. The example at the bottom of page 494 illustrates the required analysis of the item previously discussed. With a purchase price of only $1.50 per unit, the EOQ was 80 units, resulting in a total annual variable cost of $24.00. If the supplier offers a 5% discount for a purchase of 160 units or more, the order cost will decrease $6.00 (three less purchases at $2.00 each), the holding cost will increase $12.00 (40 units more in inventory at $.0142 at 20%), but the annual purchase price will decrease by $36.00 (480 unit annual usage at $.75 cost reduction per unit). The net change is a savings of $30.00 and, therefore, the order quantity should be equal to the item break point of 160 units.

FACTORS

Holding cost
Ordering cost
Purchasing price

EXAMPLES

Purchase price = $1.50

I. ORDER QUANTITY 80 units

Annual ordering cost	$12.00 (6 orders per year at $2.00)
Annual holding cost	$12.00 (4 units at $1.50 at 20%)
Total	$24.00

II. ORDER QUANTITY 120 units

Annual ordering cost	$ 8.00 (4 orders per year at $2.00)
Annual holding cost	$18.00 (60 units at $1.50 at 20%)
Total	$26.00

III. ORDER QUANTITY 60 units

Annual ordering cost	$16.00 (8 orders per year at $2.00)
Annual holding cost	$ 9.00 (30 units at $1.50 at 20%)
Total	$25.00

The formula used to arrived at the EOQ is as follows:

$$EOQ = \sqrt{\frac{2AS}{IC}}$$

$$\sqrt{\frac{2(\text{annual units}) (\text{ordering cost})}{(\text{carrying cost \%}) (\text{cost per unit})}}$$

The examples at the top of the opposite page illustrate the impact of changing the factors used in the formula. Pay particular attention to the results of the changes.

PRICE-BREAK FACTORS

Holding cost
Ordering cost
Purchase price

EXAMPLE

Normal order quantity	80 units
Normal purchase price	$ 1.50
Normal ordering cost	$12.00
Normal holding cost	$12.00

AT 5% DISCOUNT FOR 160 UNITS

Order quantity	**160**
Order cost change	**$(12)**
Holding cost change	**$ 12**
Purchase price change	**$(12)**
Net change	**$(12)**

Forecasting

The approach for forecasting supply demand or usage that is common to most inventory management systems involves the projecting of the past into the future. This approach differs from prediction, and to introduce and anticipate changes in new circumstances still remains the function of the inventory manager. To function effectively, an inventory management system must have the benefit of both forecast and prediction.

Techniques

There are several techniques that can be used to project the future on the basis of past experience. Generally, these techniques all employ the statistical concept of an average.

The Moving Average. The simplest of these approaches is the *moving average*, which produces a forecast for the future that represents the simple average of the periods encompassed by this moving or sliding approach. Each historical period is generally given equal weight. In a 5-month average, each of the 5 months contributes 20% to the forecast of the next period. When the actual experience becomes available for the next period, the oldest experience is dropped and the most current set of five experiences is again averaged. This approach is good for stable items but generally not for items with upward/downward trends.

Annual units   600
Ordering cost $8.00
Inventory carrying cost   20%
Cost per unit $30

$$EOQ = \sqrt{\frac{2(600)(8)}{(.20)(30)}} = \sqrt{\frac{9600}{.06}} = \sqrt{160,000} = 400$$

$$\sqrt{\frac{2(600)(8)}{(.20)(300)}} = \quad 13 \text{ high cost}$$

$\uparrow$

$$\sqrt{\frac{2(600)(8)}{(.10)(30)}} = \quad 565 \text{ Low carrying cost}$$

$\uparrow \quad \downarrow$

$$\sqrt{\frac{2(600)(80)}{(20)(30)}} = \quad 1265 \text{ High ordering cost}$$

$$\sqrt{\frac{2(12,000)(8)}{(20)(30)}} = 1789 \text{ high usage}$$

Regression Analysis. *Regression analysis* produces a forecast by fitting a line or curve to a series of experiences. This line is commonly called the "line of best fit." Regression, unlike the moving average, assigns a weight to each experience that varies with the amount of deviation from the average. The greater the deviation, the greater the weight assigned. Unlike the moving average, the regression approach may not be responsive to upward or downward trends.

Exponential Smoothing. *Exponential smoothing* is a moving average that assigns unique weights to a historical experience. The greatest weight is assigned to the most current experience. For this reason, the smoothing approach is more responsive to upward or downward trends than the moving average. However, the adjustment will always lag behind the trend; the lag will determine the number of periods being used. To compensate for this lag, second-order, or double, smoothing can be used. With double smoothing forecasting can be highly responsive to trend.

Figure 31-7 illustrates the weights associated with different alpha factors that are used in exponential smoothing. As the illustration shows, an alpha factor of 0.3 is equivalent to a 5-month to 7-month moving average using unequal weights, while an alpha factor of 0.5 is equivalent to a 3-month to 5-month moving average.

Exponential smoothing also has several computational advantages, which makes it desirable for use in computer applications. These advantages center around the fact that only the old forecast is required for determining the new forecast, with a simple moving average of all historical data retained.

New forecast = Alpha × Demand + (1 − Alpha) × Old forecast

The example on the following page illustrates how a single smooth forecast is computed with an alpha of 0.3 (a 5-month to 7-month moving average). With the current demand of 80 units for the first month, the new forecast becomes 66 units. For the next month only, this figure is used in determining the new forecast of 67 units. (For illustrative purposes, the calculation is also shown with additional historical data.)

Base Index. The *base index* approach is used most often in conjunction with an averaging technique to compensate for items with seasonal demands. While averaging will smooth out seasonal patterns, the base index approach attempts to reinstate these regular patterns. This approach requires substantial demand history and works by averaging the same month of the year over several years. For example, if traditionally the seasonal peak for an item is July, the July average will be greater than the smoothing or simple average, and this relationship

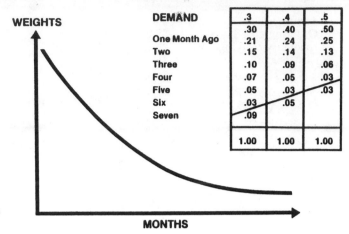

DEMAND	.3	.4	.5
	.30	.40	.50
One Month Ago	.21	.24	.25
Two	.15	.14	.13
Three	.10	.09	.06
Four	.07	.05	.03
Five	.05	.03	.03
Six	.03	.05	
Seven	.09		
	1.00	1.00	1.00

FIGURE 31-7. Exponential smoothing in forecasting.

will be used to correct the smoothed or simple average when forecasting July.

Adaptive Smoothing. An averaging approach that assigns unequal weight to past experiences, *adaptive smoothing* uses sine and cosine functions, adjusting for trends and seasonal demands while averaging. Accordingly, the weights assigned to past experiences vary considerably, depending on the number of terms employed in the calculation. This approach can be very responsive and effective but is highly sophisticated and therefore difficult to start up or adjust once in use.

Responsiveness

Throughout the discussion of various forecasting approaches, responsiveness was emphasized. *Re-*

sponsiveness means an ability to react to an indication of a shift in demand. This characteristic is desirable for forecasting. However, since trends or shifts in demands are not always readily discernible, responsiveness must be dampened so as not to cause an overreaction.

It is not uncommon for a trend to be accompanied by sporadic demands on both the high and low sides of the trend. When too few experiences are considered, the magnitude and even the direction of the trend may be misread. Likewise, the forecast approach may react to too few experiences. This applies to forecasting trends where they do, in fact, exist and, just as importantly, to not forecasting trends where they do not exist. A shift in demand based on a few unusual experiences does not make a trend.

Forecasting Error

An integral part of forecasting is measuring the forecast error. The forecast error is the difference between actual demand and forecast demand. Accordingly, the better the forecasting approach selected, the smaller the forecast error. On the other hand, a realistic understanding of the forecast error enables the inventory management system to establish a sufficient buffer or safety stock to compensate for the inability to forecast accurately. Therefore, regardless of the ability to forecast, adequate safety stock should be available to ensure satisfying supply service objectives. Obviously, it is desirable to forecast as accurately as possible, because it reduces the need for safety stock, thus minimizing inventory investment. However, because safety stock is dependent on the forecast error, the existence of the fore-

---

EXAMPLE

Old forecast	60
Demand	80
Alpha	0.3
New forecast	0.3(80) + 0.7(60)
	24 + 42 = 66

NEXT MONTH

Old forecast	66
Demand	70
Alpha	0.3
New forecast	0.3(70) + 0.7(66)
	21 + 46 = 67

or

0.3(70) + 0.7(24 + 42)
21   17   29 = 67

cast error should not necessarily affect supply service. For this reason, the measure of the forecast error is often considered more important than the forecast itself.

Forecasting Illustrated

To gain a better understanding of how forecasting is done and how responsiveness and forecasting errors are handled, let us now examine single exponential smoothing in more detail. This method is probably the one most commonly used in the health-care industry today.

The issue of responsiveness is normally handled through a method called *demand screening*. The current demand used to update the forecast is screened to minimize the effect of the new forecast on any unusual situation manifesting itself in the current demand amount. One should attempt to keep the new forecast from being too responsive to a chance event. On the other hand, if this unusual demand is the beginning of a drastic change, the screening process will retard the adjustment of the forecast to the drastic change. It is more desirable not to overreact to a chance event than it is to respond too slowly to a drastic change in an item's demand. Since the latter should be recognized by the people dealing with distribution and inventory, a manual adjustment can be made.

The screening process works by computing demand limits that range from plus four times the mean absolute deviation (MAD) to minus four times MAD. If the actual demand is outside this range, the demand limit is used instead of the actual demand in updating the forecast. The real demand should be maintained and used when it becomes necessary to reanalyze the item being forecast.

Figure 31-8 illustrates a normal distribution curve, which represents demand in relationship to the forecast. There is a 50% probability that demand will not exceed the current forecast at each level of MAD. The measure of the forecast error commonly associated with this forecasting approach is MAD. This method of error or standard deviation can be associated with any forecasting approach employing statistical averages.

Figure 31-9 illustrates that MAD is the average of the absolute forecast error. This average is commonly calculated by exponential smoothing in the same manner as the forecast. In addition to the MAD established in this illustration, there is one other factor used in measuring forecast error—the sum of errors. It is computed as MAD is, except that the signed (plus or minus) difference is used.

Reorder Point

Inventory systems should recalculate ROP and safety stocks on a periodic basis, probably once a month. As indicated below, the ROP is comprised of the average lead-time supply plus safety stock.

$$ROP = F(LT + RT) + SS$$

where

F = Forecast	RT = Review time
LT = Lead time	SS = Safety stock

ROP = (Lead time) (Demand) + Safety stock = Reasonable maximum

30 days + 40/mo
      40   + 20 = 60 *ROP*

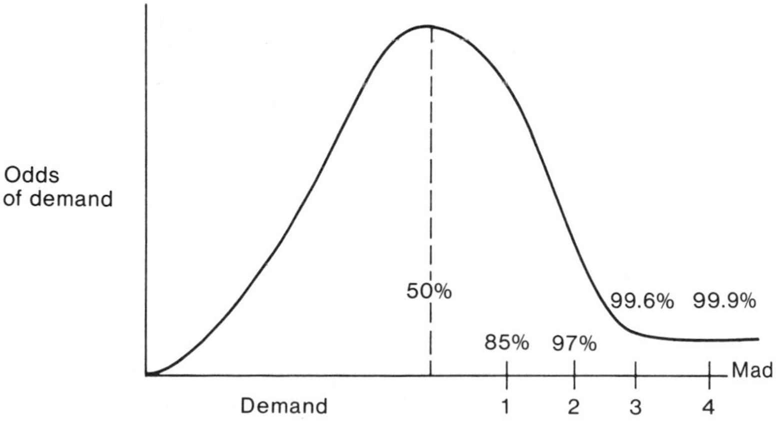

FIGURE 31-8. Demand in relation to forecast (MAD = mean absolute deviation).

Odds of demand

50%

85% 97%

99.6% 99.9%

Mad

Demand

1   2   3   4

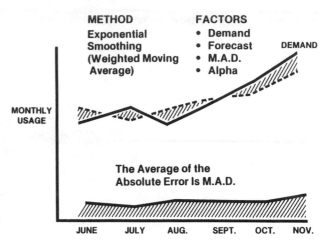

FIGURE 31-9. Mean Absolute Deviation (MAD) as the average of the absolute forecast error.

Safety stock has been previously described as the amount needed to increase the average lead-time supply to the reasonable maximum demand for the lead-time period. This reasonable maximum demand is determined by considering supply service objectives for this item. Safety stock is commonly calculated with the statistical approach that follows.

Determination of Safety Stock

FACTORS

Lead time

Demand

Forecast error during lead time (MAD_L)

Service level

EXAMPLE

Safety stock $= K\,(\text{MAD}_L)$

Where K is based on

$$F(K) = (1 - \text{service})\frac{EOQ}{MAD_L}$$

$$F(K) = (1 - \text{service})\frac{EOQ}{MAD_L}^{(80)} = 0.22$$

$K = 0.8$

$SS = K(\text{MAD}_L) = 20$

$(0.8)\ (25)$

Cost Containment

It we view the total cost of purchasing as an iceberg, we see that the unit price paid for an item is only the tip of the iceberg. Since the unit price is the most visible component, it is only logical that it would be likened to the tip or most visible part of the iceberg. However, somewhat out of sight of the users of supplies are two other costs. The middle portion of the iceberg is the cost of acquisition, the cost necessary for purchasing supplies. It is the cost of personnel involved in the paper-flow process of purchasing. Buried deeper in the iceberg is the cost of inventory. The cost of putting an item on the shelf and anticipating its use is composed of such things as shrinkage, obsolescence, depreciation, the cost of personnel to distribute or redistribute the product, and the cost of capital.

To understand more clearly the relationship between the unit price of an item and the costs of logistical support, consider the following information gathered by the American Hospital Association concerning an average 250-bed hospital in the United States. An average hospital has an operating budget of approximately $50,000 per bed per year. Of that, $10,000 per bed per year pays for the unit price of supplies, while another $10,000 per bed per year pays for the logistical support system. Clearly, there is a dollar-for-dollar relationship between the cost of supplies and the total cost of acquisition and inventory. It is also apparent that the matériel management department is clearly responsible for approximately 40% of the total operating budget of the average hospital.

With the understanding that the average health-care institution is a large business and, further, that the matériel management department is responsible for 40% of the cost of operation of this large business, it is only proper that we view the matériel management function from one of industry's measures of efficiency—return or investment. The matériel management department is definitely a business operation. The process of ordering, receiving, inventory, distributing, and reprocessing (manufacturing) is nothing more than the process of manufacturing and distribution.

Return on investment (ROI), for our purposes, is defined as earnings divided by assets. To increase ROI from the vantage point of matériel management, it is necessary to either reduce operating expenses, and thereby increase earnings, or reduce assets. To reduce operating expenses and increase earnings, matériel management has the opportunity to decrease the cost of acquisition, especially with regard to personnel productivity. Additionally, reduced expenses can originate from the reduction of inventory and thereby the reduction of inventory-holding costs. The matériel management department may also decrease assets by reducing inventory. The combination of reduced inventory and increased productivity within the cost of acquisition process will yield a twofold impact on the increasing ROI.

Cost of Acquisition

The cost of an average purchase order in a health-care institution can range from $25 to $50. Reported actual stated costs have ranged from $60 to $108. Whatever the cost of the purchase order process, it is necessary to understand that approximately 75% of cost is directly attributable to personnel, and only 25%, or even less, is attributable to the cost of supplies for the purchase-order process. Any significant impact on reducing the costs of acquisition will result directly from increasing the productivity of the people involved in the process.

For purposes of illustration, this chapter includes a case study of cost of acquisition and inventory analysis. In the case study, General Medical Center has invited a consulting team to analyze their matériel management program with specific emphasis placed upon the impact of this function on the laboratory environment.

Case Study

Cost of Acquisition Analysis

Interviews in Purchasing, Matériel Management, the Clinical Laboratory, and Accounting revealed the purchasing paper flow and accountability system to be comprehensive but overly burdened in two particular areas:

1. The requisition process
2. Documentation and accountability files

The paper-flow process was studied in detail. It should be understood that this study depicts the flow of documentation for a "clean" order, receiving, and accounting process. Various errors, either user- or vendor-induced, can cause any or all of the system to be "turned" one or more additional times.

It was found that at least two requisitions are prepared before the purchase order is actually typed. Both requisitions were also typed. From the standpoint of productivity, time is wasted in typing each order *three times* at General Medical Center. The first requisition prepared by departmental personnel is a composite for that department for all vendors. The laboratory coordinator's office then prepares from those documents individual requisitions for each department by vendor.

With respect to document files, closed-order files, which are maintained for seven years, were discovered within the medical center in Purchasing, Accounting, and Receiving. Audit accountability was the only reason given for the need for closed-order files; so, therefore, the file in Accounting was the only file necessary.

The general accountability of the system for audit purposes was found to be excellent. In fact, the mechanism established for accountability was found to be too exhaustive and produced severe limitations to purchase-order productivity. Those limitations are imposed by the following criteria established for purchase orders:

Only one account number (department) per purchase order

Only one vendor per purchase order

Only one page per purchase order with space for only four items with two-line descriptions or eight items with one-line descriptions

These restrictions result in significantly reduced purchase order productivity. For example, if two departments within the clinical laboratory order the same item from the same vendor, there will be two distinct purchase orders, receivings, invoices, and so forth. Thus, the purchasing paper-flow system will turn twice. In reality, all that is required is that each expenditure, regardless of vendor and item, be accounted for by department account number.

The Paper Flow Process — Pre-Analysis

STEPS	PROCESS	HOURS/WEEK
1.	Requisition cards are pulled once a week by the 12 departments in the lab by department heads	1/12 EA
2.	Cards are sent to lab purchasing clerk who types a three-part (white, yellow, pink) requisition form.	28
3.	Lab director reviews requisition form, assigns class code and account number, and approves.	0.5
4.	Requisition form is sent to Purchasing.	
5.	Buyer receives requisition, prices the items, and ensures that description, catalog number, and so forth are correct. Yellow and pink copies are sent back to the laboratory (filed).	40
6.	Buyer assigns vendor and purchase order number.	
7.	From the requisition, a six-part purchase order is typed.	20
8.	Purchasing director approves the purchase order.	40
9.	Purchase order is sent back to the buyer, where the purchase order is distributed as follows: two copies mailed or given to vendor; pink copy filed in Purchasing by clerk typist; blue copy sent to Accounts Payable; white and yellow copies (do not show pricing) sent to Receiving).	
10.	Accounts Payable files blue copy (notes about order made on this copy) and Receiving files white and yellow copies (pulls both when order arrives).	6
11.	When order is received, items are checked against original purchase order and two copies sent back to Purchasing; merchandise is dispersed and signed for by end-user department.	25/14
12.	Purchasing checks receiving for completeness of order (white copy). Yellow copy is matched with pink copy and filed in a "completed" file, along with any notes regarding the order.	10
13.	Purchasing sends original purchase order (white copy) to Accounts Payable.	
14.	Accounts Payable matches the original purchase order (white copy) with the blue copy and the vendor invoice. Payment is made, and two copies of the purchase order and a copy of the invoice are filled.	34/4 EA

The paper-flow system was found also to contribute to lead-time-induced inventory. The total time from recognition of a need by the end-user to vendor action (shipment, back-order, and so forth) was found to be approximately 9 working days.

One particular area inducing as much as a 2-day delay was the budget control process. While the function and purpose of this was clearly understood, in practice it was not realistic for the clinical laboratory for routine supply items. The budget-control process for such items was probably best performed "after the fact." Critical products for patient diagnosis would not, it seems, be rejected for order because of budget overrun. The budget accountability process should be managed on a periodic basis by exception.

The cost of a purchase order was calculated to be $39.84. The details of how this was calculated are found in Figures 31-10, 31-11, and 31-12.

Recommendations (General/All-Vendor Interface)

It should be understood that the recommendations that follow are suggested areas for consideration. Although potential procedural guidelines are provided, they are not totally comprehensive. They are offered within the confines of the research and thus limited to the clinical laboratory current procedures and perceived needs. Many recommendations may apply to other departmental areas or, in fact, be limited owing to restrictions imposed by other departmental purchasing areas. Figures 31-13, 31-14, 31-15, 31-16 demonstrate graphically the specific changes in the cost of acquisition process and the related financial impacts of those changes.

As regards the clinical laboratory and purchasing for routine consumables (value per unit less than $300), eliminate the budget-control process

FIGURE 31-10. Cost of acquisition. Departmental contribution—pre-analysis.

Contribution	Annual Costs	Suggested Factor	Factor	Contribution Cost
All labor costs in purchasing including fringes (excludes department managers)	167,700	100%	100%	167,700
Purchasing department— Manager's salary/ fringes		25%		
All labor costs in accounts payable attributable to payment of invoices generated through purchasing	71,510	Variable	85%	60,784
Labor for receiving and stores	247,946	25%	90%	223,151
Telephone costs for:				
—Purchasing	2,100	50%	40%	840
—Receiving	900	50%	50%	450
—Stores	—	50%	—	—
—Accounts Payable	900	50%	50%	450
Office supplies for:				
—Purchasing	—	75%	—	—
—Accounts Payable	1,416	75%	75%	1,062
—Receiving	—	75%	—	—

Total annual contribution costs (excludes end-user contribution)	$454,437.
Total number of purchase orders annually (includes end-user POs)	19,500
Departmental purchase order cost	$23.30
Average lines per order	3.4

Contribution	Annual Costs (Salary/Fringes)	% of Time Involvement* (Factor)	Contribution Cost
Laboratory director	38,000	2	$ 760
Laboratory manager			
Laboratory secretary			
Laboratory purch. clerk	12,500	70	8750
Departmental supervisors (combine all if more than one)	256,485 (12 supervisors)	3	7695
Medical technologists (combine all if more than one			
Others _____			
_____			
_____			

Total annual contribution costs	$17,205
Total number of laboratory purchase orders annually	1,040
End-user purchase order cost	$16.54

* Percent of time involvement is percent of employees' time directly related to the functions of analyzing need for products to be ordered, requisitioning, purchasing, expediting, receiving merchandise, correcting errors, and so forth.

FIGURE 31-11. Cost of acquisition. End-user contribution — pre-analysis.

FIGURE 31-12. Cost of acquisition. Total contribution cost — pre-analysis.

Contribution	Total Contribution Cost	Total Orders	Cost Per Order
All departments except requisitioning department	454,437	19,500	$ 23.30 /Purchase order (A)
Requisitioning department (end-user)	17,205	1,040	$ 16.54 /Purchase order (B)

Cost per order for orders from end-user   (A + B) = $ 39.84 /Purchase order

$$\text{Cost per order line} = \frac{\text{Cost per order}}{(A + B)} \div \frac{\text{Average lines}}{\text{per order}} = \$ \underline{11.72} /\text{line}$$

Contribution	Annual Costs	Suggested Factor	Factor	Contribution Cost
All labor costs in purchasing including fringes (excludes department managers)	167,700	100%	80%	134,160
Purchasing department— manager's salary/ fringes		25%		
All labor costs in accounts payable attributable to payment of invoices generated through purchasing	71,510	Variable	85%	60,784
Labor for receiving and stores	247,946	25%	75%	185,960
Telephone costs for				
—Purchasing	2100	50%	40%	840
—Receiving	900	50%	50%	450
—Stores	—	50%	—	—
—Accounts payable	900	50%	50%	450
Office supplies for				
—Purchasing	—	75%	—	—
—Accounts payable	1416	75%	75%	1062
—Receiving	—	75%	—	—

Total annual contribution costs (excludes end-user contribution)	$383,706.
Total number of purchase orders annually (includes end-user POs)	19,360
Departmental purchase order cost	$ 19.82
Average lines per order	4.0

FIGURE 31-13.   Cost of acquisition. Department contribution—postanalysis.

prior to the complete purchasing process. In theory the budget-control process step within the purchasing process is sound, but in practice it loses merit and is a greater limitation than its merit warrants.

Eliminate two of the three closed-order files. Three such existing files are not deemed necessary and, in fact, are potentially very counterproductive. Entries to a file after the fact for information relative to a specific order in a given file may not carry through all three files, thus creating discrepancies. The single file necessary

should be associated with the accounting department because the control/accountability of that file rests within the accounting department.

Increase the number of pages per purchase order. Productivity within the purchasing process is severely limited owing to the restrictions on the number of items on a given purchase order document (four to eight items). This increases "turns" in the paper-flow process, increases receiving, increases deliveries to the user departments, and increases the number of invoices to be processed through Accounts Payable. Second

Contribution	Annual Costs (Salary/Fringes)	% of Time Involvement* (Factor)	Contribution Cost
Laboratory director	38,000	0	0
Laboratory manager			
Laboratory secretary			
Laboratory purch. clerk	12,500	70	$8750
Departmental supervisors (combine all if more than one)	256,485 (12 supervisors)	1.5	$3847
Medical technologists (combine all if more than one			
Others _____ _____ _____			

Total annual contribution costs	$12,597
Total number of laboratory purchase orders annually	900
End-user purchase order cost	$14

* Percent of time involvement is percent of employees' time directly related to the functions of analyzing need for products to be ordered, requisitioning, purchasing, expediting, receiving merchandise, correcting errors, and so forth.

FIGURE 31-14. Cost of acquisition. End-user contribution—postanalysis.

FIGURE 31-15. Cost of acquisition. Total cost contribution—postanalysis.

Contribution	Total Contribution Cost	Total Orders	Cost Per Order
All departments except requisitioning department	383,706	19,360	$ 19.82/Purchase order (A)
Requisitioning department (end-user)	12,597	900	$ 14.00/Purchase order (B)

Cost per order for orders from end-user $(A + B) =$ $ 33.82/Purchase order

Cost per order line $=$ Cost per order $(A + B)$ $\div$ Average lines per order $=$ $ 8.46/line

Category	Existing System	Revised System	% Improvement	Dollar Impact
Paper flow process steps	14	10	—	—
Departmental contribution cost	$454,437	$383,706	15.6	$70,731
End-user contribution cost	$ 17,205	$ 12,597	26.8	$ 4,608
Total contribution cost	$471,642	$396,303	16.0	$75,339
Cost per purchase order	$39.84	$33.82	15.1	$6.02
Cost per order line	$11.72	$8.46	27.8	$3.26
Number of end-user purchase orders	1,040	900	—	—
Total number of purchase orders (all departments)	19,500	19,360	—	—

FIGURE 31-16. Comparative financial analysis—cost of acquisition.

and third pages of the original purchase order document could have the purchase order number, page number, and so forth recorded on them.

Consolidate orders to vendors across departmental lines and account numbers. All that is required is that a given item on a given purchase order have the account number for the user department associated with it. This would significantly increase the purchase system productivity but is predicated on implementation of the preceding recommendation.

Reduce or eliminate typed requisition process at the user department and laboratory coordinator level. A "card system" for requisitioning is in place for some items in the clinical laboratory. This should be expanded to include all the laboratory items purchased (at least on a routine basis). Each department would submit cards to the laboratory coordinator's office on a routine basis. These cards would be compiled by vendor within the laboratory coordinator's office (see the previous recommendation) and forwarded to Purchasing for purchase order preparation. Each group of cards would indicate a specific vendor and thereby constitute a single purchase order. The user portion of the purchase order could be returned to the laboratory coordinator's office with the cards to verify the order. Alternatively, the laboratory secretary could be charged with the responsibility of typing the actual purchase order documents and forwarding those to the purchasing department for approval and vendor submission. This would serve to decentralize the work effort of the purchase order preparation but retain centralized purchasing control

Reduce the total number of copies of the purchase order document. An inordinate amount of paper flows through the system for the relatively small order dollar volume. Eliminating Receiving's and Purchasing's closed-order file as previously recommended does away with the need for two of the copies. Receiving can function properly with only one copy of the original document. Photocopies (which exist in the system now) can be used effectively. Receiving's single copy master would be retained until all shipments against the purchase order were complete, with photocopies flowing through the system for partial shipments. With completion of the order, Receiving's master would flow through the system. The ultimate effect here is that Receiving would have no remaining paperwork on the order—no closed-order file.

Since Purchasing would not be keeping a closed order file, it is not necessary to have a Receiving copy for Purchasing notification.

Purchasing will now handle errors and expedite on a by-exception basis. The single copy file in Purchasing can be updated periodically or on an ongoing basis. For example, the final copy from Receiving indicating order completion could be routed through the Purchasing department, signaling that the order is complete. At that point it would no longer be necessary for Purchasing to retain their copy of the original purchase document.

In practice, unless Accounting is encumbering funds, it is not necessary for Accounting to receive an additional copy of the purchase order. The accounting function is to process invoices for payment based upon verification from Receiving and the user department that shipment is accurate and complete. Accounting is notified of accuracy and completeness of shipment by Receiving's copy of the original purchase document. The lack of an original purchase order copy to Accounting serves to control potential prepayment of the invoice.

If these processes are used, the original purchase order would be reduced from six to four copies: (1) Vendor, (2) Purchasing, (3) Receiving, and (4) Accounts Payable.

The paper-flow process can be significantly reduced. Not only are there fewer pieces of paper flowing through the system, but there are fewer people and less time involved in the process. These two reductions can only result in increased productivity.

The Paper Flow Process — After Analysis

STEPS	PROCESS	HOURS/WEEK
1.	Requisition cards are pulled once a week by the 12 departments in the lab by department heads	0.5/12 EA
2.	Cards are sent to lab purchasing clerk who types a four-part (white, yellow, blue, pink) purchase order form.	28
3.	Purchase order form is sent to Purchasing.	
4.	Buyer receives purchase order and pulls automated transmitter cards and transmits order. Other orders are processed as before.	20
5.	Purchase order is distributed as follows: white copy is mailed or given to vendor, blue copy sent to Accounts Payable, and yellow copy (does not show pricing) sent to Receiving.	
6.	Accounts Payable files blue copy (notes about order made on this copy), Receiving files yellow copy (pulls when order arrives), and Purchasing files pink copy.	
7.	When order is received, items are checked against yellow purchase order, which is sent back to Purchasing; merchandise is dispersed and signed for by end-user department.	25/14 EA
8.	Purchasing checks Receiving for completeness of order (yellow and pink copies).	10
9.	Purchasing sends yellow and pink copies to Accounts Payable, where three copies (yellow, pink, blue) are marked with the invoice.	
10.	Accounts Payable matches the original purchase order (yellow and pink copies) with the blue copy and the vendor invoice. Payment is made, and one copy of the purchase order and a copy of the invoice are filed.	34/4

Through a complete and thorough review and a systems approach to the acquisition process, the matériel management department can significantly affect the process and reduce the cost.

Cost of Inventory

Inventory is like a gas, in that it will expand to fill the container to which it is allotted. Historically, users of a given supply item will base judgment on the quantity of inventory on the space available for storing an item.

Especially in health-care institutions, which deal with human lives, the technical users of various items would view the ideal inventory as an almost limitless supply available at any given time. However, the product laboratory manager would argue, conversely, that the smallest possible inventory or no inventory would be ideal, because inventory is expensive. Obviously, there must be some median whereby the service level to the end-user is in harmony with the cost of maintaining the inventory. Yes, there must be trade-offs.

The laboratory manager has obviously based his desires upon the fact that inventory investment significantly affects many areas within the financial system. Inventory basically is a large nonspendable asset and as such can severely affect the cash flow system. Inventory requires handling for storage and redistribution, and it requires space for storage. Therefore, inventory affects operating revenues. Also significant is the fact that the monetary assets bound up in inventory represent an opportunity for investment income. To a cash-rich institution this income opportunity could be realized in the form of high-interest certificates of deposit. At a minimum, the cash-poor institution could use freed working capital to reduce debt. The financial implications of inventory investment clearly state that inventory is an asset worthy of strict management principles.

The following case study analyzes the inventory control mechanisms in the clinical laboratory at the mythical General Medical Center. The financial impact of the recommendations made after the analysis is shown in Figure 31-17.

Case Study

Inventory Analysis

All inventory in the clinical laboratory is classified as "unofficial," because it has been expensed to a user department instead of being maintained as an asset. As is common among clinical laboratories, there exists no inventory control system except the per-

petual-card system. The end-user ultimately controls the inventory. The only control perceived outside the stockroom is the routine schedule for the ordering process. Historically, this proves to have little or no influence in the actual controlling of inventory.

The laboratory stockroom was defined as containing items common to all user departments within the clinical laboratory. A visit to this stockroom verified that the items located there were, in part, common to more than one user department. However, much of that inventory appeared to have been there for quite some time. Some of the items could be better classified as those originally purchased in a large volume and stored there for convenience. Other items stored represent a very small dollar volume and are, in essence, not worth controlling.

The perpetual card system in place for this laboratory exists in practice but is not properly controlled. For example, EOQs were historically established and do not appear to have been periodically reviewed or changed. Each department had instances where quantity on hand far exceeded monthly usage.

In summary, the inventory control process in the clinical laboratory is determined by the end-user —not matériel management.

Recommendations

Perform ABC inventory analysis to determine how best to handle the inventory control process of various products or product groups. Analysis of order history for various items is a relatively time-consuming process and may require research of documentation from vendors but will prove to be a significant savings opportunity. ABC analysis is merely a method of determining which items require what type of inventory control. It is not in and of itself an inventory control system.

Establish an effective inventory control program for the clinical laboratory (for at least class A items as defined in the preceding recommendation). Inventory control is best defined here as determining proper EOQs and ROPs for items. Calculations of these parameters for each item would be time-consuming and an ongoing process but can be performed with a programmable calculator. (Normally attempts to institute such a system are computer based/assisted.) Effective adherence to calculated EOQs and ROPs based upon inventory reduction goals set by General Medical Center would serve to continue inventory control at the end-user level without the necessity of carrying the entire inventory in a stockroom environment and subjecting it to rou-

Department or Class	Existing System				Revised System				% Improvement	Dollar Impact
	DIOH Turn	Total Inv. Value	Holding Costs	Total Inv. Investment	DIOH Turn	Total Inv. Value	Holding Costs	Total Inv. Investment		
Chemistry	51/ 7.2	$42,006	$12,602	$54,608	30/ 12	$25,353	$7606	$32,959	39.6	$21,649
Blood bank	91/4	14,380	4314	18,694	61/6	9591	2877	12,468	33.3	6226
Cytology	65/ 5.0	4820	1446	6266	30/ 12	2256	677	2933	53.2	3333
Histology	228/ 1.6	1263	379	1642	15/ 24	35	26	111	932.0	1531
Immunology	66/ 5.5	15,919	4776	20,695	30/ 12	7301	2190	9491	54.1	11,204
Hematology Coag.	111/ 3.3	28,300	8490	36,3790	37/ 10	9334	2800	12,134	67.0	24,656
Microbiology	64/ 5.7	17,286	5165	22,471	30/ 12	8138	2441	10,579	53.0	11,892
Phlebotomy	94/ 3.9	19,273	5782	25,054	15/ 24	3139	942	4031	83.7	20,973
Urinalysis	182/ 2.0	22,400	6720	29,120	30/ 12	3798	1139	4937	83.0	24,183
Totals	76/ 4.8	165,646	49,694	215,340	32/ 11.5	68,995	20,698	89,693	58.3	125,647

Total holding cost savings	$28,996
Total reduced working capital requirement	$96,651
[Total inv. value (existing) − total inv. value (revised)]	

FIGURE 31-17. Comparative financial analysis—inventory.

tine physical inventories. As such, this system would serve to control unofficial inventory efficiently.

Use the existing stockroom space in the clinical laboratory for controlling only class A inventory items common to more than one department. To the extent that inventories become more visible, they are more readily controlled and accounted for. While it is apparent that the concept of inventorying and controlling certain items exists within the current stockroom environment, in essence the wrong items are being inventoried. ABC analysis would identify those items that should be maintained within this stockroom environment. Class A inventory should turn so rapidly that creating it as an asset would be of little significance.

ANNOTATED BIBLIOGRAPHY

Astor SD: Loss Prevention: Controls and Concepts. Los Angeles, Security World Publishing, 1978

> This text covers basic principles of loss prevention, including employee involvement and methods of distribution center security.

Compton HK: Supplies and Materials Management, 2nd ed. Estover, England, MacDonald & Evans, 1979

> A complete discussion of the maintenance of inventory and supplies is covered in this basic reference. Of particular interest are Chapters 5, 7, 9, and 10 addressing the ABC classification, storage cycle, supply flow patterns, and economic order quantity, respectively.

Fourre JP: Applying Inventory Control Techniques. New York, American Management Association, 1969

> As the name of this reference implies, this is an application monograph describing some of the basic inventory tools. The author presents several techniques with examples. The reader is appropriately cautioned that modification of some of the control techniques may be necessary before they are practical.

Larson SE: Inventory Systems and Controls Handbook. Englewood Cliffs, Prentice-Hall, 1976

> While written primarily for industry, this text has many ideas and solutions with regard to inventory maintenance that can be used in the clinical laboratory. Chapter 9 covers aspects of "what" and "when" to order. Chapter 12 describes methods for reducing the costs of material receiving, handling, and stocking.

Lewis CD: Scientific Inventory Control. New York, American Elsevier, 1970

> This reference takes a statistical look at inventory control. Of particular note are the forecasting techniques and equations for considering reorder levels and replenishment order quantities.

Spechler JW: Administering the Company Warehouse and Inventory Function. Englewood Cliffs, Prentice-Hall, 1975

> This is a practical "how to" book written with a building-block approach to the study of inventory control and cost containment. Chapter 11 deals with inventory control planning, providing examples and discussion of many of the concepts covered in laboratory inventory control.

Stafford AC: Inventory control through focus forecasting. MLO 17, No. 10:49–53, 1985

> This reference article describes four different strategies for inventory management based on the prior-use date: A—the same volume is anticipated as in prior 3 months; B—the same volume is anticipated as in the same 3 months last year; C—a 10% increase in volume is predicted for the next 3 months; and D—a 50% increase in volume is forecast for the next 3 months.

Index

Page numbers in italics indicate figures; page numbers followed by t indicate tabular material.

A

AABB. *See* American Association of Blood Banks
Absence report form, *41,* 42
ACA. *See* Automated Clinical Analyzer
Acceptance, of decision, 46
Accident reports, 336
Accountability, 34
Accounting. *See also* Cost accounting
  payroll, 455–456
  step-down method for, 416, 466–471, 467–469t
Accreditation
  definition of, 339–340
  inspection and, 341–343, 349–368
    accrediting agencies and, 349–350, 350t
    by American Association of Blood Banks, 343
    by College of American Pathologists, 341–342, 350–354
    by Joint Commission on Accreditation of Hospitals, 342–343
    preparation for, 355–356
    quality assurance and, 354–355
Acquisition costs, of personnel, 447
ACS. *See* American College of Surgeons
Activity, in network analysis, 31
Adaptiveness, of group, 95
Adaptive smoothing, forecasting and, 500
Add-air fume hood, 334–335
ADEA. *See* Age Discrimination in Employment Act of 1967
Administration. *See also* Administrators; Management; Manager(s)
  as art or science, 4
  controlling and, 9

  decision-making and, 9–10
  definition of, 5, *6*
  directing and, 9
  organizing and, 9
  planning and, 9
  transition to, 10–15
Administrative process, 7, *8,* 9–10
Administrative technologists, 6
Administrators, 6. *See also* Manager(s)
  challenges for, 16, *17,* 18
  duties of, 5–6, *7*
  educating, 15–16
Adult ego state, transactional analysis and, 80
Advertising, 399
Affirmative action, 179–180
Age Discrimination in Employment Act of 1967 (ADEA), 178, 181
Agency-shop laws, 252
Agendas, hidden, 146, *146*
Agreement, as change stratagem, 164
Airborne route of infection, 326
Algebraic apportionment, for cost-finding, 416
Alkyl ethers, 329
Allowances, 416
American Association of Blood Banks (AABB), 310, 350
  accreditation program of, 343
American College of Physicians, 342
American College of Surgeons (ACS), 342
American Dental Association, 342
American Hospital Association, 342
  rate-setting techniques recommended by, 439–442
American Medical Association, 342

American Nurses Association, compensation and, 445
American Society of Clinical Pathologists, 346
American Society of Medical Technology, 346
Analytical errors, resolving, 274–277
Antidiscrimination legislation, 446
Application form, 181–182, *186–189*
Appropriateness, 371
Appropriation budget, 423
Arbitration, 255–256
ARR. *See* Average rate of return
Association for the Advancement of Medical Instrumentation, 324
Authoritarian decision-making, 47, 49
Authority, 34, 137–142
    delegation and, 138–142
    motivation and, 69
    sources of, 137
    types of, 137
AutoAnalyzer, 302, *303*
Autocratic leader, 101
Automated Clinical Analyzer (ACA), 303
Automation, space allocation and, 26
Autonomous work teams, 123, 133–134
    limitations and, 134
    management and, 134
    structural considerations with, 133–134
Autonomy, reduction of, change and, 159
Average rate of return (ARR), 432–433, 435t

B

Bargaining unit, 251–252
Base index, forecasting and, 499–500
Behaviorally anchored rating scale, *220,* 221
Behavioral viewpoint, on conflict, 166
Benzidine, 327
Benzidine hydrochloride, 327
Billable procedure/dollar, 490
Binary code, 301
Biologic hazards, labeling and, 331, 333, *333*
Biologic variability, allowable error and, 271
Blenders, safety and, 324
Blood, precautions for laboratories and, 326–330
Blood bank
    laboratory information systems and, 309
    problems with, 384–385
Blood samples, drawn at request of police, problems associated with, 382
Blue Cross/Blue Shield, 410
Body fluids, precautions for laboratories and, 326–330
"Bottom up" change stratagem, 161
Brainstorming, 150
Break-even point, 416–417, *417*
Breathless decision, 46

Budgets, 421–429, 482–483, 483–486t, 487
    appropriation, 423
    assessing performance relative to, 426–427, 428t, 429, 429t
    capital, 430–431
    fixed forecast, 423
    forecast and narrative for, 422–423
    operating expense, 421–422, 426
    for personnel expenses, 423, 425–426, 448–449, *449*
    reasons for having, 421
    revenue, 438–439
    variable or flexible, 423
Burns, 329–330
Bypass fume hood, 334

C

Canadian Medical Association, 342
CAP. *See* College of American Pathologists
Capital decision-making, 429–438, 435t
    alternative choice financing decisions and, 436, 438
    capital budget categories and, 430–431
    data analysis techniques and, 431–434, 435t
    preliminary considerations in, 429–430
Carbon tetrachloride, 327
Carcinogenic chemicals, 327–328
Case study, for inservice education, 240
Cathode ray tube (CRT), 300
CDC. *See* Centers for Disease Control
Centers for Disease Control (CDC)
    infectious hazards and, 325
    interlaboratory survey provided by, 273
    preventive maintenance and, 316
Central processing unit (CPU), 300
Centrifuges, safety and, 324
Certification, definition of, 340
Chain of custody, 384
Change, 153–164
    change efforts and, 160–161
        selection of stratagem for, 161–164, *162,* 163t
    change process and, 157–160
        diagnosing resistance and, 158–159
        framework for analysis of, 159–160
    inevitability of, 153–154
    laboratory as organizational entity and, *154,* 154–155
    sequence of, 156–157, *157*
Change/conflict survival model, 156, *156*
Channel, in interpersonal communication, 76–77, 77
Chart of accounts, 413, 415
Checklist, for performance evaluation, 221
Chemical hazards, 327–329
Chief technologists, 6
Child ego state, transactional analysis and, 80
Chloroform, 327

Civil Rights Act of 1964, 446
  interviewing and employee selection and, 178
Civil Service Commission (CSC), 180
Civil Service Reform Act, 246
Climate, reflecting leader behavior, 95–96
Clinical Laboratories Improvement Act of 1967 (CLIA '67),
    309, 315–316
  regulation under, 341–342, 344
Clinical Laboratory Management Association, 346
COBRA. See Comprehensive Omnibus Budget Reconciliation
    Act
Coercion, as change stratagem, 164
Coercive power, 97
Collective bargaining, 252–254
  hours of work and, 253–254
  wages and, 253
  working conditions and, 254
College of American Pathologists (CAP), 310, 346
  accreditation program of, 341–342, 350–354
    goals of, 351–352
    management responsibilities under, 352
    programs/services integral to operation of, 354
    standards for, 352–353, 356–360
    steps in, 353–354
  fixed criteria for proficiency testing and, 273–274, 274t
  flammable chemicals and, 329
  interlaboratory survey provided by, 272–273
  personnel needs and, 448
  preventive maintenance and, 316
  work-load recording program of, 27, 27–28, 200, 309, 461
Commitment, to decision, 46
Communication, 73–90
  as change stratagem, 162
  conflict and, 165
  interpersonal, 73–78
    barriers to, 85–86
    definition of, 73
    improving, 86
    realistic model of, 74–78, 76
    simplistic view of, 73–74
    as transactional process, 78–81
  interviewing and, 191–192
  motivation and, 68
  nonverbal, 88
  organizational, 81–84
    barriers to, 84–85
    definition of, 73
    downward, 81–82
    horizontal, 83–84
    improving, 86–90
    informal, 84, 84
    upward, 82–83
  of performance evaluation results, 219
  of standards and criteria, 219
Communication networks, 301

Compensable factors, 450–451
Compensation. See Wage and salary administration
Competition, 4
  marketing plan and, 401–402
Complacency, change and, 157
Complementary transaction, 80, 81
Comprehensive Omnibus Reconciliation Act (COBRA), 3
Compressed gas cylinders, safety and, 324
Computers, 299–314, 300
  computer systems and, 300–301
    in-house versus vendor development of, 313
  extent of use of, 312–313
  integration of, 313–314
  laboratory information system and
    choosing, 312–314
    current and future requirements for, 308–312
    fundamental functions of, 301–308
  necessity of, 312
  problems in information handling prior to, 299–300
Conflict, 164–171
  change/conflict survival model and, 156, 156
  diagnosis of, 117–118
    coping techniques and, 167, 168–169t, 170–171
  encouraging, 170–171
  inevitability of, 153–154
  interpersonal, 165
  laboratory as organizational entity and, 154, 154–155
  sources of, 165
  viewpoints on, 166–167
Consensus decision-making, 49, 50
Consent, problems associated with, 382
Consideration, 102
Consultative leader, 101
Consumer price index (CPI), 426, 427
Contamination, 383
Contingency model, leadership styles and, 115–116, 116
Continuing education, 239–240
Continuous budget, 423
Contract administration, 254–256
Control, 9, 38, 41–42. See also Quality control
  laboratory information system and, 309–310
Co-optation, as change stratagem, 164
Corrective actions, 373–374
Corrosive chemicals, 328
Cost(s)
  of acquisition, 503–511, 505–509
  of change, 158
  of decision, 46
  direct, 412, 413, 415
  fixed and variable, 411–412, 411–413
  of health care, 407–408
  indirect, 412
  interaction and control of, 413
  of inventory, 511, 512, 513
  overhead, 468, 468t, 470

Cost(s) (continued)
    payroll-related, *450,* 455
    social, of change, 158
    standard, 415
    test, determining labor component of, 473–474
    unit, 412–413, 413t, *414*
Cost accounting
    for human resources, 446–448, *447*
    work-load statistics and. *See* Work-load analysis, work-load
        recording and
Cost centers, 4, 466, 467, 467t, 468t, 482, *482*
Cost containment, 4
    inventory and, 502–513
Cost-effectiveness
    comparing, 474t, 474–475
    of instrument operation, determining, 475–476, 476t, 477t
    of laboratory information system, 308–309
Cost-finding methods, 416
Cost-plus method, 440
Country Club leadership style, 102, 104
CPI. *See* Consumer price index
CPM. *See* Critical path method
CPU. *See* Central processing unit
Credentialing, definition of, 340
Criteria, 218–219
    communication of, 219
    monitoring and, 371
    for proficiency testing, 273–274, 274t
Criteria-based job description, 201–207, 202t
    nontechnical service duties and, 201, 203
    technical service duties and, 203–207
Critical incident performance evaluation, 222
Critical Path Method (CPM), 31
Crossed transaction, 80, *82*
CRT. *See* Cathode ray tube
CSC. *See* Civil Service Commission
Curriculum vitae, trial preparation and, 387

D

Damages, 381
Data, 301
Data collection specifications, monitoring and, 371
Decentralization, 308–309
Decision-making, 9–10, 45–56
    acceptance of and commitment to decision and, 46
    approaches and effects of, 46–50, *47,* 48t
        authoritarian, 47, 49
        consensus, 49, 50
        democratic, 48, 49
        laissez-faire, 49, 50
    breathless, 46
    capital. *See* Capital decision-making
    cost of decision and, 46

    dangerous habits in, 46, *47*
    decision strategy analysis and, 55–56
    financial ratios for. *See* Financial ratios
    hold-off, 47
    human factors in, 50
    levels of participation in, 49, *49*
    management decision styles and, 53–55, 55t
    managerial authority for, 95
    problem attributes assessment and, 53
    with proficiency data, 56
    quality of decision and, 45
    quantitative tools for, 50
    speed of decision and, 46
    steps in, *51,* 51–53
    value judgments in decision and, 46
Decision strategy analysis, 55–56
Decision support aids, 310
Decision tree, 53, *54*
Decoding, in interpersonal communication, 77
Deemed status, 342
Delegation, 138–142
    barriers to, 141
    as contract, 140–141
    manner of, 138–140, 139t
    motivation and, 69
    problems of, 141–142
    reasons for, 138
"Delta" check, 305
Democratic decision-making, 48, 49
Democratic leader, 101
Demographic variables, market segmentation and, 397
Departmental trend summary, 427, 428t
Department of Health and Human Services (DHHS), 343
    infectious hazards and, 325
    regulation and, 345
Department of Labor, infectious hazards and, 325
Dependence, conflict and, 165
Depreciation, 431
Development
    of group, 95
    of staff, 236–237
Development costs, of personnel, 447–448
DHHS. *See* Department of Health and Human Services
Diagnostic related groups (DRGs), 3–4
    financial management and, 408–409
    quality assurance and, 370
3,3-Dichlorobenzidine, 327
4-Dimethylaminoazobenzene, 327
Dinitrobenzenes, 329
2,4-Dinitrophenol, 329
2,4-Dinitrotoluene, 329
Dioxane, 329
Direct apportionment cost-finding, 416
Direct costs, 412, 413, 415
Directing, 9

Direct inoculation, as route of infection, 326
Directors, 6
  CAP requirements for, 356, 357
  duties of, 5
  medical, in organizational structure, 10
Disability income protection, 453
Disciplinary sequence, 42
Discussion, for inservice education, 240
Disease prevalence, allowable error and, 271
Disinfectant, infectious hazards and, 325
Disparate-impact doctrine, 180
Disposal, of hazardous materials, 335–336
Distributed computing systems, 310, *311,* 312
Distribution, in marketing mix, 398
Documentation
  monitoring and, 372
  preservice education and, 238–239
  preventive maintenance and, 316–317, 317t, *318–321,*
    319
Donated services, 455–456
Double step-down method, for cost-finding, 416
Downward communication, 81–82
Drawing-out stage, of interview, 190
DRGs. *See* Diagnostic related groups

E

Economic forces, in marketing environment, 397
Economic order quantity (EOQ), 496–498, *497*
Economic Stabilization Program, 445
Education, 233–243
  as change stratagem, 162
  developing activities for, 240–243
    assessing needs and, 241
    determining content and, 242
    developing objectives and, 241–242
    establishing teaching method and, 242
  inservice and continuing, 239–240
    teaching methodologies for, 240
  lifelong learning and, 234–235
  preservice, 237–239
    documentation and, 238–239
    job description and, 237
    laboratory section and, 238
    policies and procedures and, 237
    routine protocols, analytic procedures, and techniques
      and, 238
    safety equipment and procedures and, 238
    staff introduction and, 237
  staff development and, 236–237
EEOC. *See* Equal Employment Opportunity Commission
Effectiveness, in life-cycle theory, 114t, 115, 115t
Efficiency, of group, 95
Ego state, transactional analysis and, 80

Electrical hazards, 324–325
Element, monitoring and, 371
Emergency procedures, 336
Emotions, as communication barrier, 86
Empathy, improving communication and, 87–88
Employee(s). *See* Labor relations; Personnel; Scheduling;
    Staffing
Employee association, 245
Employee-involvement work groups, 123–135, *135*
  autonomous work teams and, 133–134
  quality circles and, 124–129
  quality of work life approach and, 129–133, *130*
Encoding, in interpersonal communication, 74
Environment, marketing, 397–398
EOQ. *See* Economic order quantity
Equal Employment Act, 452
Equal Employment Opportunity Commission (EEOC),
    180–181, 247
Equal Employment Opportunity for Handicapped Individuals
    Act of 1980, 178
Equal Opportunity Act of 1972, 178
Equal Pay Act of 1963, 446
Equal Pay for Equal Work Provisions, 445
Error(s)
  allowable, 269–272
    cost of missed diagnoses and, 269–271
    defining, 269
    effect of changing precision on predictive value and,
      269, 270t
    variables affecting, 271
  analytical, resolving, 274–277
  blunder detection and, 277–278
  defining blunders and, 277
  forecasting, 500–501
  of manufacturer, 383
  mathematical, 383–384
  reducing, 2778–279
  types of, 278
Esteem needs, 64
Ethical conduct, marketing and, 395
Ethyl ether, 329
Evaluation, 371. *See also* Method evaluation; Performance
    appraisal
  of education, 243
Event, in network analysis, 31
Executive Order 10925, 179
Executive Order 10988, 246
Executive Order 11246, 179
Executive Order 11491, 246
Executive Order 11749, 179
Expert power, 98
Expert witness, technologist as, 386
Explanation, monitoring and, 371
Exponential smoothing, forecasting and, 499, *500*
Extroversion/introversion, 106, *111–112*

F

Facilitation, as change stratagem, 163–164
Facilitator, quality circles and, 126
Facilities, CAP requirements for, 358
Factor Evaluation System (FES), 451
Fact witness, 386
Fainting, problems associated with, 382
Fair Labor Standards Act of 1967 (FLSA), 445
Fair-share laws, 252
Federal employees, labor relations law governing, 246–247
Federal Labor Relations Authority, 246, 247
Federal Mediation and Conciliation Service (FMCS), 247
Federal regulations, reports and, 297
Feedback
   improving communication and, 88, 89t
   in interpersonal communication, 77–78
Feeling/thinking, 113
Fee-setting
   by macro approach, 468, 469t
   by micro-approach, 468–471
FES. *See* Factor Evaluation System
Financial management, 407–419
   cost, volume, and revenue relationships and, 411–418
   financial ratios and, 479–490
   health care costs and, 407–411
   manager's role in, 418–419
   planned service capacity and, 419
Financial ratios, 479–490
Financial resources, 5
Fiscal control, laboratory information systems and, 309
Fixed forecast budget, 423
Fixed-period inventory replenishment systems, 493–494, *495*
Fixed-quantity inventory replenishment system, 493, *493, 494*
Flammable material, 328–329
   disposal of, 335
   labeling and, 333
Flexible budget, 423
Float, in network analysis, 32
Floor plan, 26–30
   space allocation and, 26–28
   structural design and, 28–30
FLRA. *See* Federal Labor Relations Authority
FLSA. *See* Fair Labor Standards Act of 1967
FMCS. *See* Federal Mediation and Conciliation Service
Followership, 103–113
   individual temperaments and, 106, *111–112,* 112–113
   participative leadership and, 105–106, *107–110*
Follow-up
   of interview, 192
   of meetings, 147–148, 148t
Forced-choice rating, for performance evaluation, 222
Forced distribution, for performance evaluation, 222

Forecasting, 498–501
   adaptive smoothing and, 500
   base index and, 499–500
   error and, 500–501
   exponential smoothing and, 499, *500*
   illustration of, 501, *501, 502*
   moving average and, 498
   regression analysis and, 499
   responsiveness and, 500
Formal groups, functions of, 69
Free-form performance evaluation, 222
Fringe benefits, 452–454
   collective bargaining and, 253
Frustration
   model of, 155, *155*
   need fulfillment and, 64–65, *65*
Full costing, 415–416
Fume hoods, 334–335

G

Game analysis, transactional analysis and, 80
Glassware, broken
   disposal of, 336
   wounds from, 330
Goals, definition of, 119
Governing board, 10–11, *11*
Grapevine, 84, *84*
Graphic rating scales, for performance evaluation, *220,* 220–221
Grievance procedure, 255–256
Gross area, 26
Group(s)
   effectiveness of, measures of, 94–95
   employee-involvement. *See* Employee-involvement work groups
   formal and informal, 69
Group dynamics, motivation and, 69–70

H

Halo effect
   as communication barrier, 85
   interviewing and, 193
Hardware, 300–301
Hazardous materials
   disposal of, 335–336
   labeling system and, 331, *332, 333, 333*
HCFA. *See* Health Care Financing Administration
Health and accident protection, 453
Health care, costs of, 407–408
Health Care Financing Administration (HCFA), 342
   preventive maintenance and, 316
   regulation and, 345

Health hazard, labeling and, 333
Health Maintenance Organization Act of 1973 (HMO), 446
Hidden agendas, meetings and, 146, *146*
HMO. *See* Health Maintenance Organization Act of 1973
Hold-off decisions, 47
Holding costs, 496
Hoods, 334–335
Horizontal communication, 83–84
Hourly-rate method, 439
House Rule 4154, 181
Human resources, 5
    cost accounting for, 446–448, *447*
    staffing and scheduling and, 210–211
Hygiene factors, motivation and, 66

I

Identification, change and, 157–158
Immigration Reform and Control Act of 1986 (IRCA), 181
Impoverished leadership style, 102, 104
Incident report form, *40*, 41–42
Income equivalent payments, 453–454
Income protection legislation, 445–446
Indirect costs, 412. *See also* Overhead costs
Infectious materials, 325–326
    disposal of, 335–336
Informal communication systems, 84, *84*
Informal groups, functions of, 69
Information power, 98
Information processing, decision-making and, 50
Information stage, of interview, 190
Ingestion, as route of infection, 326
Initiating structure, 102
Insecurity, change and, 158
Inservice education, 239–240
Inspection. *See* Accreditation, inspection and
Instruments
    preventive maintenance for. *See* Preventive maintenance
    failure of, 383
    "interfaces" and, 301
Interactionist viewpoint, on conflict, 166
Interlaboratory surveys, quality control and, 272–274
Internalization, change and, 157–158
Internal rate of return (IRR), 434
Interpersonal communication. *See* Communication, interpersonal
Interview(ing)
    analysis of resume and, 191
    communication skills and, 191–192
    conducting, 182, 190–194
    environment for, 191
    legal aspects of, 178–181
    limitations of, 192–193
    for performance appraisal, 222

    preparation for, 190
    structured, 191
    team, 193
    termination and follow-up of, 192
Introversion/extroversion, 106, *111–112*
Intuition/sensing, 106, *111–112,* 112–113
Inventory management, 491–513
    cost containment and, 502–513
    economic order quantity and, 496–498, *497*
    fixed-period replenishment systems and, 493–494, *495*
    fixed-quantity replenishment system and, 493, *493, 494*
    forecasting and, 498–501
    laboratory information systems and, 309
    mixed replenishment system and, *495,* 495–496
    reorder point and, 501–502
    scientific, 491–493
Involvement, as change stratagem, 162–163
IRCA. *See* Immigration Reform and Control Act of 1986
IRR. *See* Internal rate of return
Isopropyl ether, 329
Item for count, 462

J

Japanese management, employee involvement and, 123–124
Japanese viewpoint, on conflict, 166–167
JCAH. *See* Joint Commission on Accreditation of Hospitals
JCAHO. *See* Joint Commission on Accreditation of Healthcare Organizations
Job analysis, compensation and, 450
Job description
    criteria-based, 201–207, 202t
    preservice education and, 237
Job duties, 203
Job evaluation, factor-based, compensable, 450–451
Job relationships, 203
Job sharing, 214
Joint Commission on Accreditation of Healthcare Organizations (JCAHO), 350, 360–368
    medical staff standards of, 373
    preventive maintenance and, 316
    quality assurance and, 370
    requisitions and reports and, 285
Joint Commission on Accreditation of Hospitals (JCAH), 10, 310
    accreditation program of, 342–343
    reports and, 292
Judgment/perception, 113

L

Labeling, infectious hazards and, 325
Laboratory information cycles, 299, *300*

Laboratory information system. *See* Computers, laboratory information system and
Laboratory inspection. *See* Accreditation, inspection and
Laboratory structural design, 28–30
  modular, *28,* 28–29
  open, *29,* 29–30
Labor costs, direct and indirect, 468–469
Labor-Management Relations Act (Taft-Hartley Act), 247–248
Labor-Management Reporting and Disclosure Act, 249–250
Labor relations, 245–256
  law and
    private-sector employee and, 247–250
    public employees and, 245–247
  unions and, 250–256
    bargaining unit and, 251–252
    collective bargaining and, 252–254
    contract administration and, 254–256
    reasons for joining, 250–251
Laissez-faire decision-making, 49, 50
Laissez-faire leadership style, 101
Laws. *See* Legal forces; Legal liability; Legislation
Layout flow chart, 30, *31, 32*
LDBQ. *See* Leader Behavior Description Questionnaire
Leader
  autocratic, 101
  bases of power and influence of, 97–98
  boss versus, 7
  consultative, 101
  democratic, 101
  interpersonal relationships of, 96
  persuasive, 101
  quality circles and, 127
Leader Behavior Description Questionnaire (LDBQ), 102
Leader Opinion Questionnaire (LOQ), 102
Leadership
  definition of, 93–94
  effective, 150–151
  of quality circles, 125
Leadership skills, management levels and, 7, *7*
Leadership styles, 93–119
  climate reflecting leader behavior and, 95–96
  continuum of, *101.* 101–102
  diagnosis and, 116–118, *117*
  factors influencing, 99–100
  followership linked to, 103–113
    individual temperaments and, 106, *111–112,* 112–113
    participative leadership and, 105–106, *107–110*
  initiating structure and consideration and, 102, *102*
  laissez-faire, 101
  management by objectives and, *118,* 118–119
  managerial grid and, 102–103, *103*
  need for change and, 119
  situation and, 113–116
    contingency model and, 115–116, *116*

situational leadership theory and tridimensional model and, 113–115, *114,* 114t, 115t
  theories X and Y and, 100–101
Least-Preferred Coworker (LPC), 116
Lecture, for inservice education, 240
Legal forces, in marketing environment, 398
Legal liability, 379–385
  problem areas in, 382–385
  records and, 388–390
  subpoena and, 385
  technologist as witness and, 386–388
Legibility, 384
Legislation, 3. *See also specific legislation*
  compensation administration and, 445–448
  governing labor relations, 245–250, *246*
    private-sector employees and, 247–250
    public employees and, 245–247
    right-to-work, 249
  minimum wage, 445
Legitimate power, 98
Length of stay (LOS), 200
Levey-Jennings charts, 264–266
  criticism of method using, 267–269, *268*
  dispersion or contraction and, 265, *265*
  shifts and, *265,* 265–266, *266–267*
  stable performance and, *264,* 264–265
  tends and, 265, *265*
Liability. *See* Legal liability
License
  definition of, 340–341
  laboratory information systems and, 309–310
Life-cycle theory, *114,* 114t, 114–115, 115t
Lifelong learning, 234–235
Limited-term budget, 423
Linear programming, decision-making and, 50
Line position, 34
Listening, improving communication and, 86–87
LOQ. *See* Leader Opinion Questionnaire
LOS. *See* Length of stay
Loss-of-job income continuation, 453
LPC. *See* Least-Preferred Coworker

M

Machine code, 301
Management. *See also* Administration; Administrators; Manager(s)
  as social process, 116–118, *117*
Management by exception, 95
Management by objectives (MBO), *118,* 118–119
Management's rights clause, 256
Management support functions, *309,* 309–310
Management team, levels in, 6

Manager(s), 6. *See also* Administrators
  duties of, 6
  financial management and, 418
  leadership role of, 96–97
  "linking pin" function of, 93, *94*
Managerial grid, 102–103, *103*
Manipulation, as change stratagem, 164
Man-to-man comparison, for performance evaluation, 222
Manufacturer's error, 383
Manufacturing Chemists Association, chemical hazards and, 327
Marketing, 395–402
  definition of, 395–396
  marketing environment and, 397–397
  marketing mix and, 398–399
  marketing plan and, 399–402
  market research and, 396–397
  market segmentation and, 397
  overview of, 402, *402*
Materials, budgeting for, 426
Materials costs, indirect, 469–470
Mathematical errors, 383–384
Maturity, in life-cycle theory, 114
MBO. *See* Management by objectives
MBTI. *See* Myers-Briggs Type Indicator
Mechanical hazards, 324
Medicaid, 408–410, 446
  reports and, 297
Medical directors, in organizational structure, 10
Medicare, 408–410, 446
  quality assurance and, 370
  regulation by, 342, 343–344
  reports and, 297
Meeting(s)
  effective, 143–151
    conducting, 146–147
    follow-up and, 147–148, 148t
    leadership for, 150–151
    meeting purposes and, 143–144
    planning and, 144–146
  nonproductive
    avoiding, 149–150
    causes and solutions to,
Meeting room, 145
Merit, employee incentive systems based on, 454–455
Merit Systems Protection Board (MSPB), 246
Message, in interpersonal communication, 74, 76
Method evaluation, 279–283
  estimates of accuracy and, 281, 281t
  estimates of precision and, 281–282
  interference and recovery studies and, 282
  judging acceptability of a method and, 282–283
  method comparison studies and, 279–281, *280*
    selection of reference method and, 279

  statistical tests of comparison data and, 280–281, *281*
Microtome blades, wounds from, 330
Middle of the road leadership style, 103
Minimum wage laws, 445
Missed diagnoses, cost to society of, 269–271
Mixed costs, 411
Mixed inventory replenishment system, *495*, 495–496
Modems (modulating-demodulating devices), 300
Monitoring, 371
MONITREND report, 464–466
Motivation, 61–71
  definition of, 61–62
  group dynamics and, 69–70
    group structure and, 69–70
    motivational assumptions and, 70
  management responsibilities and, 68–69
  nature of, 61–62
  need-hierarchy theory of, 62–65
    esteem needs and, 64
    psychologic needs and, 63
    safety needs and, 63–64
    self-actualization needs and, 64
    social needs and, 64
    two-factor theory compared with, 66, 67
  into 1990's, 70–71
  personality and, 62
  preference-expectation theory and, 66–67
  process of, 62, *62*
  theories X and Y and, 67–68, 68t
  two-factor theory of, 65–66
    need-hierarchy theory compared with, 66, 67
Motivator-hygiene theory, of motivation, 65–66
Moving average, forecasting and, 498
MSPB. *See* Merit Systems Protection Board
Myers-Briggs Type Indicator (MBTI), 106

N

β-Naphthylamine, 327
Narrative, for performance evaluation, 221–222
National Cancer Institute, Safety Standards of, 327
National Fire Prevention Association (NFPA)
  chemical hazards and, 327
  hazard warning emblem of, 331, *332*
National Institute for Occupational Safety and Health (NIOSH), flammable chemicals and, 329
National Institutes of Health (NIH), chemical carcinogens and, 327
National Labor Relations Act (Wagner Act), 245, 247–249
  compensation and, 445
  Health Care Amendments to, 245, 247, 249–250, 252
  union membership and, 252
National Labor Relations Board (NLRB), 246

Natural classifications, 423, 424t
Need(s), assessing, for educational activities, 241
Need-hierarchy theory of motivation. *See* Motivation
Negligent acts, 379
Negotiation, as change stratagem, 164
Net area, 26
Net income, 416
Net present value (NPV), 434, 435t
Network analysis, work flow and, 30–32, *34*
NFPA. *See* National Fire Prevention Association
NIH. *See* National Institutes of Health
NIOSH. *See* National Institute for Occupational Safety and
    Health
NLRB. *See* National Labor Relations Board
Noise, in interpersonal communication, 78, *79*
Noncritical path, in network analysis, 31–32
Not-for-profit hospitals, 408
NPV. *See* Net present value
Nuclear Regulatory Commission, 310

O

Objectives
    definition of, 119
    developing, for educational activities, 241–242
OBRA. *See* Omnibus Budget Reconciliation Act
Occupational Safety and Health Act, 323
Occupational Safety and Health Administration (OSHA),
    63–64
    chemical hazards and, 327
    infectious hazards and, 325
Office of Federal Contract Compliance (OFCCP), 180
Office of Management and Budget (OMB), 346
Omnibus Budget Reconciliation Act (OBRA), 3
Operating expense budget, 421–422
Operating ratios, 487, 488t, 489t, 490
Operating system, 301
Operational approach, to space allocation, 26
Operational flow chart, 30, *32–33*
Operational lines, *276,* 276–277
    analysis of, *276,* 276–277, 277t
    preparation of, 276, 277t
Ordering costs, 496
Ordinary witness, 386
Organization
    ambiguous, conflict and, 165
    definition of, 32
Organizational structure, 32–38
    autonomous work groups and, 133–134
    departmentalization/specialization and, 36
    dual hierarchy and, 10–11, *11*
    flat, *37,* 37–38
    informal, 38, *38*
    planning related to, 23, *24*

quality circles and, *126,* 126–127
quality of work life approach and, 129–130, *131*
scalar principle and, 36
span of control and, *37,* 37–38
tall, *37,* 37–38
unity of command and, 37
unity of direction and, 36–37
Organization chart, 33–34, *35, 36,* 199
    administrative versus technical structure and, 34, *36*
    for hospital, *154*
Organizing, 9
OSHA. *See* Occupational Safety and Health Administration
Overhead costs, 470. *See also* Indirect costs
    allocation of, 468, 468t
Overlap, allowable error and, 271
Overtime, budgeting for, 426

P

PACE. *See* Professional Acknowledgement for Continuing Ed-
    ucation program
Paired comparison, for performance evaluation, 222
Panel discussions, for inservice education, 240
Parent ego state, transactional analysis and, 80
Participation, as change stratagem, 162–163
Participative leadership, 105–106, *107–110. See also* Em-
    ployee-involvement work groups
Part-time employees, budgeting for, 426
Patient results, control method for, *39,* 41
Payback analysis, 432, 435t
Payroll accounting, 455–456
Peer review. *See* Quality assurance, peer review and
Peer Review Improvement Act, 372
Peer Review Organizations (PROs), 201, 372–373
Pension plans, 446
People, in marketing mix, 399
Perception, decision-making and, 50
Perception/judgment, 113
Performance appraisal, 217–231
    checklist for, 221
    communication of results and, 219
    critical incident, 222
    definition and purposes of, 217–218
    designing, 219–223
        interview and, 222–223
        written component and, 220–222, 221t
    forced-choice rating for, 222
    forced distribution for, 222
    free-form, 222
    frequency of evaluation and, 219
    graphic rating scales for, *220,* 220–221
    man-to-man comparison for, 222
    narrative for, 221–222
    paired comparison for, 222

performance management and, 223–231, *230*
ranking for, 222
relative to budget, 426–427, 428t, 429, 429t
standards and criteria for, 218–219
   communication of, 219
Performance chart, 208, *209*
Personality, motivation and, 62
Personality conflict, diagnosis of, 117
Personal selling, 399
Personnel. *See also* Labor relations; Scheduling; Staffing
   budgeting for, 423, 424t, *425,* 425–426, 448–449, *449*
   CAP requirements for, 456–458
   compensation for. *See* Wage and salary administration
   disciplinary sequence and, 42
   employee selection and, 177–196
      application form and, 181–182
      interviewing and, conduction of interview and, 182, 190–194
      legal aspects of, 178–181
      legal aspects of interviewing and, 178–181
      recruitment and, 178
      reference checks and, 182
      selection process and, 194
      transfer and promotion and, 194–196
   evaluation of. *See* Performance appraisal
   interviewing and selection of, 177–196
   introduction to, 237
   JCAHO standards for, 373
   laboratory information systems and, 309
   planning for, 199–200
   size of, space allocation and, 26–28
   staff development and, 236–237
   training and experience of, quality control and, 261–262
   turnover of, 177
Persuasive leader, 101
PERT. *See* Program Evaluation Review Technique
Phlebotomists, 203, 207
   puncture wounds and, 330
PHS. *See* Public Health Service
Physical resources, 5
Physician(s), compensating, 456–457
Physician review organizations (PROs), 201
Physiologic needs, 63
Picric acid, 329
Pipetting, infectious hazards and, 325–326
Place, in marketing mix, 398
Plan, marketing, 399–402
Planned service capacity, 419
Planning, 9
   at departmental level, 23
   for effective meetings, 144–146
   organizational hierarchy related to, 23, *24*
   strategic, 21–23
Policies and procedures, 23–25
   characteristics of, 25

establishing, 23–25
origin of, 24–25
preservice education and, 237
variations among, 24
Political forces
   decision-making and, 50
   in marketing environment, 398
Position control document, 448–449, *449*
Power, 97–98
   coercive, 97
   decision-making and, 50
   expert, 98
   information, 98
   legitimate, 98
   referent, 98
   reward, 97–98
   sanctioned, 98
PPOs. *See* Preferred provider organizations
PPSs. *See* Prospective Payment Systems
Precision, changing, effect on predictive value, 269, 270t
Preference-expectation theory, of motivation, 66–67
Preferred provider organizations (PPOs), 410
Pregnancy Discrimination Act of 1978, 178
Present value, 433–434, 435t
Preservice education, 237–239
Preventive maintenance, 315–322
   benefits of, 322
   documentation and, 316–317, 317t, *318–321,* 319
   government and accrediting agency requirements for, 315–316
   instrument selection and implementation and, 316
   performance responsibility and, 319–322
Private health insurance, 410
Probability theory, decision-making and, 50
Problem attributes assessment, 53
Problem-solving
   in inservice education, 240
   monitoring and, 371–372
Procedures. *See* Policies and procedures
Procedure volume trend analysis, 421, *421*
Process, definition of, 33
Product, in marketing mix, 398
Production, of group, 95
Productivity
   evaluating with work-load analysis, 471–473
   monitoring system for, 208
   paid, 471–472
   specified, 472–473
   worked, 472
Professional Acknowledgement for Continuing Education (PACE) program, 236
Professional appearance, 388
Professional Standards Review Organizations (PSRO), 373
Proficiency Survey Program, 354
Profit and loss statement, 427, 429t

Program Evaluation Review Technique (PERT), 31
Projected workload, 210
Promotion
　in marketing mix, 398–399
　of personnel, 194–196
Property and liability protection, 453
PROs. *See* Peer Review Organizations
Prospective payment systems (PPSs), 3–4, 409
　financial management and, 408
PSRO. *See* Professional Standards Review Organizations
Psychographic variables, market segmentation and, 397
Public employees, labor relations law governing, 245–247
Public Health Service (PHS), regulation and, 345
Public relations, 399
Puncture wounds, 330
Purchase price, 496–497, *497*
Purchasing, 492–493

Q

QAS. *See* Quality Assurance Service
QCs. *See* Quality circles
Qualifications, 203
Quality, 371
Quality assurance
　CAP requirements for, 358
　definition of, 354
　laboratory information system and, 304–305, *305*
　peer review and, 369–377
　　definition of, 370–371
　　future perspectives on, 376–377
　　implementation of, 374–376
　　monitoring care and outcomes and, 371–374
Quality Assurance Service (QAS), 354
Quality circles (QCs), 70–71, 123, 124–129
　decision to implement, 127
　expectations for, 125–126
　implementation of, 127–128
　leadership of, 125
　limitations of, 128–129
　organizational structure and, *126*, 126–127
　training for, 128
Quality control, 261–279
　allowable error and, 269–272
　　cost of missed diagnoses and, 269–271
　　defining, 269
　　effect of changing precision on predictive value and, 269, 270t
　　variables affecting, 271
　CAP requirements for, 359
　definition of, 354
　determination of laboratory variation and, 264
　frequency of analysis of control sera and, 263–264
　interlaboratory surveys and, 272–274

CAP fixed criteria for proficiency testing and, 273–274, 274t
　　commercial, 273
　　government agencies providing, 273
　　professional organizations providing, 272–273
　laboratory mistakes and, 277–279
　method evaluation and, 279–283
　reference sample method of, 262–263
　resolving analytical errors and, 274–277
　Stewhart control rules and, 266–269
　training and experience of personnel and, 261–262
　use of L-J charts and, 264–266
　within-laboratory, 262
Quality of work life (QWL) programs, 123, 129–133, *130*
　implementation and training and, 130–131, *132*
　limitations of, 132–133
　memorandum of agreement and, 129
　objectives of, 129
　organizational structure and, 129–130, *131*
　training content and mechanics of, 131–132
Questions
　direct, 191
　leading, 191
　open-ended, 191
　probing, 191–192
Queuing theory, decision-making and, 50
QWL. *See* Quality of work life programs

R

Ranking, for performance evaluation, 222
Rate-setting, 438–442
　realities of, 440–442
　revenue budget and, 438–439
　techniques for, 439–442
Rating
　forced-choice, for performance evaluation, 222
　graphic, for performance evaluation, *220*, 220–221
Raw count, 462
Reactivity, labeling and, 333
Reasonable and customary charges, for physicians, 457, *458, 459*
"Reasonable man" standard, 379–380
Records, legal aspects of, 388–390
Recruitment, 178
Reference checks, 182
Reference laboratories, reports and, 297
Reference sample method of quality control, 262–263
　commercially available controls and, 262–263
Referent power, 98
Refreezing, change and, 158
Regression analysis, forecasting and, 499
Regulation
　under Clinical Laboratory Improvement Act of 1967, 344

definition of, 341
in marketing environment, 398
Medicare, 343–344
regulatory climate and, 345–346
reports and, 297
state, 345
Rehabilitation Act of 1973, 178
Reimbursement system, 409
Relative value units, 464
Relevant range, 411
Reliability, of interviewing, 193
Reorder point (ROP), 492, 501–502
Repeat, 462
Replicate, 462
Reports, 292, *293–296,* 297–298
accident, 336
monitoring and, 372
problem areas and, 384
Required rate of return, 431
Requisitions, 285, *286–290,* 291–292
Research, market, 396–397
Resistance, to change, diagnosing, 158–159
Resources. *See also* Human resources
CAP requirements for, 358
financial, 5
needed for computer system, 313
physical, 5
scarce, conflict and, 165
Resource utilization ratios, 487
Respondent superior doctrine, 381
Responsibility, 34
monitoring and, 371
motivation and, 69
Responsiveness, forecasting and, 500
Resume, analysis of, 191
Return on investment (ROI), 503
Revenue Act of 1978, 446
Revenue budget, 438–439
Revenue per billable procedure, 490
Review time, 494
Reward power, 97–98
Right-to-work laws, 249
ROI. *See* Return on investment
Role conflict, diagnosis of, 117
Role-personality conflict, diagnosis of, 117–118
Role playing, for inservice education, 240
ROP. *See* Reorder point
Rotating generalist staff, 210–211

S

Safety, 323–337
accident reports and, 336
blood and body fluids, precautions and, 326–330

disposal of hazardous materials and, 335–336
emergency procedures and, 336
fume hoods and, 334–335
hazard labeling system and, 331, *332,* 333, *333*
preservice education and, 238
safety cabinets and, 328–329, 333–334
safety committee and, 336–337
workplace hazards and, 323–326
Safety cabinets, 328–329, 333–334
Safety committee, 336–337
Safety needs, 63–64
Safety stock, 492
Salaries. *See* Wage and salary administration
Sales promotion, 399
Sanctioned power, 98
Satisfaction, of group, 95
Scheduling, 200
for efficient service, 207–208
guides for, 208, 210
historic changes in, 200–201
innovative approaches in, *211–213,* 211–214
responsibility and importance of, 200
Script analysis, transactional analysis and, 80
Segmentation, market, 397
Selection, 200
Self-actualization needs, 64
Self-esteem, motivation and, 69
Semantic Problem, as communication barrier, 85–86
Sensing/intuition, 106, *111–112,* 112–113
Sensitivity analysis, 417–418
Separation costs, 448
Sera, control, frequency of analysis of, 263–264
Shock, 324
Simulation, for inservice education, 240
Situation, leadership and, 113–116
situational leadership theory and tridimensional model and, 113–115, *114,* 114t, 115t
Situational favorableness dimension, 116, *116*
Skin contact, as route of infection, 326
SNOMED (Systematized Nomenclature of Medicine), 304
Social costs, of change, 158
Social needs, 64
Social Security Act. *See also* Medicaid; Medicare
regulation and, 345
Societal forces, in marketing environment, 398
Sodium azide, 329
Software, 301
Source, in interpersonal communication, 74, *75*
Specimens
chain of custody and, 384
incorrect identification of, 383
loss of, 383
Speed, of decision, 46
Spouse and family income protection, 453
Staff. *See* Personnel; Scheduling; Staffing

Staff development, 236–237
Staffing
  criteria-based job description and, 201–207, 202t
  determining needs for, 473
  guides for, 208, 210
  historic changes in, 200–201
  responsibility and importance of, 200
Staff position, 34
Standard(s), 218–219
  for CAP accreditation, 352–353, 356–360
  communication of, 219
  control and, 41
  for JCAH and JCAHO accreditation, 285, 292, 316, 342–343, 370, 373
  sources of, 218–219
Standard costs, 415
Standard operating procedure, 383
State employees, labor relations law governing, 247
Steering committee, quality circles and, 126
Step-down accounting method, 416, 466–471, 467–469t
Stewhart control rules
  application of, 266–269
  criticism of L-J method and, 267–269, 268
  development of model and, 267
  flow diagram of multirule procedure, 267, 268
Straight-line depreciation, 431
Strategic management, definition of, 21, 22
Strategic planning, 21–23
Structural analysis, transactional analysis and, 80
Structure. See also Organizational structure
  definition of, 32–33
  laboratory design and, 28–30
Subpoena, 385
Subpoena duces tecum, 385
Supervisor(s), 6
  circle of influence of, 14, 14–15
  duties of, 6
  leadership role of, 96–97
Supplies, budgeting for, 426
Supply cost per billable procedure, 487
Support, as change stratagem, 163–164
Surcharge method, 440
Syringe needle, breaking of, 382

T

Taft-Hartley Act (Labor-Management Relations Act), 247–248
TAR. See Time-adjusted return method
Task oriented leadership style, 102–103, 104
TAT. See Turn-around time
Tax Equity and Fiscal Responsibility Act (TEFRA), 446, 479
Tax investment legislation, 446
Team(s), quality circles and, 126–127
Team interviewing, 193

Team leader, quality circles and, 127
Team oriented leadership style, 103, 104
Technologic forces, in marketing environment, 398
TEFRA. See Tax Equity and Fiscal Responsibility Act
Temperaments, leadership styles and, 106, 111–112, 112–113
Test costs, determining labor component of, 473–474
Testimony, presentation of, 388
Test utilization ratios, 487
Tetrahydrofuran, 329
Theories X and Y
  leadership styles and, 100–101
  motivation and, 67–68, 68t
Thinking/feeling, 113
Time-adjusted return (TAR) method, 434, 435t
Time constraints, decision-making and, 50
Top down change stratagem, 161
Tort, 379
Total cost per billable procedure, 487, 490
Toxic materials, 329
  disposal of, 335
Trade-offs
  habit of, in decision-making, 46–47
  power and, 98
Training
  for quality circles, 128
  quality of work life approach and, 130–132, 132
Transactional analysis, 78–81, 81–83
  structural analysis and, 80
Transfer, 194–196
Trial, preparation for, 396–388
Tridimensional model, situational leadership theory and, 113–115, 114, 114t, 115t
Tuning Out, as communication barrier, 86
Turn-around time (TAT), 200
Two-factor theory, of motivation, 65–66
  need-hierarchy theory compared with, 66, 67

U

Ulterior transaction, 80–81, 83
Unfreezing, change and, 157
Union(s), 245, 250–256
  bargaining unit and, 251–252
  change and, 158–159
  collective bargaining and, 252–254
    hours of work and, 253–254
    wages and, 253
    working conditions and, 254
  contract administration and, 254–256
    management's rights and, 256
  quality of work life approach and, 129–133, 130
  reasons for joining, 250–251
    personal, 250

union image as, 250–251
Union-shop clause, 252
Union steward, 255
Unit costs, 412–413, 413t, *414*
Unit value per procedure, 462
Upward communication, 82–83
Use factor, 26

V

Value(s)
   conflict and, 165
   decision-making and, 50
Value judgments, in decision, 46
Variable budget, 423
Variable costs, 411, *411*
Variance analysis, 415
Venipuncture, problems in, 382
Vietnam Veterans Readjustment Act, 178
Visual aids, for meetings, 145

W

Wage and salary administration, 443–458
   benefits and services and, 452–454
   collective bargaining and, 253
   compensation and, 443, 449–452
      deferred, 454
      survey and, 451–452, 452t
   incentive systems based on merit and, 454–455
   legislation and, 445–448
   payroll accounting and, 455–456
   personnel budgeting and, 448–449, *449*
   physician compensation and, 456–457
   reward system and, 443–445, *444*

compensation and, 443
   noncompensation, 443–445
Wagner Act. *See* National Labor Relations Act
Warm-up stage, of interview, 190
Weighted-value basis, 440
Witness, technologist as, 386–388
Work aids, 203
Workers' Compensation, 445–446
Work flow design, 30–32
   layout floor chart and, 30, *31, 32*
   network analysis and, 30–32, *34*
   operational flow chart and, 30, *32–33*
Work-flow diagram, 208, *209*
Work-force analysis, 427, 428t
Work groups, employee-involvement. *See* Employee-involvement work groups
Working conditions, collective bargaining and, 254
Working hours, collective bargaining and, 253–254
Work-load analysis, 471–477
   comparing cost-effectiveness of two methods with, 474t, 474–475
   computing labor component of test costs and, 473–474
   cost accounting and, 464–471
      MONITREND report and, 464–466
      relative value units and, 464
      step-down accounting method and, 466–471, 467–469t
   determining cost-effective instrument operation with, 475–476, 476t, 477t
   determining staff needs with, 473
   evaluating productivity with, 471–473
   identifying problem areas with, 476–477, 477t
   work-load recording and, 208, 461–464
      cost accounting and, 464–471
      data collection for, 462–464
      purpose, use, and history of, 461
      terminology for, 461–462
Wounds, 330

ISBN 0-397-50857-3

90000